Smart Innovation, Systems and Technologies

Volume 45

About this Series

The Smart Innovation, Systems and Technologies book series encompasses the topics of knowledge, intelligence, innovation and sustainability. The aim of the series is to make available a platform for the publication of books on all aspects of single and multi-disciplinary research on these themes in order to make the latest results available in a readily-accessible form. Volumes on interdisciplinary research combining two or more of these areas is particularly sought.

The series covers systems and paradigms that employ knowledge and intelligence in a broad sense. Its scope is systems having embedded knowledge and intelligence, which may be applied to the solution of world problems in industry, the environment and the community. It also focusses on the knowledge-transfer methodologies and innovation strategies employed to make this happen effectively. The combination of intelligent systems tools and a broad range of applications introduces a need for a synergy of disciplines from science, technology, business and the humanities. The series will include conference proceedings, edited collections, monographs, handbooks, reference books, and other relevant types of book in areas of science and technology where smart systems and technologies can offer innovative solutions.

High quality content is an essential feature for all book proposals accepted for the series. It is expected that editors of all accepted volumes will ensure that contributions are subjected to an appropriate level of reviewing process and adhere to KES quality principles.

More information about this series at http://www.springer.com/series/8767

Yen-Wei Chen · Carlos Toro
Satoshi Tanaka · Robert J. Howlett
Lakhmi C. Jain
Editors

Innovation in Medicine and Healthcare 2015

Springer

Editors
Yen-Wei Chen
College of Information Science and Engineering
Ritsumeikan University
Kusatsu, Shiga
Japan

Carlos Toro
Vicomtech-IK4
Donostia San Sebastian
Spain

Satoshi Tanaka
College of Information Science and Engineering
Ritsumeikan University
Kusatsu, Shiga
Japan

Robert J. Howlett
KES International
Shoreham-by-Sea
UK

Lakhmi C. Jain
Faculty of Education, Science, Technology and Mathematics
University of Canberra
Canberra
Australia

ISSN 2190-3018 ISSN 2190-3026 (electronic)
Smart Innovation, Systems and Technologies
ISBN 978-3-319-37311-9 ISBN 978-3-319-23024-5 (eBook)
DOI 10.1007/978-3-319-23024-5

Springer Cham Heidelberg New York Dordrecht London

Softcover reprint of the hardcover 1st edition 2015

Printed on acid-free paper

Springer International Publishing AG Switzerland is part of Springer Science+Business Media (www.springer.com)

Preface

The third KES International Conference on Innovation in Medicine and Healthcare (InMed-15) was held during 11–12 September 2015 in Kyoto, Japan, organized by KES International and co-organized by Research Center of Advanced ICT for Medical and Healthcare, Ritsumeikan University, Japan.

InMed-15 is the third edition of the InMed series of conferences. The first and the second InMed conferences were held in Greece and Spain, respectively. InMed-15 is the first conference held outside of European countries. The conference focuses on the major trends and innovations in modern intelligent systems applying to medicine, surgery, healthcare and the issues of an ageing population. The purpose of the conference is to exchange new ideas, new technologies and current research results in these research fields.

We received 78 submissions from 16 countries. All submissions were carefully reviewed by at least two reviewers of the International Programme Committee. Finally 53 papers (including one short paper) were accepted to be presented at the proceedings. The major areas covered at the conference and presented at the proceedings include: (1) Medical Informatics; (2) Biomedical Engineering; (3) Management for Mealthcares; (4) Advanced ICT for Medical and Healthcare; (5) Simulation and Visualization/VR for Medicine; (6) Statistical Signal Processing and Artificial Intelligence; (7) Smart Medical and Healthcare System and (8) Healthcare Support System. In addition to the accepted research papers, three keynote speeches by leading researchers were presented at the conference.

We thank Dr. Xian-hua Han and Dr. Rui Xu of Ritsumeikan University for their valuable editing assistance for this book. We are also grateful to the authors and reviewers for their contributions.

September 2015

Yen-Wei Chen
Carlos Toro
Satoshi Tanaka
Robert J. Howlett
Lakhmi C. Jain

InMed 2015 Organization

General Chair

Yen-Wei Chen, Ritsumeikan University, Japan

General Co-chairs

Shigehiro Morikawa, Shiga University of Medical University, Japan
Lakhmi C. Jain, University of South Australia, Australia

Executive Chair

Robert J. Howlett, Bournemouth University, UK

Programme Chairs

Satoshi Tanaka, Ritsumeikan University, Japan
Edward J. Ciaccio, Columbia University, USA

Publicity Chair

Lanfen Lin, Zhejiang University, China

Co-Chairs of Workshop on Smart Medical and Healthcare Systems

Carlos Toro, Vicomtech-IK4, Spain
Ivan Macia Oliver, Vicomtech-IK4, Spain

Organization and Management

KES International (www.kesinternational.org) in partnership with **Ritsumeikan University, Japan** (www.ritsumei.jp) and **the Institute of Knowledge Transfer** (www.ikt.org.uk)

International Programme Committee Members and Reviewers

Sergio Albiol-Pérez, Universidad de Zaragoza, Spain
Arnulfo Alanis, Instituto Tecnológico de Tijuana, Mexico
Danni Ai, Beijing Institute of Technology, China
Tsukasa Aso, National Institute of Technology, Toyama College, Japan
Shinichiro Ataka, Osaka International University, Japan
Ahmad Taher Azar, Faculty of Computers and Information, Benha University, Egypt
Vitoantonio Bevilacqua, Dipartimento di Ingegneria Elettrica e dell'Informazione –Politecnico di Bari, Italy
Giosue Lo Bosco, University of Palermo, Italy
Christopher Buckingham, Computer Science, Aston University, Birmingham, UK
M. Emre Celebi, Louisiana State University in Shreveport, USA
Yen-Wei Chen, Ritsumeikan University, Japan
D. Chyzhyk, Ritsumeikan University, Japan
Luis Enrique Sánchez Crespo, Universidad de las Fuerzas Armadas, Ecuador
Guifang Duan, Zhejiang University, China
Nashwa Mamdouh El-Bendary, Arab Academy for Science, Technology, and Maritime Transport
Massimo Esposito, ICAR-CNR, Italy
Cecilia Dias Flores, Federal University of Health Sciences of Porto Alegre
José Manuel Fonseca, Faculty of Sciences and Technology of Universidade Nova de Lisboa, Lisbon
Amir H. Foruzan, Shahed University, Iran
Arfan Ghani, University of Bolton, Greater Manchester, UK
Manuel Graña, University of the Basque Country, Spain
Hiroshi Hagiwara, Ritsumeikan University, Japan

Xian-hua Han, Ritsumeikan University, Japan
Kyoko Hasegawa, Ritsumeikan University, Japan
Aboul Ella Hassanien, Cairo University, Egypt
Ioannis Hatzilygeroudis, University of Patras, Greece
Elena Hernández-Pereira, University of A Coruña, Spain
Yasushi Hirano, Yamaguchi University, Japan
Robert Howlett, Bournemouth University, UK
Monica Huerta, Universidad Simón Bolívar-Venezuela and Universidad Politécnica Salesiana—Ecuador
Hongjie Hu, Zhejiang University, China
Ajita Ichalkaranje, Seven Steps Physiotherapy Clinic, Adelaide, South Australia.
Nikhil Ichalkaranje, Government of South Australia, Adelaide, South Australia.
Soichiro Ikuno, Tokyo University of Technology, Japan
Ignacio Illan, Universitat Rovira i Virgili (URV), Catalonia, Spain
David Isern, Universitat Rovira i Virgili (URV), Catalonia, Spain
Sandhya Jain, Medical Practitioner, Adelaide, South Australia.
Huiyan Jiang, Northeastern University, China
Kyoji Kawagoe, Ritsumeikan University, Japan
Hiroharu Kawanaka, Graduate School of Engineering, Mie University, Japan
Takayuki Kawaura, Kansai Medical University, Japan
Akinori Kimura, Ashikaga Institute of Technology, Japan
Ziad Kobti, University of Windsor, Canada
Tomohiro Kuroda, Kyoto University Hospital, Japan
Joo-ho Lee, Ritsumeikan University, Japan
Lenin G. Lemus-Zúñiga, Universitat Politècnica de València, España
Jingbing Li, Hainan University, China
Sergio Magdaleno, Instituto Tecnologico de Tijuana
Paco Martinez, Instituto Tecnologico de Tijuana
Esperanza Manrique, Universidad Autonoma de Baja California
Takafumi Marutani, Ritsumeikan University, Japan
Yasushi Matsumura, Osaka University, Japan
Naoki Matsushiro, Osaka Police Hospital, Japan
Kazuyuki Matsumoto, University of Tokushima, Japan
Yoshiyuki Matsumoto, Shimonoseki City University, Japan
Tadashi Matsuo, Ritsumeikan University, Japan
Rashid Mehmood, College of Computer Science, King Khalid University
Nora del Carmen Osuna Millan, Universidad Autónoma de Baja California and Osuna Consultor
Hongying Meng, Brunel University London, UK
Takashi Mitsuda, Ritsumeikan University, Japan
Jose Montanana, Universidad Complutense de Madrid, Spain
Antonio Moreno, Universitat Rovira i Virgili (URV), Spain
Louise Moody, Coventry School of Art and Design, Coventry University, UK
Keisuke Nagase, Kanazawa University, Japan
Kazuo Nakazawa, National Cerebral and Cardiovascular Center, Japan

Contents

Part I
Emerging Research Leaders of Medical Informatics in KANSAI Area

Prediction of Clinical Practices by Clinical Data of the Previous Day Using Linear Support Vector Machine

Takashi Nakai, Tadamasa Takemura, Risa Sakurai, Kenichiro Fujita, Kazuya Okamoto and Tomohiro Kuroda

Abstract For preventing mistakes and guaranteeing quality, Clinical Decision Support System (CDSS) is expected to support decision-making of healthcare professionals. Until now, there had been many studies of CDSS based on rule-based production system. However practical use of CDSS had been limited because of the complexity of medical care. On the other hand, the machine learning that required huge amounts of data is used to make data-driven predictions or decisions in computer science recently. We considered that this method was effective in practical care. Firstly, we constructed a model based on the hypothesis that clinical practices of a day might determine them of next day for the same patients. Next, we created predictors using linear support vector machines and clinical actions on Diagnosis Procedure Combination/Per-Per Diem Payment System introduced for medical billing in Japan. Finally we evaluated predictive performance by cross validation. As a result, the clinical actions whose frequency of appearance were

The erratum of this chapter can be found under DOI 10.1007/978-3-319-23024-5_54

T. Nakai (✉) · T. Takemura · R. Sakurai · K. Fujita
Graduate School of Applied Informatics University of Hyogo, Kobe, Japan
e-mail: ab14h405@ai.u-hyogo.ac.jp

T. Takemura
e-mail: takemura@ai.u-hyogo.ac.jp

R. Sakurai
e-mail: ab14v403@ai.u-hyogo.ac.jp

K. Fujita
e-mail: kfujita@kuhp.kyoto-u.ac.jp

K. Fujita · K. Okamoto · T. Kuroda
Division of Medical Information Technology and Administration Planning,
Kyoto University Hospital, Kyoto, Japan
e-mail: kazuya@kuhp.kyoto-u.ac.jp

T. Kuroda
e-mail: tomo@kuhp.kyoto-u.ac.jp

Y.-W. Chen et al. (eds.), *Innovation in Medicine and Healthcare 2015*,
Smart Innovation, Systems and Technologies 45,
DOI 10.1007/978-3-319-23024-5_1

higher trend to have higher predictive performance. Thus, it was suggested that predictive performance was improved by preparing sufficient amount of data and ensuring the frequency of appearance.

1 Introduction

For preventing medical mistakes and guaranteeing medical quality, Clinical Decision Support System (CDSS) is expected to provide reference information for decision-making of healthcare professionals [1, 2]. A lot of studies have been made on CDSS based on rule-based production system that began in MYCIN in the 1970s. However, it is difficult to make rules for all clinical decision because medical care is very complicated and complex. Only a few systems are in practical use with limited condition such as irregular pulse determination system. On the other hand, in computer science, the machine learning that required huge amounts of data is used to make data-driven predictions or decisions. Recently, several these studies give high predictive performance because of development of methods of machine learning and computers. For example, several systems by applying machine learning that required huge amounts of data have beat professional players in shogi. We consider these methods would be applicable to medical care.

In this study, we examined the predictability of clinical practices to a patient of a day by using huge clinical actions and machine learning. Actual data of clinical actions was entered and accumulated into hospital information system, however we used clinical actions data of Diagnosis Procedure Combination/Per-Diem Payment System (DPC/PDPS) in this study. DPC/PDPS is a system for medical billing in Japan and the data of clinical actions based on DPC/PDPS are represented as the Combination of Diagnosis and Procedure. These data are being accumulated based on domestic standards in Japan. We constructed a model based on the hypothesis that clinical practices can be predicted from the data of clinical practices done on the day before for the same patient. We predicted all clinical actions appeared in the future by machine learning and evaluated the results. Concretely we created predictors by using linear support vector machines and 6 months of the DPC data as clinical actions on all admission at a large-scale university hospital. We evaluated predictive performance by cross validation.

2 Background and Related Work

2.1 Proposed Model for Prediction of Clinical Actions

In this paper, we propose the model based on the hypothesis that clinical practices can be predicted from the data of clinical practices done on the day before for the

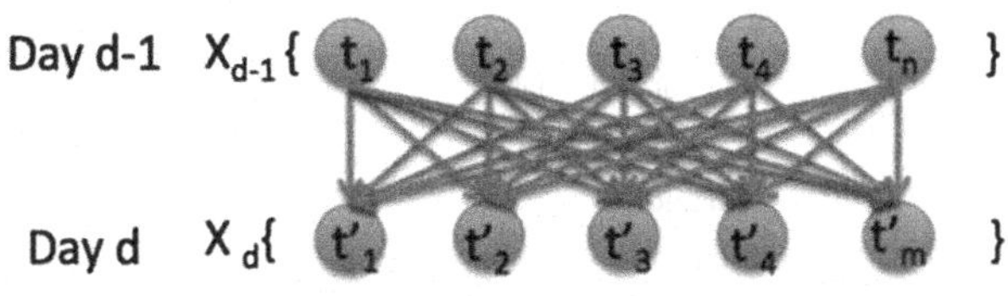

Fig. 1 Concept of prediction model

same patient. Figure 1 shows the concept of this model. We examined that clinical practice set $X_d(t'_1,t'_2,\ldots t'_n)$ on a day d can be predicted from clinical practice set $X_{(d-1)}(t_1, t_2,\ldots,t_m)$ done on the day before for the same patient. Concretely, we created predictors by applying machine learning to clinical practice sets of all d and d-1 in clinical action data. We examined predictability of appearance of the clinical practice using this predictor.

In this paper, we used Diagnosis Procedure Combination (DPC) data as clinical actions data. DPC data is accumulated by Diagnosis Procedure Combination/Per-Diem Payment System (DPC/PDPS) in Japan, and used linear support vector machine as the machine learning method.

2.2 *Diagnosis Procedure Combination/Per-Diem Payment System*

Diagnosis Procedure Combination/Per-Diem Payment System (DPC/PDPS) is the flat-rate payment system based on Diagnosis Procedure Combination (DPC) [3]. DPC was made considering clinical circumstance in Japan based on Diagnosis Related Group (DRG) of USA. The purposes of DPC and DPC/PDPS are the improvement of medical costs and services. DPC/PDPS was first introduced to 82 advanced treatment hospitals that had 66,497 beds totally in April 2003, and introduced to 1585 hospitals that had 492,206 bets totally in April 2014 [4].

The files of DPC are easy handle format for computer such as “style 1”, “D file”, “E file” and “F file”. For medical service comparison, clinical actions for patients are accumulated. E and F file include details of clinical actions. On these file, clinical actions to patients are represented as the data category code and the unified electronic receipt code. Particularly the data category code shows the rough category of the clinical actions and indicates if the clinical action is practiced in any situation. Table 1 shows examples of data category code.

2.3 *Linear Support Vector Machines*

Linear support vector machine (Linear SVM) is the methods of machine learning and one kind of supervised learning [5]. Linear SVMs are mainly used as 2 class

Table 1 Examples of data categories

Data category code	Data category name
11	First consultation fee
13	Education
14	Home care
21	Medicines for internal use
22	Potion
23	Medicine for external use
24	Drug compounding = hospitalization
26	Narcotic drug and so on
27	Basic technical fee for dispensing
31	Intramuscular injection
32	Intravenous infusion
33	others (injection)
40	Procedures
50	Operation
54	Anesthesia
60	Examination
70	Radiology and image diagnosis
80	Others (rehabilitation, radiation therapy and so on)
90	Basic fee for hospitalization = hospitalization
92	Specific hospital charges = hospitalization
97	Hospital meals standard obligation fees = hospitalization

classifier for data whose class is not known. In linear SVM, data is handled as feature vectors. If the feature vectors are m-dimensional vectors, linear SVM determines a class of data using separating hyperplane expressed as the following.

$$f(x) = w^T x + b$$

w is a m-dimensional vector and b is a bias term. There are innumerable separating hyperplane. Linear SVM uses the maximum margin separating hyperplane which has the maximum distance (margin) to teacher data of each class because the maximum margin separating hyperplane is expected to have good classification accuracy for unknown data.

3 Experiment of Prediction of Clinical Practices

This chapter describes the experiment of prediction of clinical practices as previously explained.

Table 2 Summary of E files and F files

Item	Number of data
Number of hospitalizations	6,445
Total number of days of hospitalizations	118,150
"data category code" + "receipt computerized system code" Combinations	5,279
Number of records of F files	2,543,205

3.1 Target Data

We used the E and F files about the patients who had admitted and discharged in the large-scale university hospital within the period from 2006/4 to 2006/6 for the experiment. These files included the data of 6,445 hospitalizations and 118,150 days as shown in Table 2.

In these files, a clinical practice is represented as receipt computerized system code. However, if two practices have same unified electronic receipt code and different data category code, it is possible to consider different clinical practice. For example, we can separate that "medicine (name)" is used "operation" and "medicine for external use" using the date category code. So, if two clinical practices had different data category code, we considered these clinical practices were different in this study. Therefore we regarded 5,279 combinations of "data category code" and "unified electronic receipt code" as targets of prediction.

3.2 Experiment

The purpose of the proposed model is the clinical practices a day could determine the clinical practice next day. Linear SVM handles data as vector as described in Sect. 2.3, therefore we handle data as 5279-dimensional vectors in this experiment. Each element of the vector is mapped to 5279 clinical practices as shown in Table 3.

We make the experimental data set for each clinical practice. We evaluate the predictive performance.

1. Make lists of clinical practices for each patient by the day from DPC data

Make vectors from lists of step 1 as shown in Fig. 2. The value of vector elements is 1 if the clinical action is done. The value of vector elements is 0 if the clinical action is not done.

2. Classify vectors of step 0 into class 1 if the target clinical practice is done on the day after. Classify vectors into class 0 if not. For example, Table 4 shows the

Table 3 Elements of vector for linear svm

Element number of feature vector	Data category code	Receipt computerized system code	Medical specification name
1	11	111000110	first consultation fee (hospital)
2	11	111000370	first consultation fee (infants)
3	11	111000570	first consultation fee (overtime)
4	11	111000670	first consultation fee (holiday)
:			
4543	60	160101210	Arterial blood sampling
:			
5278	97	197000470	special diet fee (per one meal)
5279	97	197000570	diet fee in dining room

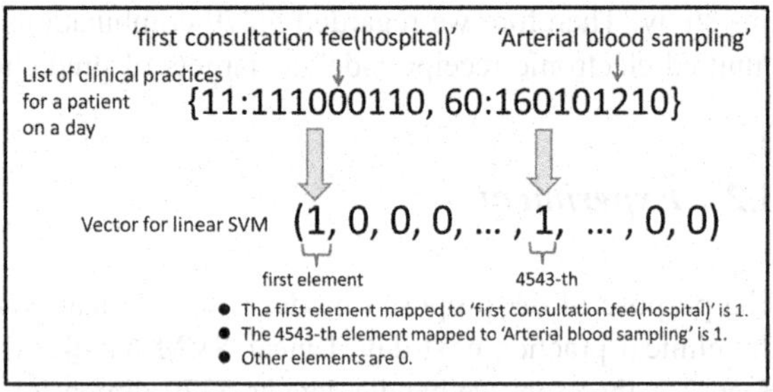

Fig. 2 Conversion of list of clinical practices to vectors

example of experimental data whose target clinical practice is 'Arterial blood sampling'. The 4543-th element is mapped to 'Arterial blood sampling' as shown in Table 3. Therefore we classify the vector into class 1 if the 4543-th element of vector of the day after is 1. We classify the vector into class 0 if not. We remove the vectors for discharge date from the experimental data because none of clinical practices on the next day. As a result we got 111,705 vectors as experimental data of each clinical practice of prediction target.

3. Divide experimental data into 10 parts. Use one of parts as test data in rotation and use other parts as teacher data. Create the classifier by using teacher data, and evaluated prediction performance for teacher data by 10-fold cross validation [5]. We used Liblinear [6] to create classifiers and to predict for test data.

Table 4 Image of experimental data for 'Arterial blood sampling'

Patient ID	Date	List of clinical actions provided (feature vector)	Whether 'Arterial blood sampling' has been practiced on the next day	Class
α	dα (admission date)	(1,0,0,0,...,0,...,0,0,0)	Not practiced	0
α	dα+1	(0,0,0,0,...,0,...,0,0,0)	Practiced	1
α	dα+2	(0,0,0,0,...,1,...,0,0,0)	Not practiced	0
		:		
α	dα+x-1	4543-th element 0,0,0)	Not practiced	0
α	dα+x (discharge date)	remove the vectors for discharge date from th		
β	dβ (admission date)	(1,0,0,1,...,0,...,0,0,1)	Practiced	1
β	dβ+1	(1,0,0,1,...,1,...,0,0,1)	Not practiced	0
		:		
β	dβ+x-1	(1,0,0,1,...,0,...,0,0,1)	Not practiced	0
β	dβ+x (discharge date)	remove the vectors for discharge date from the experimental data		
		:		

If 'Arterial blood sampling' practiced on the next day, the vector is classified into class 1. If not, the vector is classified into class 0.

3.3 Result

Table 5 shows the result of experiment about 'Arterial blood sampling' by the method described in Sect. 3.2. 'True Positive' is the number of test data of class 1 predicted correctly. 'False Positive' is the number of test data of class 0 predicted to be class 1 by mistake. 'False Negative' is the number of test data of class 1 predicted to be class 0 by mistake. 'True Negative' is the number of test data of class 0 predicted correctly. We calculated precision and recall rate for each 10 test data. Based on cross validation, the average values of these rates are final precision

Table 5 Results of prediction for "Arterial blood sampling"

Target test data	True positive (TP)	False positive (FP)	False negative (FN)	True negative (TN)	Precision = TP/(TP + FP)	Recall = TP/(TP + FN)
1	66	26	186	10893	0.717	0.262
2	99	43	140	10889	0.697	0.414
3	55	25	149	10942	0.688	0.270
4	92	57	161	10861	0.618	0.364
5	68	29	147	10927	0.701	0.316
6	73	37	167	10893	0.664	0.304
7	124	81	207	10758	0.605	0.375
8	97	37	168	10868	0.729	0.366
9	47	19	163	10941	0.712	0.224
10	49	30	134	10957	0.620	0.268
The average precision and recall (result of 10-folds cross validation)					0.675	0.316

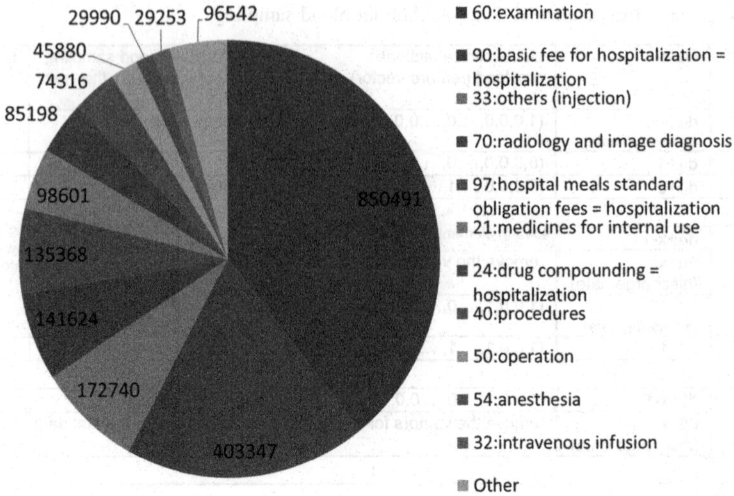

Fig. 3 Number of clinical actions by clinical data category

and recall rate of 'Arterial blood sampling' in this paper. As a result, precision rate was 0.675 and recall rate was 0.316.

We predicted 5279 kinds of clinical practices by the same steps. Figure 3 shows number of clinical actions by clinical data category in experimental data. The number of appearances of clinical actions can be restated as the number of vectors classified into class 1 by the step 4 of 0, and was divided by data category code and by unified electronic receipt code.

The 235 clinical practices only appeared on the first day of admission in total 5279 practices, so this system did not predict these admission date practices. In addition, few clinical practices appeared in this data could not be fitted SVMs because this machine learning method needs a certain amount data to learn and judge the correct answers. Therefore, on 10-fold cross validation, we omitted clinical practices that did not appear on all validation from the total practices. As a result, there were 657 clinical practices could be calculated on 10-fold validation this time. Figure 4 shows a scatter diagram of precision rate versus recall rate. The sizes of circle are proportional to the frequency of appearance.

We shows examples of clinical practices and their precision rate and recall rate of '33 others (injection)' as Table 6 and '21 medicines for internal use' as Table 7. In addition, Fig. 5 shows a scatter diagram of precision rate versus recall rate of '33 others (injection)' as well as Fig. 4. Figure 6 is the same diagram of '21 medicines for internal use'.

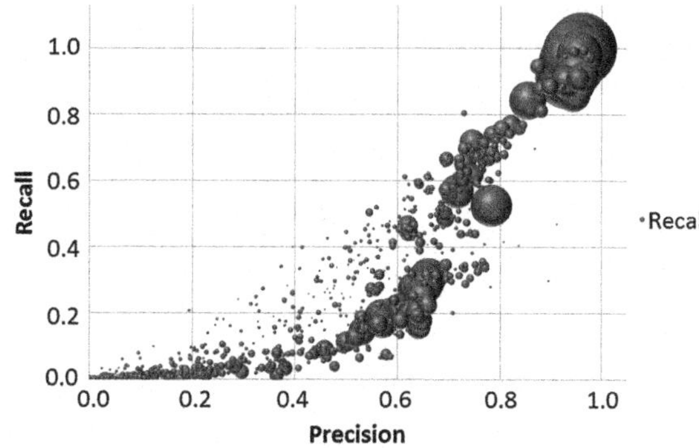

Fig. 4 Scatter diagram of precision rate versus recall rate

Table 6 Examples of precision and recall of others (injection)

Receipt computerized system code	Medical specification name	Number of appearance	Precision	Recall
130004410	Central venous injection	6249	0.896	0.885
640451009	Omepral 20 mg	2862	0.836	0.758
643910067	Stronger Neo-Minophagen C 20 mL	1595	0.806	0.680
620002258	Twinpal 500 mL	1204	0.805	0.721
130000210	Precise continuous intravenous infusion	5797	0.801	0.758
620002191	Glyceol 200 mL	744	0.796	0.624
620001934	Neoparen No. 2 1000 mL	1207	0.790	0.722
620001933	Neoparen No. 1 1000 mL	870	0.789	0.706

Table 7 Examples of precision and recall of medicines for internal use

Receipt computerized system code	Medical specification name	Number of appearance	Precision	Recall
616130532	Cefzon 100 mg	891	0.519	0.167
612320346	Selbex 50 mg	2162	0.435	0.077
611140694	Loxonin 60 mg	1215	0.383	0.043
610411058	Flomox 100 mg	1209	0.377	0.053
612520024	Methergin 0.125 mg	109	0.318	0.108
620003469	Plavix 75 mg	242	0.305	0.093
613330003	Warfarin 1 mg	1494	0.290	0.047
610451009	Prograf 0.2 mg	425	0.227	0.082

Fig. 5 Scatter diagram of precision rate versus recall rate of others (injection)

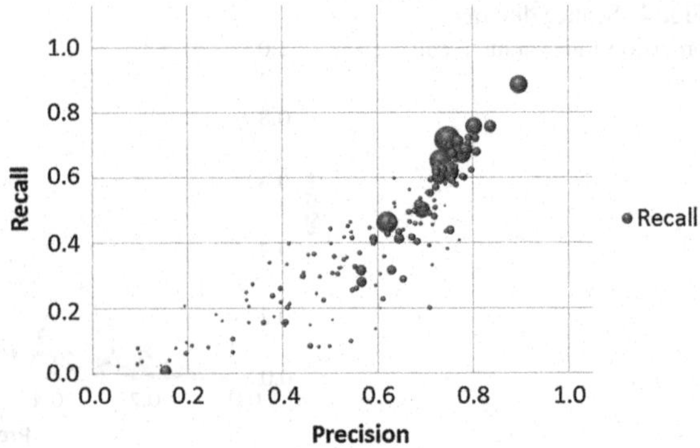

Fig. 6 Scatter diagram of precision rate vs. recall rate of medicines for internal use

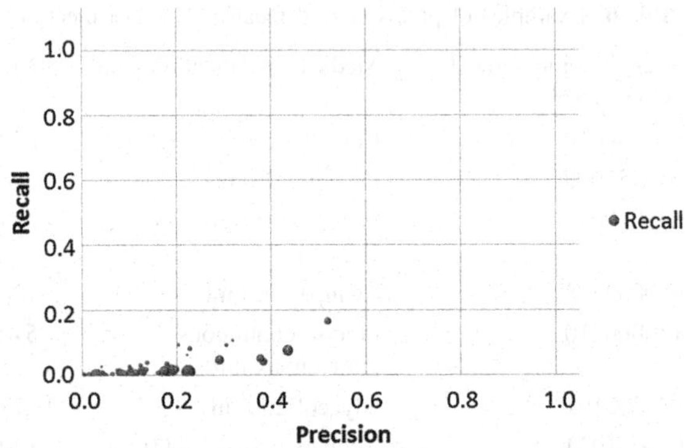

3.4 Discussion

In this study, we used machine learning and all clinical practice data of the day before as teacher data, and evaluated predictability of clinical practices for a patient of a day. Although there are some differences in each data category, some clinical practices have high precision rate and recall rate and others have low precision rate and recall rate. Generally, recall rate seems to be positively correlated with precision rate especially when precision rate is more than 0.4 as shown in Fig. 4. On the other hand, when precision rate is less than 0.4, recall rate trends to be low. Furthermore, from the aspect of the number of data included in each data category (i.e. the number of times that is appeared as a clinical action), the precision rate of the practice with higher frequency tends to be higher. It is assumed that larger amount of data improves the prediction performance. Additionally, the basic codes for medical calculation appear almost every day. It is assumed that it is easy to predict these codes. Concretely, data categories such as 'injection' and 'procedures' have relatively high precision rate and recall rate as shown in Table 6 and Fig. 5. It is seems that this is the result of prediction by learning quantitatively patterns of practices as training data. On the other hand, data categories such as 'medicines for internal use', 'potion', 'medicine for external use' and 'examination' have relatively low precision rate and recall rate as shown in Table 7 and Fig. 6. Especially, a lot of medicines are included in categories such as 'medicines for 'internal use', 'potion' and 'medicine for external use'. Therefore, the frequency of appearances of individual code is not relatively high. As a result, it seems that linear svm was not been able to learn in the 10-fold cross-validation sufficiently. In fact, codes for medicine was 1163 types, whereas, codes that were able to be calculated precision rate were only 65 types. The linear svm could predict more types of medicine if we could get more data. On the other hand, the precision rate and recall rate of the codes of 'examination' with high frequency are high relatively but the precision rate and recall rate of the practice which appears rarely is low relatively.

As a result, we consider that the precision rate is high when the frequency of appearance is increased. We intend to improve the prediction performance for more clinical practices by using larger data.

References

1. Bates, D., et al.: Reducing the frequency of errors in medicine using information technology. J. Am. Med. Inform. Assoc. **8**(4), 299–308 (2001)
2. Jensen, P.B., Jensen, L.J., Brunak, S.: Mining electronic health records: towards better research applications and clinical care. Nat. Rev. Genet. **13**(6), 395–405 (2012)
3. DPC System (Summary and Basic concept DPC/PDPS). http://www.mhlw.go.jp/stf/shingi/2r985200000105vx-att/2r98520000010612.pdf (in Japanese)
4. Summary of a revision of payment for medical services in Heisei 26. http://www.mhlw.go.jp/file/06-Seisakujouhou-12400000-Hokenkyoku/0000039616.pdf (in Japanese)
5. Abe, S.: Approach support vector machines for pattern recognition. Morikita Publishing Co., Ltd. 55, 16–26 (2013) (in Japanese)
6. LIBLINEAR—A Library for Large Linear Classification from http://www.csie.ntu.edu.tw/~cjlin/liblinear/

Method for Detecting Drug-Induced Interstitial Pneumonia from Accumulated Medical Record Data at a Hospital

Yoshie Shimai, Toshihiro Takeda, Shirou Manabe, Kei Teramoto, Naoki Mihara and Yasushi Matsumura

Abstract Drug-induced interstitial pneumonia (DIP) is a serious adverse drug reaction. The occurrence rete of DIP was evaluated by clinical trial before available in the market. However, due to limited number of cases in clinical trials, it may be inapplicable to the real market. We aimed to seek a method to evaluate the occurrence rate of DIP using clinical data warehouse at a hospital. Initially we developed a method that assesses whether presence of IP was written in reports by natural language processing. Next we detected DIP by estimating IP before, during and after the drug administration. Presence of IP was determined according to the reports of CT if CT was performed, otherwise it was determined based on the changes in the results of chest X-ray, level of KL-6 or SP-D. DIP was determined according to the pattern of presence of IP in each phase. In this study we chose amiodarone as a target drug. The number of patients who suffered from IP caused by amiodarone was 16 (3.9 %), including one definitively diagnosed and 15 strong doubt cases. Most of them could be validated by medical record chart. Using this method, we were able to successfully detect occurrence of DIP from accumulated data in a hospital information system.

1 Introduction

Various adverse events occur related to medication use. Information regarding the risk of adverse events for each medicine is important for clinical practice. The safety of medicines is evaluated in clinical trials before the drugs are introduced into the market. However, because the number of subjects in clinical trials is limited, information regarding adverse events generated in clinical trials may be inadequate [1].

Y. Shimai (✉) · T. Takeda · S. Manabe · K. Teramoto · N. Mihara · Y. Matsumura
Medical Informatics, Osaka University Graduate School of Medicine, Osaka, Japan
e-mail: shimai@hp-info.med.osaka-u.ac.jp

Y.-W. Chen et al. (eds.), *Innovation in Medicine and Healthcare 2015*,
Smart Innovation, Systems and Technologies 45,
DOI 10.1007/978-3-319-23024-5_2

Therefore, post-market pharmacovigilance is required for drug safety. Under the present circumstances, spontaneous reporting is the major method for gathering information about adverse events. This method is effective for detecting signals of the side effects of a drug; however, it is impossible to estimate the rate of occurrence of each side effect.

Recently, many hospitals have introduced electronic medical record systems, especially in Japan. Some of these systems include a clinical data warehouse (CDW) for the secondary use of the clinical data. Data relating to drug safety are expected to be included in CDW [2–6]. However, the raw data contained in the CDW are difficult to handle with respect to detecting adverse events.

In this study, we focused on drug-induced interstitial pneumonia which is one of the serious adverse drug reactions potentially terminated in death. Interstitial pneumonia (IP) is mainly diagnosed by chest CT, while chest X-ray, the sialylated carbohydrate antigen KL-6 (KL-6) and surfactant protein D (SP-D) levels are useful adjuncts to the diagnosis. We developed a method that detects the occurrence of IP using these data contained in CDW. Next, we devised a method to detect drug-induced IP (DIP) based on the timing of administration of the drug and occurrence or remission of IP. In this study, we chose amiodarone as a causal medicine of DIP. Amiodaron is one of the effective anti-arrhythmic drugs susceptible to DIP.

2 Methods

2.1 Subject Data

We used the text data of chest CT and chest X-ray reports and data of the KL-6 and SP-D levels contained in the CDW of Osaka University Medial Hospital from January 1, 2010 to March 31, 2013. The study protocol was approved by the Ethics Review Board of Osaka University Medical Hospital (Approval No. 13531, May 8th, 2014).

2.2 Analysis of Chest CT and Chest X-Ray

Each report of chest CT and chest X-ray consist of finding field and diagnosis field. Free text data are written in these fields. A radiologist inferred the diagnosis based on the findings of abnormalities. Initially we evaluated the data in diagnosis field and subsequently assessed the data in finding field when no definitive diagnosis could be obtained from data in the diagnosis field. The diagnostic data were searched for the keyword “interstitial pneumonia”. If IP was definitively diagnosed,

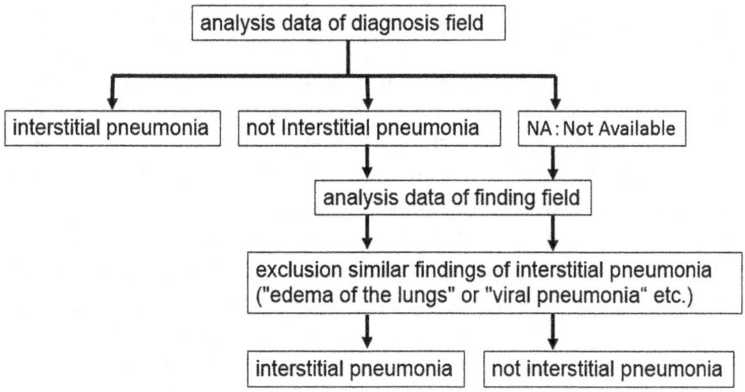

Fig. 1 Algorithm for detecting interstitial pneumonia using chest CT or X-ray reports

a flag for IP was set on the report. A synonym or detailed diagnosis of IP, such as "usual interstitial pneumonia (UIP)" or "acute interstitial pneumonia (AIP)", was regarded as IP. When there was no definitive diagnosis, we then evaluated the data in the finding field. We searched for keywords in the finding data. Likelihood ratios of founded keywords are multiplied to obtain an IP score. A flag was set when IP score exceeded the cut-off value. There are some disease which have similar findings to those of IP, such as "edema of the lung" and "viral pneumonia". There also are the cases of IP but not DIP, such as "lymphocytic interstitial pneumonia (LIP)" and "respiratory bronchiolitis-associated interstitial lung disease (RB-ILD)". In these cases DIP should be denied, hence lower the flag if a flag for IP was set on the report (Fig. 1).

2.3 Likelihood Ratios and Cut-off Values for Chest CT and X-Ray

We selected 400 patients with interstitial pneumonia and 400 patients without interstitial pneumonia diagnosed by a radiologist using chest CT images from January 1, 2011 to March 31, 2013. Among these cases, 300 in each group were allocated to the learning dataset and 100 were allocated to the testing dataset (test data1). In addition, we selected 100 cases at random (test data2), which were not used for the learning data or test data1 sets. We also selected the data for chest X-ray obtained within three months from the chest CT. The learning data, test data1 and test data2 sets for chest X-ray (patients with and without interstitial pneumonia) included 354 cases (133, 221), 66 cases (24, 42) and 35 cases (4, 31), respectively. We extracted keywords from text data in the field of the chest CT reports for the training dataset. We used KHCoder to collect keywords [7] and selected words appeared in more than 10 reports of IP. We calculated the likelihood ratio for a positive finding based on the frequency of each keyword. We also calculated the likelihood ratio for the learning dataset for chest X-ray. We handled abbreviations and detailed words, such as "UIP" (usual interstitial pneumonia) and "AIP" (acute interstitial pneumonia), and synonymous words, such as "frosted glass" and "ground glass", as the same keywords. In cases that negative words, such as "not accepted" or "not confirmed", in the neighborhood of a keyword, it was regarded as absence. Furthermore, in cases that there is a keyword but whose modifier is different from lung, such as "liver cyst" or "aortic calcification", the keywords were regarded as absence. The likelihood ratios of the keywords appeared in a report were multiplied to determine IP score. We plotted ROC curve by changing cut-off point and obtained the nearest cut-off value to point (0, 1) on the ROC curve using test data1. We also evaluated the precision of the findings for detecting interstitial pneumonia using test data2.

2.4 Detection of DIP

We sought to detect cases of DIP caused by amiodarone in order to evaluate the proposing method. We used the reports of CT, X-ray and the level of KL-6 and SP-D obtained under treatment with amiodarone in the period from January 1, 2010 to December 31, 2013. The reports of chest CT and X-ray were judged to be positive or negative by the above-mentioned method. The KL-6 and SP-D levels were judged to be positive or negative according to the upper limit of normal values of each test. We then devised a method to determine the presence of IP before, during and after administration of amiodarone. The presence of IP was determined based on the reports of CT if CT was performed, otherwise it was determined according to the changes in the results of chest X-ray, the level of KL-6 or SP-D. In cases in which a judgment resulting from any of the reports of chest X-ray, the level of KL-6 or SP-D was the same as that of chest CT in a given phase, and the test judgement changed in another phase in which no chest CT findings, the test judgement was used as the judgement in its phase. For example, if the judgements of both chest CT and chest X-ray were "positive" during drug administration and "negative" by chest X-ray before drug administration, we noted that the assessment of chest X-ray was changed from "negative" before drug administration to "positive" during drug administration and judged the case as being "negative" before drug administration. The occurrence of DIP was judged using the five categories of "definitive", "strongly suspected," "weakly suspected," "negative" and "judgment difficulty" based on the "positive," "negative" and "not available" patterns of IP observed before, during and after drug administration (Table 1). For example, DIP was judged as being "strongly suspected" when the patterns of IP before, during and after drug administration were "negative," "positive" and "positive".

Table 1 Judgement of DIP based on the pattern of IP before, during and after drug administration (+: positive, −: negative, NA: not available)

Drug administration			Judgement
Before	During	After	
−	−	−	Negative
−	−	+	Negative
−	+	−	Definitive
−	+	+	Strongly suspected
+	−	−	Negative
+	−	+	Negative
+	+	−	Negative
+	+	+	Negative
NA	−	−	Negative
NA	−	+	Negative
NA	+	−	Strongly suspected
NA	+	+	Judgement difficulty
−	NA	−	Judgement difficulty
−	NA	+	Judgement difficulty
+	NA	−	Negative
+	NA	+	Negative
−	−	NA	Negative
−	+	NA	Strongly suspected
+	−	NA	Negative
+	+	NA	Negative
NA	NA	+	Judgement difficulty
NA	NA	−	Judgement difficulty
NA	+	NA	Weakly suspected
NA	−	NA	Negative
+	NA	NA	Negative
−	NA	NA	Judgement difficulty
NA	NA	NA	Judgement difficulty

2.5 Validation of DIP According to the Medical Records

We collected and checked the subjects' medical records as to whether doctors thought DIP was induced by amiodarone. We therefore assessed the medical records of the patients who received amiodarone and checked whether "IP" was written in the medical records. We classified the case as involving "no description" if this information was not written. If the information for IP was provided, we checked the medical records as to whether IP was caused by amiodarone and classified the cases as "DIP". "DIP suspected", "DIP negative" or "no description".

3 Results

3.1 Analysis of Chest CT and Chest X-Ray

The likelihood ratios for positive and negative findings for keywords related to chest CT using the learning data set are shown in Table 2. The keywords of "honeycombing", "collagen" and "interstitial pneumonia" showed higher positive likelihood ratios. The likelihood ratios for positive and negative findings for keywords on chest X-ray using the learning dataset are shown in Table 3. The keywords of "reticular", "interstitial pneumonia", "ground-glass" and "dot-like" showed higher positive likelihood ratios. The cut-off value for chest CT using test data1 was 0.06 (sensitivity: 0.95, specificity: 0.98) and the cut-off value for chest X-ray was 0.012 (sensitivity: 0.83, specificity: 1). In addition, we assessed the detective precision of chest CT and chest X-ray for IP using test data2. The sensitivity was 0.89 and the specificity was 0.99 for the detective precision of chest CT, which were high. In terms of the detective precision of chest X-ray, the sensitivity was 0.67 and the specificity was 1.

Table 2 Keywords and likelihood ratios for chest CT

Keywords	Frequency of keywords			Likelihood ratio	
	Interstitial pneumonia		Total		
	Positive	Negative		Positive	Negative
Honeycomb	74	0.1	74	740.00	0.75
Collagen	14	0.1	14	140.00	0.95
Interstitial pneumonia	281	5	286	56.20	0.06
Traction bronchiectasis	140	3	143	46.67	0.54
Reticular	229	8	237	28.63	0.24
Diffuse	232	13	245	17.85	0.24
Reactivity	35	11	46	3.18	0.92
Convergence	17	6	23	2.83	0.96
Ground-glass	287	113	400	2.54	0.07
Cyst	44	23	67	1.91	0.92
Inspiratory	12	8	20	1.50	0.99
Infection	16	14	30	1.14	0.99
Curve linear	80	71	151	1.13	0.96
Calcification	57	52	109	1.10	0.98
Consolidation	29	27	56	1.07	0.99
Lymph node	35	33	68	1.06	0.99
Infiltration	22	21	43	1.05	1.00
Emphysema	52	53	105	0.98	1.00
Swelling	27	28	55	0.96	1.00
Nodular density	99	165	264	0.60	1.49
Band	48	81	129	0.59	1.15

(continued)

Table 2 (continued)

Keywords	Frequency of keywords			Likelihood ratio	
	Interstitial pneumonia		Total		
	Positive	Negative		Positive	Negative
Tuberculosis	11	19	30	0.58	1.03
Inflammatory	90	180	270	0.50	1.75
Heterogeneity	5	11	16	0.45	1.02
Cancer	23	59	82	0.39	1.15
Thick	23	59	82	0.39	1.15
Dot like	16	46	62	0.35	1.12
Cavity	3	9	12	0.33	1.02
Lung edema	4	12	16	0.33	1.03
Mass	15	51	66	0.29	1.14
Metastasis	7	41	48	0.17	1.13
Tumor	2	13	15	0.15	1.04
Atelectasis	4	49	53	0.08	1.18

Table 3 Keywords and likelihood ratios for chest X-ray

Keywords	Frequency of keywords			Likelihood ratio	
	Interstitial pneumonia		Total		
	Positive	Negative		Positive	Negative
Reticular	106	6	112	30.95	0.21
Interstitial pneumonia	86	6	92	25.11	0.36
Ground-glass	121	32	153	6.62	0.10
Dot like	13	13	26	1.75	0.96
Band	20	25	45	1.40	0.95
Curve linear	21	34	55	1.08	0.99
Permeability	7	14	21	0.88	1.01
Infiltration	5	11	16	0.80	1.01
Postoperative	11	25	36	0.77	1.03
Thick	14	40	54	0.61	1.08
Nodular density	14	42	56	0.58	1.09
Atelectasis	3	11	14	0.48	1.03
Calcification	2	10	12	0.35	1.03
Metastasis	2	10	12	0.35	1.03
Inflammatory	8	58	66	0.24	1.25

Table 4 Detection of DIP caused by amiodarone

Detection of DIP by this study	Chest CT	Chest CT, chest X-ray, KL-6, SP-D
Definitive	0 (0 %)	1 (0.2 %)
Strongly suspected	9 (2.2 %)	15 (3.6 %)
Weakly suspected	18 (4.4 %)	16 (3.9 %)
Negatively suspected	0 (0 %)	96 (23.2 %)
Negative	161 (39.0 %)	162 (39.2 %)
Judgement difficulty	225 (54.5 %)	123 (24.0 %)
Total	413 (100.0 %)	413 (100.0 %)

3.2 *Determination of DIP*

The number of patients who received amiodarone was 413 (prescription: 187, injection: 120, both: 106). The rate of "judgment difficulty" was 54.5 % when CT only was used, which was reduced to 24 % when added the results of chest X-ray, the level of KL-6 and SP-D secondarily. The judgement of DIP caused by amiodarone was "definitive" in one case (0.2 %), "strongly suspected" in 15 cases (3.6 %), "weakly suspected" in 16 cases (3.9 %), "negatively suspected" in 96 cases (23.2 %), "negative" in 162 cases (39.2 %) and "judgment difficulty" in 123 cases (24.0 %) (Table 4).

3.3 *Validation of DIP According to the Medical Records*

DIP descriptions in the medical records in each pattern of IP are shown in Table 5. Regarding the one patient who was judged as "definitive" based on the pattern of IP "negative", "positive", "negative" in phase of before, during and after drug administration respectively, "no description" was found in the medical record. In two of the three patients judged as "strongly suspected" with the pattern of "negative", "positive" and "positive", "DIP" was written in the medical records, while in the other case "DIP suspected" was written. In two of the three patients judged as "strongly suspected" with the pattern of "not available", "positive" and "negative", "DIP suspected" was written in the medical records; in the other case "no description" was written. For two of the nine patients judged as "strongly suspected" with the pattern of "not available", "positive" and "negative," "DIP suspected" was written in the medical records, whereas in the other case "no description" was found. Regarding the patients with a status of "negatively suspected" or "negative" with the pattern of "not available" in 3 phases, we considered these cases not to be DIP. The rate of DIP by amiodarone was 3.9 % if the "definitive" or "strongly suspected" cases assumed to be DIP.

Table 5 Validation of DIP according to the medical records (+: positive, −: negative, NA: not available)

Drug administration			Judge	The number of patients	DIP by medical records			
Before	During	After			DIP	DIP suspect	Negative	No description
−	+	−	Definitive	1				1
−	+	+	Strongly suspected	3	2	1		
NA	+	−	Strongly suspected	3		1		2
−	+	NA	Strongly suspected	9		2		7
NA	+	NA	Weakly suspected	16		4	4	8
−	−	−	Negative	16				16
−	−	+	Negative	1				1
+	−	−	Negative	3				3
+	−	+	Negative	2				2
+	+	−	Negative	0				0
+	+	+	Negative	0				0
NA	−	−	Negative	11				11
NA	−	+	Negative	1				1
+	NA	−	Negative	1				1
+	NA	+	Negative	1				1
−	−	NA	Negative	39			2	37
+	−	NA	Negative	6				6
+	+	NA	Negative	3				3
NA	−	NA	Negative	68			2	66
+	NA	NA	Negative	10				10
NA	+	+	Difficulty	1		1		
−	NA	−	Difficulty	23				23
−	NA	+	Difficulty	2				2
NA	NA	+	Difficulty	2				2
NA	NA	−	Difficulty	7				7
−	NA	NA	Difficulty	70				70
NA	NA	NA	Difficulty	114		1	3	110

4 Discussion

Because Image reports are written in free text, it is difficult to analyse these. We estimated certainty factor for IP of a reports by multiplying the likelihood ratios of the keywords appeared in a report. As the number of words characteristic of IP increased, the certainty factor for IP increased.

In order to detect DIP, it is necessary to estimate the presence of IP in phase of before, during and after drug administration. However, CT examinations were not so frequently performed, it is impossible to estimate the presence of IP in every phase only by CT. Thus we used the results of X-ray, the level of KL-6 or SP-D to estimate the presence of IP in each phase.

According to the package insert of amiodarone, the rate of DIP as a serious side effect in the field of internal medicine is 1.9 %; the rate for injections is unknown based on spontaneous reports. According to the results of this study, the rate of DIP induced by amiodarone is estimated to be 3.9 %, which is higher than the values shown in the package insert.

5 Conclusion

Using the method described in this study, we were able to successfully detect the occurrence of drug-induced interstitial pneumonia by using accumulated medical record data in a hospital information system.

References

1. Bates, D.W., Evans, R.S., Murff, H., et al.: Detecting adverse events using information technology. J. Am. Med. Inform. Assoc. **10**, 115–128 (2003)
2. Harpaz, R., Vilar, S., DuMouchel, W., et al.: Combing signals from spontaneous reports and electronic health records for detection of adverse drug reactions. J. Am. Med. Inform. Assoc. **20**, 413–419 (2013)
3. Coloma, P.M., Schuemie, M.J., Ferrajolo, C., et al.: A reference standard for evaluation of methods for drug safety signal detection using electronic healthcare record databases. Drug Saf **36**, 13–23 (2013)
4. Strom, B.L.: Overview of automated databases in pharmacoepidemiology. In: Pharmacoepidemiology, 5th edn, pp. 158–182. Wiley, New York (2005)
5. Bates, D.W., Evants, R.S., Murff, H., et al.: Detecting adverse events using information technology. J. Am. Med. Inf. Assoc. **10**, 115–128 (2003)
6. Cheetham, T.C., Lee, J., Hunt, C.M., et al.: An automated causality assessment algorithm to detect drug-induced liver injury in electronic medical record data. Pharmacoepidemiol. Drug Saf. **23**, 601–608 (2014)
7. KHCoder v2.0, 29 October 2013 http://khc.sourceforge.net/en/. Accessed 15 April 2015

Visualization and Quantitative Analysis of Nursing Staff Trajectories Based on a Location System

Kikue Sato, Tomohiro Kuroda and Akitoshi Seiyama

Abstract We sought to clarify the impact of information communication technology (ICT) on hospital management. We used a real-time location system for nurses' workload assessment. First, we introduced a Bluetooth-based real-time location system into a hospital and visualized the trajectories of the nursing staff from the data obtained. Next, we conducted a quantitative analysis of the data to estimate the workloads of nursing staff from the duration of stay at each bedside. We found clear differences in the time spent on care between patients in general patient rooms and those in critical care rooms. These results show the potential of using the data obtained by ICT tools to support hospital management.

Keywords Staff trajectory · Workload · Location system

1 Introduction

Innumerable applications of mobile devices now use global positioning system (GPS) data to provide useful information outdoors. Recently, advances in sensor technology have enabled location measurement indoors as well. Thus, many previous studies have proposed various medical applications based on location systems using radio frequency identifiers (RFID) or Wi-Fi.

Although most such applications, such as instrument finders [1] or outpatient navigators [2], were meant to support daily clinical activities, the benefits of such

K. Sato (✉) · A. Seiyama
Graduate School of Medicine, Kyoto University, Kyoto, Japan
e-mail: kikue@gifu-u.ac.jp

T. Kuroda
Division of Medical Information Technology and Administration Planning, Kyoto University Hospital, Kyoto, Japan

Y.-W. Chen et al. (eds.), *Innovation in Medicine and Healthcare 2015*,
Smart Innovation, Systems and Technologies 45,
DOI 10.1007/978-3-319-23024-5_3

location systems are considerable. The data obtained are expected to be useful for hospital management, such as clinical safety assessments and appropriate staff assignments.

Kyoto University Hospital (KUHP) has introduced a real-time location system (RTLS) [3]. The RTLS employs Bluetooth-based proximity sensing technology, named BTID [4]. KUHP installed BTID beacons next to each bed in all wards. The nursing staff use a Bluetooth-based barcode reader to perform safety check-ups at the bedside using an auto-id/barcode-enabled medical administration (ABMA) system [5], allowing the locations of all nurses to be obtained through BTID. In a previous study, we evaluated the accuracy of location sensing in daily clinical activities in KUHP. The results showed that the system provided sufficient accuracy to perform time-and-motion studies [6].

In this paper, we analyzed the trajectories of the nursing staff based on location data obtained by the RTLS to visualize their workload and processes. The hypothesis of the study is that nursing staff spend more time on patients with relatively serious conditions. Thus, we investigated the relationship between the condition of a patient and the duration of stay.

2 Method

2.1 Data Collection

Among the four inpatient ward buildings and 1121 beds in KUHP, we selected the SEKITEI ward building as the target for data collection. It consists of eight floors of wards with approximately 40 beds on each. Location data were collected during the following periods.

(1) June 4–8, 2012
(2) September 27–28, 2012
(3) February 25—March 1, 2013

2.2 Data Analysis

This study employed a cross-sectional design. A descriptive statistical analysis was performed using the SPSS software (ver. 21). Average times spent in general patient rooms and in critical-care patient rooms were compared and the differences were assessed using statistical tests.

3 Result

3.1 Data Visualization and Rough Analysis

To analyze workload changes within 1 day, we prepared a graph to show completed visits to patients' rooms within each time period during 1 day.

Figure 1 shows a dot plot for period 1. The horizontal axis shows the time of day (from zero o'clock to 24 o'clock). As the dot plot shows, nursing staff visited patients frequently around 9 am and 2 pm.

Figure 2 shows a histogram of the total time spent in patients' rooms during each period of 1 day. Again, the chart shows that nurses spent more time at the bedsides of patients at around 9 am and 2 pm.

Figure 3 shows a breakdown of the data in Fig. 2. Each colored segment indicates time spent in a certain patient's room. This detailed analysis shows that a longer time was spent in the critical care rooms. As shown in Fig. 4, the critical-care rooms are usually placed in front of nursing staff stations and are intended for patients with relatively serious conditions.

The room with the asterisk had the longest duration of stay on the eighth floor. It is a critical-care room. Similarly, when the durations of stay on each floor were compared, the critical-care rooms on the fourth, sixth, and seventh floors had the longest stay durations.

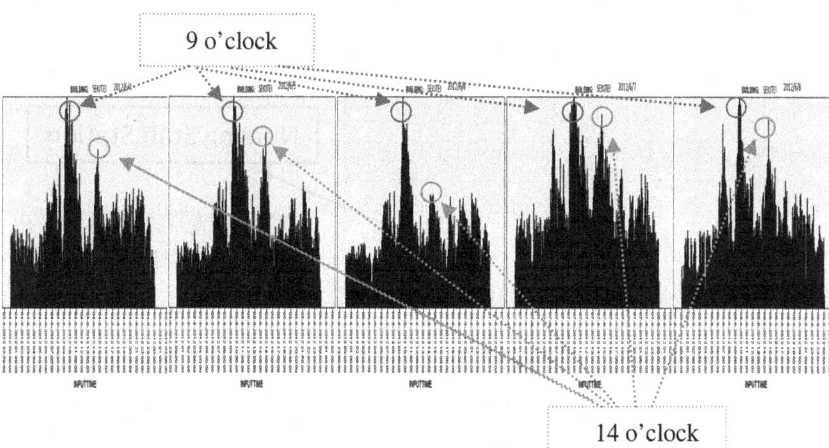

Fig. 1 Visit frequency by time band. This is the frequency distribution graph for nursing staff visiting a bed on June 4, 5, 6, 7, and 8, 2012; from the left, the x-axis is from 0:00, at 1-h intervals

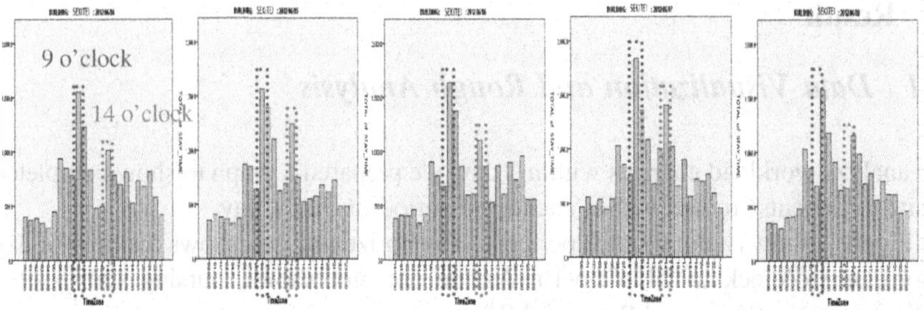

Fig. 2 Total duration of stays in various time bands. This bar chart totals the nursing staff's duration of stay at a bed on June 4, 5, 6, 7, and 8, 2012; from the left, the x-axis is from 0:00, at 1-h intervals

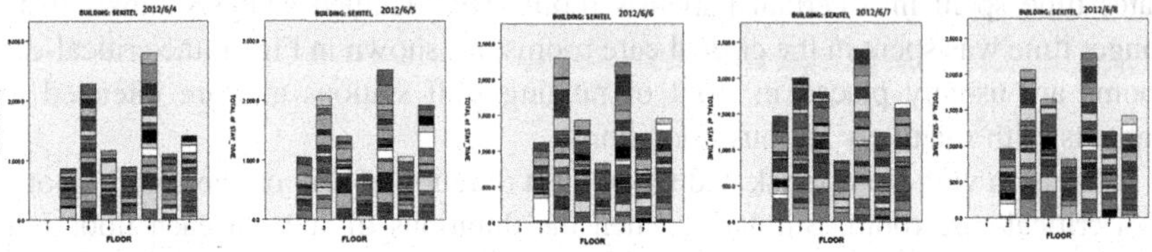

Fig. 3 Total duration of stay in various rooms. This is a cumulative bar chart showing the total duration of stay by nursing staff in each room on June 4, 5, 6, 7, and 8, 2012; from the left, the x-axis indicates floor

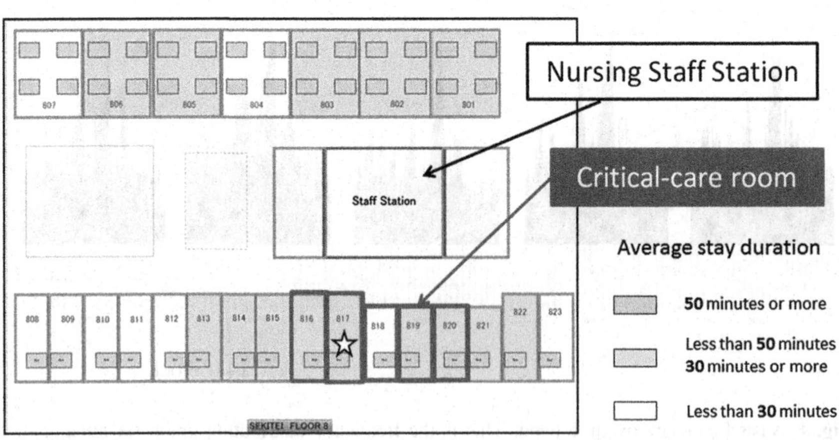

Fig. 4 The SEKITEI ward 8 floor plan

The nursing staff had a tendency to stay much longer at the bedsides of patients requiring critical care or rooms near staff stations. There was a correlation between the duration of stay and patient condition.

3.2 Relation Between the Time Spent for Patient and the Condition of Patient

To confirm the hypothesis, we conducted statistical tests. We divided patient rooms into two groups: general and critical-care rooms. The average duration of stay in each room in each hour in each survey period is shown in Figs. 5, 7, and 9 and average duration of stay in each room in each hour in each survey period on each floor is shown in Figs. 6, 8, and 10.

Table 1 shows a summary of the average duration of stay in each survey period shown in Figs. 5, 7, and 9. The Welch test (period 1: $t(67.00) = 7.93$, $p < 0.001$, period 2: $t(43.58) = 5.79$, $p < 0.001$, period 3: $t(127.23) = 9.00$, $p < 0.001$) was used to evaluate differences between the groups. The differences were significant; there was a clear relationship between patient condition (critical or not) and time spent with the patient.

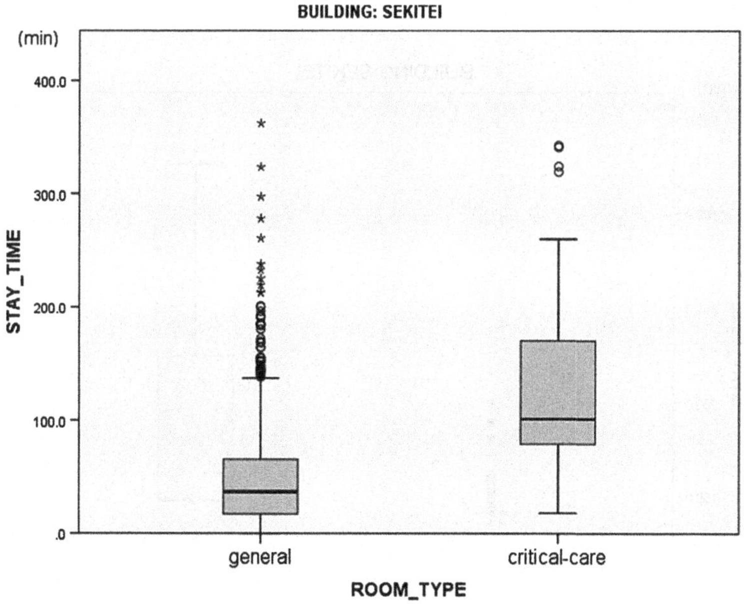

Fig. 5 Box plot of duration of stay in general and critical-care rooms during survey period 1

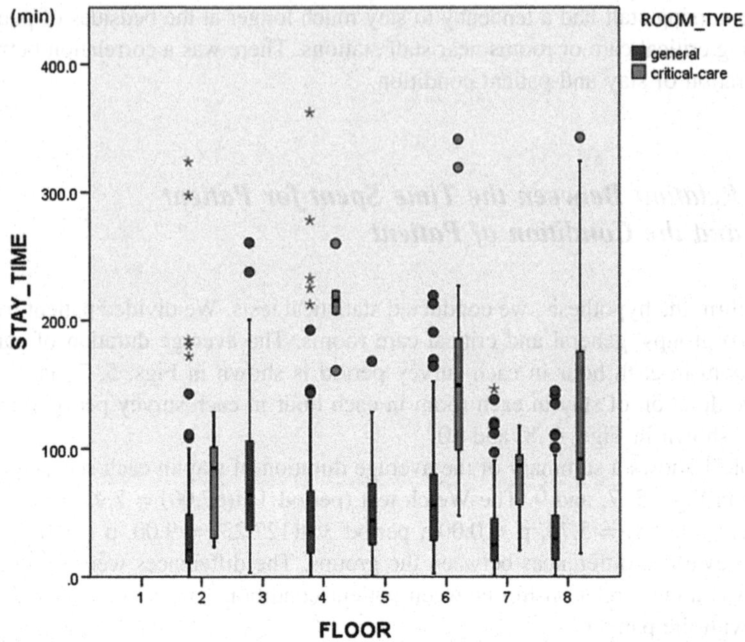

Fig. 6 Box plot of duration of stay in general and critical-care rooms on each floor during survey period 1

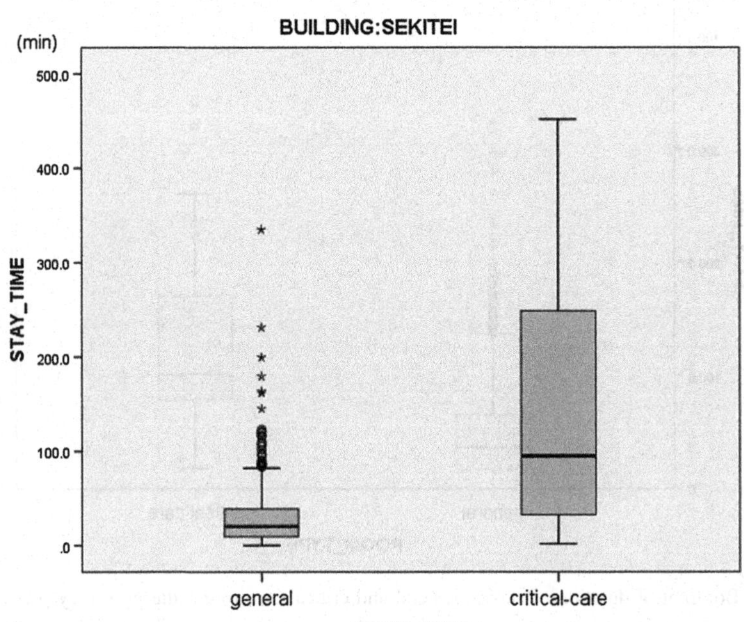

Fig. 7 Box plot of duration of stay in general and critical-care rooms during survey period 2

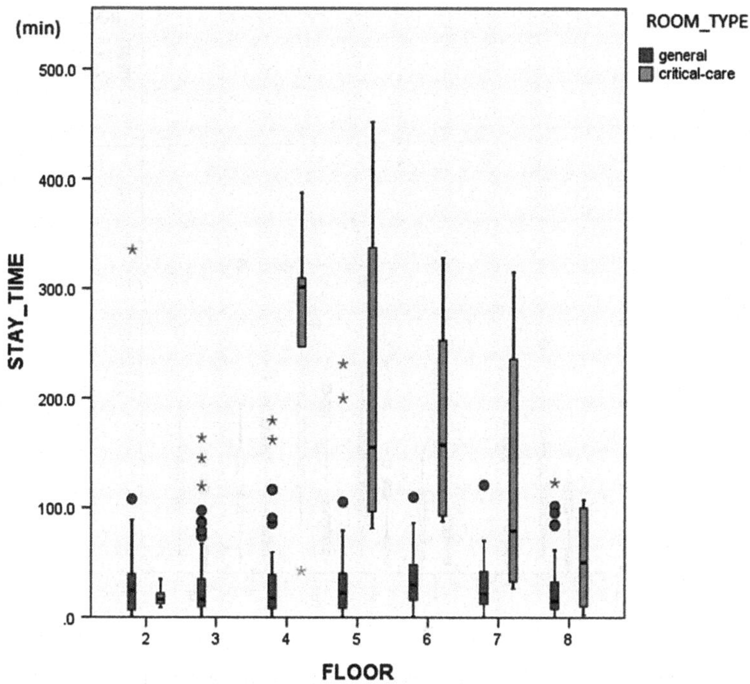

Fig. 8 Box plot of duration of stay in general and critical-care rooms on each floor during survey period 2

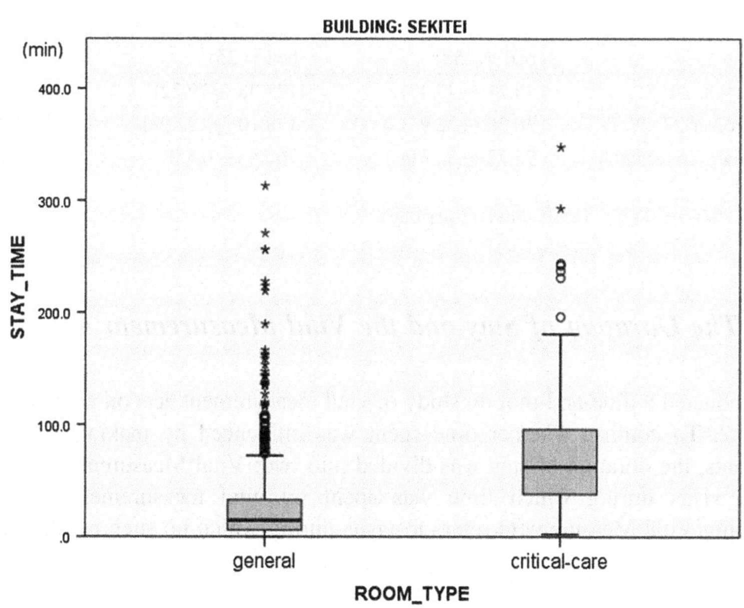

Fig. 9 Box plot of duration of stay in general and critical-care rooms during survey period 3

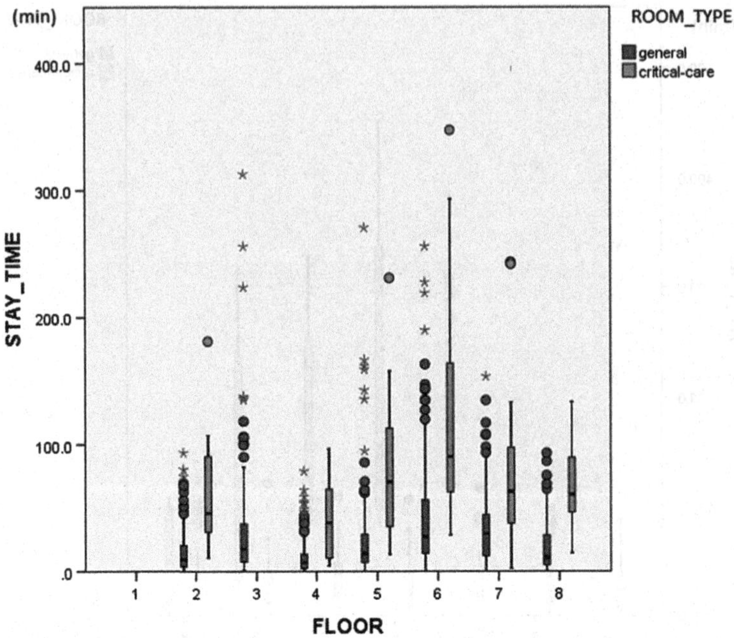

Fig. 10 Box plot of duration of stay in general and critical-care rooms during survey period 3

Table 1 Results of Welch test of relationship between room types

	General (number of bed = 258)	Critical-care (number of bed = 25)	P value
1 June 4–8, 2012	49.21 (±45.47)	127.98 (±79.22)	< 0.001
2 September 27–28, 2012	30.36 (±32.93)	138.10 (±122.98)	< 0.001
3 February 25—March 1, 2013	25.72 (±35.31)	76.58 (± 0.85)	< 0.001

(MEAN (SD) of STAY TIME min/bed per day)

3.3 The Duration of Stay and the Vital Measurement Act

We conducted a time-and-motion study of vital measurement acts on a ward during period 2. To confirm whether time spent was influenced by making vital measurements, the duration of stay was divided into two: Vital Measurement refers to patient visits during which time was spent on vital measurement acts, and Excluding Vital Measurement refers to visits during which no such measurements were made.

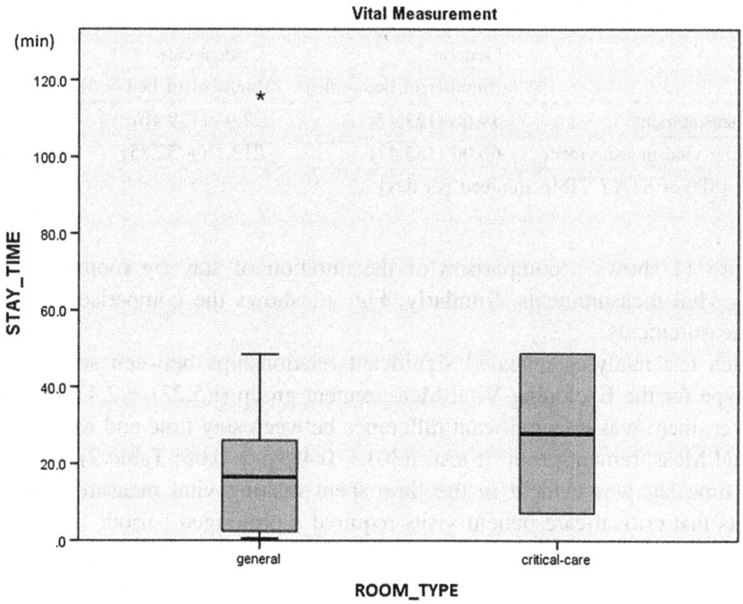

Fig. 11 Box plot of duration of stay in general and critical-care rooms for making vital measurements

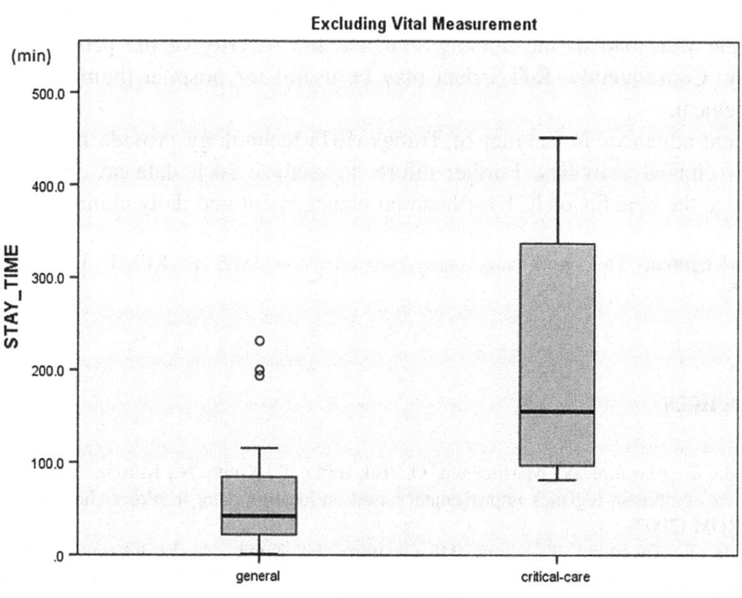

Fig. 12 Box plot of duration of stay in general and critical-care rooms excluding vital measurements

Table 2 Relationship between room type and time-and-motion study item

	General	Critical-care	P value
	(number of bed = 40)	(number of bed = 4)	
Vital measurement	19.60 (123.47)	27.96 (129.40)	0.63
Excluding vital measurement	60.96 (155.47)	213.1 (± 52.85)	<0.05

(MEAN (SD) of STAY TIME min/bed per day)

Figure 11 shows a comparison of the duration of stay by room type when making vital measurements. Similarly, Fig. 12 shows the comparison excluding vital measurements.

Welch test analyses revealed significant relationships between stay time and room type for the Excluding Vital Measurement group ($t(5.22) = 2.41$, $p < 0.05$). However, there was no significant difference between stay time and room type for the Vital Measurement group (t-test: $t(30) = 0.48$, $p > 0.05$; Table 2).

No time lag was evident in the time spent making vital measurements. This suggests that critical-care patient visits required a prolonged period.

4 Conclusions

The results described herein support the initial hypothesis; nursing staff spend more time with patients with serious conditions. The location data provided by RTLS show the workload of the nursing staff and the severity of the patient simultaneously. Consequently, RTLS data may be useful for hospital (human resource) management.

Recent advances in Internet of Things (IoT) technology provide much data to support clinical activities. Further efforts to analyze such data are important to maximize the benefits of ICT for hospital management and daily clinical activities.

Acknowledgment This work was partly supported by JSPS KAKENHI Grant Number 10304156.

References

1. Kuroda, T., Alasalmi, A., Martikainen, O., Takemrua, T., Kume, N., Kuroda, Y., Oshiro, O.: Medical equipment logistics improvement based on location data. In: Proceeding of ISMICT, CD-ROM (2007)
2. Kuroda, T., Takemura, T., Noma, H., Okamoto, K., Kume, N., Yoshihara, H.: Impact of position tracking on the outpatient navigation system. In: Proceeding of IEEE EMBC, pp. 6104–6106 (2012)
3. Noma, H., Tada, M., Kuroda, T., Takemura, T.: Development of real-time location system using bluetooth. IEICE Tech. Rep Cloud Netw. Robot. **111**(446), 29–34 (2012)

4. Naya, F., Noma, H., Ohmura, R., Kogure, K.: Bluetooth-based indoor proximity sensing for nursing context awareness. In: Proceeding of IEEE ISWC, pp. 16–18, (2006)
5. Takemura, T., Noma, H., Kuroda, T., Tada, M.: Development of bluetooth barcode system to ordering check under Wi-Fi network. Jpn. J. Med. Inform. 31(Suppl.), 986–987 (2011)
6. Sato, K., Kuroda, T., Takemura, T., Seiyama, A.: Feasibility assessment of bluetooth based location system for workflow analysis of nursing staff. In: Proceeding of IEEE EMBC.51 (Suppl), pp. 314 (2013)

A Web-Based Stroke Education Application for Older Elementary Schoolchildren Focusing on the FAST Message

Shoko Tani, Hiroshi Narazaki, Yuta Ueda, Yuji Nakamura, Tenyu Hino, Satoshi Ohyama, Shinya Tomari, Chiaki Yokota, Naoki Ohboshi, Kazuo Minematsu and Kazuo Nakazawa

Abstract It is necessary to identify the symptoms of a transient ischemic attack (TIA) quickly and provide treatment at special medical facilities to prevent stroke. All family members need to learn stroke signs. Specialists are spreading the face, arm, speech, time (FAST) message for identifying typical TIA symptoms to teens as part of stroke education activity in schools. To support these activities, we developed stroke education for older elementary schoolchildren outside of a school environment using information and communication technology. We utilized HTML5 and JavaScript to make a web-based application using on the FAST message. We provided an example of our application program at an event held at

S. Tani (✉) · K. Nakazawa
National Cerebral and Cardiovascular Center Research Institute, Suita, Japan
e-mail: t-shoko@ncvc.go.jp; tani.shoko.5s@kyoto-u.ac.jp

K. Nakazawa
e-mail: nakazawa@ncvc.go.jp

S. Tani
Center for Medical Education, Kyoto University, Kyoto, Japan

H. Narazaki · T. Hino · S. Ohyama · S. Tomari · C. Yokota · K. Minematsu
National Cerebral and Cardiovascular Center Hospital, Suita, Japan
e-mail: narazaki.hiroshi@ncvc.go.jp

T. Hino
e-mail: tenyu0405@ncvc.go.jp

S. Ohyama
e-mail: oyama.satoshi.hp@ncvc.go.jp

S. Tomari
e-mail: sny1139@ncvc.go.jp

C. Yokota
e-mail: cyokota@ncvc.go.jp

Y.-W. Chen et al. (eds.), *Innovation in Medicine and Healthcare 2015*,
Smart Innovation, Systems and Technologies 45,
DOI 10.1007/978-3-319-23024-5_4

the National Cerebral and Cardiovascular Center in Japan, 2014. On average, 83 % of older children answered questions about the FAST message correctly. Our application might be useful as a stroke education support tool.

Keywords Stroke education · Senior children at elementary school · Web-based application

1 Introduction

1.1 Background

Stroke patients often suffer from sequelae. For earlier detection and treatment of stroke, it is important to find symptoms of transient ischemic attack (TIA) quickly, and to visit a special medical facilities [1]. Stroke education for the youth is anticipated to contribute to stroke prevention. Campaigns using mass media [2–4] aimed at the population at high risk of stroke [5], have improve the knowledge of warning signs and risk factors of stroke, and have increased the number of emergency department visits or corresponding frequencies of using emergency medical service for patients suspected with acute stroke. However, these studies were intended for adults, and there are a few studies targeted at younger individuals. Williams et al. [6] reported the results of an intervention involving schoolchildren living in a community with a high stroke risk. The stroke educational program used music and dance. Wall et al. [7] evaluated the stroke awareness animation from the Stroke Heroes Act FAST campaign in Massachusetts. They found that the campaign was effective in increasing and sustaining knowledge of stroke signs and symptoms.

Amano et al. [8, 9] showed that stroke education performed by a stroke neurologist using the "FAST" mnemonic, derived from the Cincinnati Prehospital Stroke Scale (F = facial drooping, A = arm numbness or weakness, S = slurred speech or difficulty in speaking or understanding, T = time), improved stroke

K. Minematsu
e-mail: kminemat@ncvc.go.jp

Y. Ueda · N. Ohboshi
Graduate School of Science and Engineering Research, Kinki University, Higashi-Osaka, Japan
e-mail: 1433340404r@info.kindai.ac.jp

N. Ohboshi
e-mail: stern@info.kindai.ac.jp

Y. Nakamura
Faculty of Science and Engineering, Kinki University, Higashi-Osaka, Japan
e-mail: sigetige115@gmail.com

knowledge for junior high school students and their parents. We developed an online support system for schoolteachers to provide stroke education in junior high schools using information and communication technology (ICT). A schoolteacher can use our system to lecture students on stroke signs, risk factors, symptoms, and the FAST message to identify typical symptoms of a TIA. In a paper published in 2014 [10], we also confirmed that a schoolteacher could deliver the FAST message lesson to junior high school students using our system with a similar outcome to a stroke neurologist. Because this system required use in the school, it is not usable in other environments. Moreover, the content is somewhat difficult for elementary schoolchildren.

1.2 Purpose and Method

Based on this background, we developed stroke education outside of a school environment using ICT for older elementary schoolchildren as part of stroke educational activities. This is a new approach. We provided educational content about stroke that was interesting for older elementary schoolchildren focusing on the FAST message. We investigated the first impressions of our content by the older elementary schoolchildren.

In the first step, we created a simulation game on stroke education for Android. This was a stand-alone application program. An Android-based device was necessary. Next, we re-created a web application based on the Android version. Additionally, the application investigated the first impressions of the elementary schoolchildren. We utilized HTML5 and JavaScript to create the web application to run on the web browser. The web server used Apache Tomcat (version 8.0. 9). Panasonic's notebook computer was used as a server for development. The web application outline is explained in the next chapter.

2 Outline of Our Web-Based Application

In our application, stroke education flows through conversation with the mascot character. The character appears on the main screen and the window and sentences are displayed below the main screen. Actual sentences are in Japanese. When the application is first executed, users' attributions (i.e., gender, grade, etc.) are confirmed. Application content comprises explanations of stroke and FAST, a mini game, and a FAST message quiz. A function to collect logs of user information and quiz responses was added. When stroke and FAST are explained, as described above, the FAST message describes the typical symptoms of a TIA, such as facial drooping, arm numbness or weakness, slurred speech or difficulty in speaking or

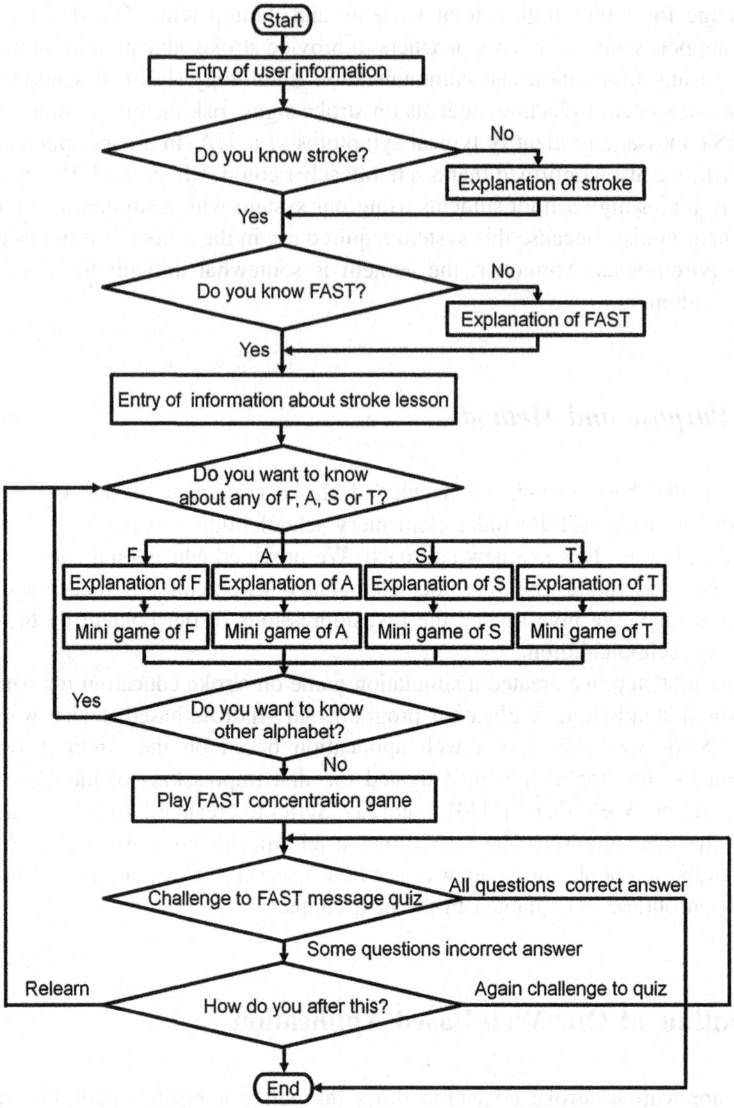

Fig. 1 Flow of our application

understanding, and time of emergency call (119 in Japan). After the explanation of one symptom, the related mini game is run. Figure 1 shows the flow of our application.

2.1 Mini Games

Mini game 1: Face. This game emphasizes the importance of distinguishing facial drooping as a stroke symptom. Two face icons (facial drooping and normal) were prepared. Each icon comes forward on the screen at random within 30 s. The remaining time is displayed at the bottom left of the screen (Fig. 2(1)). To clear the game, users need to maintain heart points by touching only the facial drooping icon (Fig. 2(2)). If the user touches the normal icon or passes over the facial drooping icon, heart points are decreased (Fig. 2(3)). There are three total heart points. When the heart points are zero, the game is over.

Mini game 2: Arm. This game emphasizes the importance of detecting arm numbness or weakness as a stroke symptom. Six elderly characters are arranged in two rows. They move their arms up and down. Four characters move both arms and two characters move only one arm. The user detects the two characters moving one arm up and down to clear the game. The character is enclosed with a red circle when answered correctly. If the user touches the remaining four incorrect characters, this mini game is over.

Mini game 3: Speech. This game emphasizes the importance of distinguishing slurred speech as a stroke symptom. A character is displayed on the screen and its voice flows. The voice data is not an actual patient's voice, but the voice of a specialist pronounced like an actual patient. Two kinds of voice flow randomly when the game starts. The speech content is "today is good weather" and "good morning" in Japanese. If the speech is normal, the user touches the button indicating the speech is fine. If the speech is slurred, the user touches the button indicating that the speech has a problem. If the user chooses the wrong answer, the game is over.

Mini game 4: Time. Thrombolytic therapy with intravenous recombinant tissue-type plasminogen activator (t-PA) can lessen stroke incidence. However, the treatment must occur within 4.5 h of the onset of an acute ischemic stroke [11]. It's important to call an ambulance and to visit special medical facilities quickly. The

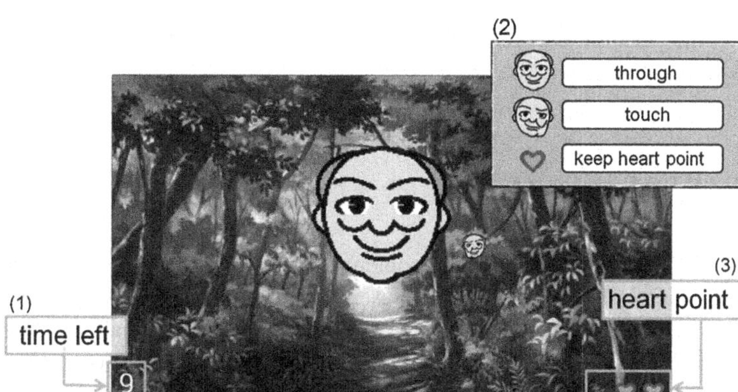

Fig. 2 How to play the face mini game

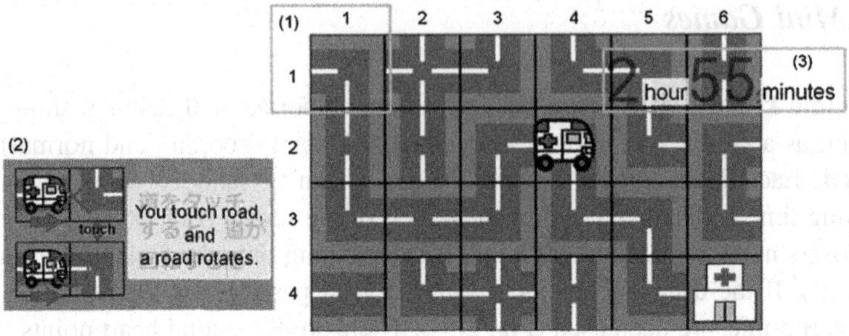

Fig. 3 How to play time mini game

mini game of Time takes the ambulance to the hospital within the time limit. The straight lines, intersections, curved roads or no roads are allocated randomly in a block of four by six cells (Fig. 3(1)). The road rotates clockwise around the ambulance when touched (Fig. 3(2)). The road is then connected and the ambulance is led to the hospital. If the ambulance reaches the hospital within the time limit, the game is successful. If it takes a road not connected on the way or the time limit expires, the user fails the game. The time limit display starts at four hours and 30 min to emphasize this is the time limit of t-PA treatment effectiveness; the time is reduced at the speed of 5 min/s (Fig. 3(3)).

2.2 FAST Concentration Game

This game is modeled on card concentration. It begins after the FAST mini games end. There are eight cards total (four pairs); the design of each card is related to FAST. T-PA was adopted for the card design because it was related to the valid time of the t-PA treatment. The back of the card displayed first was a design of the enlightenment character with the clock. In this game, neither a time limit nor game end is set; the design is seen until the cards are arranged by pairs. If every card can be opened, the game clears.

2.3 FAST Message Quiz

The FAST message quiz reviews the content explained in all of the games prior to this point. This menu is displayed after users finish the mini games and the FAST concentration game. One quiz item asks the meaning of the initials of the FAST acronym and about stroke. There are nine multiple-choice questions with three choices. Quiz responses are registered in the database.

3 Prior Evaluation

3.1 Method

We investigated the reaction of the targets to the application. We provided an example of our web-based application program at an event held in the National Cerebral and Cardiovascular Center on November 8, 2014 in Japan. Everyone was able to freely participate in this event. Children and others who attended this event played our game and quiz; we collected free opinions, grade level, and gender from them with freehand sticky notes. Additionally, users' attributes and the quiz log were collected by the web application. The application was limited to one play including the mini game so that many could participate. The FAST message quiz was a short version. Questions and choices follow.

- FAST is a word that shows symptoms of what? (Choices: influenza, cancer, or stroke).
- What does the "F" in FAST show? (Choices: face, fantastic, food).
- What does the "A" in FAST show? (Choices: apple, arm, attack).
- What does the "S" in FAST show? (Choices: sleep, sweet, speech).
- What does the "T" in FAST show? (Choices: time, tomorrow, tea).

Two laptops and one iPad device were used to connect to a monitor equipped with multi-touch function. Google Chrome (39.0. 2171.95 m) was used as a web browser.

3.2 Result

Free opinions were collected from 115 participants: elementary school students (n = 92), junior high school students (n = 3), kindergarteners (n = 5), and adults (n = 15). Focusing particularly on the elementary schoolchildren, 60 children were in the lower grades (1 to 3) and 32 children were in higher grades (4–6).

Opinion results: Table 1 shows the opinions from elementary schoolchildren. Opinions were classified into three groups: "difficult," "amusing/diverting," or "informative/educational." Multiple opinions from one subject were permitted. For example, one user stated "it is a little difficult, but amusing and informative." In the lower grades, 27 % children answered "difficult," 52 % children answered "amusing/diverting," and 42 % children answered "informative/educational." In the higher grades, 16 % children answered "difficult," 41 % children answered "amusing or diverting," and 66 % children answered "informative or educational."

Log results: There were 54 usable logs of elementary school pupils. There were 31 from lower grades and 23 from higher grades. Table 2 shows correct answer rates for the FAST message quiz. Of all elementary schoolchildren, 67 % understood the FAST message correctly. By grade, 55 % of the children in lower grades

Table 1 Opinions collected from elementary schoolchildren using freehand sticky notes

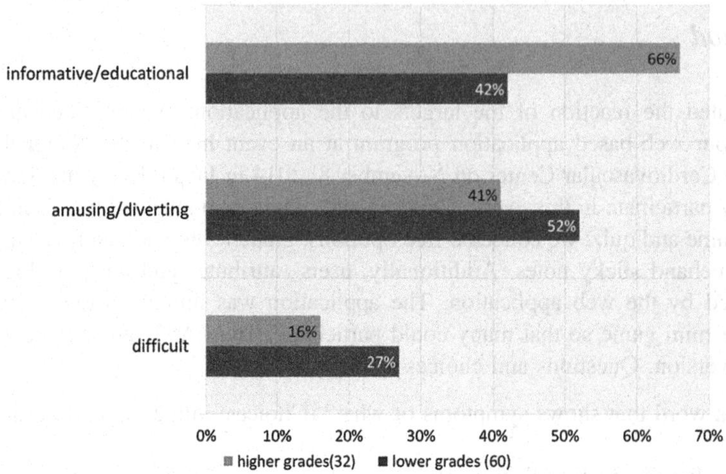

and 83 % of the children in higher grades answered correctly. In the past, stroke education was implemented in several elementary schools in Suita. In addition, a stroke lesson was implemented the day of the event. We then counted number of children who did not know stroke or FAST symptoms or did not receive the stroke lesson. Table 3 extracted only the elementary schoolchildren who answered, "I don't know a stroke," "I don't know FAST," or "I didn't receive a stroke lesson" prior to using the application.

Thirty-five elementary schoolchildren did not know stroke symptoms, FAST, or had not received past stroke education. There were 22 in lower grades and 13 in higher grades. Of the total, 74 % of children understood the FAST message correctly. By grade, 64 % of the children in lower grades and 92 % of the children in higher grades answered correctly.

4 Discussion

Many Japanese elementary schoolchildren might think that stroke is irrelevant to them. The National Cerebral and Cardiovascular Center (NCVC) in Suita, Japan began a stroke educational activity intended for elementary and junior high school pupils in 2010. As part of a series of educational activities, a stroke neurologist developed stroke educational lessons for elementary and junior high schools. A cartoon booklet, a pen, a magnet, a DVD, and other items were published and distributed by the NCVC for distribution to schools [12]. These activities aim to prevent strokes, focusing on older elementary schoolchildren, junior high school

Table 2 Correct answer rates of FAST message quiz for elementary school pupils

		Meaning of FAST (Stroke)		F (Face)		A (Arm)		S (Speech)		T (Time)		FAST (all)	
Elementary school pupil (Grade)		Correct answers	Rate (%)	Correct answers	Rate (%)	Correct answers	Rate (%)	Correct answers	Rate (%)	Correct answers	Rate (%)	Correct answers	Rate (%)
Lower (1–3)	31	29	94	28	90	25	81	23	74	26	84	17	55
Higher (4–6)	23	21	91	21	91	23	100	22	96	22	96	20	87
Total	54	50	93	49	91	48	89	45	83	48	89	37	69

Table 3 Elementary schoolchildren users who did not know stroke or FAST symptoms or who did not receive stroke education

		Meaning of FAST (Stroke)		F (Face)		A (Arm)		S (Speech)		T (Time)		FAST (all)	
Elementary school pupil (Grade)		Correct answers	Rate (%)	Correct answers	Rate (%)	Correct answers	Rate (%)	Correct answers	Rate (%)	Correct answers	Rate (%)	Correct answers	Rate (%)
Lower (1–3)	22	21	95	20	91	18	82	18	82	21	95	14	64
Higher (4–6)	13	13	100	12	92	13	100	13	100	12	92	12	92
Total	35	34	97	32	91	31	89	31	89	33	94	26	74

students, and their families. The lessons developed by the stroke neurologist are visually pleasing and interesting [8, 9]. However, they have some limitations, including a shortage of physicians to present the information. Therefore, we thought that it was important to first increase their interest in stroke. We thought a game that was executable not only in school but also at home should be offered as one of the above education items.

Prior evaluation confirmed that many children found our application to be amusing or informative as a first impression. Therefore, we thought that our application might be able to increase interest in stroke education. In the higher grades, many children (66 %) felt the application was amusing/diverting. In lower grades, that percentage was 52 %. In terms of understanding the FAST message, 55 % of lower grade and 83 % of higher grade children answered correctly. Even with those results, as the grade increases, willingness to study might also increase, though children mainly enjoy playing games in lower grades.

In terms of features, it may help to read sentences on the screen verbally and not advance to the following sentence during the fixed time. For both higher and lower grade children, a further effect can be expected by doing so to improve the application.

Our study goal was to assist patients' families to notice stroke onset quickly and handle it appropriately. Our application might be useful as a stroke education support tool.

Acknowledgement We express our deepest gratitude to Professor Keiko Takemiya (Department of Manga, Kyoto Seika University, Kyoto, Japan). This study was supported in part by Research Grants for Cardiovascular Diseases (22-4-1) from the Ministry of Health, Labor and Welfare, Japan.

References

1. American Heart Association/American Stroke Association.: Together to End Stroke. http://www.strokeassociation.org/STROKEORG/
2. Miyamatsu, N., Kimura, K., Okamura, T., et al.: Effects of public education by television on knowledge of early stroke symptoms among a Japanese popu1ation aged 40 to 74 years: a controlled study. Stroke **43**, 545–549 (2012)
3. Silver, F.L., Rubini, F., Black, D., et al.: Advertisings strategies to increase public knowledge of the warning signs of stroke. Stroke **34**, 1965–1968 (2003)
4. Hodgson, C., Lindsay, P., Rubini, F.: Can mass media influence emergency department visits for stroke? Stroke **38**, 2115–2122 (2007)
5. Kleindorfer, D., Miller, R., Sailor-Smith, S., et al.: The challenges of community-based research: the beauty shop stroke education project. Stroke **39**, 2331–2335 (2008)
6. Williams, O., Noble, J.M.: 'Hip-hop' stroke: a stroke educational program for elementary school children living in a high-risk community. Stroke **39**(10), 2809–2816 (2008)
7. Wall, H.K., Beagan, B.M., O'Neill, J., Foell, K.M., Boddie-Willis, C.L.: Addressing stroke signs and symptoms through public education: the Stroke Heroes Act FAST campaign. prev. Chronic Dis. **5**(2), A49 (online) http://www.cdc.gov/pcd/issues/2008/apr/07_0214.htm (2008)

8. Amano, T., Yokota, C., Shigehatake, Y., et al.: A stroke campaign of act FAST for junior high school students and their parents. Surg. Cereb. Stroke. **39**, 204–210 (2011). (in Japanese)
9. Amano, T., Yokota, C., Sakamoto, Y., et al.: Stroke education program of act FAST for junior high school students and their parents. J. Stroke Cerebrovasc. Dis. **23**(5), 1040–1045 (2014)
10. Miyashita, F., Yokota, C., Nishimura, K., et al.: The effectiveness of a stroke educational activity performed by a schoolteacher for junior high school students. J. stroke Cerebrovasc. Dis. **23**(6), 1385–1390 (2014)
11. Del Zoppo, G.J., Saver, J.L., Jauch, E.C., Adams Jr, H.P.: Expansion of the time window for treatment of acute ischemic stroke with intravenous tissue plasminogen activator. Stroke **40**(8), 2945–2948 (2009)
12. Shigehatake, Y., Yokota, C., Amano, T., et al.: Stroke education using an animated cartoon and a manga for junior high school students. J. Stroke Cerebrovasc. Dis. **23**(6), 1623–1627 (2014)

Part II
Biomedical Engineering, Trends, Research and Technologies

A Review of Mobile Apps for Improving Quality of Life of Asthmatic and People with Allergies

Miguel A. Mateo Pla, Lenin G. Lemus-Zúñiga, José-Miguel Montañana, Julio Pons and Arnulfo Alanis Garza

Abstract The quality of life of people with allergies to airborne substances can be improved if they are able to avoid areas with allergens. Airborne allergens information systems have become an important area of research and development. Systems that allow allergic people to know about the presence of allergens are in constant development. This is especially true in systems that report about airborne allergens, such as pollen. The massive deployment of Information and Communication Technologies makes this kind of systems available to anyone in the form of mobile applications. This paper reviews the available mobile applications for pollen information. After performing this analysis, we concluded that there is scope for research into new information systems for airborne allergens' information. These new systems could be based on technologies such as distributed intelligent systems, the Internet of Things and Smart Cities initiatives, aimed to solve problems of nowadays systems, such as internationalization and interoperability.

Keywords Airborne allergens · Mobile pollen application · Smart-cities · Personal pollen information

M.A. Mateo Pla (✉) · J. Pons
Department of Computer Engineering of the Universitat Politècnia de València, 46021 Valencia, Spain
e-mail: mimateo@disca.upv.es

J. Pons
e-mail: jpons@disca.upv.es

L.G.Lemus-Zúñiga
RIS-Itaca, Universitat Politècnia de València, 46021 Valencia, Spain
e-mail: lemus@disca.upv.es

J. Montañana
Universidad Complutense de Madrid, 28040 Madrid, Spain
e-mail: jmontanana@fdi.ucm.es

A.A.Garza
Instituto Tecnológico de Tijuana, Calzada Tecnológico S/n Unidad Tomás Aquino, 22414 Tijuana, México
e-mail: alanis@tectijuana.edu.mx

Y.-W. Chen et al. (eds.), *Innovation in Medicine and Healthcare 2015*,
Smart Innovation, Systems and Technologies 45,
DOI 10.1007/978-3-319-23024-5_5

1 Introduction

The population in the cities has increased, from beginning of the last century. It had been due different reasons such migration processes due to wars or uunemployment, [8].

Recent studies sponsored by the United Nations [6], state that from the year 1950 to the year 2014, the global urban population has increased by a factor of five (from 0.7 to 3.9 billlion). Those studies consider that the urban population will increase by a factor of 9 by the year 2050 (becoming to 6.3 billion humans).

In other words, the cities are becoming megacities with a lot of big problems such as: How to provide fresh water, how to process trash and where to put the trash, or how to evaluate and control air pollution.

To solve these problems and make cities more efficient and sustainable, the concept of smart cities was raised. This concept has evolved from gathering and storing information, to an efficient use of the resources of the city. The paper [2] provides a good approach to defining the concept of smart city and presents a framework which shows the relationships and influences between a smart city and the following factors: (i) management and organization, (ii) technological resources requirements, (iii) governance, (iv) policies, (v) people and communities, (vi)economy, (vii) built infrastructure and (viii) natural environment.

It is well accepted that ICT are key drivers of smart city initiative. The actual model Internet of Things (IoT) based on Cloud Computing makes not only possible to gather, store and process data but also to enhance the management and functioning of a city [9, 20].

One of the problems that should be solved is the prevention and control of chronic respiratory diseases [5]. These diseases not only reduce of quality of life of inhabitants, but also have an economic impact in medical costs or lost hours of work. In [4] is concluded:

- 300 million people worldwide suffer from asthma, with 250,000 annual deaths attributed to the disease.
- The number of people with asthma will grow by more than 100 million by 2025.
- About 70 % of asthmatics also have allergies.
- Approximately 250,000 people die prematurely each year from asthma. Almost all of these deaths are avoidable.

Respiratory allergy cases happen in cities at any time of the year, increasing in number year by year. Common symptoms of a respiratory allergy are red and/or watery eyes, breathing problems, skin itching and runny nose. The causes of these allergies are mainly pollen from trees such as olive trees, cypresses, plantain plants and cultivated grasses such as wheat, rye, rice, corn, barley, oats, shrubs and weeds. They affect the population of large cities in any season (even in winter) and the number of cases continues to grow. Recently, there has been found a relationship between the increase of pollution and the increase in allergies cases [7]:

"Diesel emissions together with pollen proteins cause allergies to be more virulent. Thus, the number of pollen allergy cases in cities heavily contaminated is three times higher than in rural areas with a lower level of pollution", said Dr. Subiza, through EFE agency.

The most effective way to reduce allergic symptoms is to avoid the exposure to that specific allergen [18, 21]. All the information that can be sent to those affected by the allergy is of great importance. Information on pollution and presence of pollen has proved to have an important weight. In the last years it has been gaining ground in traditional social media, up to a point where many meteorological information services include it.

On other hand, today ICT has a great impact in the way of life of citizens worldwide. Although worldwide Internet penetration rate average is under 50 %, it is more than 75 % for Europe, North American and other developed or developing countries (source http://www.internetworldstats.com/stats.htm). Moreover, more than 34 % of Internet's traffic is generated in mobile platforms and tablets (http://gs.statcounter.com/).

Thus, we have found interesting and useful at the same time to help to improve the quality of life of people with asthma and/or allergies by developing some mobile applications that can be used daily on mobile devices to gather information about airborne allergens. These applications will be based on our previous knowledge and skills on distributed and intelligent systems. At the same time, we believe that these systems could be a practical application of our research on the Internet of Things and Smart Cities initiatives.

Before developing such app, we considered necessary to study the actual solutions and the existing apps. In order to compare them, we defined which should be the most relevant aspects. The aim of this study is to provide information on the available apps for users and researchers, and define their advantages and disadvantages, while opening new developing lines for future works.

In this article, we start presenting some background material and related works. Then, the methods used to select the applications evaluated and their main characteristics are presented. After defining the application characteristics, the obtained results are summarized and analyzed. Finally, some conclusion and future work are exposed.

2 Background

The first concept we want to emphasize is air quality in cities. Air quality is a fundamental parameter in evaluating the quality of life in cities and there exists regulation regarding it. For example, EPA in the USA http://www.epa.gov/air/criteria.html. However, the common mechanism to measure air quality is based on pollutants that result from human activity. This parameter is made public in many countries as part of their regulation [12, 17]. Nowadays there are several different measurement systems for users available in the market [19].

It is particularly significant, in this aspect, the work of aqicn.org and their application for mobile devices. This application allows the users to know the air quality of a great number of cities from all around the world. In addition, the information sources for each city are shown.

Regarding natural allergens such as pollen and mold, there are no existent regulations about the measuring mechanisms or the publication of results [14]. As it is described in the article, this situation may change in the next years with new regulations at European level.

The most common method for measuring pollen is manual counting [16], which requires specialized personnel to spend a great amount of time and has a high latency to obtain the results. This high latency has made that the most popular method for warning is by "prediction", obtained from models based on the last measurements available, flowering times, the historical data of pollen levels in the same dates and weather forecast [10, 13]. The automation of the counting pollen process is an open field of research. In [3] a method based on computer vision and DNA identification [16] is described.

Two systems that offer and alternative approach are outlined in [1, 15, 22]. Both show the results of the use of the allergic people as sensors. In these cases, the input parameter for the measurement of the allergen is the effect perceived by the allergic: the onset and evolution of their symptoms, the medication taken, their general state, etc. To perform these tests, specific web pages were used where the study subjects had to fill in forms about their physical situation. In Fig. 1 it can be seen the information supplied by the application described in [15].

3 Procedures and Methods

As introduced in previous sections, there are a lot of web pages that can be used to get information about many kinds of allergens, including pollen, which is also true for mobile applications. In this section, we will describe the method we used to select the applications' essential characteristics and later the applications to test. A summary of these steps is shown in Fig. 2.

3.1 Application Selection

The main objective of this paper is to describe the main characteristics of mobile applications related to airborne allergens. We have used Google Play as the main tool for application search. Within Google play, applications that included the words "pollen", "air quality" and "allergy" have been searched. From these results, games and similar applications were removed and the rest were unified in a single list.

After downloading five applications, studying their references and consulting other websites, we designed the questionnaire that will be later used to evaluate the applications.

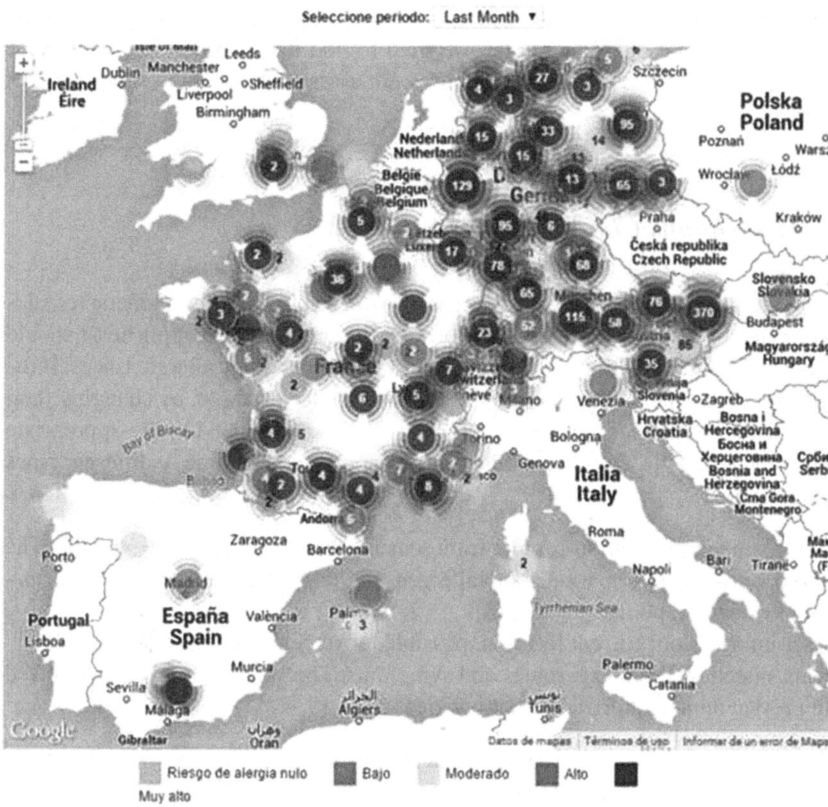

Fig. 1 An example of allergic symptoms map from polleninfo.org

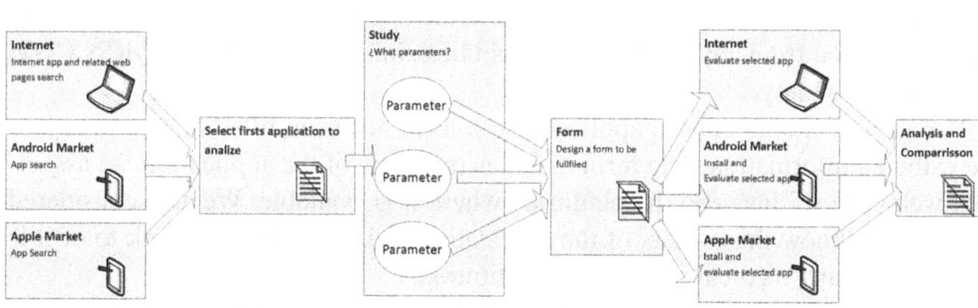

Fig. 2 Summary of the method steps

Due to the limited time available, we decided to select only 25 applications. When selecting the applications we have set a filter where the 25 applications studied must be free and capable of offering real time information to the user about the situation of allergens. In other words, free applications that obtain data from some kind of online service which measures or predicts the pollen concentration. Afterwards, it was decided not to evaluate some applications as it was impossible to understand their user environment due to language problems.

For each application, we installed it, checked its correct functioning and visited its website if it had one. In addition, we tried to find the source of data where the online information is obtained, but this was not always easy and in some cases not possible.

3.2 Applications Characteristics Selection

Once selected the applications, it is necessary to establish the set of characteristics to compare and to analyze them. A priori, we thought the ideal application should be able to alert the user of the risks in the near future caused by allergic issues. If the user knows these risks, they are able to avoid them, for example, by changing their daily route to work, and reduce its effects by, for example, taking the appropriate medication [15, 18] . To achieve this goal, the application uses three different types of information:

- Environment information coming from sensors installed in the user's vicinity. The sensors provide information about allergens in the air and other relevant information as weather, pollution, etc. [13].
- User information: current location, possible movements, allergies,etc.
- Data shared by users, e.g. routes and symptoms. This data should be anonymized to prevent an unauthorized use of personal data [15, 22].

In addition, the application should make suggestions, which are not substitutive of advice given by appropriate medical personnel. The inclusion of health professionals in the development of these applications should be an important characteristic to consider.

Regarding the environmental information, the app should be capable of showing this information from anywhere in the world in a similar way to what AQICN.COM does with air quality.

For each of the 25 chosen applications, a form has been filled that summarizes the gathered information. The form includes the name of the application, an associated web page (if any) and the platforms where it is available. We also considered important to know the owners of the application and if it provides a link to or it is supported by any medical or scientific institution.

The type of applications is also something important to consider. We have determined that the applications should have one or more of the following main objectives:

1. To provide information about allergens. The application downloads an index of one or more types of allergens. The source of information can be selected according to the location of obtained from the GPS or defined by the user. Although all the application offer a summary of the current situation and some short-term forecast, the forecasting models are not specified.
2. To ease the keeping of a history of symptoms. Such applications allow users to describe the situation of their allergy. These apps are most useful to people with

multiple or unknown allergies, or with a difficult "prophylaxis". The data about the evolution of the disease can be used by medical staff.
3. To offer value-added services. Some applications offer additional services such as prediction of allergens along a route or a reminder of prescriptions.

The key element of the applications analyzed is the user's ability to obtain information on allergens. The most useful information about allergens is the one concerning the atmosphere, such pollen and pollution levels. We have collected the following data:

- Type of information provided. Some applications designed for allergy problems with the respiratory tract don't display the current information but are based on historic data.
- Source of data. It is important to know the accuracy and validity of the information sources. For us, it is also useful to know if this data is open to new research or not.
- Geographical scope. Applications are able to get information only from one geographical area. This area can vary in size, ranging from a city to a continent.

Finally, it is evaluated if the application allows the user to register and then:

- To store their preferences on location and/or allergens.
- To share their personal information in order to improve the information provided by the application to other users. This is the most advanced option and it is present only in few applications. In any case, as discussed in [15], this option seems a very promising way of improving the quality of life of people with allergies.

When this set of characteristics was defined, a form was prepared. Then this form was filled for each of the 25 applications selected.

4 Results

The obtained data are summarized in Table 1.

5 Discussion

The analysis of the applications shows that the majority provide national coverage. The three applications with the coverage limited to a city are exceptional cases (e.g. RAllergo).

The only two applications with a range of use greater than a country correspond to neighboring countries that have in common their official language (Germany and Austria on one side, Belgium and Luxemburg on the other side).

The importance given to the trustworthiness that users give to medical and scientific based-applications can be checked in the fact that only 4 out of 25 apps don't

Table 1 Obtained data summary

App. name	Web page	Platform	App main objectives			App. responsible	Medical or scientific institution
			Allergen info	Diary	Other		
RALERGO	www.ralergo.com	Web	X		X	IIS/HUP La Fe and UPV	HUP La Fe Valencia
Hooikoorts PollenRadar	www.allerfre.nl	Android	X			Reckitt Benckiser Healthcare BV	
Pollen	www.pollenwarndienst.at	Web, Android, iOS	X			pollenwarndienst	Medizinische Universitat Wien
POllenweerbericht	www.avogel.be	Web, Android, iOS	X			Avogel	Biohorma Belgium N.V.
Pollen-Vorhersage	www.allergie.hexal.de/pollenflug/pollenflug-mobil	Android, iOS	X			Hexal AG	Entwickler: Hexal AG
Pollen forecast		Android	X				
Control de polen	www.almirallmed.es	Android, iOS	X	X	X	Almirall	SEAIC
Alerta Polen		Android, iOS	X			AstraZeneca Respiratorio	AstraZeneca Farmacéutica Spain S.A
Alergo Alarm		Android, iOS	X			Almirall	SEAIC
Polen Argentina	www.facebook.com/polenargentina	Android	X				
e-symptoms	www.aha.cg	Android, iOS	X	X		aha! Swiss Allergy Centre	
Pollen-News	www.aha.ch	Android, iOS	X			aha! Swiss Allergy Centre	
Austin Allergy	www.kvue.com	Android	X			kvue-TV	

(continued)

Table 1 (continued)

App. name	Geographical region	Data URL	User profile	If user Profile is present, app allows to			
Allergy Pollen Count	www.toledoallergy.com	Android, iOS	X			Dr. Safadi & Associates, Inc.	
Allergy Alert	www.pollen.com	Android, iOS	X			IMS Health	IMS Health
AccuWeather	www.accuweather.com	Web	X			AccuWeather	
PolliniItalia	www.ilpolline.it	Android, iOS	X			Associazione Italiana di Aerobiologia	
Meteo Allergie	www.pollinieallergia.net		X			Associazione Allergologi ed Immunologi Territoriali ed Ospedalieri	
Dagens Pollental	www.astma-allergi.dk/ ditmobilepollental	Android, iOS	X	X		Astma-Allergi Danmark	
Alergia.sk	www.alergia.sk	Android	X			C4P Ltd.	
Gary C. Steven, MD, PhD	www.myaasc.com	Android, iOS	X			http://www.myaasc.com/	
Alergo Alert	www.stampar.hr		X			Dr. Andrija Stampar Institue	
Pollen Info	www.pollen-info.be	Web, Android, iOS	X			MSD Belgium	MSD Belgium
Canberra Pollen Count	www.canberrapollen.com.au	Web, Android, iOS	X			Australian National University	Dept. of Archaeology and Natural History
APCYL		Android	X	X			
				Share info	Pos. log	Refine allergies	Rec. 'feels'

(continued)

Table 1 (continued)

App. name	Geographical region	Data URL	User profile	If user Profile is present, app allows to			
RALERGO	Valencia (ES)	www.valencia.es/ayuntamiento/datosabiertos.nsf					
Hooikoorts PollenRadar	Netherlands	www.zakelijk.meteovista.nl					
Pollen	Austria, Germany		X	X	X	X	X
POllenweerbericht	Belgium	www.zakelijk.meteovista.nl					
Pollen-Vorhersage	Germany						
Pollen forecast	Sweden						
Control de polen	Spain		X		X	X	X
Alerta Polen	Spain	www.polenes.com					
Alergo Alarm	Spain	www.polenes.com	X				
Polen Argentina	Argentina						
e-symptoms	Switzerland						
Pollen-News	Switzerland						
Austin Allergy	Austin, Texas (US)						
Allergy Pollen Count	Ohio (US)						
Allergy Alert	USA	www.bonap.org	X			X	X
AccuWeather	USA						
PolliniItalia	Italy	www.pollnet.it					
Meteo Allergie	Italy	www.pollinieallergia.net					
Dagens Pollental	Denmark		X			X	X

(continued)

Table 1 (continued)

App. name	Geographical region	Data URL	User profile	If user Profile is present, app allows to			
Alergia.sk	Slovenia						
Gary C. Steven, MD, PhD	South Wisconsin (US)	www.milwaukeepollen.com	X		X	X	
Alergo Alert	Croatia	www.stampar.hr					
Pollen Info	Belgium, Luxembourg	www.meteovista.com					
Canberra Pollen Count	Canberra (AU)	www.canberrapollen.com.au					
APCYL	Castilla y León (Spain)	www.datosabiertos.jcyl.es	X			X	X

make any explicit reference to any supporting entity. These cases correspond to applications developed specifically for a country (Sweden) or a region (Castilla y León), a value added service included in an existing application (Accuweather) and a service to attract the attention from a mass media (K4VUE in Austin).

Related to data sources, only in 13 applications it has been possible to find out the URL from which data was obtained. From these 13, only Valencia and Castilla y León appear as places where it is possible to obtain the information in an open way. In all the other cases no specific authorizations exist for this particular action. The access to this information is an open issue and relevant regulations are evolving towards its openness and standarization [13].

Regarding the ownership of the application, 9 of them have been financed by a pharmaceutical company. In other 7 applications, it's been a public entity related with the research or treatment of allergies (universities, hospitals and research societies) the one who has created or financed it. The other cases are more difficult to classify.

6 Conclusions and Future Work

In this paper have been studied 25 mobile applications whose main goal is to report the presence of airborne allergens. This information is very useful since the most effective way of not suffering an allergy is to avoid the allergen.

In our study it has been impossible to find any application that offered information at a global scale. In fact, they all had the same main problemi. They report information about a particular geographical region only in the language of that region (locality).

The lack of a global system that enables sharing data between different agencies researching on this subject, entities that are currently publishing information indexes and the applications that show it up makes things worse. Moreover, data is not always found in a format legally usable, which makes its use even more difficult.

Another aspect that should be highlighted is that most applications are unidirectional, meaning they offer information only to the end user.

We can conclude that new applications should help to solve the lack of up-to-date data about allergens. Pollen collection systems have a high cost and a high latency. The information provided by the users of a new generation of applications can generate allergens impact indexes with a much lower response time. There already exist prototypes of it. We want to stand out the work described in [11] where an impact index of the allergy is tried to be built using as a source of information the searches people carried out on the Internet.

References

1. Bastl, K., Kmenta, M., Jäger, S., Bergmann, K.C., Berger, U., et al.: Development of a symptom load index: enabling temporal and regional pollen season comparisons and pointing out the need for personalized pollen information. Aerobiologia **30**(3), 269–280 (2014)
2. Chourabi, H., Nam, T., Walker, S., Gil-Garcia, J.R., Mellouli, S., Nahon, K., Pardo, T.A., Scholl, H.J.: Understanding smart cities: an integrative framework. In: Proceedings of the 45th Hawaii International Conference on System Science (HICSS'12), pp. 2289–2297. IEEE (2012)
3. Costa, C.M., Yang, S.: Counting pollen grains using readily available, free image processing and analysis software. Ann. Bot. **104**(5), 1005–1010 (2009). http://aob.oxfordjournals.org/content/104/5/1005.abstract
4. Cruz, A.A., Bousquet, J., Khaltaev, N.: Global surveillance, prevention and control of chronic respiratory diseases: a comprehensive approach. World Health Organization (2007)
5. D'amato, G., Cecchi, L., Bonini, S., Nunes, C., Annesi-Maesano, I., Behrendt, H., Liccardi, G., Popov, T., Cauwenberge, P.V.: Allergenic pollen and pollen allergy in europe. Allergy **62**(9), 976–990 (2007)
6. Division, P.: Our urbanizing world (2014). http://www.un.org/en/development/desa/population/publications/pdf/popfacts/PopFacts_2014-3.pdf
7. Division, P.: Por qué está aumentando la alergia al polen? (2014). http://encuentralainspiracion.es/por-que-estan-aumentando-la-alergia-al-polen/
8. Fields, G.S.: Rural-urban migration, urban unemployment and underemployment, and job-search activity in ldcs. J. Dev. Econ. **2**(2), 165 – 187 (1975). http://www.sciencedirect.com/science/article/pii/0304387875900140
9. García, A.V., Soria-Rodriguez, P., Bisson, P., Gidoin, D., Trabelsi, S., Serme, G.: Fi-ware security: future internet security core. Towards a Service-Based Internet, pp. 144–152. Springer, Berlin (2011)
10. Gonzalo-Garijo, M., Tormo-Molina, R., Silva, P., Pérez-Calderon, R., Fernández-Rodríguez, S.: Use of a short messaging service system to provide information about airborne pollen concentrations and forecasts. J. Investig. Allergol. Clin. Immunol. **19**(5), 418 (2009)
11. Kang, M.G., Song, W.J., Choi, S., Kim, H., Ha, H., Kim, S.H., Cho, S.H., Min, K.U., Yoon, S., Chang, Y.S.: Google unveils a glimpse of allergic rhinitis in the real world. Allergy **70**(1), 124–128 (2015)
12. Karatzas, K.: State-of-the-art in the dissemination of AQ information to the general public. Proc. EnviroInfo **2**, 41–47 (2007)
13. Karatzas, K.: Informing the public about atmospheric quality: air pollution and pollen. Allergo J. **18**(3), 212–217 (2009)
14. Karatzas, K.D., Riga, M., Smith, M.: Presentation and dissemination of pollen information. Allergenic Pollen, pp. 217–247. Springer, Berlin (2013)
15. Kmenta, M., Bastl, K., Jäger, S., Berger, U.: Development of personal pollen information-the next generation of pollen information and a step forward for hay fever sufferers. Int. J. Biometeorol. **58**(8), 1721–1726 (2014)
16. Kraaijeveld, K., Weger, L.A., García, M.V., Buermans, H., Frank, J., Hiemstra, P.S., Dunnen, J.T.: Efficient and sensitive identification and quantification of airborne pollen using next-generation dna sequencing. Mol. Ecol. Res. **15**(1), 8–16 (2015)
17. Kukkonen, J., Klein, T., Karatzas, K., Torseth, K., Fahre, V., José, R.S., Balk, T., Sofiev, M.: Cost es0602: towards a european network on chemical weather forecasting and information systems. Adv. Sci. Res. **3**(1), 27–33 (2009)
18. Lau-Schadendorf, S., Wahn, U.: prevention of exposure in respiratory allergies. Therapeutische Umschau. Revue therapeutique **51**(1), 61–66 (1994)
19. Magazine, W.V.O.: New air quality sensors aim to track the air you breathe in a simple way (2015). https://wtvox.com/2015/02/new-air-quality-sensors-aim-to-track-the-air-you-breathe
20. Odendaal, N.: Information and communication technology and local governance: understanding the difference between cities in developed and emerging economies. Comput. Environ. Urban Syst. **27**(6), 585–607 (2003)

21. Reiss, M.: allergic rhinitis–is allergen elimination a useful form of therapy?. Wiener medizinische Wochenschrift (1946) **147**(14), 328–332 (1996)
22. Weger, L., Hiemstra, P., den Buysch, E.O., Vliet, A.: Spatiotemporal monitoring of allergic rhinitis symptoms in the netherlands using citizen science. Allergy **69**(8), 1085–1091 (2014)

Physical Implementation of a Customisable System to Assist a User with Mobility Problems

Sandra López, Rosario Baltazar, Miguel Ángel Casillas, Víctor Zamudio, Juan Francisco Mosiño, Arnulfo Alanis and Guillermo Méndez

Abstract The implementation of technology at home has caught the attention of many people, especially if elderly, handicapped or disable people are living on it. It is important to consider that the technology must be friendly with users, and even adapt to their needs and desires [1]. In this research, we present the physical implementation of a general system to assist users and patients in daily activities or duties. The system was implemented in a room and include sensors, actuators and wireless agents. This research is focused on people with some movement restrictions. The results are very promising, the user was successfully able to move several elements in the room (like windows or blinds) using only a mobile device as a tablet or a smart phone. Additionally, in order to see his potential adaptation and versatility, several devices where connected successfully to give comfort to the users.

Keywords Assistance to people · Assist in daily activities · Movement restrictions · Embedded agents · Sensors · Actuators

1 Introduction

In 2011 there were approximately 647 million people aged 65 years and over in the world and is expected to accelerate to 1.91 billion people in 2050 [2]. Majority of elderly people prefer to remain in their own homes for as long as possible [3], because these people are independent persons, and want to keep their independence as much as possible.

S. López · R. Baltazar (✉) · M.Á. Casillas · V. Zamudio · J.F. Mosiño · G. Méndez
Instituto Tecnológico de León, León Guanajuato, Mexico
e-mail: r.baltazar@ieee.org

A. Alanis
Instituto Tecnológico de Tijuana, Tijuana, Mexico
e-mail: alanis@tectijuana.edu.mx

Y.-W. Chen et al. (eds.), *Innovation in Medicine and Healthcare 2015*,
Smart Innovation, Systems and Technologies 45,
DOI 10.1007/978-3-319-23024-5_6

In home, the people with difficult to move or make several task is a problem, because they cannot be independent and always need of somebody. Due this reason, it is necessary a friendly system to manipulate the environment.

In this work, an intelligent system is applied, to help user to manipulate a room and at the same time collect information that are stored on a data base. This information can be used for two cases, in one hand for monitoring for a doctor, nurse or a relative of the user, on the other hand to be used for intelligent algorithms (in future applications).

The major contribution of our work is the application of a robust system of agents, sensors and actuators located in a room in a discreet and natural way. The difference with other physical system is: The actuators, sensors, agents (with an operating system developed by us) were designed to be installed quickly and without any modification or adaptation in this. Thus the system can be placed in any environment where it is needed.

2 State of Art

At the present, there are a number of off-the-shelve products available in the market e.g. fall monitoring system on mobile phone, emergency alarm, etc. Usually they are closed, stand-alone systems with limited ability to describe actual situations, often too difficult for elderly people to use and ineffective in emergency situations [4].

Ambient intelligence is a new vision for electronic environments that are sensitive and responsive to human presence [5]. Inside these environments, the electronic devices are virtually invisible and are able to respond to the user needs. The systems learn the user behaviour using the information collected from users' daily activities, always following the principles of ubiquity, transparency and intelligence [5].

The implemented system includes sensors, as Aztiria, Izaguirre and Augusto explain in [6]; the first step in the process of providing the environment with intelligence is to know the state of the user or users as well as the state of the environment itself. Sensors are a key technology that allows linking the real world with the reasoning algorithms. Following the decision making process the system may decide that some conditions needs adjustment (for example, closing the curtains or starting the heating) or interaction with humans is needed (for example, to alert a carer if a person in the house has fallen). The most natural way of acting is by means of actuators integrated in standard devices [6].

An important work for help wheelchair user people, in [7] the author show a prototype powered wheelchair system that are easy to use and safe. They use a simple system with ultrasonic sensor to assist users. In application for remote healthcare system, in [8] the users can monitor their healthy lifestyle through daily check-ups and make changes based on the prescription provided. In [9], the authors propose a system that has been designed to monitor elders which live alone and want to keep living independently. An important contribution in this work is related with the capability of the system to adapt its behaviour to that of the monitored elder. In [10] and [11], the authors developed a framework where the agent agents adapt the environment depending on the user's emotions.

Other authors, as [12], have already developed a system that consists of two basic modules. At the lower level, Wireless Sensor Network (WSN) capture the sensor data based on the usage of house-hold appliances and store the data in the computer system for further data processing. The monitoring of health patient in the home in [13], describes the implementation of a complete wireless body-area network (WBAN) system to deploy in medical environments. The wireless system in the WBAN uses medical bands to obtain physiological data from sensor nodes.

The aim of our work goes far beyond implementing specific applications such as those mentioned above in state of art. The aim is to present a robust system that allows applications, including health monitoring, activity monitoring, intelligent learning, optimization of comfort, detection of accidents, etc. Without having to worry about physical layer.

The system has the ability to connect 127 different types of sensors, 127 different types of actuators (considering that the amount of devices is not the same that the number of types of devices) and the agents can be connected in a central or distributed way. Besides it include a Middleware that was designed by members of the team [14]. That mean that the system can be used constantly, can include new actuators and sensor without problem.

In other words the system has easy installation and failsafe detection, because it can identify faults in the system (link issues, identification of disconnected devices, etc.). Besides it has flexibility, because it was designed as a platform for be used for many future applications and designs. And finally due of its management, operation and performance, this work surpasses other hardware (used in assisting users with mobility problems).

The paper is structured as follows. Considering that an important part is the physical system, because it supports people to perform daily activities in a simple and friendly way, in Sects. 2 and 3, the technology, design and hardware structure will be explained. In Sect. 4 we show the application layer of the system. And finally in Sect. 5 we present possible future work and conclusions.

3 System Description

The general vision model for the system, is composed of three layers, see Fig. 1, the physical layer, link layer and application layer. The physical layer is the hardware of the system and include the design and installation of sensors (temperature, light, humidity) and actuators (windows, blinds, lamps and air conditioning) in the room. As well as the hardware of the agents. The link layer is where are connected the devices with agents, in which were installed an operative system. And finally in the

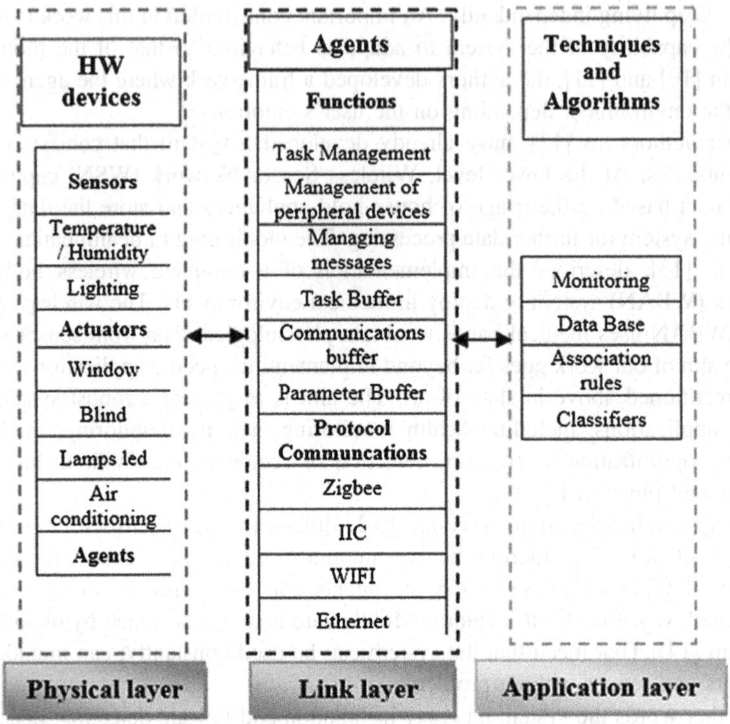

Fig. 1 Overview of the proposal system

application layer is where the user interacts with the system. Also in this last layer is where it can program the intelligent algorithm(s).

4 Physical Layer

The system includes especially environment sensors, the assistance for the user is help him to complete tasks in a room. In the Table 1, it's shown the features of the sensors. As it can see, we use 8 temperature/humidity sensors and 8 light sensors with wide range of operation. All the sensors are communicated in wired way with IIC protocol, in the Fig. 2, we present the sensors conditioned for communicate with agents.

In the same layer there are different actuators. Each actuator have a control stage, a power stage and its own power supply voltage. All the actuators can installed in rooms, offices, clinic room, etc. in an easy way, see Table 1.

The window actuator allow open or close the windows gradually, in Fig. 3 it is shown its parts and the installation in a window.

Table 1 Devices features of the system

Devices features			
Name of device	Operating range	MCU	Amount installed
Sensors			
AM2303 temperature/humidity	−40, 80 (C) 0, 100 (RH)	MSP430g2553	8
BH1750FVI lighting	0, 65535 (Lux)	MSP430g2553	8
Actuators			
Window	0, 255 (Positions)	MSP430g2553	4
Blind	0, 10 (Positions)	MSP430g2553	4
Lamp led	0, 255 (Levels)	MSP430g2553	21
Air conditioning	16–32 (Degrees)	MSP430g2553	1
Agents			
Agent with operative system	–	TM4C123G	12
Gateway	–	TM4C123G	2

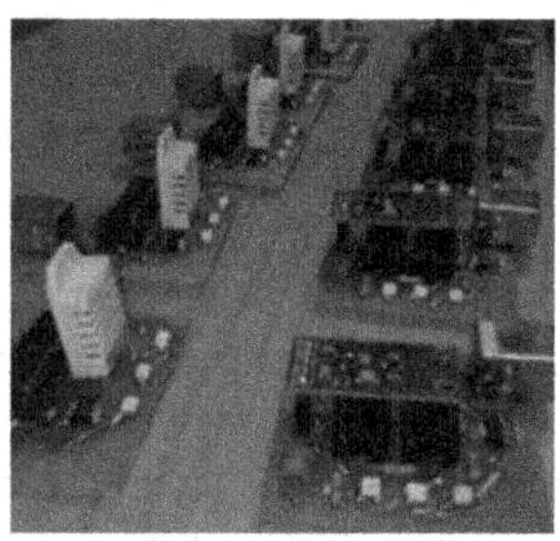

Fig. 2 Electronic boards of sensors

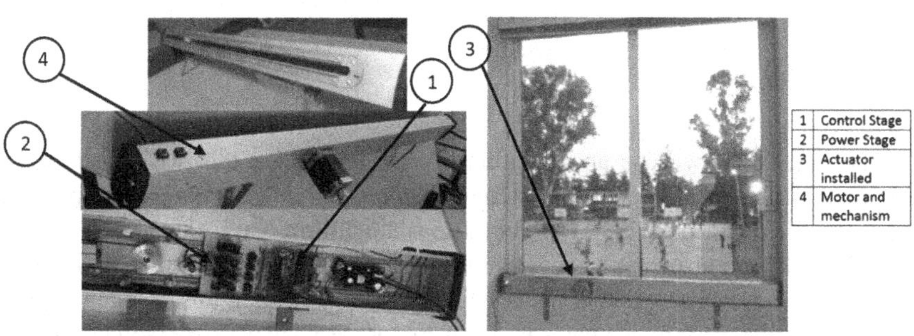

Fig. 3 Implementation of our window actuator

The actuator of motorized blind, allows obstruct or leave introduce light natural external, include an optical sensor for counting the number of turns. In this way the system know the position of the blind actuator, see Fig. 4.

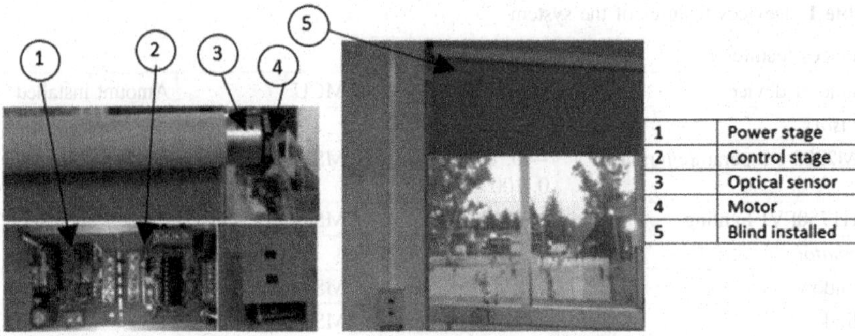

Fig. 4 Implementation of our actuator: window blind

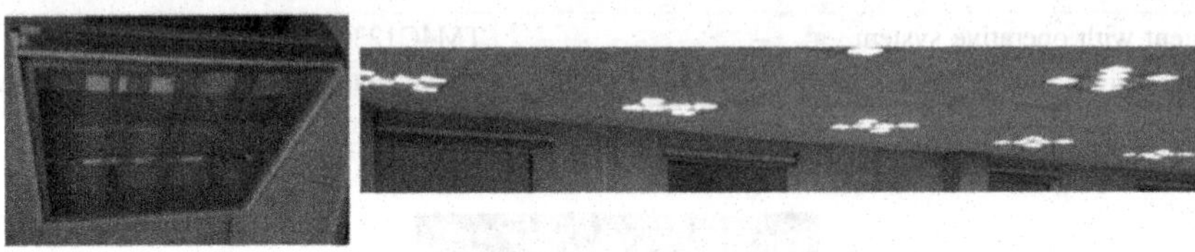

Fig. 5 Implementation of actuator: LED lamps

The light actuator comprises a led lighting system, which can be controlled gradually, see Fig. 5, and the air conditioning actuator can be controlled in a range of 16 °C, via an infrared light transmitter. All the actuators can be communicated wired way (protocol IIC) to the agents. Each agent can be interconnected with four devices locally, and wirelessly using ZigBee protocol can be communicated with other agents.

5 Link Layer

For the link layer, we use an operating system embedded that we called AIOS (Ambient Intelligence Operative System) on embedded devices that was appointed as agents. We decided to use AIOS, because is a platform that is developing by our team of work, and also each agent have the goal of manage task. It is possible that an agent have own task or other agent planting external task in this. A main feature of the operative system is that can interrupt process, in case of some cyclical instability between agents.

Each agent have a ZigBee, a TM4C123G microcontroller, core ARM Cortex-M4 (Tiva C Series Texas Instruments) and a power stage, see Table 1 for the feature of agent and the Fig. 6 for see the agent implemented. We use ZigBee because this technology include low complexity, low energy consumption, slow data rate and low cost, and it is based on IEEE 802.15.4 Standard. Today organizations use

Fig. 6 Implementation physical Agent

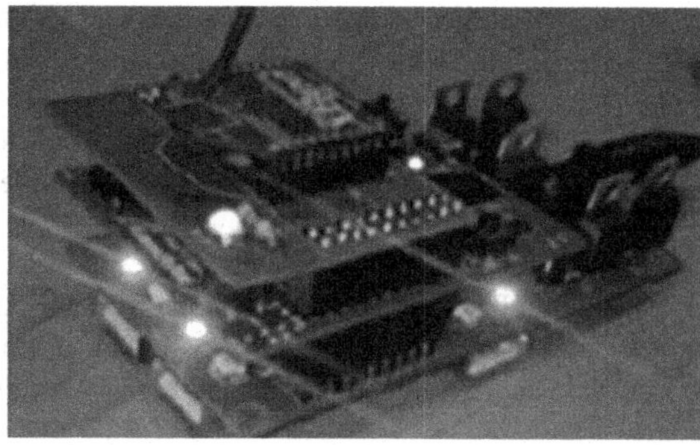

IEEE802.15.4 and ZigBee to effectively deliver solutions for a variety of areas, such as consumer electronic device control, energy management and efficiency home and commercial building automation as well as industrial plant management.

The devices-agent communication is with IIC protocol. The agent can send a frame for write, read or synchronized with the device. The devices can send a frame for answer the petition of the agent, see Fig. 7.

The agent-agent communication is in wireless way using ZigBee. Each agent have a set of tasks destined, but other another agent can sow different tasks to it.

The main point of the operative system on agent is the task management, through the main buffers, that are core elements of its structure. The three buffers are:

- *Task Buffer*: memory space reserved, for storing and organizing tasks like read a sensor, write in actuators, to consult type device, create new task,etc.
- *Message Buffer*: memory space reserved, to manage the sending and receiving of messages transmitted by different channels of communication in the agent.
- *Parameter Buffer*: memory space reserved, for storing received parameters necessary for achieving tasks.

These buffers are only storage elements, so that different modules, processes elements of a buffer to another. These modules are managers:

- *Task Manager*: creates to-do items, deletes items from tasks, creates message elements and analyzes each element of task buffer.

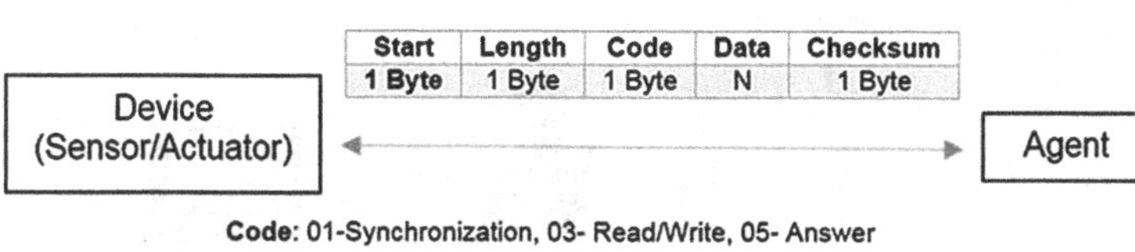

Fig. 7 Agent-Device communication

- *Message Manager*: extracts elements of message buffer, processes elements of message buffer, creates elements for parameter buffer and modifies elements of the parameter buffer.
- *Parameter Manager*: extracts elements of parameter buffer, deletes elements of parameter buffer, modify elements of the task buffer and buffer elements creates tasks.
- *Comm Manager*: extracts elements of message buffer, creates elements of message buffer, creates elements for communications buffer of outgoing and extracts elements of communications buffer of input.
- *Network Manager*: controls the sending and receiving information via ZigBee network.
- *Device Manager*: control the communication, receive and management of connected devices (sensors and actuators).

In our implementation the user send a task using a mobile device to the agent, this is communicated with the system and with a computer (serial communication between agent and computer), see the Fig. 8. The agents are connecting in a central way, but the system could change in a distributed manner without any problem.

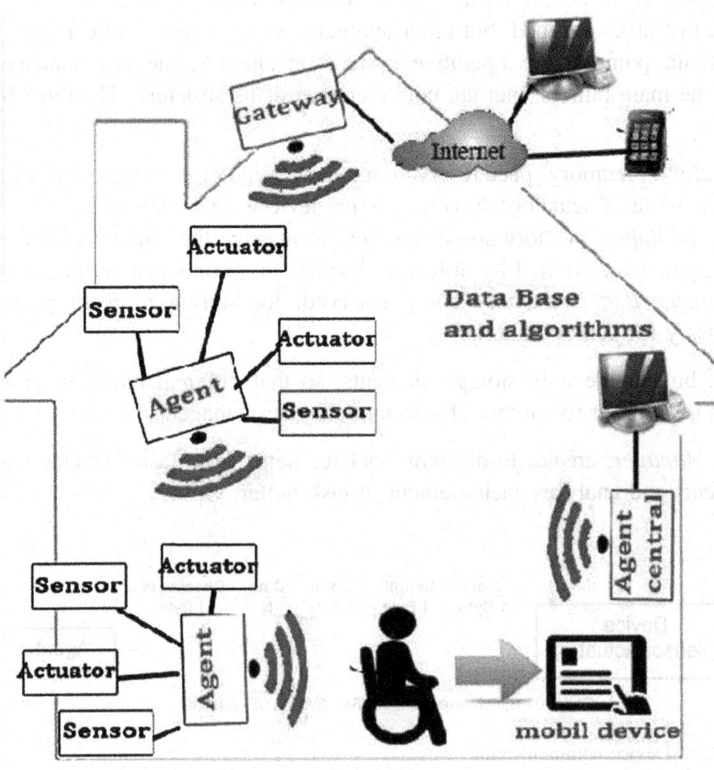

Fig. 8 Overview of link layer

In this layer also the programmer can manipulate the system and adapt it to the desired application. All this by changing the connection of agents and devices, and setting the distribution.

6 Application Layer

The application layer is where the user interacts with the system via a graphical interface in a mobile device. In this way the user can manipulate the room since the bed or a wheelchair. The mobile device is connected by Bluetooth protocol through the gateway agent to the rest of the system, then every agent is ready to control the actuators as the user requirements.

The actions is collected by the Customisable System through the sensors and the state of the actuators in a data base. Then a nurse or a relative of the patient can be monitoring the activities.

7 Conclusion and Future Work

In this work, it is presented a system to help people with a physical disability to get comfort in any room of a house, this due to the actuators can be controlled by a mobile device. All the sensors and actuators are agents and are connected to a central agent by the wireless x-bee protocol and are controlled by an embedded operating system called AIOS. This system proved to be customisable, efficient, and versatile for to be used in user assistance for do his daily activities. Because of this result, the system will be used in a platform, in order to develop intelligent services for elderly, handicapped or/and disable people. Particularly will be used to learn the user's behavior and to react automatically in function of this learning (for a personalized service).

Future research can be performed adding sensors to help monitor the health of the user, developing learning behavior of users for personalized assistance, optimization of comfort as a second stage of learning of patients, adding security systems and identification of users accidents.

Acknowledgments The authors want to acknowledge the kind and generous support from CONACyT and DGEST to this project.

References

1. Aztiria, A., Augusto, J.C., Basagoiti, R., Izaguirre, A., Cook, D.J.: Learning frequent behaviors of the users. In: IEEE Transactions on Intelligent Environments Systems, Man, and Cybernetics Systems, vol 43, no. 6 (2013)

2. United Nations, D. o. E., Social Affairs, P. D: World population prospects, CD-ROM edition (2011)
3. Bayer, A., Harper, L., Greenwald, M. of Retired Persons A.A.: Fixing to Stay: A National Survey of Housing and Home Modification Issues. American Association of Retired Persons, Washington (2000)
4. Kleinberger, T., Becker, M., Ras, E., Holzinger, A., Muller, P.: Ambient intelligence in assisted living: enable elderly people to handle future interfaces. In: Stephanidis, C. (ed.) Universal access in human-computer interaction: ambient interaction UAHCI'07. Springer, Heidelberg (2007)
5. Ducatel, K., Bogdanowicz, M., Scapolo, F., Leijten, J., Burgelman, J.C.: Scenarios for ambient intelligence in 2010. IST Advisory Group. Tech. Rep. (2011). ftp.cordis.lu/pub/ist/docs/istagscenarios2010.pdf
6. Aztiria, A., Izaguirre, A., Augusto, J.C.: Learning patterns in ambient intelligence environments: a survey. In: Springer Science + Business Media B. V., pp. 35–51 (2010). doi:10.1007/s10462-010-9160-3
7. Sanders, D., Stott, I.: A new prototype intelligent mobility system to assist powered wheelchair users. Ind. Robot Int. J. **26**(6), 466–475 (1999). ISSN 0143-991X
8. Youm, S., Lee, G., Park, S., Zhu, W.: Development of remote healthcare system for measuring and promoting healthy lifestyle. Expert Syst. Appl. **38**, 2828–2834 (2011)
9. Botia, J.A., Villa, A., Palma, J.: Ambient assisted living system for in-home monitoring of healthy independent elders. Expert Syst. Appl. **39**, 8136–8148 (2012)
10. Mowafey, S., Gardner, S., Patz, R.: Development of an ambient intelligent environment to facilitate the modelling of well-being. In: IET Seminar on Assisted Living 2011, pp. 1–6 (2011)
11. Sherief, M., Steve, G.: Towards ambient Intelligence in assisted living: the creation of an intelligent home care. In: Science and Information Conference, pp. 51–50. London, U.K (2013)
12. Suryadevara, N.K., Gaddam, A., Rayudu, R.K., Mukhopadhyay, S.C.: Wireless sensors network based safe home to care elderly people: behaviour detection. Sens. Actuators A **186**, 277–283 (2012)
13. Yuce, M.R.: Implementation of wireless body area networks for healthcare systems. Sens. Actuators A **162**, 116–129 (2010)
14. Barrón, T.J., Baltazar, R., Casillas, M.A., Zamudio, V.M., Martínez, B.: Diseño de un middleware basado en agentes para la creación de inteligencia ambiental. In: XI Congreso Internacional sobre Innovación y Desarrollo Tecnológico. CIINDET, México (2014)

Mobile Applications in Health, Competitive Advantage in the State of Baja California Mexico

Nora del Carmen Osuna Millán, Margarita Ramírez Ramírez, María del Consuelo Salgado Soto, Bogart Yali Márquez Lobato and Arnulfo Alanís Garza

Abstract The review of the status of the medical device sector in Mexico and its relationship or development support through mobile devices is the main objective of this research where the main objective is to determine the major players in the sector, success stories, frame regulatory or corporate governance of IT in the health sector, for the opportunity areas that allow redirect joint efforts of government, universities, private sector, foundations, associations and everyone involved in general. Was detected that Baja California has a fundamental role in the development and export of medical devices in the region but still not much with a representative level in mobile health oriented applications which creates an area of missed opportunity by the state and country. That is why it is necessary to explore a collaboration agreement with the main players and the agency will direct these efforts.

Keywords Health · Mobile health · Medical device

N. del Carmen Osuna Millán (✉) · M. Ramírez Ramírez · M. del Consuelo Salgado Soto
Facultad de Contaduría y Administración, Universidad Autónoma de Baja California, Calzada Universidad 14418, Parque Industrial Internacional Tijuana, C.P. 22390 Tijuana, BC, Mexico
e-mail: nora.osuna@uabc.edu.mx

M. Ramírez Ramírez
e-mail: maguiram@uabc.edu.mx

M. del Consuelo Salgado Soto
e-mail: csalgado@uabc.edu.mx; mary_sevilla@uabc.edu.mx

B.Y. Márquez Lobato
Instituto Tecnológico de Tijuana, ITT, Calzada Tecnologico S/N, Unidad Tomas Aquino, Tijuana, BC, Mexico
e-mail: bmarquez@tectijuana.edu.mx

A. Alanís Garza
Departamento de Sistemas y Computación, Instituto Tecnológico de Tijuana, ITT, Calzada Tecnologico S/N, Unidad Tomas Aquino, Tijuana, BC, Mexico
e-mail: alanis@tectijuana.edu.mx

Y.-W. Chen et al. (eds.), *Innovation in Medicine and Healthcare 2015*,
Smart Innovation, Systems and Technologies 45,
DOI 10.1007/978-3-319-23024-5_7

1 Introduction

Mexico has distinguished itself by its participation in export of medical devices, primarily our neighboring country United States, but still has areas of opportunity that should be exploited to develop another sector strengthened research and development and innovation in the medical sector, and not only manufacturing, universities will participate with companies, associations, and government, to strengthen technological capabilities acquired by the operation of the processes in each institution and obtain a shared development to innovate the way of working of the main actors.

The main actors their roles, responsibilities and functions to achieve a common objective health support through IT (Information Technology) are defined, which represents and has represented throughout history progress more agile on the findings, testing, monitoring, knowledge bases, technological learning in the health sector.

2 Mobile Applications in Health, Opportunity Area in Mexico

The percentage of exports from Mexico by the Medical Devices sector has doubled to 2.7 billion dollars in 2003 to 5,800,000,000 in 2010 dollars shown in Figure which determines a representative growth in the analyzed area, Baja California captures over 50 % of export earnings from medical devices [1]; where the geographical location plays a very important role and is benefited by the proximity to the center of global innovation located in Silicon Valley; Tijuana, Baja California Mexico located a mile from the California border, has become the center of manufacturing for medical devices.

Mexico exported nearly six billion dollars in 2010, which was placed in eleventh place as exporter of medical devices globally. Were obtained about three billion dollars surplus 2003 [2]. Exports of medical device sector grew at an average annual rate of 11.4 % in 2003–2010, which shows the area of opportunity in collaboration for the health sector and you (Fig. 1).

3 Main Stakeholders Involved in Promoting the Advancement of ICT in the Health Sector

For an objective of common good compliance should be the main players and each of them establish, identify and develop some roles and responsibilities of its technological capabilities, acquired through the processes of knowledge acquisition,

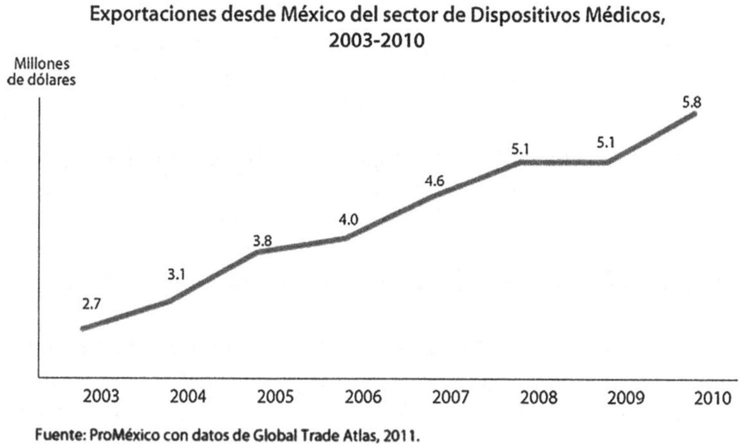

Fig. 1 Revenue from export of medical devices

technological learning, arising from the activities developed in the everyday operation as well as Research & development and Innovation.

Therefore there needs to be a regulatory framework, a guide to good practice enabling us know and identify those involved, areas of interest, history, current status, specific requirements of the health sector in order to deliver added value in the desired results.

3.1 Government Ministries of Economy and Health

The main entities and government agencies responsible for regulating Mexico economic, human and research resources are: Ministry of Economy, Health and CONACYT (National Council of Science and Technology).

3.1.1 Ministries of Economy (SE)

The SE is the one responsible for managing financial resources derived from local taxes and export prices also mentioned and consumer advocacy with their commercial suppliers and other activities [3].

According to Article 34 of the Basic Law of the Federal Public Administration (LOAPF) [4]. The Ministry of Economy is responsible clearance of the following matters, among others:

I. formulate and conduct the general policies of industry, trade, interior, supply and prices in the country; except for the prices of goods and services of the Federal Public Administration;

Regular
XXIII promote, guide, encourage and stimulate domestic industry;
XXV Promote and, where appropriate, organize technical and industrial research,

These sections among others are to support regulation, consulting, development and strengthening momentum of development of IT applications in health industry.

3.1.2 Ministrie of Health (SE)

The secretary of state of the federal executive, is responsible for the nation's health; as well as their education and care; as well as in relevant aspects of the sector. Manages, regulates and directs public and private health centers; among other activities [5]. According to Article 39 of the LOAPF Secretary of Health [4] is responsible enters others, the following functions:

- Conduct national policy on social assistance, medical services and general health, except as on the improvement of the environment; coordinate programs and services to the health of the federal public administration as well as groupings of functions and related programs to be determined.
- Create and manage local health, welfare and social therapy anywhere in the country and organize public assistance in the Federal District.
- To plan, regulate, coordinate and evaluate the NHS and provide adequate participation of the agencies and public entities providing health services to ensure compliance with the law.
- Execute control over dispensing, possession, use, supply, import, export and distribution of drugs and medicinal products, except for veterinary use are not covered by the Geneva Convention.
- Implement measures to preserve the health and lives of farmworkers and city and industrial hygiene, except as it relates to the social security system at work.

These functions among others are related to the application of mobile devices as a support tool to manage better efficiency, effectiveness and productivity in the scope and coverage of health, achieving if being competitive in both the national level and international.

3.1.3 Conacyt

National committee on Science and Technology (CONACYT) is a public agency Mexican government functions promotion, dissemination and stimulation of science and technology in the country. You are responsible for developing policies governing the optimal and efficient operation of science and technology [6].

The main functions of Conacyt driving the development of ICT oriented particular case are:las principales funciones de Conacyt:

- Develop and propose to the National Government national policies and strategies for science, technology and innovation quality for the country, in line with the policy of economic and social development of the State. In coordination with related institutions monitor and evaluate the implementation of these policies and strategies.
- Make science, technology, innovation and national quality efforts with those made abroad by promoting research networks and their development.
- Determine criteria and/or principles of science, technology and innovation and quality to be incorporated into the formulation of national policies.
- Sponsor training and specialization of human resources for the development of the National Quality System and the National Science, Technology and Innovation.
- Coordinate and support the work of national public authorities, civil associations and nongovernmental organizations on matters within its competence.
- Define the concepts related to the areas of competence, in accordance with criteria established and accepted internationally.
- To establish standing committees or ad hoc committees for the treatment and study of specific topics, as well as for the evaluation of specific projects within the areas of competence.
- Encourage the development of science, technology, innovation and quality through incentive mechanisms to institutions, companies and individuals.

3.1.4 FUMEC

The US-Mexico Foundation for Science (FUMEC) is a nongovernmental organization created during preparations for the signing of the North American Free Trade Agreement, based on a bilateral agreement to promote and support collaborative science and technology between the two countries [7].

The niches or areas of opportunity detected for FUMEC are grouped by Table 1 showing us among the leading IT and Technology Health immersed TI which the current topic of study is relevant to the country, state and society overall, since it provides a guide of interest to business creation, sectors, occupations, specialization, etc.

Table 1 áreas de oportunidades detectadas por FUMEC

Sector	Opportunity
Information technology	Cloud computing, mobile technologies, multimedia
Automotive	Advanced manufacturing
Aerospace	Advanced manufacturing, maintenance and repair, airport services
Health technologies	Clinical trials, new drugs, health IT
Food technology	Nutraceuticals, manufacturing processes
Sustainability	Clean technologies (air, water, land) alternative energy
Microsystems	Embedded systems FPGAS

3.1.5 TechBA Inistrie of Health (SE)

The TechBA program is an international business accelerator which was created in 2004 by WSCF in conjunction with the Ministry of Economy [8], allows the realization of strategic alliances and linkages with innovation networks to facilitate access to international network of consultants and senior experts, which will allow the company to improve its value offer and ensure success internationally, to ensure their permanence. Currently has offices located in Arizona, Austin, Madrid, Michigan, Montreal, Seattle, Silicon Valley and Vancouver. TechBA aims to support the internationalization of small and medium-sized Mexican technologies where their development proposals are innovative addition to the potential to compete in global markets [9].

3.1.6 AMIM

It is a civil association that aims to be an organization with its own academic and professional legal personality in order to integrate, coordinate, support, disseminate and develop the different technological and application of information technology in health sciences areas and science related in the United States of Mexico. It also seeks to integrate professional country's participation in various national and international forums in the field of Medical Informatics and promote participation of the groups represented [10].

3.1.7 Clusters de Dispositivos Médicos en México

Mexico has seven clusters sector comprising about 130 companies within them is the cluster of Baja California that captures more than 50 % of national exports of the sector. The Fig. 2 identifies those referred clusters [8], and the Fig. 3 identifies Medical device products.

4 Case Studies in Mexico

Through the coordination of Technologies for Health (hereinafter TecSalud) WSCF in 2012 supporting 88 companies in the states of Baja California, State of Mexico, Federal District, Jalisco and Nuevo Leon; of which 56 were trained in order to obtain certifications in ISO 9100 and ISO 13485 (oriented medical devices), and about a dozen have benefited in calls for innovation funds from CONACYT, the SE or state governments [8].

Approximately 30 companies served by this program between 2011 and 2012 traveled to the United States, Canada, Spain and Germany to meet business

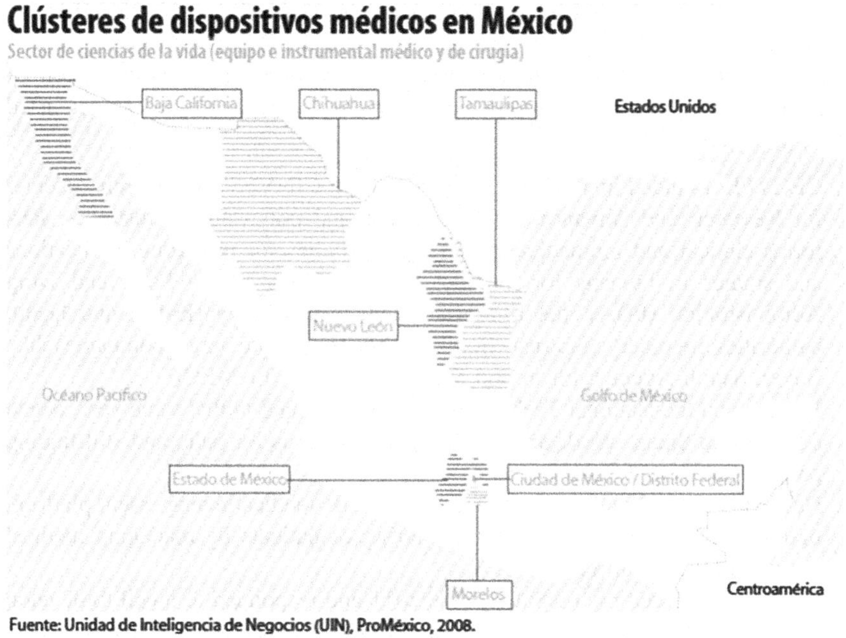

Fig. 2 Ubicación geográfica de los clústeres de dispositivos médicos en México [1]

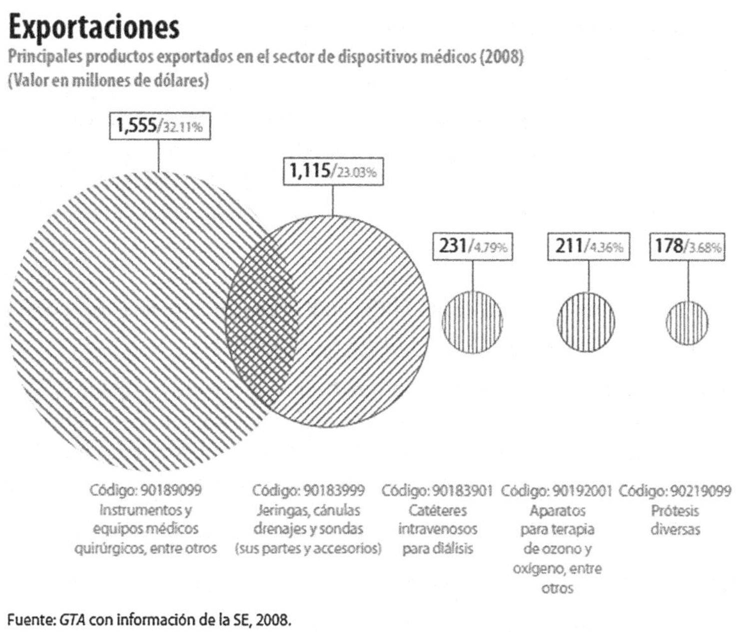

Fig. 3 Medical device products are mainly exported to the United States [1]

ecosystems of these countries and to assess the possibilities of expanding its operations.

Derived from these jobs and promotion, distribution and administration of FUMEC some companies are addressed example to follow as success stories listed below are a few:

1. CECYPE, founded in 1995 by researchers from CINVESTAV Morelia (Center for Research and Advanced Studies of national polytechnical institute). Performs clinical and biomedical research and studies for new drug applications and studies in humans for the first time recording in the Food and Drug Administration (FDA), the European Medicines Agency (EMA) and health authorities in other countries. Some of his clients are large companies like Bayer, Sanofi-Aventis, Pfizer and Schering Plough. [FUMEC]
   He received the National Technology Award 2010 and in that same year, began operating in Spain. Work on new therapeutic options for pain, and still finding partners for joint developments.
2. Neoteck, Aguascalientes, developed Virtumedik, medical management platform based on internet, which allows monitoring of patients by managing medical records and medical reports.
   Neoteck is advised by TecSalud since 2011 and responded to a call to develop mobile applications for the Ministry of Health of Oaxaca. The company was the winner with a project based on the use of tablets to integrate information locally (images, text and video), record the location of the patient and their health. The project includes tablets to take advantage of self-care information on prenatal care, immunization, diabetes mellitus and cervical cancer.
   In late 2011, Neoteck agreed to Technological Innovation Funds issued by the Ministry of Economy and CONACYT and continue the development of new medical monitors for monitoring patients in areas of difficult access.
3. Alandra Medical is one of the companies attracted by the TecSalud program. This company offers outsourcing services to develop medical devices and supports companies to turn their ideas into commercial applications through its acceleration services. TecSalud helped to expand its network of contacts with companies and stakeholders inside and outside the country. Also supported in implementing the Standard ISO13485, and organize projects to access funds innovation CONACYT and the Ministry of Economy.

In order to strengthen the work that has been done with companies, TecSalud organized the Mexican delegation who attended Biospain in September 2012, a leading biotechnology meeting internationally and one of the participants of representation fu the CISESE (Ensenada Center for Scientific Research and Higher Education) located in Baja California.

5 Cluster of Medical Devices in Baja California and Competitive

The Cluster of medical devices Baja California, is a regional cluster concentrating the development and manufacture of medical devices Baja California, and is made by companies like Medtronic, Welch Allyn, Greatbatch Medical, Care Fusion, which are related to the sector manufacturing of medical products also linked with sectors of government, universities and suppliers.

Within the strategic plan Cluster is the increasing competitiveness of the medical products industry. Some of the benefits accruing to firms to become members of this cluster are the link between companies, organizations and government; The impetus for the development of suppliers and new businesses; promoting the training of specialized human resources.

Currently, the state has 66 manufacturers of medical products, of which 39 are located in Tijuana (location near Silicon Valley), representing up to 42,000 direct jobs, making Baja California, the state with the highest concentration of industry Medical nationwide [11].

6 Conclusion

According to the status of the medical device sector in Mexico, significant annual growth of 11 % in export revenues related to the period from 2003 to 2010 products, determines an area that requires attention, advice and regulatory guidelines that help to greater efficiency and effectiveness in the sector, and to enable an agile innovation that responds to the requirements and needs of all stakeholders at national and international level.

Baja California is the state with the highest concentration of companies and direct jobs in the medical device sector nationally, which predicts further growth in the area; provided it is administered correctly, the real needs of the sector. Therefore it is also necessary to generate state-level regulatory framework that promotes State Route Map in partnership with key stakeholders and agency efforts lead them.

References

1. Route map device health. https://www.promexico.gob.mx. Accessed 6 April 2015
2. Internal expansion services. http://es.intexser.com/industrias/dispositivos-medicos. Accessed 10 April 2015
3. Ministry of Economy. www.economia.gob.mx. Accessed 2 April 2015
4. http://www.normateca.gob.mx/Archivos/66_D_3632_22-01-2014.pdf. Accessed 10 April 2015
5. Ministries of Economy and Health. www.salud.gob.mx. Accessed 13 April 2015

6. National Committee on Science and Technology. www.conacyt.gob.mx. Accessed 6 April 2015
7. http://fumec.org/v6/index.php?lang=es
8. TechBA: International Technology Business Accelerator. http://fumec.org/v6/index.php?option=com_content&view=category&layout=blog&id=40&Itemid=443&lang=es. Accessed 12 April 2015
9. TechBA. http://techba.org. Accessed 10 April 2015
10. Mexican Association of Medical Informatics. http://amim.mx/portal/. Accessed 15 April 2015
11. Cluster of medical devices in Baja California and competitive www.industriamedica.org/. Accessed 24 April 2015

Mental Activation of Seniors Incorporating ICT in Their Daily Lives

Maricela Sevilla Caro, María del Consuelo Salgado Soto, Margarita Ramírez Ramírez, Esperanza Manrique Rojas, Hilda Beatriz Ramírez Moreno and Lenin G. Lemus Zúñiga

Abstract This paper aims to know the impact of the use of computers in everyday life for older adults. The results of the investigation confirm that seniors were not prepared to deal with information and communication technologies, moreover, that many of them are not active in the technological society, creating feelings of loneliness, fear and ignorance. The aim of the study was to determine the changes in mood and mindset to incorporate older adults today's technological society through a process of learning of ICT. The training workshop for older adults achieved an increase of motivation toward learning and use of ICT and reducing loneliness and isolation, promoting communication through the use of new technologies.

Keywords Seniors · Mental activation · Digital age

M.S. Caro (✉) · M. del Consuelo Salgado Soto · M.R. Ramírez · E.M. Rojas · H.B.R. Moreno
Facultad de Contaduría y Administración, UABC, Calzada Universidad 14418, Parque Industrial Internacional Tijuana, 22390 Tijuana, BC, Mexico
e-mail: mary_sevilla@uabc.edu.mx

M. del Consuelo Salgado Soto
e-mail: csalgado@uabc.edu.mx

M.R. Ramírez
e-mail: maguiram@uabc.edu.mx

E.M. Rojas
e-mail: emanrique@uabc.edu.mx

H.B.R. Moreno
e-mail: ramirezmb@uabc.edu.mx

L.G.L. Zúñiga
RIS-Itaca, Universitat Politècnia de València, Camino de Vera, s/n, 46022 València, Spain
e-mail: lemus@upv.es

Y.-W. Chen et al. (eds.), *Innovation in Medicine and Healthcare 2015*,
Smart Innovation, Systems and Technologies 45,
DOI 10.1007/978-3-319-23024-5_8

1 Introduction

The digital age was seen as technological revolution has definitely installed between us, and as such, generates fears, hopes encourages creates industries and generates new words. Critically examine the promises that bring new technologies seems a prudent way of entering in the information society. The Information and Communications Technology, also known as ICT, are a set of technologies developed to manage and send information from one place to another. They cover a very wide range of solutions. They include technologies to store information and retrieve it later, send and receive information from one place to another, or process information to calculate and report results. He is currently very high, and increasing the rate of Internet penetration globally. Thus was created the term "Digital Divide" to define the differences and separation between countries with access to new technologies and countries that do not have access to them. The term "digital divide" also refers to the differences between social groups in using ICTs, taking into account different levels of literacy in addition to the technological capacity.

2 Research Background

In Mexico, the Institute of Statistics, Geography and Informatics (INEGI) [1], published in December 2014 that the population using the computer in the range of 55 years or more, total 2,171,169 users of 49,448,510 of the rest of the population. On the use of internet, INEGI reports that the 47,441,244 users only 4.4% (2,066,906) are older than 55 years old. The above data show that this sector of the population not using technology to communicate, socialize, or find updated information are isolated from their families and society triggering emotions that increase the feeling of loneliness.

Manrique [2] indicates that older adults cannot stay out of the information society and knowledge that every day becomes, evolving high-tech environment that generates new ways of creating and maintaining social relationships and the production of knowledge.

2.1 Seniors

According to Belsky [3], in most cultures it is considered as an adult to every person who has more than 18 years. Even after 60 years people call them seniors, elders or seniors, and adults remain, there are differences between those who are over 18 and under 60. The adult does not start or end exactly at these limits chronological.

In traditional societies the elderly had a prominent position and leading role in the orientation of their societies. They are respected, revered and obeyed in its role as counselors and guides the community; were considered repositories of accumulated wisdom gained throughout his life.

Gómez [4] mentions in his article that this situation changed radically.

In the current technologized consumer societies, particularly in developing countries, the vast majority of elderly people are victims of neglect. From the moment they cease to be part of the production system or have an active professional life, it seems to stop being part of society.

From that moment, a huge percentage of them and they are not considered valuable, these people who were once so revered, seem now take place in a technology-driven and market society, where things change increasingly rapidly and the pursuit of wisdom has given way on the road of life to other seemingly more pressing issues, such as consumption and accumulation of material goods.

For these reasons, older people are often considered a burden to his family, particularly when health questions fall into a situation of dependence and should be left to caregivers or be confined in nursing homes.

The WHO (World Health Organization) reports that in 2025 there will be a total of about 1.2 billion people over 60 years. And by 2050, there will be two billion people over that age, with 80 % of them living in developing countries. Therefore, the WHO stresses the need for all countries, especially in developing countries, measures are working to help older people remain healthy and active, participating actively in society so independent.

2.2 Emotions Esteem

Abud and Bojórquez [5], consider self-esteem as a concept, an attitude, a feeling, an image; the ability to assess and treat me with dignity, love and reality.

It has been shown that humans of all ages to have a good family relationship and significant sources of support, is kept in optimum psychological conditions and thus easily overcome the tensions or the disease itself; On the contrary, according to Lopez [6], those seniors with absent or poor quality bonding are affected, yielding to the disease, so the social support makes a noticeable difference between the desire to continue living. By going to lose their emotional ties, the elderly also lose the social roles that for some time took place, which affects their self-esteem in the design of their future life and the way in which you must socialize with their environment.

2.3 Depression and Anxiety

Martinez [7] quotes that depressive states are the major causes of suicidal reactions since all depressed there is a potential suicide. It is said that there is depression whenever a fault appears in the neuro psychic tone, either passenger or enduring. Depression can range from mild depression to stupor; in its lightest form, an unhappy person of the third age has a feeling of helplessness, despair, worthlessness has a feeling of helplessness, despair, worthlessness and loss of interest in usual activities. In the slightly deeper depression there is a constant unpleasant tension; every experience is accompanied by sorrow, and the patient may be fearful, worried, anxious, restless and suffer physical or emotional suffering. A depressive episode in a person seniors can sometimes be difficult to differentiate from dementia, as both may coincide with symptoms such as apathy, difficulty concentrating and memory disturbances.

Anxiety is a signal or fairly common general reaction in humans, Kaplan and Sadock [8] mentioned that the experience of anxiety has two components: awareness of physiological sensations (such as palpitations and sweating) and the awareness of being nervous or scared. The feeling of shame can increase anxiety. Anxious people are predisposed to select certain things around and neglecting others in their effort to prove that this justified to consider a situation as threatening, if falsely justify their fear, anxieties increase by selective response and create a vicious circle anxiety, distorted perception and increased anxiety.

2.4 *Loneliness and Isolation*

According Montero and Sanchez [9], loneliness has been conceived as a subjective state that arises as a response to the lack of a particular relationship, the consequences can be addressed in a negative or positive way. You can think of the causes of loneliness in elderly people and those associated with aging according Laforet [10]. These crises focus on experienced losses that undermine self-esteem; in the physical deterioration and relationship independently perform daily activities; crisis and loss of roles in their social group and decreased physical abilities.

On the issue of isolation, according Pisa [11] is a contemporary, observable and measurable phenomenon refers to the lack of company and meaningful encounters with others. Keep in mind that the human being can be isolated not feel lonely or otherwise may have many contacts and lonely.

Loneliness and isolation can be considered as one of the main features of the way of life in elderly people.

2.5 *Theories of Socialization in the Elderly*

It is necessary to consider two theories that influence the socialization of aging, following the approach of Salvarezza [12], there are two predominant approaches to the issue of aging:

Theory of detachment: This theory suggests that as you get older and lose interest in activities and surrounding objects, isolated over the environment, other people's problems and reduces interaction with others. This detachment generates to stay away from social interaction, leads to emotional loneliness, feelings of anxiety and isolation can only be relieved by finding other as suppliers of needed relationship (Amico) [13].

Activity theory or addiction, maintaining that adults older must remain active as long as possible, further indicates that they should seek substitutes for those activities that no longer can perform (Amico) [13]. This theory, as discussed in the publication Montero and Sanchez [9], indicating that attachment is provided by the relationship that makes the person feel safe and is provided in most cases by a spouse or partner; what characterizes centrally an attachment figure is perceived and feels like providing security, as someone who cares to listen, accessible, reliable, interested and sympathetic.

2.6 *Mental Activation*

Mental activation is related to the current applied to perform a specific action. This energy level is related to motivation and character of each person.

Luque [14] mentioned that the lack of cognitive mental activity explains the decreased learning ability in old age, and the relevance of training and stimulation to activate and reactivate the mental energies, is to guide behavior towards new roads, unknown and challenging.

2.7 *Active Ageing*

As defined OMS, Active aging is the "process of optimizing opportunities for health, participation and security in order to improve the quality of life as people age".

The active term refers to a continuous participation in social, economic, cultural, spiritual and civic affairs, not just the ability to be physically active or participate in the workforce. Adults seniors who retire, are ill or in disability may remain active in society.

Active aging is to extend the life expectancy in health and quality of life for all people as they age, including those frail, disabled or need assistance.

Galarza [15] mentioned that the concept of active aging also implies that aging takes place within the context of others: friends, coworkers, neighbors and family members. Interdependence and intergenerational solidarity (give and receive reciprocally between individuals and between generations of old and young) are important principles of active aging.

As we age, our body undergoes various modifications of morphological type (in form), physiological (operation), psychological and social, which are generated by own age changes and accumulated wear.

During the normal aging process, some cognitive abilities (as the speed in learning and memory) decreases with age. However, these losses can be offset by an increase of knowledge and experience. Deterioration of cognitive performance is often caused by disuse (lack of practice), illness (depression), behavioral factors (alcohol and drugs), psychological factors (lack of motivation) and social factors (loneliness and isolation), rather than aging itself.

In Mexico demographic transition is occurring resulting in a significant increase in the elderly population. In fact, in 1950 the number of people aged 60 and over amounted to 1,419,685 (5.5 % of the total), a figure that rose to 8,364,334 in 2005 (8.1 %). It is also expected that by 2025 will increase to 17,512,000 (12.4 %) (Galarza) [15].

The primary objectives of active aging are achieving maximum health, wellness, quality of life and social development of older adults, considering their physical and intellectual potential and the opportunities offered by the company.

The Gerontology indicates that the positive aspects of active aging for older people emphasize the following:

- Increased social contact and perception of well-being.
- Ability to improve their income through productive projects.
- Prevention and control of chronic diseases.
- Conservation, extension and recovery of physical, mental and social functioning.
- Increased psychosocial development.
- Improvement of self-esteem, quality of life and wellbeing.

3 Methodolical Framework

The research methodology in this study was qualitative, through the modality of case study, according to Sandín [16], the focus is on the investigation of a phenomenon, population or general condition. The study does not focus on a specific case, but in a certain set of cases. This is not a collective study, but the study of several cases.

The case study is a research method for the analysis of social reality, and represents the most relevant and naturally oriented research from a qualitative perspective. According to Martinez Migueles [17], the case studies focus on a situation, event, program or particular phenomenon. The case itself is important for what it reveals about the phenomenon and what it may represent. This specificity makes it suitable for practical problems, issues and situations or events that arise in daily life.

The qualitative sampling is purposeful. The first actions to choose the sample occur from the same approach as the context in which we expect to find cases that interest in qualitative research in selected instead of asking: Who will be measured?, are questioned: Which cases initially interested in and where to find?

Also conducted literature review, observation, informal interviews plus. Data were analyzed qualitatively. The sample was taken from the School of Accounting and Administration of the Autonomous University of Baja California, the course entitled "Seniors learning new technologies".

The sources of information gathering are the testimonies of the elderly participants and attendees of the course taught at the School of Accounting and Administration, UABC, Tijuana, Mexico. The techniques of data collection for this study were the interview and observation. The sample is 20 seniors, who participated in a course designed under the assumptions of gerontology, which is the science that studies the elderly.

4 Analysis of Results

The interest of this research was focused on mental activation of older adults to incorporate ICT into their daily lives. It is noteworthy that the first day presented the course; adults come with high expectations and no confidence in them for fear of the unknown, in this case, in the use of technologies.

In the first phase of the study were interviewed 20 adults before starting the course entitled "Seniors learning new technologies" where most responses focus on the need to learn to use the computer as it is the media today days, the desire to know to use the medium that gives the computer to access the current technology, and, most mentioned the desire to keep up and not get help to do things, expressing the desire to excel; another common response was achieved communicate with family and friends.

The second phase of the investigation was to finish the aforementioned course, where he met the same group of participants and the responses is summarized in the experience of each of the adults:

At the end of the course feel more confident in the use of new technologies relating it to the job performance and personal.

Adults feel fully at the forefront in computing and cyber world, which broadens the mind activation and consequently the adult enters the process of active aging.

They feel sad, because they will no longer see their fellow students and new friends for a while, indicating that before coming to the course felt isolated and alone.

Adults conclude that they are motivated to keep going, safe for every day of his life by entering a new world considered impossible, the above can relate raise self-esteem and confidence, and reduce the possibility that the people of the Seniors come into states of depression.

References

1. INEGI. Institute of Statistics, Geography and Informatics. Accessed April 15 2015. http://www.inegi.org.mx/default.aspx
2. Manrique Rojas, E.: Impacto de la incorporación de las TIC en la vida de los adultos mayores de 60 años de edad, en Tijuana, B.C, Ph.D. thesis (2011)
3. Belsky, J.K.: Psicología del envejecimiento. Masson, Barcelona (1996)
4. Gómez Vecchio, R.: Tercera Edad y TICs. Una sociedad positiva. Writing in Digital City, magazine reporting on Knowledge Society, Citizen Participation and ICTs. July 1, (2014). Accessed April 16 2015. http://www.usuaria.org.ar/noticias/tercera-edad-y-tics-una-sociedad-positiva
5. Abud, C.: Bojórquez : Efectos psicológicos: ansiedad, depresión, autoestima y relación de pareja. Tesis de licenciatura en psicología, Mérida Yucatán (1997)
6. López, C.: Diferencia de autoestima entre ancianos institucionalizados y no institucionalizados en la ciudad de Mérida. Thesis in psychology, Mérida (1998)
7. Martínez, M.: El paciente con enfermedad en estado terminal y el rechazo a la eutanasia. Tesis de licenciatura. Toluca, Edo. De México (2003)
8. Kaplan, H.Y., Sadock, B.: Sinopsis de psiquiatría. Ediciones científicas y médicas, Barcelona (1998)
9. Montero, L.L.M., Sánchez, S.J.J.: La soledad como fenómeno psicológico: un análisis conceptual. Salud Mental, febrero, 19–27. Royal Spanish Academy (2001). Accessed April 15 2015. http://www.rae.es/
10. Laforet, J.: La Necesidad de pertenencia. En Introducción a la Gerontología. Editorial Herder, Barcelona (1991)
11. Pisa, H.: Accessed April 5 2015. http://www.psicogeriatria.net/2011/05/16/soledad-depresi%C3%B3n-y-aislamiento/
12. Salvarezza, L.: (Compilador): La vejez: Una mirada gerontológica actual. Buenos Aires, Paidós (2000)
13. Amico Lucía del Carmen.: Envejecer en el siglo XXI. No siempre Querer es Poder. Hacia la de-construcción de mitos y la superación de estereotipos en torno a los adultos mayores en sociedad. Theories of aging in Socialization.Edición No. 55 (2009). Accessed April 17 2015. http://margen.org/suscri/margen55/amico.pdf
14. Luque, L.E.: Aprender informática en la tercera edad. Institution: Universe Program. Aging—Maest. Gerontología—UNC. Thematic Area: Technology. Accessed April 5 2015. www.fimte.fac.org.ar/doc/15cordoba/Luque.doc
15. Galarza Vásquez, K.: Envejecimiento activo, mejor vida en la tercera edad (2014). Accessed April 12 2015. http://www.saludymedicinas.com.mx/centros-de-salud/climaterio/prevencion/envejecimiento-activo.html
16. Sandín, E., Paz, M.: Investigación Cualitativa en educación. MacGraw-Hil, México (2003)
17. Martínez Migueles, M.: Ciencia y arte de la Metodología cualitativa. México: Trillas (2007)

Quality of Life and Active Aging Through Educational Gerontology in Information Technology and Communication

Esperanza Manrique Rojas, Hilda Beatriz Ramírez Moreno, Margarita Ramírez Ramirez, Nora del Carmen Osuna Millan, Arnulfo Alanís Garza and José Sergio Magdaleno Palencia

Abstract This research was conducted through action research; was through training course information technologies to incorporate into the daily life of an older adult use computers. The sample consisted of 20 elderly who participate in a course designed low assumptions of gerontology, which is the science that studies the changes in old age and during aging. The study was justified because most seniors are not prepared to deal with these technologies and as a result many of them are not active in the technological society, this creates feelings of loneliness, fear, ignorance and forgetfulness, among others. In addition, there is a profound shift in values and social attitudes, changes capable of causing a major rift between young people and their ancestors. The aim of this study was to determine the impact of the inclusion of the elderly to today's technological society, through the process of learning technologies in Baja California, México.

Keywords Gerontology · Older adults · Communication technologies

E.M. Rojas (✉) · H.B.R. Moreno · M.R. Ramirez · N. del Carmen Osuna Millan
Facultad de Contaduría y Administración, UABC, Calzada Universidad 14418,
Parque Industrial Internacional Tijuana, 22390 Tijuana, BC, Mexico
e-mail: emanrique@uabc.edu.mx

H.B.R. Moreno
e-mail: ramirezmb@uabc.edu.mx

M.R. Ramirez
e-mail: maguiram@uabc.edu.mx

N. del Carmen Osuna Millan
e-mail: noraosuna@uabc.edu.mx

A.A. Garza · J.S.M. Palencia
Departamento de Sistemas y Computación, Instituto Tecnológico de Tijuana,
Calzada del Tecnológico S/N, Tomas Aquino, 22414 Tijuana, BC, Mexico
e-mail: alanis@tectijuana.edu.mx

J.S.M. Palencia
e-mail: jmagdaleno@tectijuana.edu.mx

Y.-W. Chen et al. (eds.), *Innovation in Medicine and Healthcare 2015*,
Smart Innovation, Systems and Technologies 45,
DOI 10.1007/978-3-319-23024-5_9

1 Introduction

The period of the Digital Era begins in the second half of the twentieth century, were installed abruptly technological tools in the daily lives of people. In this sense, Area Moreira [1] indicates that the demand for mastering the Information Technology and Communication has quickly become a problem, nationally and globally, and that adults who were born in the decade previous generations of the 90s y not know how to use these resources are called 'digital immigrants' being phased out by a system that is perceived naturally by the 'digital natives', composed of young people who interact extensively with reality through technological supports whole.

The right to education should not be limited to age or social status, for the elderly, to exercise this right means a chance to upgrade, social participation and reaffirmation of their potential. For people who are in this stage of life, education can help the development of a culture of aging and enhancing the quality of life, which translates into improved health, welfare and happiness.

Notes Vallejo [2], seniors cannot stay out of the information society and knowledge that every day becomes, evolves and creates new ways of creating and maintaining social relationships and knowledge. Thus the need for the elderly, incorporated into your daily life, the use of the computer as a tool to be attuned to the XXI century increase their active aging, continuously enriching the argument.

Older adults through participation in a process of teaching and learning have the opportunity to learn to use a computer with support of gerontological strategies and a methodology based on the Andragogic model of teaching-learning [3] may develop creativity and practice active aging for better quality of life.

2 Overall Objective

Understanding the impact of the incorporation of adults older than 59 years today's technological society, through a process of teaching and learning communication technologies, in the community of Tijuana, Baja California, Mexico.

2.1 *Specific Objectives*

Evaluate the results obtained in the teaching-learning of computer use, through the design of a computer course, focused on developing technological skills of older adults, with bases in andragogy and gerontology.

Analyze the experiences and impact of adults who participated in the course to complete the process.

3 Research Background

Technological advances presented in recent decades, are evident; daily activities are increasingly linked, mostly with the use of technology [4]. The main objective of the emergence of new technology is to facilitate and improve the activities for which they were designed.

The use of information technology is not only to meet the needs of future generations and the majority of seniors (over 60 years) are not prepared to deal with these technologies and as a result many of them are not active within this technological society, generating feelings of loneliness, fear, ignorance and forgetfulness, among others. In addition, there is a profound shift in values and social attitudes, changes capable of causing a major rift between young people and their ancestors.

Some seniors feel alienated from society, family and friends for not knowing how to use a computer, and not just because of no use, but the computer becomes a social mediator that guarantees a space and virtual presence users within the world community and this represents for the elderly is a huge possibility for social inclusion or exclusion.

The elderly population has experienced remarkable growth in response to numerous factors have combined to support a longer life expectancy, the Naciones Unidad has considered, through various agencies, general policies directly benefit conditions lives of these people. Plans and programs undertaken worldwide by UNESCO in the area of culture and education, and developed by the World Health Organization (WHO), who have placed special emphasis on preventive health benefit of stand a higher quality of life.

Older adults in Mexico are catered for with programs of economic self-sufficiency (pantries and medical consultations), although these do not solve the problem of discrimination and backwardness, many people seniors who have physical and mental strength to be efficient workers, thanks to their experience and wisdom.

A study by Sancho [5] to the Jaume I, Spain University, Adults older graduates who studied at the University for Older determined that these courses promote the welfare of the people involved in them, and as a result, intellectual activities that they perform, strengthen their self-esteem. It also found that the motivation is not altered by the fact of aging, both older students and young people have very high scores for motivation in the study. The other was identified that retirement does not involve the decreased motivation for conducting social and educational activities, so that the fact that retirement is not a factor which reduce the motivation to study.

3.1 Gerontology

Giraldo [6] defines the gerontology, the science dealing with old age and aging in all its dimensions: biological, psychological, sociological, anthropological, economic, political and social.

Cervera and Sainz [7] define social gerontology as the science that most concerned the study of aging from the perspective sociocultural or anthropological partner.

Some factors that influence the development in most adulthood, are subject to individual conditions, family and sociocultural conditions. It is important that the elderly recognize their potential, enabling a more positive perception of the stage that passes, greater acceptance of it; that meet their communication needs and transmission of accumulated experience, this is accomplished with the support of family, friends and potential of educational spaces.

3.2 Educational Gerontology

According to Bartholomew [8], education plays a very important role in human life, education for adults is andragogy with the support of gerontology as a science that deals with the aging people. In converge knowledge of psychology, medicine, education, sociology, and all with the goal of making the experience of aging in a less negative adventure, and why not, even positive.

This science is based on four assumptions, taking into account the adult learner: self-concept, experience, willingness to learn and perspectives and learning orientation. Gerontology is an opportunity and a right of humans to permanently internalized in what to do with their personal fulfillment through a scientific and comprehensive preventive knowledge of their life cycle.

For Diaz Barriga and Hernandez [9], learning not only fulfills a function of biological adaptation, but responds to the need to mean the physical and social world in which he lives. This new way of learning required in the elderly necessarily an active attitude.

Giraldo [10] that 'pleasure, interest in what is done, motivation, depend on the power we have over what we say. Not having to be manipulated, dominated, crushed, leading to passivity, disinterest and, eventually, to a psychic degradation and deadly petrification of personality or develop power over our actions, in our private lives, in our work, in society, and take initiatives in existence, or our personality dies before our physical death'.

Education should serve to form a social ethic that responds to the requirements of development planning; at the individual level should be practical purposes such as providing knowledge, skills, abilities and habits either for insertion into economic activity, the exercise of a trade, or the compliance with the conditions and transformations of the productive system and everyday life.

Active aging from the point of view of social gerontology allows people to realize their potential for physical, social and mental well-being throughout the life cycle and participate in society according to their needs, desires and capabilities, while that provides protection and safety [11].

Quality of life is a social construct that exists only through the experience of people in their interactions with all elements of their environment, enabling you to meet your expectations and needs. Has different definitions and two dimensions: the objective when discussing health, physical functioning, economic status; and subjective when taking into account the appreciation of feeling good and satisfied.

Retain autonomy and interdependence as you age is a task of the whole society, as aging occurs within society, work, friends, neighbors and family. Because of this interdependence and solidarity between generations are important principles of active aging WHO [12].

4 Issues

The social environment surrounding the elderly has changed aggressively in recent decades. Technological advances have brought about a radical change in the forms of production, dissemination and knowledge acquisition.

Current forms of communication and activities are conducted through various technological devices like mobile phones, ATMs, home computers and computerization of most of the commercial and industrial activities, causing new training needs and knowledge on citizens. Intelligent Access and use of this set of technologies require a person with a different level were trained older adults. Interact with menu systems or options, navigate without getting lost through hypertext documents, access e-mail to communicate, receive instant messages via different devices, facing a flood of images, audio and audiovisual sequences, etc., are among other new skills to be mastered anyone to be able to function autonomously in society Marzal [13] digital information.

Studies show that most seniors need help with processes that were created to simplify, not complicate; for this need to be surrounded by family and young people to help them in this task of renewing and those in nursing homes and lack the support of loved ones, are neglected by society (Monzón, Stanislavsky, Urrutia, [14]).

This research indicates that older adults cannot stay out of the information society and knowledge to daily changes. Thus the need for older adults, especially the computer as a tool to be in tune with the demands of the XXI century increase their active aging, continuously enriching the argument.

5 Methodological Framework

This model describes action research and reflective action cycles:

Phase 1: a course was designed with the aim of incorporating older adults to use ICT, developing skills in handling computer, based on the characteristics of the andgragogía and gerontology.

Phase 2: the course was provided to a group of seniors, opportunity areas were detected, the necessary adjustments were made and finally the lessons learned during this process was collected. The name of the course 'assets Elderly Learning New Technologies'.

Phase 3: After a lapse of three months that ended the course by telephone was conducted a survey in order to identify the impact of the use of computers in everyday life of adults.

Group shows: In the Autonomous University of Baja California, Tijuana Campus, Faculty of Accounting and Administration, took out the course called Active Seniors Learning New Technologies, where participating seniors. Distributed 35 each of the five computer laboratories. Hence a group of 20 adults was selected to conduct this research [15].

6 Analysis of Results

The results of the investigation are presented in each of the phases:

Phase 1: the content of the course with practical issues in the area of ICT is design, teaching strategies and learning, where it was considered to be remembered with clarity and for a longer period of time which has been repeated and exercised were applied especially was linked with topics of general interest to seniors, thus ensured that they are active participants in the process.

To know the reason why they decided to participate in the ICT course underwent an interview with each of the participants and in response to the question Why did you decide to participate in the introductory course to tick?: The results indicate that participated for Interest in learning, not to be dependent on others, to communicate, self-improvement, are aware of the need to learn. It is observed that older adults have clear objectives, know what they want to achieve, have a desire for self-improvement. Do not want to be outside current context, are interested in keeping in touch with others and now they want to do through the computer. They recognize the importance of addressing some fears and break barreas between them and computers.

Phase 2: At the end of the course, conducts a survey where one of the questions was how you feel today is the last day of course again? Some of the most significant responses are:

'We integrate into modern life and take us out of isolation giving us opportunities we had no'.

'Today I feel great and motivated to continue, it gave me a lot of security for all the days of my life, because I could enter a new world that made it impossible for me and I learned that nothing is impossible when time is spent what you proposed to us, thank you for thinking of us. Thanks for helping young people to both get this dream come'.

'I'm not afraid to use the PC, I feel safer to go to some of the programs taught in class because I have carefully with practice I got to read the instructions on the PC and taking into account the guidance given to me in using the UABC advisors. Very grateful to the UABC'.

'Happy to finish the course for learning how to use the computer, sad to have finished, the time for me is very little, and hopefully the following courses last a little longer, no matter if they raise the price of it, it is fair and I think everyone would agree, thank you again'.

Phase 3: After 3 months ending on course, was done via phone, a survey of adults who participated in the course, to identify if they use the computer or not, that activities performed in it, and the impact of the use of computers in everyday life of adults. They commented that increased security in themselves, some of them joined the working life, were able to be contacted his distant family and have the opportunity to share images and photos, the possibility for them to see their programs and movies when they can.

Welcome the opportunity to incorporate technological life, now have access to information of interest through the use of a computer to help them in their daily lives.

7 Conclusions

Carrying out research with older adults allowed demystify seniors as passive. Contrary to this after meeting their needs, their fears, live with them, the experience of learning, are characterized as active, willing to learn about ICT, and with great ability to develop their cognitive processes.

The experiences of each of the seniors at the end of the course, demonstrated the importance for this population knowledge of computer use and internet. For not only was possible that they felt able to learn something new-a benefit in itself important, but this learning, hopefully, contribute to the extension and maintenance of cognitive processes during aging, which are fundamental premises Gerontology and active

Similarly it is noteworthy that managed to break the stereotype of fear of using technology as a senior you are, it was shown that making adjustments in forms and assistance in the process, it is possible to develop self-confidence, motivation and interest in access to ICT.

Another important achievement was the coexistence and intergenerational learning, for the opportunity to interact both with older adults and youth who supported, provided an atmosphere to socialize, improve their communication skills and develops appropriate measures to resolve the problems that arose social networks by use of the computer.

The discovery that made use of the network exceeded expectations since realized the type and amount of information they can access, taking the basic tools of network access.

This research helps to ensure that seniors who learn and apply ICT in their daily life will bring many benefits rather than impediments exercise their creativity and develop memory (cognitive level); were given a new tool for interaction and communication with the social environment for intergenerational communication; and they will practice active aging.

References

1. Area, M.: Manuel, introduction to educational technology. University of La Laguna, Spain (2009)
2. Vallejo, E., Article Conception Andragogic Of Higher Education. http://andragogos.blogspot.mx/2010/08/articulo-concepcion-andragogica-de-la.html (2010). Accessed March 2012
3. Knowles, M.: Andragogía, el aprendizaje de los adultos. Holton, E y Swanson R. Traducido de la quinta edición en inglés de The Adult Learner. Oxford University Press, México, D.F (2001)
4. Sevilla, M., María Del, C.S.: Terminology of information technology and communication, ILCSA S.A. de C.V (2011)
5. Sancho, C., Blasco, M.J., Martínez-Mir, R. Palmero, F.: Analysis of the reasons for the aging study, University Jaume I. http://reme.uji.es/articulos/apalmf8342905102/texto.html (2000). Accessed March 2012
6. Giraldo, A., Gerontologist, Never too late to learn. http://www.enplenitud.com/nota.asp?articuloID=7219#ixzz1Fh5HULi8 (2008). Accessed March 2011
7. Cervera, C., Sainz, J.: Actualización en Geriatría Y Gerontología. http://www.librosaulamagna.com/ENFERMERIA-GERIATRIA-y-GERONTOLOGIA/898/ (2006). Accessed February 2012
8. Bartolomé, A.: Preparando para un nuevo modo de conocer. En: Gorreta, Rosa (coord.). Desenvolupament de capacitats: Noves Estraègies. Hospitalet de Llobregat: Centre Cultural Pineda, págs, 69–86 (1997)
9. Díaz Barriga, A.F.Y., Hernández, G.: Teaching Strategies for Meaningful Learning, a Constructivist Interpretation. Edition Mc Graw Hill, México (2001)
10. Giraldo. A.: Never too late to learn. http://www.emigracionlegal.com/nota.asp?articuloID=7219 (2011). Accessed March 2012
11. Forttes, A.: Introduction to social gerontology. In: Program for the Elderly, A.C. (pp. 1–17). Diploma in social gerontology distance for municipal managers. Pontificia Universidad Católica de Chile, Santiago (2007)
12. OMS. Active aging: a policy framework. In: International Plan on Aging. Second World Assembly on Ageing. World Health Organization, Madrid (2002)
13. Marzal, M.A., Calzada, J., Cuevas, A.: Development of a metadata schema for describing educational resources. The profile of the MiMeta application. Span. J. Sci. Document. **29**. 4 Oct–Dec 2006

14. Monzón, A., Stanislavsky, P., Urrutia, M.: The elderly and technology: stay out? http://fido.palermo.edu/servicios_dyc/publicacionesdc/vista/detalle_articulo.php?id_libro=34&id_articulo=4371 (2008). Accessed Feb 2012
15. Manrique Rojas, E.: Impact of the incorporation of ICT in the lives of adults 60 years of age in Tijuana, BC Thesis, University Northern Pacific, Mazatlan, Sinaloa (2012)

Simulation of Cervical Cord Compression Using Finite Element Method (FEM)

Nur Fadhlina Binti Shaari, Junji Ohgi, Norihiro Nishida, Xian Chen, Itsuo Sakuramoto and Toshihiko Taguchi

Abstract Cervical myelopathy results in loss of nerves functions along the spinal cord below the damage area as it is the result of spinal cord compression which nowadays always occur during traffic accidents. Patients with cervical myelopathy do not necessarily share the same symptoms. These vary according to the degree of cervical cord compression and cross sectional shape at every segment of cervical cord which caused difficulties in diagnosis. In this study, two dimension model of every cervical cord segment were built. Then, differences of compression results in every segment were verified. After that, to verify the effects of compression to other segments, three dimensions model of cervical cord model is built. From this study, we can see that cervical cord with flat shaped gray matter have higher stress distribution than cervical cord with hill shaped grey matter. Other than that, the injury start occurred in ventral column of white matter instead of gray matter during early injury stage.

Keywords Spinal cord · Cervical spine · White matter · Gray matter · Finite element method · Stress distribution · Spinal cord compression

N.F.B. Shaari (✉) · J. Ohgi · X. Chen
Department of Applied Medical Engineering Science, Yamaguchi University, Yamaguchi, Japan
e-mail: u016uf@yamaguchi-u.ac.jp

J. Ohgi
e-mail: ohgi@yamaguchi-u.ac.jp

X. Chen
e-mail: xchen@yamaguchi-u.ac.jp

N. Nishida · T. Taguchi
Department of Orthopedic Surgery, Yamaguchi University, Yamaguchi, Japan
e-mail: nishida3@yamaguchi-u.ac.jp

T. Taguchi
e-mail: taguchi@yamaguchi-u.ac.jp

I. Sakuramoto
Tokuyama National College of Technology, Yamaguchi, Japan
e-mail: sakuramo@tokuyama.ac.jp

Y.-W. Chen et al. (eds.), *Innovation in Medicine and Healthcare 2015*,
Smart Innovation, Systems and Technologies 45,
DOI 10.1007/978-3-319-23024-5_10

1 Introduction

Cervical myelopathy is the result of spinal cord compression in the cervical spine, disrupt the normal transmission of the neural signals involve the arms, legs and bowel functions. As cervical myelopathy occur, there are reports on compression form and shape based on static factor and dynamic factor. However, patients with cervical myelopathy do not necessarily share the same symptoms. These differ according to the degree of compression and cross sectional shape of cervical cord, thus caused difficulties in diagnosis. Therefore, in this study, using pathological model, pia mater, gray matter and white matter of every segments of cervical cord were plotted. From simulation results of built models, differences in stress values at every cross section which have different shape of gray matter and white matter were verified. It will be related with patients' symptoms and the results will make patients diagnosis easier.

2 Methods

2.1 Building Two Dimension (2D) Model

In this study, Simple Digitizer software was used in plotting coordinates from cervical cord cross section images from C2 to C8. Magnetic Resonance Imaging (MRI) images of cervical cord as shown in Fig. 1 from journal entitled Morphologic Features of the Human Cadaveric Spinal Cord by Takeshi Kameyama [1] were inserted in Simple Digitizer. This journal studied about the cross sectional area and diameter of the normal cadaveric spinal cord at each segment from C2 to S3 level in 12 cadaveric specimens and their orphologic features. As a result, it is found that relative ratio of the cross sectional area of each segment to that of C3 segment was similar in all the specimens examined despite a large individual variation in absolute cord size and also each segment had distinct qualitative and quantitative morphologic features. Then, coordinates of every segment were then taken from the images. Actual sizes of transverse diameter and sagittal diameter of every segment from the journal as shown in Table 1 were used. Coordinate (0,0) was made as the central canal. Then, the coordinates of pia mater, gray matter and white matter were used to build model using ANSYS software. All 2D models then were meshed in ANSYS. Figure 2 below shows meshed 2D model of cervical cord, C2 to C8 built in ANSYS with pia mater at the outer layer, white matter in the middle and gray matter at the inner layer.

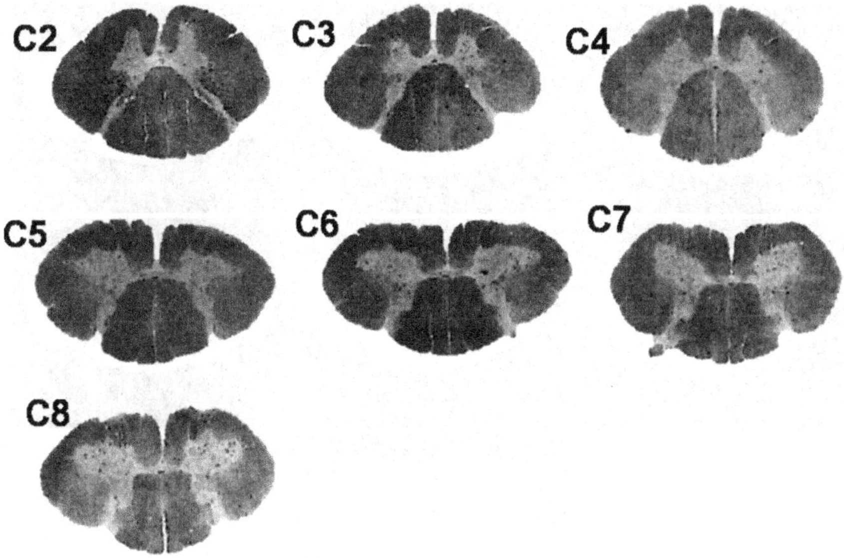

Fig. 1 MRI images of cross sections of cervical cord

Table 1 The average cross-sectional measurement at each spinal cord segment

Cervical segment	Transverse diameter (mm)	Sagittal diameter (mm)
C2	10.5 ± 0.8	6.4 ± 0.4
C3	10.7 ± 0.7	6.2 ± 0.4
C4	11.3 ± 0.9	6.1 ± 0.6
C5	12.2 ± 0.8	6.0 ± 0.4
C6	12.6 ± 0.7	5.8 ± 0.5
C7	12.3 ± 0.7	5.8 ± 0.5
C8	11.7 ± 0.6	5.6 ± 0.4

2.2 *Materials Mechanical Properties*

The mechanical properties of every elements from previous research [2] were adopted. Young modulus, poisson's ratio and hyperelastic data for each pia mater, white matter and gray matter were inserted in each segment of cervical cord. The data were taken from previous research results.

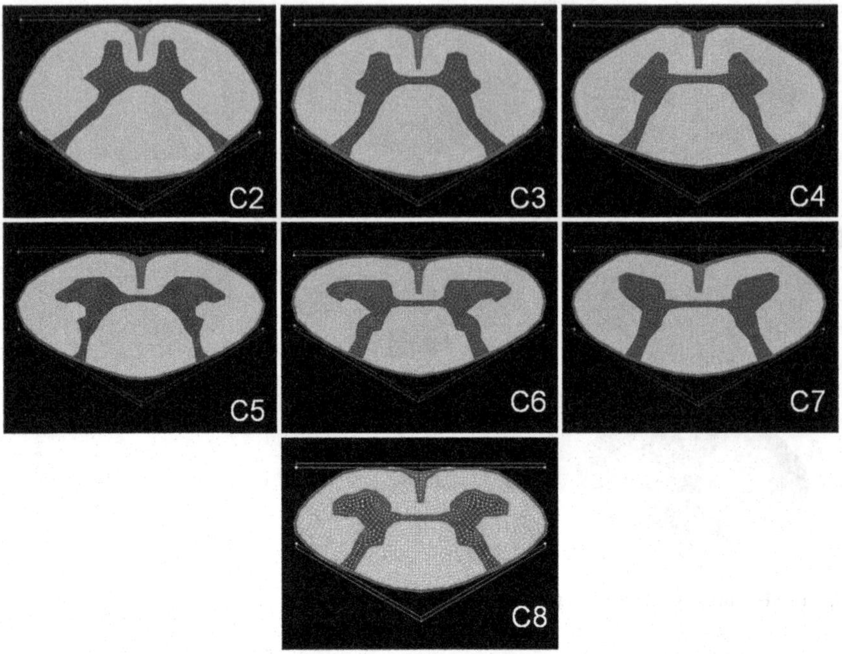

Fig. 2 Meshed cervical sections from C2 to C8 built in ANSYS

2.3 Boundary Condition

Simulation boundary conditions of every segments of cervical cord are shown in Fig. 3. At the anterior side of the cervical cord which is at the upper part of the segment, the rigid body represent bone and at the posterior side represent ligament. The rigid body at the posterior side was set 30° symmetrically as it is the shape of the yellow ligament. The compression angle at cervical anterior side was 180° and 30° symmetrically at posterior side. Then, during simulation, bone at anterior side was set fixed and compression displacement of ligament at posterior side was from 10 up to 30 % from every cervical segment's sagittal diameter from C2 until C8. Figure 4 shows the compression condition as in three dimension image. For horizontal direction, the displacement is zero which mean fixed.

2.4 Building Three Dimension (3D) Model

Cervical cord compression sometimes involves more than one cervical segments. To verify the effects of compression to other segments when one segment is compressed, simulation using three dimension model is needed. Other than that, 3D

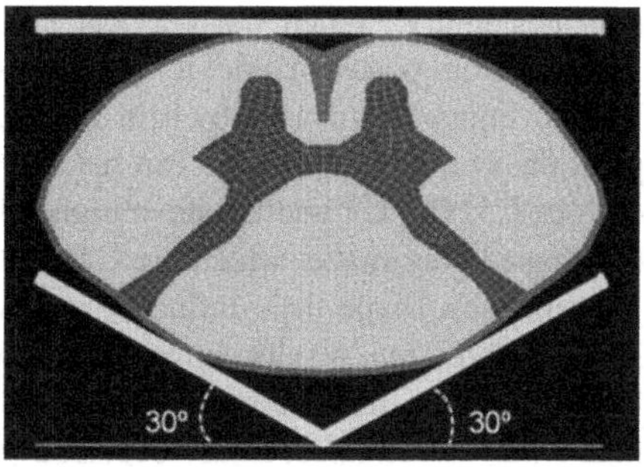

Fig. 3 Boundary conditions

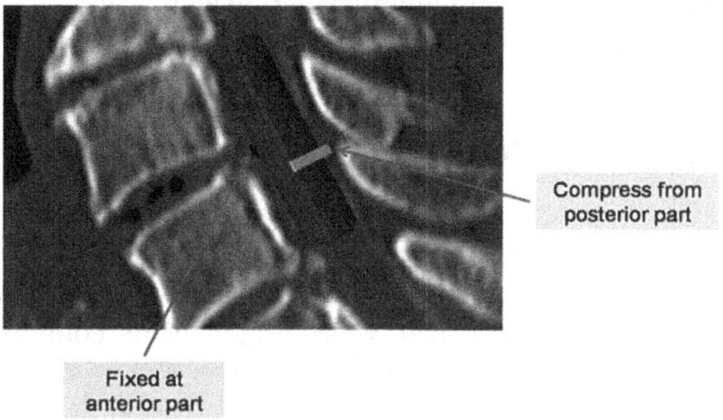

Fig. 4 Compression condition in three dimension image

model also needed because even only one segment got injured or compressed, sometimes bone and ligament of other segment will get involve during treatment. Therefore, three dimensions model of cervical cord model is built in this study. For building three dimension model of cervical cord, the model was first built by connecting C2 until C8 segments by plotting coordinates in software called Shade for both gray matter and white matter. Pia mater was not inserted in this early stage. The distance between segments is 14 mm. Then, the data was exported to Mesh lab for smoothing and after that to ScanIP software for meshing. From ICEM, the model then exported to ANSYS for calculation. For time being, the step is only until meshing. The calculation is still on progress.

3 Results and Discussions

3.1 Two Dimension (2D) Model Simulation

Calculation was made by inserted allowable stress for every element; pia mater, white matter and gray matter which is 3, 0.015 and 0.043 MPa respectively. Results were recorded when the compression percentage is 10, 20, 30 % and when injury occured. Results shows stress distribution in equivalent stress form and red part indicates injury. When the cervical cord was compressed by 10 % of sagittal diameter from posterior side, it shows no similar tendency in all segments and there was no injury occur as shown in Fig. 5. Figure 6 shows results for 20 % compression. From this result, we can see that cervical cord with flat shaped gray matter such as C5, C6, C7 and C8 have higher stress distribution than cervical cord with hill shaped gray matter which are C2, C3 and C4. From here, we can conclude that gray matter's shape does influence stress distribution in every cervical cord. For 30 % compression, results shows almost all segments had complete injury as shown in Fig. 7. After that, the state of cervical cord and compression percentage during injury was investigated. Injury occurred when the compression was 15–18 % varies from C2 to C8 as shown in Fig. 9. Also, for all segments, it shows that the injury started at ventral column of white matter as shown in Fig. 8.

3.2 Three Dimension (3D) Model

Figure 10 shows the results; both gray matter and white matter built in Shade from C2 to C8. The model is built half as we assume that cervical is symmetry. Then both white matter and grey matter were combined in ScanIP for meshing.

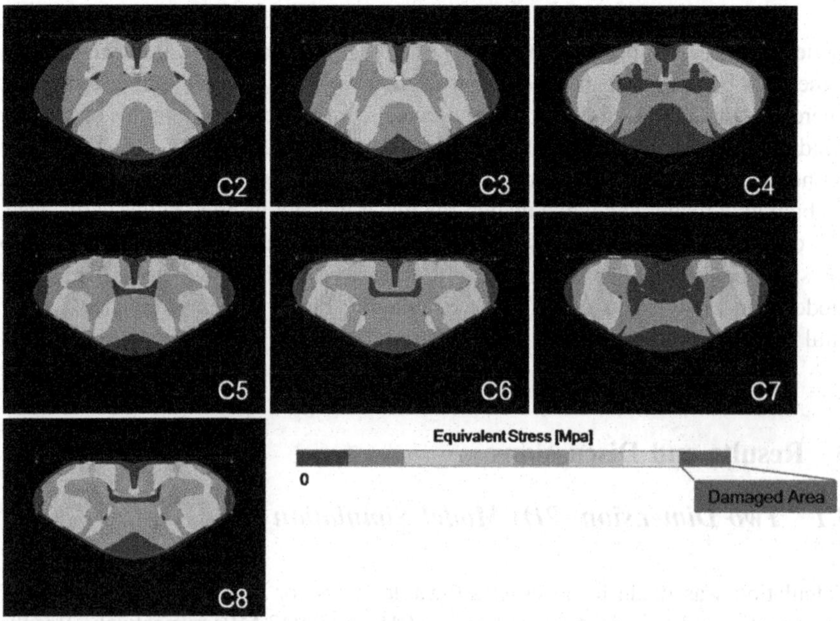

Fig. 5 Results for 10 % compression

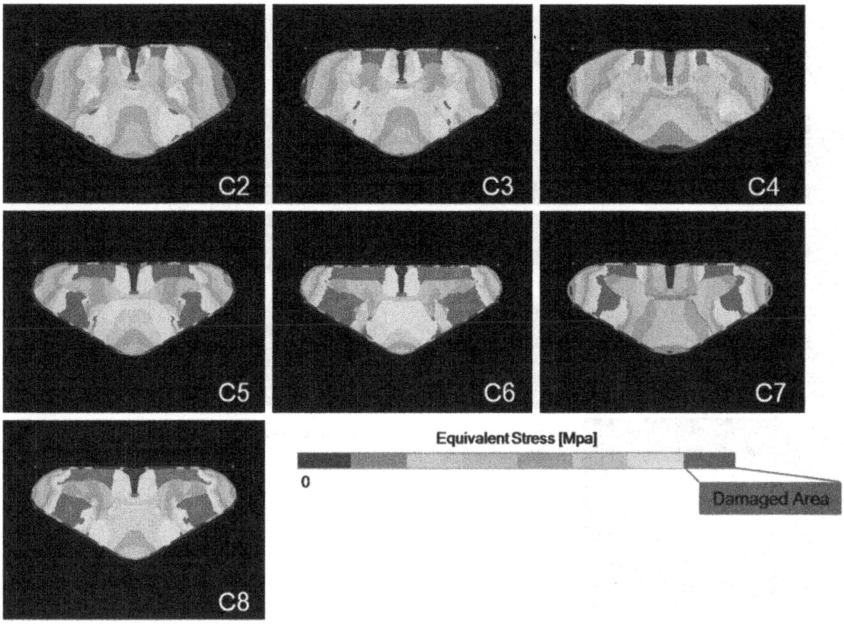

Fig. 6 Results for 20 % compression

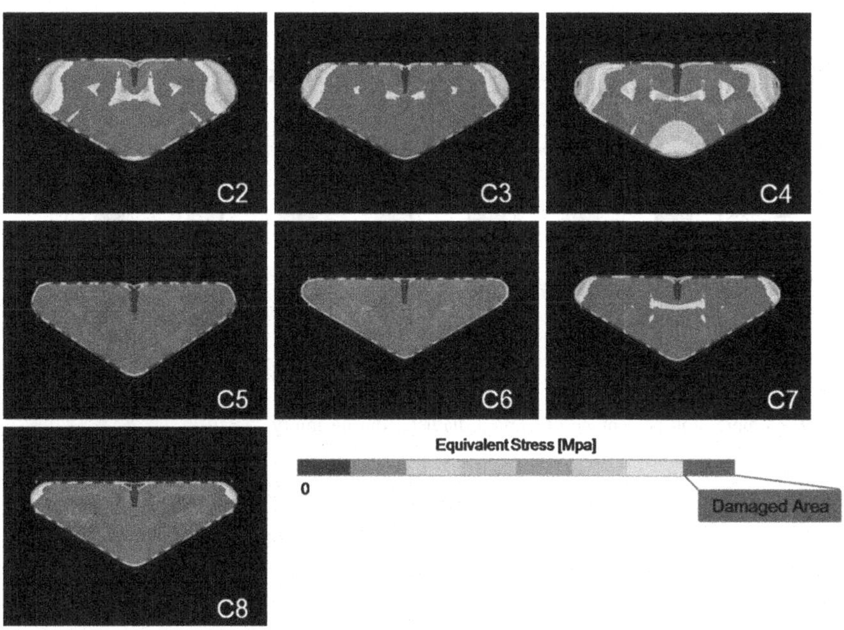

Fig. 7 Results for 30 % compression

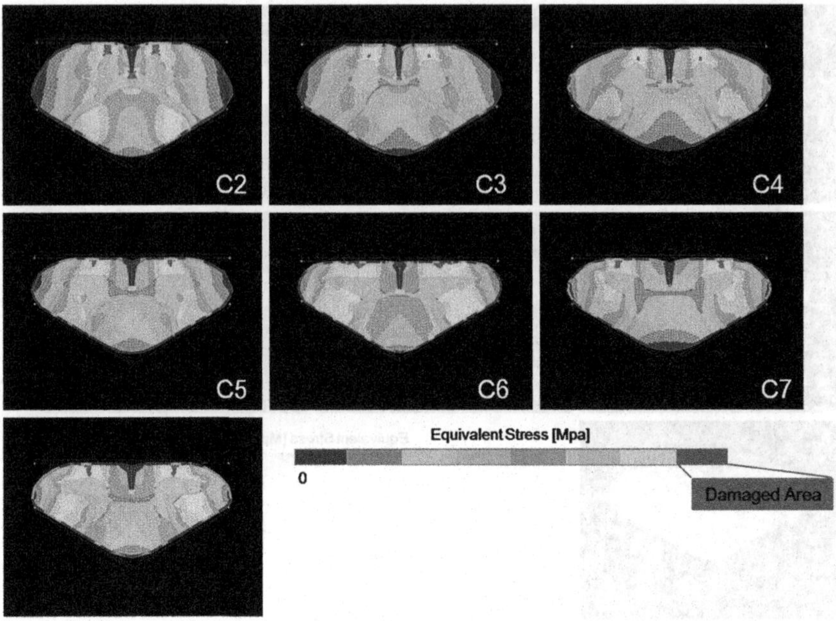

Fig. 8 Cervical cord condition during injury

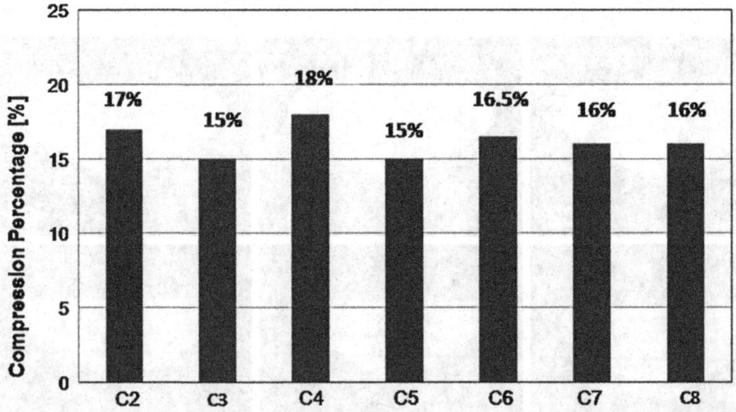

Fig. 9 Compression percentage of sagittal diameter during injury

Figures 11 and 12 shows meshed model. Figure 11 shows cervical from C2 direction and Fig. 12 from C8 direction. The model element number is 213, 106. The calculation process is still in progress and done in ANSYS software.

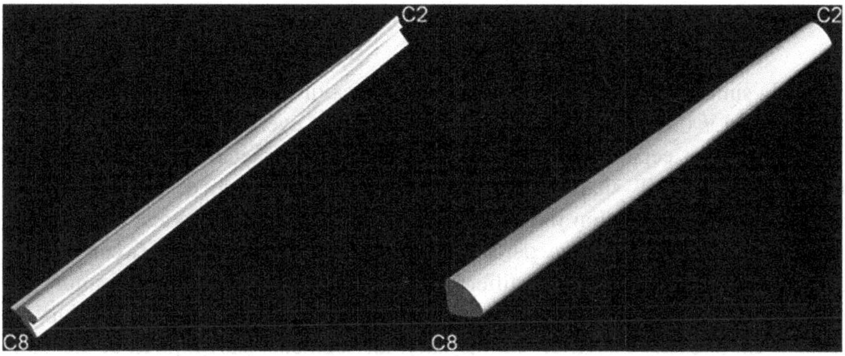

Fig. 10 *Gray* matter at the *left* and *white* matter at the *right*

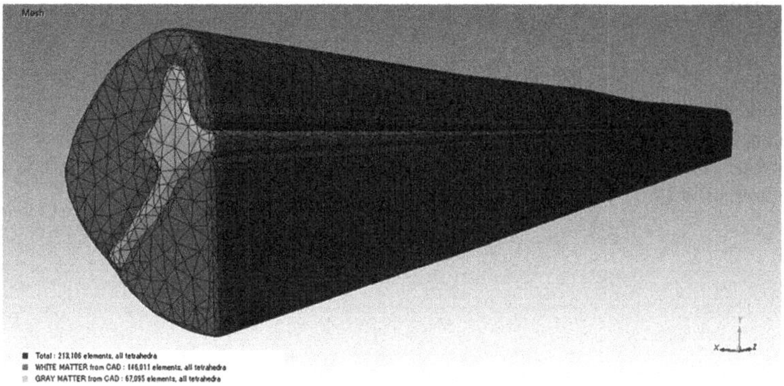

Fig. 11 Meshed 3D model from C2 direction

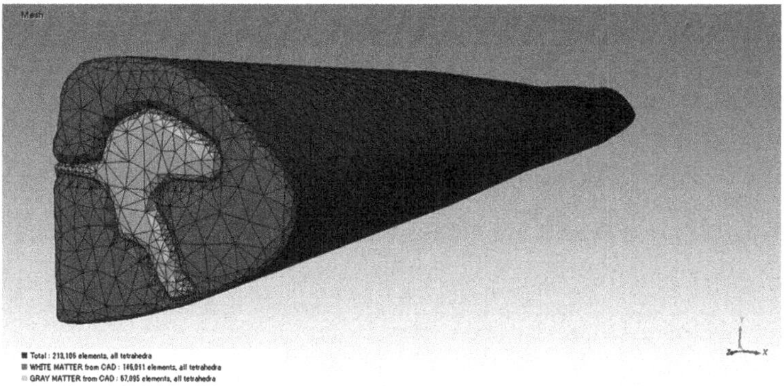

Fig. 12 Meshed 3D model from C8 direction

4 Conclusion

From 2D simulation results, we can see that stress distribution in each segment of cervical cord is different and the stress distribution of every elements also different. Other than that, cervical cords with flat shaped gray matter have higher stress distribution than hill shaped gray matter shows that shape of gray matter do influence stress distribution in spinal cord. Every segment of cervical cord start to injure when the compression percentage of sagittal diameter is between 15 and 18 %. This results shows a little difference from actual percentage in real injury but we assumed that this is because the simulation is done in two dimension thus the plane strain is easily increase. Additionally, all segments start injured at the same place which is ventral column of white matter with this static analysis.

References

1. Kameyama, T., Hashizume, Y., Sobue, G.: Morphologic features of the normal human cadaveric spinal cord. SPINE **21**(11), 1285–1290 (1996)
2. Ichihara, K., Taguchi, T., Shimada, Y., Sakuramoto, I., Kawano, S., Kawai, S.: Gray matter of the bovine cervical spinal cord is mechanically more rigid and fragile than the white matter. J. Neurotrauma **18**(3), 361–367 (2001)

Part III
Management for Healthcare

A Study of Older People's Socializing Form with Others: Comparative Analysis of "Living Alone" and "Living with a Spouse" Using Quantification Theory Type II

Takayuki Kawaura and Yasuyuki Sugatani

Abstract The Comprehensive Survey of Living Conditions conducted by Ministry of Health, Labor and Welfare has announced households with elderly people aged 65 years old and over increased to 44.7 % of all households in 2013. Furthermore, the population of elderly people living alone increased to 17.7 % of the all households in 2013. According to preceding studies and surveys, in the case of elderly people living alone, illness and loneliness lead to stress and other illnesses, and these people experience various difficulties in their everyday life. Although some local governments support elderly living alone, it is important to understand the psychological characteristics of the elderly is important. In this paper, we analyze the results of a survey of elderly people using a questionnaire based on L. Tornstam's theory of Gerotranscendence. In this analysis, we analyze the questionnaire using quantification theory type II. An elderly living alone is focused on, and we compare "elderly living alone" with "elderly living with a spouse" in order to find utilizing ways to support elderly people.

1 Introduction

The population census reported by the Statistics Bureau of the Ministry of Internal Affairs and Communications, as of October 1, 2014, has announced the number of people aged 65 years and over in Japan was 33 million and it is 26.3 % of the total population [1]. The population aged 65 years and over has grown by 1.1 million compared to the same month last year [1]. In 1950, the population aged 65 and over

T. Kawaura (✉)
Department of Mathematics, Kansai Medical University, Moriguchi, Japan
e-mail: kawaurat@hirakata.kmu.ac.jp

Y. Sugatani
Center for Medical Education, Kansai Medical University, Moriguchi, Japan
e-mail: sugatani@hirakata.kmu.ac.jp

Y.-W. Chen et al. (eds.), *Innovation in Medicine and Healthcare 2015*,
Smart Innovation, Systems and Technologies 45,
DOI 10.1007/978-3-319-23024-5_11

was under 5 % of the total population. However, it increased to 7 % in 1970, and to more than 14 % in 1994. Thus, Japan has been well on the way to an aging society. Apparently Japanese society is significantly aging, so that aged 65 or over is currently accounted for 26.0 % of the total population and aged 75 or over is 12.5 % [1, 2]. Therefore, Japanese society is entering a super-ageing society.

Furthermore, the number of households with elderly people aged 65 and over is increasing. According to the 2013 Comprehensive Survey of Living Conditions by the Ministry of Health, Labour and Welfare, as of 2014, the number of households in Japan with elderly people aged 65 and over was 22 million, it accounts for 44.7 % of all 50 million [3]. Moreover, households with elderly people aged 65 years old and over increased to 38.6 % of all households in 2004, 40.1 % in 2007, 42.6 % in 2010, and 44.7 % in 2013. Households with elderly people comprise 40 % of the total, of which "One-person only households" and "households with only a married couple" comprise the majority of households with elderly people. Furthermore, single-person households has increased 14.7 % of all households in 2004, 15.7 % in 2007, and 16.9 % in 2010.

By the way, previous studies and surveys have warned the possibility that elderly living alone can cause illness and loneliness, and they lead to stress and other illnesses [4, 5]. Elderly living alone experience various difficulties in their everyday life. According to the 2001 Survey of Old-Age Persons' Attitude about economic conditions conducted by the cabinet office of the government of Japan, the percent of people with "nobody to rely on when in trouble" to the total population is 2.4 %, however approximately 20 % of males living alone and 8.5 % of females living alone [6]. Although some local governments support elderly living alone, it is important to understand the psychological characteristics of the elderly is important.

According to preceding studies, the tendency towards depression of elderly people who live alone is stronger than those who live with other, and their satisfaction with their lives is low [7].

Furthermore it is necessary to understand that elderly people's living situations related to their psychological conditions.

In this paper, we analyze changing a way to interact with others using the results of a survey of elderly people using a questionnaire based on L. Tornstam's theory of Gerotranscendence [8–10]. In this analysis, we analyze the questionnaire using quantification theory type II. An elderly living alone is focused on, and we compare "elderly living alone" with "elderly living with a spouse" in order to find utilizing ways to support elderly people.

2 Data

We performed a questionnaire survey of 56 elderly people living in pay nursing homes of Hyogo, Chiba, Shizuoka, Kanagawa and Ehime Prefectures through May 2010 to March 2011. We analyze the results of this survey based on L. Tornstam's theory of Gerotranscendence. We categorized 35 questions into the following five categories:

(A) Change of feelings to oneself
(B) Change in how to deal with other people
(C) Change of feeling toward own family
(D) Change in transcendentalism such as breaking free from own obsession and loosing own religion
(E) A negative change caused by old age

We use seven items as attributes of respondents as the followings:

- Age classification > Young old (65–74 years old), Old-old (75-84 years old), Oldest-old (over 85 years old)
- Sex > Male, Female
- Child > Child, No child
- Health consciousness > High, Usual, Low
- Treatment by a doctor > Always, Not always
- Life circumstances > Rich, Common, Poor
- Frequency of care and support > Always, Not always

3 Analysis

The respondents are classified into two groups: 37 people of "living alone" and 19 people of "living with a spouse." In this paper, we analyze the only question B and the influence of the above mentioned 7 items on external criteria for each residential style using quantification theory type II [11–14]. The question B is shown in Table 1.

Table 1 Question B

B-1: Do you feel that your socializing with others has decreased?
B-2: Do you feel that you avoid contact with others more than before?
B-3: Do you feel that time spent alone has increased?
B-4: Do you feel that you enjoy spending time alone more than before?
B-5: Do you feel that compared to before you pay less attention to how others perceive you when you are doing something?
B-6: Would you like to make new friends?
B-7: Would you like to strengthen your communal and social ties?

4 Result

Table 2 shows the correlation ratio of the question B: "Do you have changed the way of dealing with others by aging?" Although the correlation ratio of the "elderly living with a spouse" group is relatively large, that of the "elderly living alone" group is small. In addition, since B-4 has unusual values, B-4 is omitted from this analysis.

4.1 Discriminant of B-1

We analyzed our data using the question B-1 as an external criterion. Table 3 shows the category scores, the range of the category scores, and the partial correlation coefficients according to the living situations. The negative values mean that the respondents feel that their socializing with others has decreased. The explanatory variables which have a wide range have a large contribution ratio of the variable to the external criterion. Besides, the partial correlation coefficients represent the relationship between the external criterion and each explanatory variable. Table 3 shows, when B-1 was used as external criterion, the explanatory variable which has a large contribution ratio are "Frequency of care and support" in the "elderly living alone" group and "Age classification" in the "elderly living with a spouse" group; these values are 1.4599 and 2.3274, respectively. Moreover, the explanatory variables which has a large partial correlation coefficient are "Age classification" in the group concerned living together; these values are 1.4599 and 2.3274, respectively.

The explanatory variable "Frequency of care and support" shows the respondents who answered "Not always" have a strong correlation with the answer of B-1, compared to answered "Always" in the "elderly living alone" group. The signs of the values in the all category scores for the explanatory variable "Frequency of care and support" are same between the "elderly living alone" group and the "elderly living with a spouse" group.

Next, in terms of the explanatory variable "Age classification," "Old-old" and "Oldest-old" have a strong correlation with the answer of B-1, compared to "Young old" do in the "elderly living with a spouse" group. The sign of the category scores

Table 2 The correlation ratio of the question B

	Liviing alone	Living with a spouse
B-1	0.2202	0.6530
B-2	0.3107	0.8052
B-3	0.4246	0.9033
B-4	0.2309	–
B-5	0.2969	0.6552
B-6	0.3239	0.7132
B-7	0.3541	0.6649

Table 3 Result of B-1

B-1		Category score		Range		Partial correlation	
		Liviing alone	Living with a spouse	Liviing alone	Living with a spouse	Liviing alone	Living with a spouse
Age classification	Young old	−0.1012	1.1142	1.3365	2.3274	0.2863	0.6448
	Old-old	0.6663	−0.7208				
	Oldest-old	−0.6702	−1.2132				
Sex	Male	0.6490	0.3887	0.7746	0.6714	0.1382	0.3169
	Female	−0.1256	−0.2827				
Child	Child	−0.1718	−0.0141	0.4237	0.0448	0.1030	0.0258
	No child	0.2519	0.0306				
Health consciousness	High	−0.3007	0.0518	1.2117	1.7903	0.1497	0.5991
	Usual	0.1344	0.3651				
	Low	0.9110	−1.4252				
Treatment by a doctor	Always	0.1126	−0.1555	0.6941	0.9847	0.1249	0.3965
	Not always	−0.5816	0.8292				
Life circumstances	Rich	−0.1415	0.6926	0.5351	0.9399	0.0764	0.3814
	Common	0.0853	−0.2473				
	Poor	0.3937	0.6926				
Frequency of care and support	Always	1.0653	0.8127	1.4599	1.0294	0.2802	0.3801
	Not always	−0.3946	−0.2167				

of "Young old" and "Old-old" in the categories for the explanatory variable "Age classification" are different between groups the "elderly living alone" and the "elderly living with a spouse."

4.2 *Discriminant of B-2*

We analyzed our data using the question B-2 as an external criterion. Table 4 shows the category scores, the range of the category scores, and the partial correlation coefficients according to the living situations. The negative values mean that the respondents feel that they avoid contact with others more than before. Table 4 shows, the explanatory variables which has a large contribution ratio are "Age classification" in the "elderly living alone" group and "Life circumstances" in the "elderly living with a spouse" group; these values are 2.0292 and 3.0866, respectively. Moreover, the explanatory variables which have a large partial correlation coefficient are also "Age classification" in the group concerned living together; these values are 0.4330 and 0.8366, respectively.

Table 4 Result of B-2

B-2		Category score		Range		Partial correlation	
		Liviing alone	Living with a spouse	Liviing alone	Living with a spouse	Liviing alone	Living with a spouse
Age classification	Young old	−1.2837	1.1530	2.0292	2.1943	0.4330	0.8366
	Old-old	0.7456	−1.0413				
	Oldest-old	−0.2818	0.0740				
Sex	Male	−0.1675	0.9160	0.1999	1.5822	0.0417	0.7972
	Female	0.0324	−0.6662				
Child	Child	0.1537	−0.3391	0.3790	1.0738	0.1188	0.6776
	No child	−0.2254	0.7347				
Health consciousness	High	0.0464	0.0431	0.5491	2.1373	0.0736	0.7322
	Usual	0.0155	0.4426				
	Low	−0.5027	−1.6947				
Treatment by a doctor	Always	0.2058	−0.1294	1.2693	0.8196	0.2809	0.4797
	Not always	−1.0635	0.6902				
Life circumstances	Rich	0.0733	0.2102	1.2335	3.0866	0.1938	0.7098
	Common	−0.2642	−0.2618				
	Poor	0.9693	2.8248				
Frequency of care and support	Always	0.6197	0.5775	0.8492	0.7314	0.2169	0.4173
	Not always	−0.2295	−0.1540				

The explanatory variable "Age classification" shows the respondents who answered "Young old" and "Oldest-old" have a strong correlation with the answer of B-2, compared to answered "Old-old" in the "elderly living alone" group. The signs of the category score of the "Young old" and "Old-old" in "Age classification" are different between groups the "elderly living alone" and the "elderly living with a spouse."

Next, in terms of the explanatory variable "Life circumstances," "Common" has a strong correlation with the answer of B-2, compared to "Rich" and "Poor" does in the "elderly living with a spouse." The signs of the values in the all category scores for the explanatory variable "Life circumstances" are same between the "elderly living alone" group and the "elderly living with a spouse" group.

4.3 Discriminant of B-3

We analyzed our data using the question B-3 as an external criterion. Table 5 shows the category scores, the range of the category scores, and the partial correlation

Table 5 Result of B-3

B-3		Category score		Range		Partial correlation	
		Liviing alone	Living with a spouse	Liviing alone	Living with a spouse	Liviing alone	Living with a spouse
Age classification	Young old	−0.2099	1.0881	1.0037	2.4316	0.3450	0.8637
	Old-old	0.5263	−0.6686				
	Oldest-old	−0.4774	−1.3436				
Sex	Male	1.6365	0.3066	1.9532	0.5295	0.5015	0.4690
	Female	−0.3167	−0.2229				
Child	Child	0.1062	−0.3209	0.2619	1.0161	0.1035	0.7970
	No child	−0.1558	0.6953				
Health consciousness	High	0.2653	0.3939	1.5112	1.6855	0.2634	0.7473
	Usual	−0.0743	0.1732				
	Low	−1.2459	−1.2916				
Treatment by a doctor	Always	−0.1316	−0.0202	0.8114	0.1277	0.2319	0.1214
	Not always	0.6798	0.1076				
Life circumstances	Rich	−0.3972	−1.0990	1.0426	2.1050	0.2960	0.6728
	Common	0.3259	0.2421				
	Poor	0.6454	1.0061				
Frequency of care and support	Always	1.0285	2.1003	1.4095	2.6604	0.4108	0.8533
	Not always	−0.3809	−0.5601				

coefficients according to the living situations. The negative values mean that the respondents feel that time spent alone has increased. Table 5 shows, when B-3 was used as external criterion, the explanatory variables which has a large contribution ratio are "Sex" in the "elderly living alone" group and "Frequency of care and support" in the "elderly living with a spouse" group; these values are 1.9532 and 2.6604, respectively. Moreover, the explanatory variables which have a large partial correlation coefficient are also "Sex" in the "elderly living alone" group and "Age classification" in the "elderly living with a spouse" group; these values are 0.5015 and 0.8637, respectively.

The explanatory variable "Sex" shows who answered "women" in the "elderly living alone" group tend to feel that time spent alone has increased, more than answered "men". The signs of the values in the all category scores for the explanatory variable "Sex" are same between the "elderly living alone" group and the "elderly living with a spouse" group.

Next, in terms of the explanatory variable "Frequency of care and support," "Not always" has a strong correlation with the answer of B-3, compared to "Always" do in the "elderly living with a spouse" group. The signs of the values in the all category scores for the explanatory variable "Frequency of care and support" are not related to the number of living together.

4.4 Discriminant of B-5

We analyzed our data using the question B-5 as an external criterion. Table 6 shows the category scores, the range of the category scores, and the partial correlation coefficients according to the living situations. The negative values in each category means that the respondents feel that compared to before they pay less attention to how others perceive they when they are doing something. Table 6 shows, the explanatory variables which have a large contribution ratio are "Life circumstances" in the group concerned with living together; these values are 2.7643 and 4.0847, respectively. Moreover, the explanatory variables which have a large partial correlation coefficient are "Age classification" in the "elderly living alone" group and also "Life circumstances" in the "elderly living with a spouse" group; these values are 0.4101 and 0.7614, respectively.

Table 6 Result of B-5

B-5		Category score		Range		Partial correlation	
		Liviing alone	Living with a spouse	Liviing alone	Living with a spouse	Liviing alone	Living with a spouse
Age classification	Young old	0.9185	0.2616	1.8265	2.2475	0.4101	0.5850
	Old-old	0.5068	−0.5989				
	Oldest-old	−0.9080	1.6485				
Sex	Male	1.6359	−0.0491	1.9525	0.0849	0.3628	0.0516
	Female	−0.3166	0.0357				
Child	Child	0.1591	0.2915	0.3924	0.9231	0.1158	0.4932
	No child	−0.2333	−0.6316				
Health consciousness	High	−0.5668	−0.1036	0.9747	0.9186	0.2786	0.3597
	Usual	0.4079	−0.1599				
	Low	0.1720	0.7588				
Treatment by a doctor	Always	−0.1164	0.2119	0.7176	1.3422	0.1577	0.4887
	Not always	0.6012	−1.1303				
Life circumstances	Rich	0.0423	3.1639	2.7643	4.0847	0.3822	0.7614
	Common	0.3964	−0.9209				
	Poor	−2.3679	0.2364				
Frequency of care and support	Always	0.8100	−2.2428	1.1100	2.8408	0.2760	0.6485
	Not always	−0.3000	0.5981				

The explanatory variable "Life circumstances" shows the respondents who answered "Poor" have a strong correlation with the answer of B-5, compared to answered "Rich" and "Common" in the "elderly living alone" group. The signs of the category score of the "Common" and "Poor" in "Life circumstances" are different between groups the "elderly living alone" and the "elderly living with a spouse."

Next, in terms of the explanatory variable "Age classification," "Oldest-old" has a strong correlation with the answer of B-5, compared to "Yong old" and "Old-old" does in the "elderly living with a spouse" group. The signs of the category score of the "Old-old" and "Oldest-old" in "Age classification" are different between groups the "elderly living alone" and the "elderly living with a spouse."

4.5 *Discriminant of B-6*

We analyzed our data using the question B-6 as an external criterion. Table 7 shows the category scores, the range of the category scores, and the partial correlation coefficients according to the living situations. The negative values in each category

Table 7 Result of B-6

B-6		Category score		Range		Partial correlation	
		Liviing alone	Living with a spouse	Liviing alone	Living with a spouse	Liviing alone	Living with a spouse
Age classification	Young old	0.4807	0.6226	1.0491	1.3806	0.3051	0.5832
	Old-old	−0.5684	−0.7038				
	Oldest-old	0.4140	0.6768				
Sex	Male	−0.3691	−0.1912	0.4406	0.3303	0.1007	0.2135
	Female	0.0714	0.1391				
Child	Child	−0.0257	−0.2926	0.0634	0.9266	0.0203	0.5286
	No child	0.0377	0.6340				
Health consciousness	High	−0.8559	−0.9167	1.4929	1.5534	0.4217	0.7251
	Usual	0.5783	0.6367				
	Low	0.6370	−0.8066				
Treatment by a doctor	Always	0.0468	−0.0583	0.2885	0.3693	0.0686	0.1709
	Not always	−0.2417	0.3110				
Life circumstances	Rich	0.3493	0.6303	0.8346	1.0079	0.2495	0.3603
	Common	−0.4627	−0.2353				
	Poor	0.3719	0.7726				
Frequency of care and support	Always	−0.8903	−0.5871	1.2201	0.7436	0.3228	0.3381
	Not always	0.3298	0.1566				

mean that the respondents make new friends. Table 7 shows, the explanatory variables which have a large contribution ratio are "Health consciousness" in the group concerned with living together; these values are 1.4929 and 1.5534, respectively. Moreover, the explanatory variables which have a large partial correlation coefficient are also "Health consciousness" in the group concerned with living together; these values are 0.4217 and 0.7251, respectively.

The explanatory variable "Health consciousness" shows the respondents who answered "High" have a strong correlation with the answer of B-6, compared to answered "Usual" and "Low" in the "elderly living alone" group. The signs of the category score of the "Low" in "Age classification" are different between groups the "elderly living alone" and the "elderly living with a spouse."

4.6 Discriminant of B-7

We analyzed our data using the question B-7 as an external criterion. Table 8 shows the category scores, the range of the category scores, and the partial correlation

Table 8 Result of B-7

B-7		Category score		Range		Partial correlation	
		Liviing alone	Living with a spouse	Liviing alone	Living with a spouse	Liviing alone	Living with a spouse
Age classification	Young old	0.1495	−0.9393	0.4336	2.8210	0.1400	0.6589
	Old-old	−0.2387	0.4168				
	Oldest-old	0.1948	1.8817				
Sex	Male	−0.0900	−0.6653	0.1074	1.1491	0.0268	0.4932
	Female	0.0174	0.4838				
Child	Child	0.2509	−0.0792	0.6190	0.2509	0.2063	0.1489
	No child	−0.3681	0.1716				
Health consciousness	High	−0.3296	−0.0792	0.5999	1.7333	0.1974	0.4659
	Usual	0.2703	0.3997				
	Low	−0.2306	−1.3336				
Treatment by a doctor	Always	0.0348	−0.3440	0.2146	2.1789	0.0546	0.6742
	Not always	−0.1798	1.8349				
Life circumstances	Rich	0.3450	−1.7516	0.7740	5.2560	0.2457	0.6296
	Common	−0.4290	0.2501				
	Poor	0.2177	3.5044				
Frequency of care and support	Always	−1.4738	1.2590	2.0196	1.5947	0.5069	0.4012
	Not always	0.5458	−0.3357				

coefficients according to the living situations. The negative values in each category means that the respondents strengthen your communal and social ties. Table 8 shows, the explanatory variables which have a large contribution ratio are "Frequency of care and support" in the "elderly living alone" group and "Age classification" in the "elderly living with a spouse" group; these values are 2.0196 and 2.8210, respectively. Moreover, the explanatory variables which have a large partial correlation coefficient are also "Frequency of care and support" in the "elderly living alone" group and "Treatment by a doctor" in the "elderly living with a spouse" group; these values are 0.5069 and 0.6742, respectively.

The explanatory variable "Frequency of care and support" shows the respondents who answered "Always" have a strong correlation with the answer of B-7, compared to answered "Not always" in the "elderly living alone" group. The signs of the values in the all category scores for the explanatory variable Frequency of care and support" are different between the "elderly living alone" group and the "elderly living with a spouse" group.

Next, in terms of the explanatory variable "Age classification," "Yong old" has a strong correlation with the answer of B-7, compared to "Old-old" and "Oldest-old" does in the "elderly living with a spouse" group. The signs of the category score of the "Yong old" and "Old-old" in "Age classification" are different between groups the "elderly living alone" and the "elderly living with a spouse."

The explanatory variable "Treatment by a doctor" shows who answered "Always" in the "elderly living with a spouse" group tend to "have more involvement with your community and society" more than answered "Not always". The signs of the values in the all category scores for the explanatory variable "Treatment by a doctor" are difficult between the "elderly living alone" group and the "elderly living with a spouse" group.

5 Conclusion

In this paper, we analyzed changing a way to interact with others using the results of a survey of elderly people using a questionnaire based on L. Tornstam's theory of Gerotranscendence. In this analysis, we analyzed the questionnaire using quantification theory type II. Classified two groups living alone and living with a spouse have been compared, and the relation and influence between the explanatory variables on the external criteria.

In next study, the questionnaire will be considered such as variable selection and other explanatory variables will be employed. Consideration about this result is required. However the result of this analysis should be utilized to the elderly support. In addition, although our questionnaire has more questions except the seven above mentioned, we will analyze data using all question.

References

1. The Statistics Bureau of the Ministry of Internal Affairs and Communications: The population statistics released in October 2013 (2014)
2. Director General for Policy on Cohesive Society: The white paper on aging society in 2014 (2014)
3. Ministry of Health, Labour and Welfare: Comprehensive survey of living conditions in 2014 (2014)
4. Hasebe, M.: A study of autobiographical memory functions in elderly people who live alone. The Study of Social Work, No.48, 111–114 (2009)
5. Mizuho Information & Research Institute: Business report on surveys and research of community infrastructure and its plan to support in elderly people who live alone and aged household (2012)
6. Cabinet Office, Government of Japan.: Old-Age Persons' Attitude about Life Finance FY2001 (2012)
7. Yamashita, K., Kobayashi, S., Tsunematsu, T.: Depressed mood and subjective sensation well-being in the elderly living alone on Oki Island in Shimane Prefecture, Nippon Ronen Igakkai Zasshi. Japan. J. Geriatr. **29**(3), 179–184 (1992)
8. Tomizawa, K.: Gerotranscendence as an adjustment outcome in the ninth stage of life cycle: a case study of the oldest old in the Amami Archipelago. Bulletin Graduate Sch. Human Dev. Environ. **2**(2), 111–119 (2009)
9. Tsukuda, A.: One consideration for the re-formulation of successful aging, Ritsumeikan review of industrial society. Ritsumeikan Soc. Sci. Rev. **43**(4), 133–154 (2008)
10. Tornstam, L.: Gerotranscendence. Springer Publishing Company, New York (2005)
11. Kan, T., Yasunori, F.: Quantification Theory Type II. Gendai-Sugakusha, Kyoto (2011)
12. Fujii, Y.: Vol.1 Categorical Data Analysis, Data Science Learning Through R, Kyoritsu Shuppan (2010)
13. Watada, J., Tanaka, H., Asai, K.: Analysis of purchasing factors by using fuzzy quantification theory type II. J. Japan Ind. Manag. Assoc. **32**(5), 385–392 (1981)
14. Kusunoki, M.: The sensibility to cold in female students: the quantification method entitled II. J. Yasuda Women's Univ. **39**, 193–200 (2011)

Analysis of Japanese Health using Fuzzy Principal Component Analysis

Yoshiyuki Yabuuchi and Takayuki Kawaura

Abstract Japanese population is 128 million, and the population of younger than 15 years old is less than elderly people at least 65 years old. Then, Japanese population pyramid is distorted. While the population under 65 years old has reduced, the population 65 years old and above have increased. Japanese major health insurance society has reported that lifestyle-related medical costs are about 1,791 billion yen in fiscal medical expenses total about 1,184 billion yen. It becomes about 15 % of the total. This is a great amount of costs which is able to be ignored. Therefore, we analyzed the relation between the medical expense and food intakes by a regression model, and the results have been reported in InMed-14. In addition, we have analyzed the relation between the numbers of outpatient and food intakes in five years by a regression model. It is because lifestyle is made by continuing food intakes. Although we have obtained the results by these analyzes, however we need to analyze the relationships between factors.Therefore, in this paper, we analyze the relation between these factors by a principal component analysis.

Keywords Health care · Medical care cost · Lifestyle-related disease · Fuzzy regression model · Fuzzy principal component analysis

1 Introduction

Japanese population is 128 million, and the population of younger than 15 years old is less than elderly people at least 65 years old. Then, Japanese population pyramid is distorted. While the population under 65 years old has reduced, the population 65 years old and above have increased.

Y. Yabuuchi (✉)
Shimonoseki City University, 2-1-1 Daigaku-cho, Shimonoseki,
Yamaguchi 751-8510, Japan
e-mail: yabuuchi@shimonoseki-cu.ac.jp

K. Kawaura
Kansai Medical University, Hirakata, Osaka, Japan
e-mail: kawaurat@hirakata.kmu.ac.jp

Y.-W. Chen et al. (eds.), *Innovation in Medicine and Healthcare 2015*,
Smart Innovation, Systems and Technologies 45,
DOI 10.1007/978-3-319-23024-5_12

In 2012, 15.13 % of the total fiscal medical care expenditure was for lifestyle-related health care costs. This represents a significant cost burden.

The Ministry of Health, Labour and Welfare stated that lifestyle-related diseases are not only the biggest factor in reducing healthy life expectancy but also have the most significant impact on national medical care expenditure [4]. Lifestyle-related diseases can be prevented by moderate daily exercise, a well-balanced diet, and not smoking.

Therefore, we discussed the relation between medical care costs and factors such as the number of medical checkup examinees and diet by prefecture using Annual Health, Labour and Welfare reports 2008 of the Ministry of Health, Labour and Welfare [17]. In addition this, we discussed the relation between the numbers of patients and factors such as body mass index, foods intake by prefecture [18].

Generally, the statistical data concerned with a person has a wider spread distribution. And it is difficult to accurately describe the features of a target system. Therefore, our fuzzy robust regression model was used for these analyses, as this model can illustrate a possibility of a target system even if data have a large vagueness. These analyses taught two things to us; Japanese-style meal is good nutritional balance, and nutrition obtained from it just enough. It means that food items, such as meal and dairy products, which are increased opportunity to eat by the westernized of foods is lead to consume nutrition in excessive quantities. As the result, it becomes one of the reasons of lifestyle-related diseases.

We remain the task to analyze the relationship between these factors still. Therefore, in this paper, we analyze the relation between these factors by a fuzzy principal component analysis [13].

This paper is consisted as follows: Sect. 2 presents the definition of our fuzzy robust regression model. A fuzzy robust regression model is able to remove an influence of unusual samples and to illustrate a possibility of focal system. Section 3 presents the results of two analyses. The first analysis discussed the relation between medical care costs and factors that express our personal life such as the number of medical checkup examinees and diet by prefecture. The second analysis discussed the relation between the number of outpatient and lifestyle factors. In Sect. 4, we discuss the relation between the lifestyle factors using a fuzzy principal component analysis.

2 Fuzzy Robust Regression Model

The objective of an interval-based fuzzy regression model is to describe the possibilities of a system. Possibilities are represented by an interval that includes the whole data observed from the system in this model [9, 10]. Samples separated far from the center of data distort the shape of the model.

The pivotal role of the center position of the system is emphasized when building a possibilistic regression model instead of using an interval to describe the possibility of a focal system. Tanaka and Guo use an exponential possibility distribution for their model [10], whereas Inuiguchi et al. [1] and Yabuuchi and Watada [14–16] are independently working on making the centers of a possibility distribution and the center of a possibilistic regression model coinciding.

The model by Yabuuchi and Watada describes the possibility of a system using the center of a fuzzy regression model. The proposed model fits intuitive understanding because it makes the center of the model and the center of the system coincide. This model is built by maximizing the sum of possibility grades derived from model estimates and data. Therefore, this model can be built using granule or fuzzy data, as the model can deal with both granule and fuzzy data.

When the model is constructed, outlier samples greatly influence fuzzy coefficients. Heuristically, we can employ the following objective function for a linear programming.

$$\max . Z = \alpha \sum_{i=1}^{n} \mu'(y_i, \mathbf{x}_i) - (1-\alpha)\gamma \sum_{i=1}^{n} W_i, \tag{1}$$

where α, $0 \leq \alpha \leq 1$, is the parameter reflecting the decision between maximizing possibility grades and minimizing the vagueness of the model. γ is the tuning parameter for the difference between the total sum of possibility grades and the vagueness of the model. And, the following possibility grade $\mu'(y_i, \mathbf{x}_i)$ is employed in the objective function (1):

$$\mu(y_i, \mathbf{x}_i) = \sum_{i=1}^{n} \max \left\{ 0, \delta - \frac{|Y_i^C - y_i|}{W_i} \right\}$$

where, the positive real value δ is heuristically decided. After coefficients are obtained, the possibility grade should be reduced in scale $0 \leq \mu(y_i, \mathbf{x}_i) \leq \delta$ to $0 \leq \mu(y_i, \mathbf{x}_i) \leq 1$. As a result, some data is outside the a possibility interval.

Here, when $\alpha = 0$ and $\gamma = 1$, we obtain a conventional fuzzy regression model.

3 Analyses of the Relation Between Medical Care and Lifestyle

3.1 Analysis of Medical Care Cost by Japanese Prefecture

According to the Ministry of Internal Affairs and Communications Statistics Bureau population estimates as of October 1, 2013, the total Japanese population is approximately 128 million. Compared with the previous year, changes in the three population age groups were as follows: children under 14 years old decreased by 0.160 million, the working-age population aged between 15 and 64 years decreased by 1.17

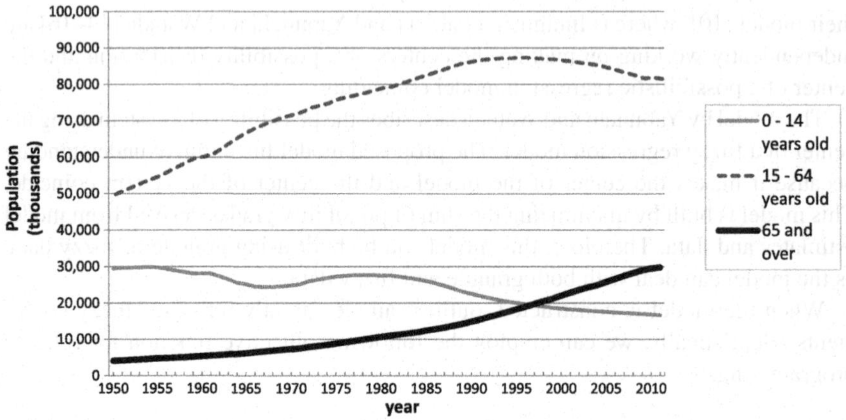

Fig. 1 Japanese population by age group between 1950 and 2010

million, and the population aged over 65 years increased by 1.04 million. At October 1, 2013, the over 1965s population exceeded 30 million.

Figure 1 shows the changes in Japanese population for three age groups between 1950 and 2010. The older population exceeded the child population in 1997. Since then, the 65 and over population has increased, and the 0–14 population has decreased. Thus, in structure of the Japanese population has changed, and the population pyramid is distorted. Although this is changing society's structure, it has not yet been able to respond to the change in conditions. Under such conditions, the health of the older population is economically critical. In 2010, the Ministry of Health, Labour and Welfare has reported the national health medical care expenditure, the total amount of medical expenses for treating illness or injury paid to medical institutions, was 38 trillion, 585 billion yen [4]. This is approximately 300 thousand yen per capita. National medical care expenditure has increased for five consecutive years from 2006.

Lifestyle-related diseases are familiar to us, as medical cost of lifestyle-related diseases in national medical care expenditure is too large to be ignored. In 2012, the total fiscal medical care expenditure was 1.184 trillion yen, and lifestyle-related health care costs were 1.791billion yen or 15.13 %. Inpatients accounts for 19.35 % of total, and outpatients accounts for 80.65 %. They account for 80 % of lifestyle-related health care costs. Health care costs per capita of lifestyle-related diseases are 14,407 yen.

Knowing the number of patients enables us to estimate the scale of medical costs because the correlation coefficient between medical costs and number of patients is approximately 0.996. Unfortunately, this is not the objective of our analysis. The objectives of this analysis are to understand the effects of the number of medical care check-ups and diet on citizens' health, using prefectural data.

National medical care expenditure can be used as a proxy for health impact. The number of medical checkup examinees and number of 37 foods such as fresh fish, shellfish, meat, vegetables, oils, and seasonings are used for the regression analysis.

Although Japan has 47 prefectures, there are 38 explanatory variables. Therefore, not all explanatory variables were used for this analysis; appropriate explanatory variables were selected from these 38 for the regression analysis. Although we should consider nutritional balance, the relation between medical cost and food intake by prefecture are discussed. Cluster analysis was used to divide the explanatory variables into three groups: consumption of five foods, tuna, sea bream, butter, fresh fruits, and edible oil were selected for their correlation coefficients and its features. In addition to these five foods, the number of health checkup examinees was used for the regression analysis. Medical care expenditure is the objective variable Y. The regression model explanatory variables are as follows: the number of health checkup examinees is X_1, tuna consumption is X_2, sea bream consumption is X_3, butter consumption is X_4, fresh fruit consumption is X_5, and edible oil consumption is X_6. The averages of these variables are shown in Table 1.

A statistical regression model using the least squares method and our fuzzy robust regression model using these variables were built. The statistical model Y_{S1} is as follow:

$$Y_{S1} = 5.998 - 0.025X_1 - 0.237X_2 + 0.267X_3 - 0.234X_4 + 0.149X_5 + 0.081X_6.$$

A prefecture with a large number of medical checkup examinees has smaller medical care expenditure. Tuna contains EPA, DHA, niacin, minerals that are said help prevent lifestyle-related diseases. However, in Japan, tuna is mainly eaten raw and not in great quantities. Butter contains a lot of calories and cholesterol. However, the Japanese population does not consume much butter so the health impact is small. Also, butter contains many vitamins and minerals; its nutrition value is reaffirmed. Medical care expenditure for prefectures that eat a lot of tuna and butter is low, which is intuitively correct. Sea bream contains high levels of EPA, DHA, inosinic acid, and taurine, which can reduce cholesterol. Fruits include both vitamins and sugar. Edible oil is indispensable in the modern diet; however, health problems caused by excessive intake are serious. Considering these facts, we can understand that prefec-

Table 1 Variable averages used in regression analysis

Medical care expenditure	6.579 (100 thousand yen)
Health examination examinees	7.307 (10 thousand people)
Tuna consumption	2.221 (Kg)
Sea bream consumption	0.849 (Kg)
Butter consumption	4.526 (100g)
Fresh fruit consumption	9.494 (Kg)
Edible oil consumption	8.809 (Kg)

Table 2 Difference between two fuzzy regression models

	Y_{S1}	Y_{R2}
Sum of widths of fuzzy regression coefficient	–	0.101
Sum of possibility grades by model and data	–	23.312
The correlation coefficient of observed data and the center of model	0.789	0.771

tures that consume plenty of sea bream, fresh fruits, and edible oil have large medical care expenditure.

Next, let us describe the data using our fuzzy robust regression model Y_{R1}.

$$\begin{aligned} Y_{R1} = &(4.929, 0, 0) + (-0.020, 0.000, 0)X_1 + (-0.175, 0, 0)X_2 + (0.517, 0, 0)X_3 \\ &+ (-0.289, 0, 0)X_4 + (0.242, 0.045, 0.056)X_5 + (0.076, 0.000, 0.000)X_6 \end{aligned}$$

where, the coefficient of a fuzzy robust regression model is an asymmetric triangular fuzzy number, the parameter α employed was 0.7 and δ employed was 3 in Eq. (1). A fuzzy robust regression model was built in order to maximize the sum of the possibility grade by the model and data, the centers of the model and data distribution coincided. In this analysis, the inclusion relation between the model and data is reduced because the ambiguity of the model increased. Therefore, the vagueness of the model is not large.

In comparison with the statistical model, there are some differences for each coefficient; however the centers of the fuzzy robust regression model and statistical model are not far away from each other. In addition, the ambiguity of edible oil and fresh fruits is demonstrated by the increased the vagueness of the model.

Our fuzzy robust regression model was adjusted to reduce the ambiguity of the model in order to describe the data distribution.

Table 2 shows the sum of fuzzy regression coefficients, sum of the possibility grades using the data and model, and correlation coefficients of observed values and centers of the models. Our model describes the medical care expenditure with substantially the same accuracy as the statistical model. Therefore, the relation between medical care expenditure, food consumptions, and the number of medical examination examinees were discussed using the fuzzy robust regression model.

The number of medical examination examinees, tuna and butter consumption decrease medical care expenditure, while consumption of sea bream, fresh fruits, and edible oils increases the medical care expenditure.

3.2 Analysis of Lifestyle Behavior

In the previous section, the relation between our lifestyle and medical care expenditure by prefecture was analyzed. In this analysis, it became apparent that consumption of sea bream, fresh fruits and edible oils increases the medical care expenditure and the number of medical examination examinees and consumption of tuna and butter decrease medical care expenditure, while consumption of sea bream, fresh fruits, and edible oils increases the medical care expenditure.

Generally speaking, our health is obtained by the daily life. In other words, since the continuing lifestyle affects health, bad lifestyle causes a health hazard. Therefore, we analyze the relation between lifestyle and health by a regression model in this section. Data about lifestyle from the National Health and Nutrition Survey of 1995 to 1999 by the National Institute of Health and Nutrition [7] are employed as an explanatory variable that indicates the lifestyle. And the number of patients from Patient Survey 1999 by Japanese Ministry of Health, Labour and Welfare [3] are employed as an objective variable that indicates health state.

In other words, we discuss the relation between the number of patients and the lifestyle of five years by prefecture. In this regression analysis, we employ normalized values of outpatient as Y, body mass index (BMI, kg/m^2) as X_1, rice intakes (g/day) as X_2, meats intakes (g/day) as X_3, milk and its products intakes as X_4, respectively.

A statistical regression model using the least squares method and our fuzzy robust regression model using these variables were built. The following statistical model Y_{S2} using the least squares method was obtained:

$$Y_{S2} = -0.362X_1 - 0.389X_2 + 0.205X_3 + 0.175X_4.$$

BMI and rice intake reduces the number of outpatients of prefectures.

BMI is a measure of body based on height and weight. BMI score is well known as an index that defines a body type; BMI of 18.5–24.9 is ideal; below 18.5 is underweight; 25.0–29.9 is overweight; over 30.0 is obesity. The BMI score is greatly affected by a terrible diet, imbalance between weight and height and so on. The BMI score of 18.5–24.9 is ideal; however the BMI is not an ideal value by constitution. Although BMI is associated with body fat in general, BMI is not a measure of body fat directly.

Furthermore, the relation between BMI and heart disease is a U-shaped curve, the death rate of the ideal BMI score 22.5–25.0 is the lowest [11]. In the BMI of over 25.0, obesity and cardiovascular disease increases both.

Additionally, meats intake and milk intake increase the number of outpatients of prefectures. The staple food of the Japanese diet is rice, protein and carbohydrate ware received from rice until about 1955 [6, 8]. After that, the consumption of rice as staple food was reduced; the intake of animal protein was increased from side dishes such as meat and dairy products.

From above, the obtained statistical model is acceptable.

Next, let us describe the data using our fuzzy robust regression model. The following fuzzy robust regression model Y_{R2} was obtained:

$$\begin{aligned} Y_{R2} = {} & (0.297, 0.363, 0.388) + (0.430, -0.464, 0.315)X_1 + (0.282, -0.300, 0.341)X_2 \\ & +(0.371, 0.273, 0.300)X_3 + (0.310, 0.206, 0.292)X_4, \end{aligned}$$

Table 3 Difference between two fuzzy regression models

	Y_{S2}	Y_{R2}
Sum of widths of fuzzy regression coefficient	–	2.217
Sum of possibility grades by model and data	–	20.751
Sum of widths of forecasted values	–	87.443
The residual sum of squares of observed data and the center of model	22.163	29.046
The correlation coefficient of observed data and the center of model	0.720	0.712

where parameters α, γ and δ are employed 0.3, 40 and 1.5, respectively. The BMI has a large impact on the number of outpatients than the rice intake in our model compared to the statistical model. However, center of our coefficients of X_3 is larger than the statistical model. L-carunitine that is included in the meat cause of arteriosclerosis and cardiovascular disease [2]. In addition, the survey for the Japanese, while the risk of cerebral infarction and stroke is reduced by calcium intake from daily products, the risk of ischemic heart disease in increased [12].

Our fuzzy robust regression model was adjusted to reduce the ambiguity of the model in order to describe the data distribution.

Table 3 shows the features of these two models. The parameter δ of our model is the same as the α-cut of the membership function. Therefore, some data locates outside of the possibility interval of our model, the sum of possibility grade by the model and data is small. However, the residual sum of squares of our model is not large, the multiple correlation coefficients is almost same value. Statistical evaluation of center of our model is not high compared with the statistical model; however the forecast accuracy is good as a possibility model.

In our model, the effect of BMI reduces the outpatients is the largest; the effect of rice intake is the second largest factor to reduce the outpatient. Meat intake, milk and daily intake increases outpatients.

In other words, prefecture which BMI score is small and Japanese diet is taken has small number of outpatients. In addition, there is a tendency prefectures which takes many meats intakes, milk and a dairy products intakes has many outpatients.

4 Analysis of Lifestyle Factors

In the previous section, two analyses concerned with a lifestyle have presented. The first analysis used medical care costs as objective variable and lifestyle factors as explanatory variables for a regression analysis. In the same way, the second analysis use number of outpatients as objective variable and lifestyle factors as explanatory variables for a regression analysis.

In these two analyses, we also considered correlation coefficients with variable selections. However, we did not discuss the relationships between the variables.

Since we discussed the lifestyle in two analyses, we analyze the relationship between variables indicating a lifestyle using a fuzzy principal component analysis in this paper. In other words, since we are focusing on findings the factors that lead to lifestyle-related diseases, we analyze the factors that show the lifestyle of the people of obesity.

Here, it is hard to obtain the factors that show the lifestyle of the people of obesity. In this case, a fuzzy principal component analysis helps us to analyze these.

Therefore, in this paper, we discuss the relationship between the variables using a fuzzy principal component analysis. A fuzzy principal component analysis is an approach to analyze the fuzzy set that is considered.

Let $X_{\omega,i}(\omega = 1, 2, \dots, n; i = 1, 2, \dots, p)$ denote samples. A fuzzy set A defined by its membership function $\mu_A(\omega)$. Power $N(A)$ of the fuzzy set A, a fuzzy mean m_i of ith variable and a fuzzy co-variance v_{ij} between ith and jth variables are respectively writtens as follows:

$$\left.\begin{aligned} N(A) &= \sum_{\omega=1}^{n} \mu_A(\omega), \\ m_i &= \frac{1}{N(A)} \sum_{\omega=1}^{n} X_{\omega,i}\mu_A(\omega), \\ v_{ij} &= \frac{1}{N(A)} \sum_{\omega=1}^{n} (X_{\omega,i} - m_i)(X_{\omega,j} - m_j)\mu_A(\omega). \end{aligned}\right\} \quad (2)$$

Eigen values and eigen vectors are obtained using fuzzy variance co-variance matrix or fuzzy correlation matrix which obtained by Equations (2).

Data which will be analyzed seven variables from Japan National Health and Nutrition Survey 2012 by Japanese Ministry of Health, Labour and Welfare are shown in Table 4 [5]. In this analysis, we analyze samples by age bracket shown in Table 4, and the percentage of obesity by age bracket is set the fuzzy set. Here, we set the BMI of 25 or greater as obesity.

Table 4 Standardized variables

	Variable	Unit
X_1	Alcohol consumption per day	180cc of sake/day
X_2	Percentage of habitually smoking person	%
X_3	The number of steps per day	steps
X_4	Animal food intakes per day	g/day
X_5	Vegetable food intakes per day	g/day
X_6	Per-capita dental expenditures	a thousand yen
X_7	Per-capita national medical care expenditures	a thousand yen

Table 5 Eigen values and proportions

	PC1	PC2	PC3	PC4	PC5	PC6	PC7
Eigen value	4.961	1.406	0.621	0.012	0.000	0.000	0.000
proportion	0.709	0.201	0.089	0.002	0.000	0.000	0.000
Accumulated proportion	0.709	0.910	0.998	1.000	1.000	1.000	1.000

PC: Principal component

Table 6 Eigen vectors and factor loadings

	Eigen vectors		Factor loadings	
	PC1	PC2	PC1	PC2
X1	−0.444	−0.043	−0.988	−0.051
X2	−0.441	−0.039	−0.982	−0.047
X3	−0.437	0.186	−0.974	0.220
X4	0.053	0.710	0.119	0.842
X5	0.137	0.661	0.305	0.783
X6	0.447	−0.054	0.997	−0.064
X7	0.442	−0.135	0.985	−0.160

Table 5 shows obtained eigen values and proportions. Since accumulated proportion of the second principal component (PC) is larger than 0.8, only the first PC (PC1) and the second PC (PC2) almost can explain the data vary. Table 6 shows the Eigen vectors and the factor loadings. Moreover, Table 7 shows the sample scores.

First, in the first PC, the positive large factor loadings are a dental care costs and a national medical expenditure, the negative large factor loadings are the smoking rate, the number of steps and the amount of drinking. Since it divided into activities and health care costs by age, the first principal component demotes the lifestyle by age.

Next, in the second PC, there is only the positive large factor loading, these are animal food intakes and vegetable food intakes. Since the intake is increase by biased diet, it can consider the second PC denotes a balanced diet.

We can confirm these by samples scores. In the first PC, sample scores of the twenties, the thirties and the forties are a negative large value, they are enjoying

Table 7 Sample socres

Age bracket	PC1	PC2
Twenties	−4.538	−0.269
Thirties	−3.958	−1.602
Forties	−3.423	−1.122
Fifties	−2.035	1.130
Sixties	0.891	2.210
Seventies and above	9.508	−0.924

drinking, smoking and walking. On the other hand, the seventies and above has a positive large sample score; they have paid a lot of medical expenses. At the same time, in the second PC, the fifties and the sixties have a positive large sample scores, they have a meal that is biased in any of the animal food or vegetable food. On the other hand, the thirties has a negative large sample score; they ate eating meat and vegetables without the bias.

The purpose of this analysis was to consider the relationship between the lifestyle factors. The characteristics of expected was not obtained because the samples by age bracket used. However, we could confirm the difference in the age track of behavior.

5 Concluding Remarks

We confirmed previous two analyses using a regression model; the first analysis is the relation between the medical care expenditure and food intakes, and the second analysis is the relation between the number of outpatients and food intakes for 5 years. In these analyses, since we did not discuss the relationship between variables, we have discussed it using a fuzzy principal component analysis in this paper.

This analysis teaches us two conspicuous features; they are that the seventies and above markedly require medical expenses, and the seventies and above do not have the trend of the diet although the fifties and the sixties review their diet according to age.

References

1. Inuiguchi, M., Tanino, T.: Interval linear regression methods based on Minkowski difference: a bridge between traditional and interval linear regression models. Kybernetika **42**(4), 423–440 (2006)
2. Koeth, R.A., et al.: Intestinal microbiota metabolism of l-carnitine, a nutrient in red meat, promotes atherosclerosis. Nat. Med. **19**(5), 576–585 (2013)
3. Ministry of Health, Labour and Welfare: Patient Survey (1999)
4. Ministry of Health, Labour and Welfare: Overview of 2011 national health expenditure (2013)
5. Ministry of Health, Labour and Welfare: The National Health and Nutrition Survey in Japan, 2012 (2014)
6. Morita, A., et al.: Dietary reference intakes for japanese 2010: lifestage. J. Nutr. Sci. Vitaminol. **59**(Supplement), S103–S109 (2013)
7. National Institute of Health and Nutrition: the National Health and Nutrition Survey (1995–1999)
8. Sasaki, S.: Dietary Reference Intakes for Japanese 2010: Basic Theories for the Development. Journal of Nutritional Science and Vitaminology **59**(Supplement), S9–S17 (2013)
9. Tanaka, H., Watada, J.: Possibilistic linear systems and their application to the linear regression model. Fuzzy Sets Syst. **27**(3), 275–289 (1988)
10. Tanaka, H., Guo, P.: Possibilistic Data Analysis for Operations Research. Phisica-Verlag, Heidelberg (1999)
11. Whitlock, G., et al.: Body-mass index and cause-specific mortality in 900 000 adults: collaborative analyses of 57 prospective studies. Lancet **373**(9669), 1083–1096 (2009)

12. Umesawa, M., et al.: Dietary Calcium Intake and Risks of Stroke. Its Subtypes, and Coronary Heart Disease in Japanese: The JPHC Study Cohort I, Stroke **39**(9), 2449–2456 (2008)
13. Yabuuchi, Y., Watada, J.: Fuzzy principal component analysis and its application. J. Biomed. Fuzzy Syst. Assoc. **3**(1), 83–92 (1997)
14. Yabuuchi, Y., Watada, J.: Fuzzy regression model building through possibility maximization and its application. Innovat. Comput. Inf. Control Express Lett. **4**(2), 505–510 (2010)
15. Yabuuchi, Y., Watada, J.: Fuzzy robust regression model by possibility maximization. J. Adv. Comput. Intell. Intell. Inf. (JACIII) **15**(4), 479–484 (2011)
16. Yabuuchi, Y., Watada, J.: Japanese economic analysis by possibilistic regression model which built through possibility maximization. JACIII **16**(5), 576–580 (2012)
17. Yabuuchi, Y., Kawaura, T., Watada, J.: Analysis of medical care expenditure by japanese prefecture using fuzzy robust regression model. In: Proceedings of InMed-14 (2014)
18. Yabuuchi, Y., Kawaura, T., Watada, J.: Analysis of Medical Care Expenditure by Japanese Prefecture using Fuzzy Robust Regression Model, CD-ROM. In: Proceedings of the 17th Czech Republic and Japan Seminar 2014, 16–20 September (2014)

Analysis of Time-Series Data Using the Rough Set

Yoshiyuki Matsumoto and Junzo Watada

Abstract Rough set theory was proposed by Z. Pawlak in 1982. This theory has high capability to mine knowledge based on decision rules from a database, a web base, a set and so on. The decision rule is widely used for data analysis as well. In this paper the decision rule is employed to reason for an unknown object. That is, the rough set theory is applied to analysis of economic time series data. An example shown in the paper indicates how to acquire knowledge from time series data. At the end we suggest its application to predictions.

1 Introduction

As changes in economic time-series data influence on the profits of a corporation, analyzes of such changes are widely pursued. Especially, technical and fundamental analyzes are employed as a method to analyze stock prices and dealing rates. The technical analysis is to analyze stock prices based on the time-series changes of stock prices through graphical expression of market prices. On the other hand, the fundamental analysis is to analyze stock prices based on various indices of corporate achievements and economical environments. As well, a chaotic method is also employed in forecasting of a stock [1].

The objective of this paper is to acquire knowledge from economical time-series data and forecast its change in terms of rough set theory [2, 3]. At the end, we will analyze real time-series values of TOPIX (Stock Market Index for the Tokyo Stock Exchange) and show what kind of knowledge acquisition and forecast will be done.

Y. Matsumoto (✉)
Shimonoseki City University, 2-1-1, Daigaku-Cho, Shimonoseki, Japan
e-mail: matsumoto@shimonoseki-cu.ac.jp

J. Watada
Waseda University, 2-7 Hibikino, Wakamatsu, Kitakyushu, Japan
e-mail: junzow@osb.att.ne.jp

Y.-W. Chen et al. (eds.), *Innovation in Medicine and Healthcare 2015*,
Smart Innovation, Systems and Technologies 45,
DOI 10.1007/978-3-319-23024-5_13

2 Rough Set Theory

A rough set has been proposed by Z. Pawlak in 1982 [2] and is employed to analyze various applications widely [4]. It is possible to roughly express elements in a set of considered objects according to the recognizable scale. The rough set theory denotes such rough representation as approximation. This is a method of knowledge acquisition. There are two kinds of approximations: one is an upper approximation to take an element of a rough set into consideration from possibility points of view and the other is a lower approximation to take an element of a rough set from viewpoints of necessity. The visual illustration of upper and lower approximations is shown in Fig. 1.

It is named "reduction" to obtain a subset of minimal number of features that equivalently discriminate objects with all plural features that characterize some set. General speaking, there can exist plural reductions.

It is possible to decide a decision table, if features of a set can be divided into two subsets of condition features and decision features, respectively. The decision table can be understood as decision rules that correspond to a value of conditional feature to a value of decision feature. For instance, a decision table shown in Table 1 illustrates a decision rule for sample x1.

$$\text{If } a = 1 \text{ and } b = 1 \text{ and } c = 1 \text{ then } d = 1$$

This decision table has 3 conditional features and 5 samples. It is possible to derive 5 rules with 3 conditions. But the decision rules have redundancy in the conditional portion. By employing a reduction method in the rough set theory, it is possible to derive the minimal rules required for expressing the same decision rules.

Fig. 1 Upper and lower approximations

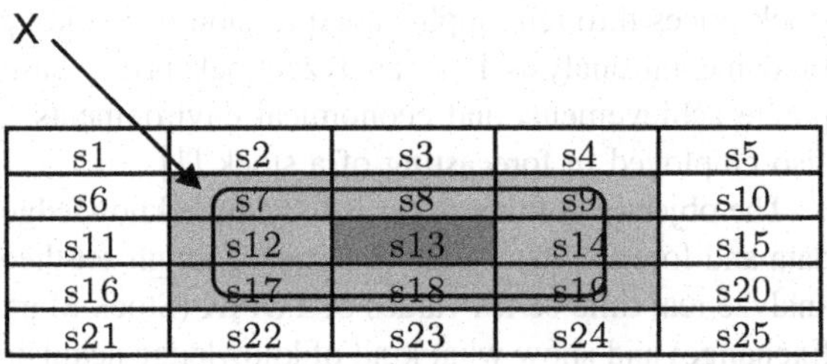

Table 1 Decision table

Sample	Conditional feature			Decision feature
	a	b	c	d
x1	1	1	1	1
x2	2	1	2	2
x3	2	1	1	1
x4	2	2	1	2
x5	1	1	2	1

In the case of a decision table shown in Table 1, rules illustrate the decision feature d = 1 as follows:

$$\text{If } a = 1 \text{ then } d = 1$$

$$\text{If } b = 1 \text{ and } c = 1 \text{ then } d = 1$$

As the same, the rule that illustrates the decision feature d = 2 can be written as follows:

$$\text{If } b = 2 \text{ then } d = 2$$

$$\text{If } a = 2 \text{ and } c = 2 \text{ then } d = 2$$

3 Determination of Decision Rules

It is required to build up a decision matrix in extracting decision rules from a decision table. For instance, the decision matrix for decision class d = 1 in Table 1 results in Table 2. This decision matrix is obtained using the lower approximation of decision class d = 1 and discriminate object d = 2.

The decision matrix is a table that describes feature value between samples. For example, on the case of x1 and x2, as a = 1 and c = 1 are deferent from x1, this value is denoted in the table. Therefore, the table explains that a = 1 or c = 1 can discriminate between x1 and x2. In the same way, x4 can be discriminated from x1 using a = 1 or b = 1.

$$\begin{aligned} &x1\text{: (a1 or c1) and (a1 or b1)} \\ &= \text{(a1) or (a1 and b1) or (a1 and c1) or (b1 and c1)} \\ &= \text{(a1) or (b1 and c1)} \end{aligned}$$

In the same way, x3 and x5 can be described as follows:

$$\begin{aligned} &x3\text{: (c1) and (b1) = (b1 and c1)} \\ &x5\text{: (a1) and (a1 or b1 or c2)} \\ &= \text{(a1) or (a1 and b1) or (a1 and c2)} \\ &= \text{(a1)} \end{aligned}$$

Table 2 Decision matrix

$A_*(d = 1)\backslash d = 2$	x2	x4
x1	a1, c1	a1, b1
x3	c1	b1
x5	a1	a1, b1, c2

As the feature results in d = 1 to discriminate x1, x3 and x5, we have a decision rule that x1, x3 or x5 result in d = 1.

$$(a1) \text{ or } (b1 \text{ and } c1) \text{ or } (b1 \text{ and } c1) \text{ or } (a1)$$
$$= (a1) \text{ or } (b1 \text{ and } c1)$$

On this case as shown in the previous section, the decision rule can be obtained as follows:

$$\text{If } a = 1 \text{ then } d = 1$$

$$\text{If } b = 1 \text{ and } c = 1 \text{ then } d = 1$$

It is possible to derive decision rules for decision class = 2 in the same way.

4 Analysis of Decision Rules

Only decision rules that are obtained rough set theory and have high C.I. are employed in reasoning. C.I. is an abbreviation of Covering Index that is a rate of objects that can sufficiently reach the same decision feature by the rule out of the whole objects [5].

Generally speaking, decision rules with high C.I. are highly reliable and results in good reasoning. In real situations, the number of obtained decision rules is often more than several hundreds. In these cases, reasoning does not employ almost all decision rules. That is, reasoning scattered almost decision rules.

It is necessary to make decision rules effective so as to combine decision rules by means of decision rule analysis [4]. Decision rule analysis enables us to obtain new combined decision rules by means that premises of decision rules are decomposed and given some points depending on their C.I. value. This method enables us to take all decision rules into consideration even if rules have a low C.I. value. In this paper, decision rules are combined and applied to forecasting.

Let us explain the detail of decision rule analysis. The decision rule analysis determines rules by calculating their column scores. The column score can be calculated in the following:

Let us consider the following three rules.

IF a = 1 and b = 1 then d = 1	(C.I. = 0.4)
IF b = 2 then d = 1	(C.I. = 0.3)
IF a = 2 and b = 2 and c = 1 then d = 1	(C.I. = 0.6)

The column score can be obtained using combination table as shown in Table 3. The combination table is an n x n matrix consisting of all features. The element of the combination table is a score of combination of two features.

Table 3 Combination table

	a = 1	a = 2	b = 1	b = 2	c = 1	c = 2	Column score
a = 1			0.2				0.2
a = 2				0.1	0.1		0.2
b = 1	0.2						0.2
b = 2		0.1		0.3	0.1		0.5
c = 1		0.1		0.1			0.2
c = 2							

For example, the first rule has a = 1 and b = 1 as its premises. On this case, the vertical column has a = 1 and the horizontal row has b = 1, and the vertical column has b = 1 and horizontal row has a = 1. We describe two scores in these elements. The score value is one or C.I. value divided by the written score value.

On this case, two elements have each score value.

$$0.4/2 = 0.2$$

On the case of the second rule, as the premise has one feature, the column and row are written 0.3 for b = 2.

On the case of the third rule, as the premise has 3 features, 6 elements (3C2 = 6) should be written scores. The written score is

$$0.6/6 = 0.1.$$

The column score is the total value of scores in each column. For example, on the case of a = 2 we obtain

$$0.1 + 0.1 = 0.2.$$

This calculation results in Table 3. Using this combination we can derive a decision table. For example, on the case of column b = 2, since there is a score in a = 2, b = 2 and c = 1, the rule of this column results in as follows:

$$\text{IF } a = 2 \text{ and } b = 2 \text{ and } c = 1 \text{ then } d = 1.$$

Usually, scores under the some threshold are not accepted. For instance, when the threshold is 0.2, the rule is written in the following:

$$\text{IF } b = 2 \text{ then } d = 1.$$

5 A Rough Set Approach to Analyzing Time-Series Data

In this paper, a rough set is applied to time-series data employing the focal time-series data and changes of related data that influence on the focal data.

Table 4 Only one time-series data

No	Conditional feature			Decision feature
	1 period previous	2 period previous	3 period previous	Present period
1	+	–	–	–
2	+	–	+	+
3	+	–	–	–
4	+	+	–	+
5	–	–	+	–

Table 5 Including related data

No.	Conditional feature						Decision feature
	Target data			Related data			
	1PP	2PP	3PP	1PP	2PP	3PP	Present period
1	+	–	–	–	–	–	–
2	+	+	–	+	+	+	+
3	+	–	–	+	–	–	–
4	+	–	+	–	–	+	+
5	–	+	–	–	+	+	–

PP: Period previous

General speaking, data treated in a rough set are categorical. In this paper, the change of the value is calculated from its single period previous value and two categories: plus and minus are defined by its going up or down changes, respectively. Such categorical data are analyzed by a rough set.

For instance, when the information of three past periods is analyzed, let us select going up or down movements from first to third periods for a conditional feature and the present change for a decision feature. That is, the present change is decided using the increasing and decreasing movement in the three past periods as shown in Table 4.

When employing other time-series data that may influence on the decision feature, such time-series data is additionally taken as a conditional feature as well and the present movement is decided depending on these features as shown in Table 5.

6 Analysis of TOPIX

The method described above is employed to analyze TOPIX time-series data. Dollar-Yen exchange rates, NY Dow-Johns Industrial Average of 30 stocks (DJIA) and NASDAQ Index are employed as a related time-series data. Let us forecast the changes of TOPIX based on the knowledge acquisition from these changes. The data employed is monthly values from 1995 to 2003. The first half 50 samples are employed for knowledge acquisition and the latter half 50 samples are employed for verifying the model.

Increasing and decreasing movements in 6 periods (half a year) are employed in the knowledge acquisition. That is, these changes of increasing and decreasing movements from the first to sixth periods are taken for a conditional feature, the change of the present period is taken for a decision feature. Analysis was done for four combinations of the above-mentioned data as (1) TOPIX, (2) TOPIX and Dollar-yen exchange rates, (3) TOPIX and NY Dow-Johns Industrial Average, and (4) TOPIX and NASDAQ index. In the 1st case TOPIX is calculated changes from the first period to sixth period, and in other cases the other data as well as TOPIX are calculated these changes and taken for conditional features (Figs. 2, 3, 4, 5, Table 8).

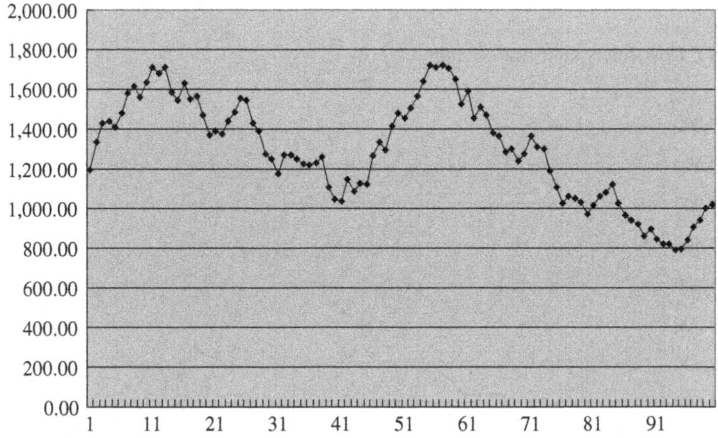

Fig. 2 TOPIX

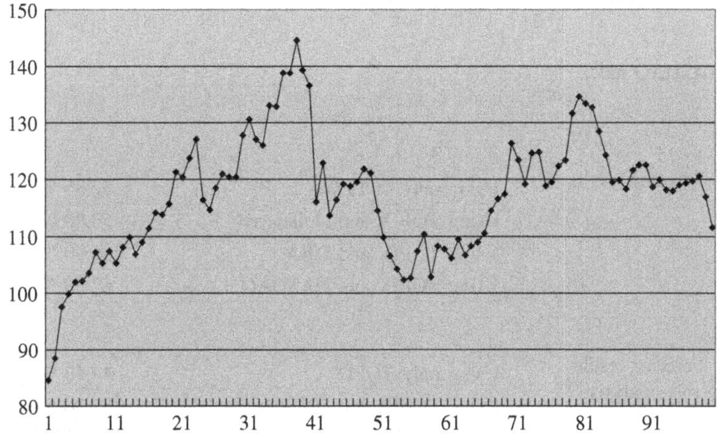

Fig. 3 Dollar-yen exchange rates

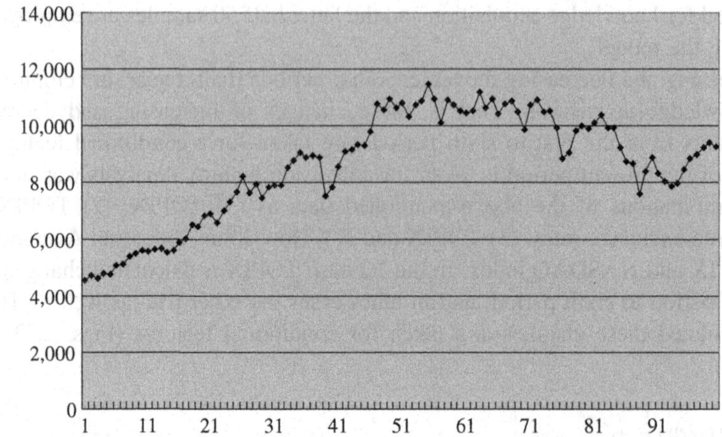

Fig. 4 NY Dow-Johns industrial average

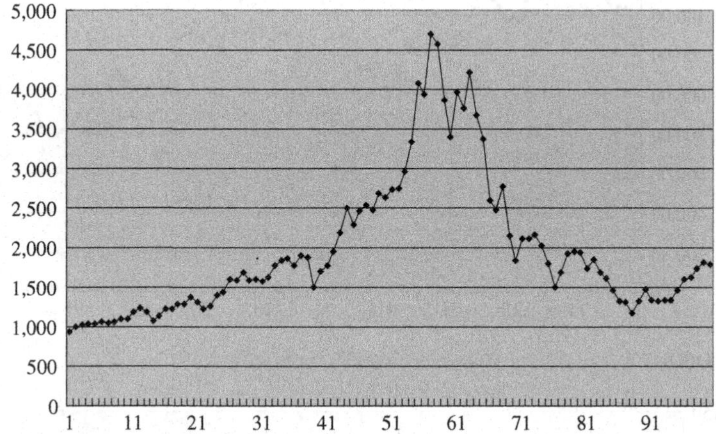

Fig. 5 NASDAQ index

Table 6 Forecast results

Using only TOPIX	52.85 %
Using TOPIX and Dollar-yen	53.80 %
Using TOPIX and DJIA	66.90 %
Using TOPIX and NASDAQ	62.50 %

Table 7 Forecast results (Decision rule analysis method)

Using only TOPIX	44.40 %
Using TOPIX and Dollar-yen	51.30 %
Using TOPIX and DJIA	54.50 %
Using TOPIX and NASDAQ	53.30 %

Table 8 Conform rate

Using only top 3 rules	32.3 %
Using decision rule analysis method	77.3 %

7 Results

Table 6 illustrates forecasted results based on these rules. Using three top rules in a C.I. value, the last half 50 values are forecasted.

Regarding C.I. values of obtained rules, the rule obtained using related data is better than the one obtained only from TOPIX. This result shows that related data could acquire better rules that cover wider range. It was the rule of (-) movement based on TOPIX and Dollar-Yen Exchange Rates that showed the best C.I. value. It can cover 40 % of the whole range.

Regarding the forecasted results using rules obtained, it is better using related data than using only TOPIX times-series data.

Considering the result of all increasing and decreasing movements, the NY Dow-Johns Industrial Average is the best effect in forecasting among all combinations.

Table 7 shows the result obtained by forecasting using the decision rules acquainted from the decision rule analysis. It is frequent that the forecasting precision becomes worse than the result using the 3 rules of the highest C.I. values. Since decision rules with low a C.I. value are employed in forecasting, the forecasting precision should be worsened. Nevertheless, the number of objects that fit to obtained decision rules is larger on the case of the decision rule analysis. That is, even though the forecasting precision is worsened, the number of forecastable objects increases.

On the case where we use three rules with higher C.I. values, there are one third less objects fitting to rules than the number of the total 50 objects. On the other hand, it is about 80 % our of the whole objects that fit to rules obtained by decision rule analysis.

8 Concluding Remarks

In this paper, we proposed a method based on a rough set to analyze time-series data. As its application we analyzed TOPIX time-series data and forecasted future changes. As data related to TOPIX, Dollar-Yen Exchange Rate, NY Dow-Johns Industrial Average of 30 stocks and NASDAQ index are employed. For these data, decision rules are acquainted in terms of a rough set theory. Employing rules with higher C.I. values, the related data could obtain better results than TOPIX without any related data. The combination of TOPIX with NY Dow-Johns Industrial Average resulted totally in the highest precise forecasting.

Also, we forecast using rules obtained by decision rule analysis. Even if the forecasting precision was worse than on the case of using three rules with highest C.I. values, the number of objects that fit to rules is more than on the case of using C.I. values. Therefore, it is effective when we forecast data that are not fit to rules with high C.I. values.

On the other words, if we forecast using rules with higher C.I. values when objects are fit to such rules and using rules obtained by decision rule analysis for the other case, the forecasting can be compensated mutually.

In this application, we employed two categories of increasing and decreasing movements of the time-series data. If we will categorize more dementedly into several ones, it may be possible to obtain more knowledge. It should be also examined to obtain decision rules that cover whole states.

References

1. Matsumoto, Y., Watada, J.: Improvement of Chaotic Short-term Forecasting on Fuzzy Reasoning and Tuning on Genetic Algorithm. J. Jpn Soc. Fuzzy Theor. Intell. Inform. **16**, 44–52 (2004)
2. Pawlak, Z.: Rough Sets. Int. J. Comput. Inf. Sci. **11**, 341–356 (1982)
3. Tsumoto, S.: Rough sets: past, present and future. J. Jpn Soc. Fuzzy Theor Syst. **13**, 552–561 (2001)
4. Mori, N., Tanaka, H., Inoue, K.: Rough sets and Kansei: knowledge acquisition and reasoning from Kansei data. Kaibundo, Tokyo (2004)
5. Tanaka, H., Tsumoto, S.: Rough sets and expert system. Math. Sci. **378**, 76–83 (1994)
6. Watada, J., Li, H.: A rough set approach to building association rules and its applications. In: 3rd International Conference on Artificial Intelligence in Engineering and Technology, Kota Kinabar, Malaysia, 22–24 Nov 2006

Study on Multi-Period Transportation Problem Considering Opportunity Loss and Inventory

Shinichiro Ataka and Hisayoshi Horioka

Abstract Transportation Problem (TP) is a well-known basic network model that can be defined as a problem to minimize the total delivery cost. But when we apply to real world, the TP model should be extended to satisfy other additional constraints. In addition, traditional TP model does not treat the concept of opportunity loss and customer demand is always satisfied. In the real world, there are many cases where customer demand is not satisfied, and opportunity loss occurs. In this paper, we formulate a multi-period transportation problem with opportunity loss and inventory cost. To solve the problem, we designed Differential Evolution (DE) with random key-based representation as efficient solution method for proposal TP model.

1 Introduction

In recent years, the management concept of company is greatly reformed by rapid development of information technologies and spread of the Internet. By this transition, the role of Supply Chain Management (SCM) in production and logistic information systems is ever becoming more important, at the same time production and logistics model designs renovation requirements. The transportation is one of the most important roles for economic goals such as expansion of the market, balancing of physical distribution and production activity.

Now a days, diversification of demand has changed from the process of trading products after finished mass-production to using high-mix low-volume production. Currently, the problem that many companies need to deal with is to quickly and

S. Ataka (✉)
Osaka International University, Tohdacho, Moriguchi, Osaka 570-8555, Japan
e-mail: s-ataka@oiu.jp

H. Horioka
Osaka International University, 3-50-1 Sugi, Hirakata, Osaka 573-0192, Japan
e-mail: m11m05@oiu.jp

Y.-W. Chen et al. (eds.), *Innovation in Medicine and Healthcare 2015*,
Smart Innovation, Systems and Technologies 45,
DOI 10.1007/978-3-319-23024-5_14

flexibly satisfy various needs of the customers. Therefore, the just-in-time delivery or deliveries with multi-product, small-lot, high frequency are important subjects with a physical distribution.

The transportation problem (TP) has been discussed in the field of Operations Research. The objective is to determine delivery amounts with minimizing the total delivery cost and satisfying all customer demands. However, the general TP model cannot be applied to the real world. More concrete constraints and extension of the model are needed. Although various extended models and their solution methods have been proposed, the extended models could not deal with various elements of the real world such as inventory [1–6]. Traditional TP models treat only one-stage (from plants to DC (Distribution Center) s) and it only considers the delivery cost in every delivery stage. Other issues such as weather or traffic condition, and drivers' physical condition are not considered.

2 Proposal TP Model

In this research, we propose multi-product two-stage transportation problem including opportunity loss and Inventory. This TP model includes several important subjects. The general TP model will always meet the customer demand. In the real world, there are many cases where customer demand is not satisfied, and opportunity loss occurs. So, proposal model designs delivery plan for multiple periods considering inventory cost and opportunity loss. When we try to sell certain goods, it is necessary to keep a certain quantity until they sold. If there are no goods to satisfy consumer demands, the opportunity for business is lost. However, if storage space for inventory is required, inventory cost occurs. Therefore, inventory costs and we must keep inventory amounts as small as possible without inventory shortage. On the other hand, a concept of time factor is needed to calculate a carrying cost in certain time. Although the company has introduced the various demand-forecasting techniques, there is no positive technique. The main reasons are short product life cycle (PLC) and diversification of demand (Fig. 1).

Indices:

I: plant, $i = 1, 2, \ldots, I$
j: DC, $j = 1, 2, \ldots, J$
k: customer (or store), $k = 1, 2, \ldots, K$
t: time period, $t = 1, 2, \ldots, T$
I: total number of plants
J: total number of DCs
K: total number of customers (or stores)
T: total number of periods

Parameters:

a_i: capacity of i-th plant
b_j: capacity of j-th DC

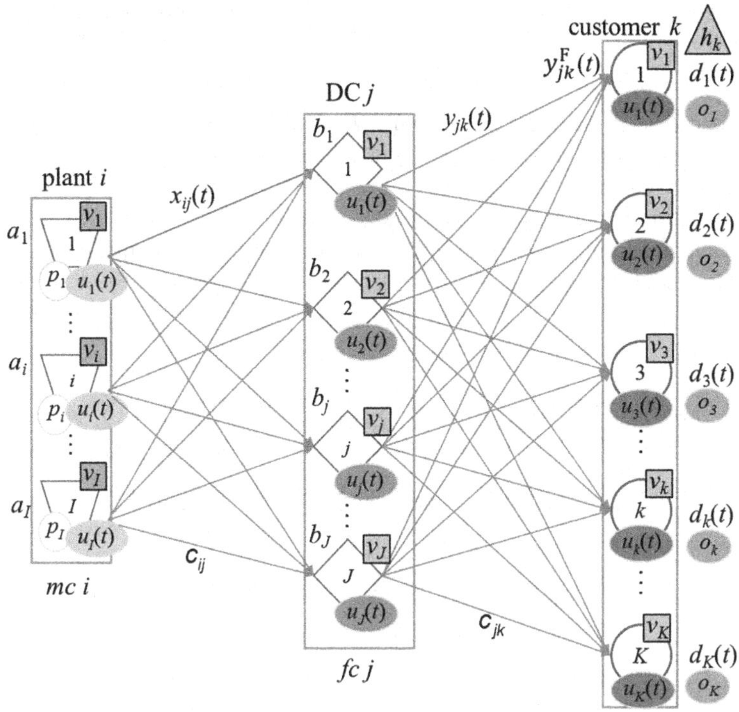

Fig. 1 Proposal TP model

$d_k(t)$: demands of customer k in period t
c_{ij}: delivery cost from plant i to DC j in period t
c_{jk}: delivery cost from DC j to customer (or store) k in period t
v_i: inventory cost of plant i
v_j: inventory cost of DC j
v_k: inventory cost of customer (or store) k
h_k: opportunity loss for customer (or store) k
mc_i: manufacture cost for plant i
fc_j: fixed administrative cost for DC j
$o_k(t)$: deficient supply quantity
$p_i(t)$: amount of production of plant i in period t
$u_i(t)$: inventory quantity of plant i in period t
$u_j(t)$: inventory quantity of DC j in period t
$u_k(t)$: inventory quantity of customer (or store) k in period t

Decision variables:
$x_{ij}(t)$: shipment amount from plant i to DC j in period t
$y_{jk}(t)$: shipment amount from DC j to customer k in period t

We assume the following assumptions for formulating proposal mathematical model.

A1. Capacity of Plant and DC are known.
A2. It is not necessarily the all customer demands are met.
A3. Arrangement place of each facility is known.
A4. Delivery cost is known at each stage.
A5. Production is performed in an instant.
A6. Delivering from the plant to the customer is carried out immediately.
A7. This model draws up a delivery plan for multiple periods.

$$\min \quad z = \sum_{t=1}^{T}\left(\sum_{i=1}^{I}\sum_{j=1}^{J} c_{ij}x_{ij}(t) + \sum_{j=1}^{J}\sum_{k=1}^{K} c_{jk}y_{jk}(t) + \sum_{i=1}^{I} v_i u_i(t) + \sum_{j=1}^{J} v_j u_j(t) + \sum_{k=1}^{K} v_k u_k(t) + \sum_{k=1}^{K} h_x o_k(t) + \sum_{i=1}^{I} mc_i p_i(t) + \sum_{j=1}^{J} fc_j\right) \quad (1)$$

$$\text{s.t.} \quad u_i(t) = a_i - \sum_{j=1}^{J} x_{ij}(t-1), \quad \forall t, i, j \quad (2)$$

$$u_j(t) = b_j - \sum_{k=1}^{K} y_{jk}(t-1), \quad \forall t, j, k \quad (3)$$

$$u_k(t) = \max\left(\sum_{j=1}^{J} y_{jk}(t) - d_k(t), \quad 0\right) \quad \forall t, j, k \quad (4)$$

$$\sum_{j=1}^{J} x_{ij}(t) \leqq a_i, \quad \forall t, i, j \quad (5)$$

$$\sum_{k=1}^{K} y_{jk}(t) \leqq b_j, \quad \forall t, j, k \quad (6)$$

$$o_k(t) = \max\left(d_k(t) - \sum_{j=1}^{J} y_{jk}(t), \quad 0\right) \quad \forall t, j, k \quad (7)$$

$$p_i(t) = a_i - u_i(t-1) \quad \forall t, i \quad (8)$$

$$x_{ij}(t), y_{jk}(t) \geq 0, \quad \forall t, i, j, k \quad (9)$$

Equation (1) is objective function for minimizing total cost. Constraints (2) and (3) show the inventory for the plant and DC in period t, respectively. Constraints (4) means the customer demands. Constraints (5) and (6) represent the capacity constraints of plants and DCs. Constraint (7) shows deficient supply quantity and (8) represent amount of production of plant i in period t.

3 Differential Evolution

Differential Evolution (DE) is one of the Evolutionary Algorithms (EA) that proposed by Storn and Price [7, 8]. This algorithm is population-based stochastic search method for optimization problem. In DE, each variable's value is represented by a real number. The advantages of DE are its simple structure, ease of use, speed and robustness. Moreover, DE has few parameters that a user must set from experience. In timetabling problem, several solution methods using EA techniques have been proposed [3–6].

Here, DE is a population based search method which utilizes *NP* variables as population of *D* dimensional parameter vectors in each generation. The initial population is chosen randomly if no information is available about the problem. In the case of the available preliminary solution, the initial population is often generated by adding normally distributed random deviations to the preliminary solution. DE generates new parameter vectors by adding the weighted difference vector between two population members to third member. And, the resulting vector yields a lower objective function value than a predetermined population member; the newly generated vector replaces the vector with which it was compared. In addition, the best parameter vector is evaluated for every generation. DE maintains two arrays, each of which holds a population size *NP* and *D* dimensional, real-valued vectors. The primary array holds the current vector population, while the secondary array accumulates vectors that are selected for the next generation. In each generation, *NP* competitions are held to determine the composition of the next generation. In mutation process, every pair of vectors (x_a, x_b) defines as a differential vector: ($x_a - x_b$). When x_a and x_b are chosen randomly, their weighted differential is used to perturb another randomly chosen base vector x_c. This mutation process can be mathematically expressed as:

$$x_c^{'} = x_c + F(x_a - x_b) \tag{10}$$

The scaling factor F is a user supplied constant in the optimal range between 0.5 and 1.0. In every generation, each primary array vector x_i is targeted for crossover with a vector $x_{c'}$ to produce a trial vector x_t. This trial vector x_t is the offspring which generated from parent vectors x_i and $x_{c'}$. The uniform crossover is used with a crossover rate (CR) which actually represents the probability that the child vector inherits the parameter values from the random vector. If trial vector x_t has better value compare with parent vector, parent vector is replaced with child vector.

So far, several kinds of DE have been proposed, such as "DE/best/1/bin" and "DE/rand/1/exp" are well known. This notation method has rule as DE/*base*/*num*/*cross*. For example, the part of "*base*" represents the selection method of the parent and "*num*" part represents the number of differential vector respectively. If "*base*" part is *best*, the algorithm selects individual as a parent having a best fitness value. On the other hand, if individual is chosen as a parent at randomly, this part is describe "rand". The last part of "*cross*" means crossover method for generates offspring. For example, DE/*base*/*num*/*bin* uses binomial crossover to replace the gene with a certain probability, and DE/*base*/*num*/*exp* uses exponential crossover to replace the gene based on probability decreasing exponentially. The basic DE process is shown as Fig. 2.

In this research, we adopt an effective solution method that is robust and able to fast convergence compared with other evolutionary strategy for TP. It called random key-based representation [9]. It is one of Individual expression for Genetic Algorithm (GA). Because this method is excellent at designing the delivery route (network model of TP), we applied in this study.

Figure 3 is example of random key-based representation for basic TP. This figure shows cost matrix and TP model, and individual representation. The length of Individual equals to total number of plants and DCs. The numbers above indicate node IDs on the network model. The decimal numbers are their priority and we use these priority values in the design of the delivery pattern.

Step1. Initial populations are generated.

Step2. DE evaluates the all individuals, if the termination condition is satisfied calculation process is finished.

Step3. The trial vector is generated from mutation process.

Step4. The child vector is generated form crossover process.

Step5. If trial vector has better value compare with parent vector, parent vector is replaced with child vector.

Step6. If the termination condition is satisfied, calculation process is finished, otherwise go back to Step 2.

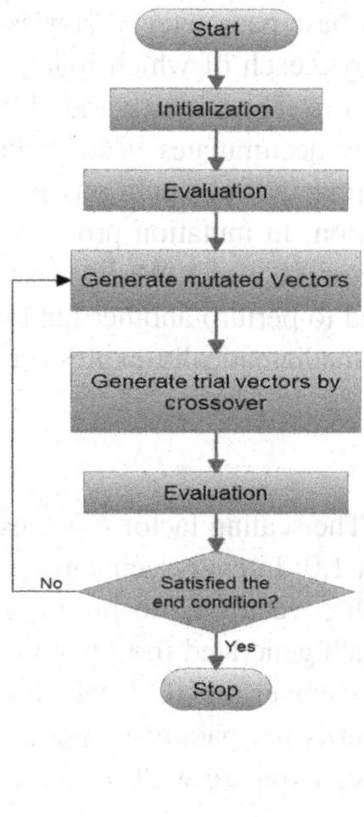

Fig. 2 Flowchart of DE

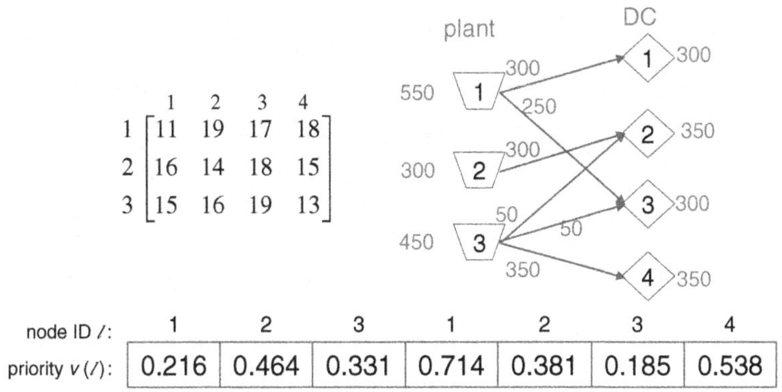

Fig. 3 A sample of random key-based representation

Step 1. Initial populations are generated.
Step 2. DE evaluates the all individuals, if the termination condition is satisfied calculation process is finished.
Step 3. The trial vector is generated from mutation process.
Step 4. The child vector is generated form crossover process.
Step 5. If trial vector has better value compare with parent vector, parent vector is replaced with child vector.
Step 6. If the termination condition is satisfied, calculation process is finished, otherwise go back to Step 2 (Table 1, Fig. 4).

As the trace table shows, in the first step, DC 1 has the highest priority in the individual and the lowest cost is between Plant 1 and DC 1. Then, an arc between DC 1 and plant 1 is added to transportation tree. After determining the amount of shipment that is $g_{11} = \min\{550, 300\} = 300$, the capacity of the plant and the demand of the DC are updated as $a_1 = 550–300 = 250$, $b_1 = 300–300 = 0$, respectively. Since $b_1 = 0$, the priority of DC 1 is set to 0, and DC 4 with the next-highest priority is selected. After adding an arc between DC 4 and plant 3, the amount of the shipment between them is determined and their capacity and demand are updated as explained above.

Usually, these processes repeat until the demands of all DCs are satisfied. However, our proposal model has realistic rule that is not satisfy customer demands. Therefore, the main purpose of using this technique is for generating initial solutions (i.e. If demand is not satisfied, it can design as much as possible low cost delivery route).

Table 1 Trace table of decoding procedure

Step	Priority value	Plant	DC
0	[0.216 0.464 0.331 I 0.714 0.381 0.185 0.538]	(550, 300, 450)	(300, 350, 300, 350)
1	[0.216 0.464 0.331 I 0.000 0.381 0.185 0.538]	(250, 300, 450)	(300, 350, 300, 350)
2	[0.216 0.464 0.331 I 0.000 0.381 0.185 0.000]	(250, 300, 100)	(300, 350, 300, 300)
3	[0.216 0.000 0.331 I 0.000 0.381 0.185 0.000]	(250, 300, 100)	(300, 350, 300, 300)
4	[0.216 0.000 0.331 I 0.000 0.000 0.185 0.000]	(250, 390, 350)	(300, 300, 300, 300)
5	[0.216 0.000 0.000 I 0.000 0.000 0.185 0.000]	(250, 300, 300)	(300, 300, 250, 300)
6	[0.000 0.000 0.000 I 0.000 0.000 0.000 0.000]	(300, 300, 300)	(300, 300, 300, 300)

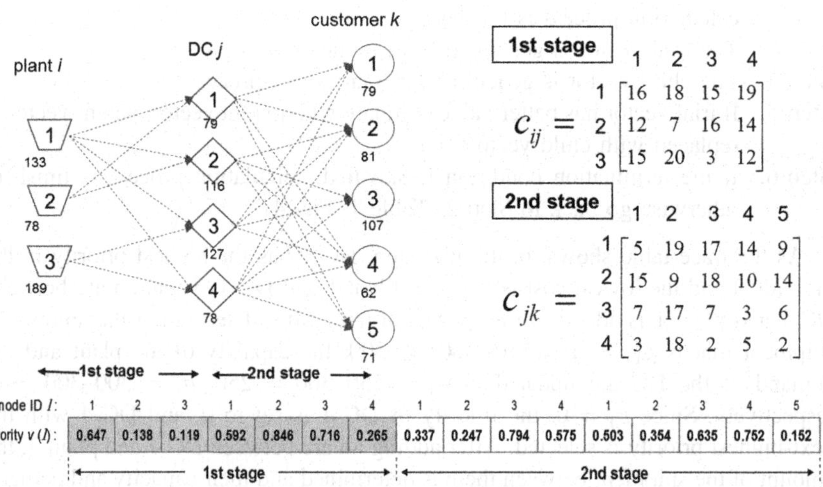

Fig. 4 A sample of Individual expression for proposal model

Table 2 Each parameter setting

Problem No.	No. of plants (i)	No. of DCs (j)	No. of customers (k)	Initial total demand
1	2	5	8	1300
2	3	7	12	2700
3	5	3	12	3000
4	6	8	20	3500

4 Numerical Experiment

In numerical experiments, we compare 10 DE strategies as follows. We have applied the random key-based representation to all of DEs.

1: DE/rand/1/bin,	6: DE/rand/1/exp,
2: DE/best/1/bin,	7: DE/best/1/exp,
3: DE/best/2/bin,	8: DE/best/2/exp
4: DE/rand/2/bin,	9: DE/rand/2/exp,
5: DE/rand-to-best/1/bin,	10: DE/rand-to-best/1/exp

In this time, we have set the parameters as follows:

- Number of population (NP): 100 • crossover rate (CR): 0.5
- Max generation: 1000 • Scaling factor (F): 0.5

We prepared four problems; in addition we set the number and initial demand of each facility as follows (Table 2).

Inventory of each facility, delivery cost, cost of product manufacturing each plant, management fixed costs of each DC were generated randomly from 1 to 30. This time we was multiplied by the opportunity loss costs (randomly caused from 1 to 30) to deficient supply quantity. Actually, lost opportunities are to be set in consideration of the size and location and reliable of the store. Total demand of after the second period is randomly generated in 0.5–1.5 times the range of the previous fiscal year.

In Fig. 5, we show the results of numerical experiments. All of DE including random key-based representation could solve these problems. DE2, 3 and 5 ware obtained better results than other methods. So, we show the results of these three DEs.

In the table, “No.” is the generation number, “avg.” the average value of 100 individuals, and “div” represents the standard deviation respectively. In addition, the figures on the right side show state of evolution. We can see that seven approaches other than de2, 3 and 5, the evolution converged at a relatively early stage. We have speculated that the cause is a difference of crossover technique.

Problem 1:

DE/best/1/bin	NP= 100	CR= 0.5	F= 0.5
No.= 0	avg= 158964.7	div= 5503.6	
No.= 1000	avg= 141637.6	div= 344.1855	mut= 0
DE/best/2/bin	NP= 100	CR= 0.5	F= 0.5
No.= 0	avg= 158964.7	div= 5503.6	
No.= 1000	avg= 141714.8	div= 365.9739	mut= 0
DE/rand-to-best/1/bin	NP= 100	CR= 0.5	F= 0.5
No.= 0	avg= 158964.7	div= 5503.6	
No.= 1000	avg= 141701.2	div= 326.4766	mut= 0

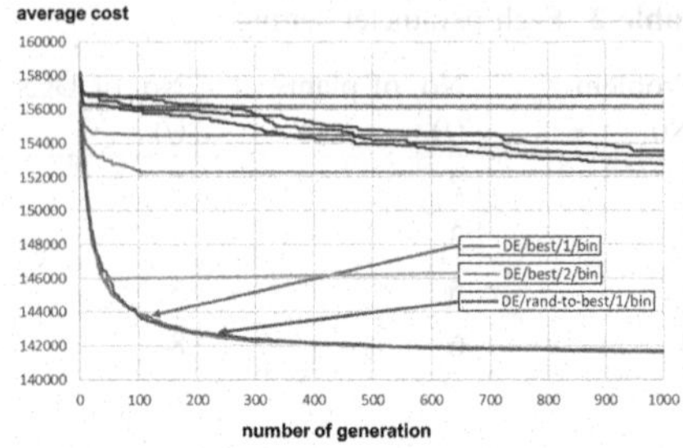

Problem 2:

DE/best/1/bin	NP= 100	CR= 0.5	F= 0.5
No.= 0	avg= 360148.7	div= 20728.79	
No.= 1000	avg= 331120.3	div= 6470.048	mut= 0
DE/best/2/bin	NP= 100	CR= 0.5	F= 0.5
No.= 0	avg= 360148.7	div= 20728.79	
No.= 1000	avg= 330421.9	div= 5511.218	mut= 0
DE/rand-to-best/1/bin	NP= 100	CR= 0.5	F= 0.5
No.= 0	avg= 360148.7	div= 20728.79	
No.= 1000	avg= 330587.3	div= 5460.012	mut= 0

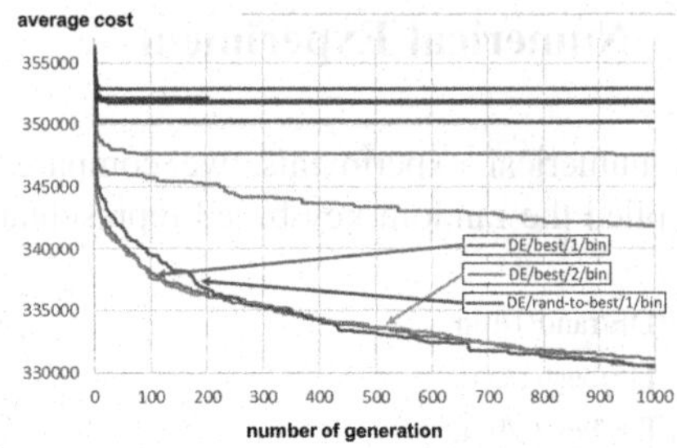

Problem 3:

DE/best/1/bin	NP= 100	CR= 0.5	F= 0.5
No.= 0	avg= 349872.5	div= 12617.48	
No.= 1000	avg= 323385.2	div= 4039.659	mut= 1
DE/best/2/bin	NP= 100	CR= 0.5	F= 0.5
No.= 0	avg= 349872.5	div= 12617.48	
No.= 1000	avg= 323850.8	div= 3684.077	mut= 0
DE/rand-to-best/1/bin	NP= 100	CR= 0.5	F= 0.5
No.= 0	avg= 349872.5	div= 12617.48	
No.= 1000	avg= 323546.8	div= 3903.49	mut= 0

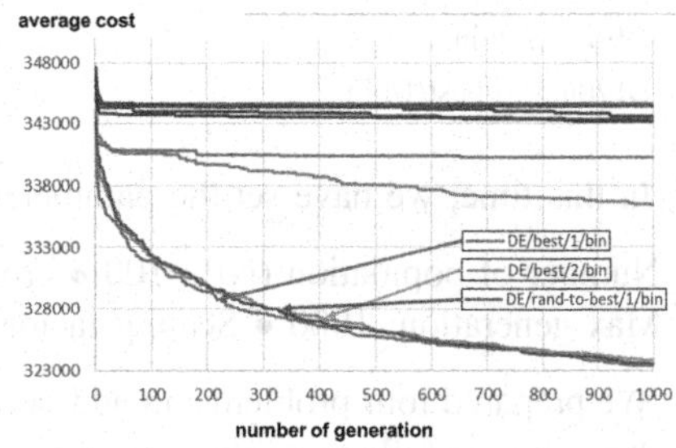

Problem 4:

DE/best/1/bin	NP= 100	CR= 0.5	F= 0.5
No.= 0	avg= 266541.7	div= 18080.24	
No.= 1000	avg= 304326.3	div= 4941.2368320	mut= 0
DE/best/2/bin	NP= 100	CR= 0.5	F= 0.5
No.= 0	avg= 266541.7	div= 18080.24	
No.= 1000	avg= 238671.6	div= 5840.986	mut= 1
DE/rand-to-best/1/bin	NP= 100	CR= 0.5	F= 0.5
No.= 0	avg= 266541.7	div= 18080.24	
No.= 1000	avg= 239623.7	div= 5131.976	mut= 0

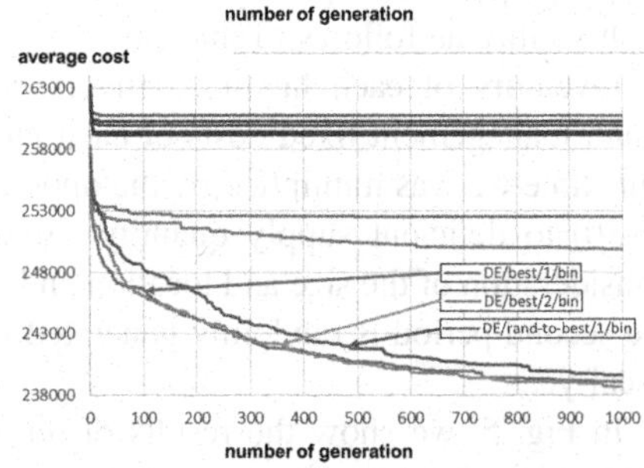

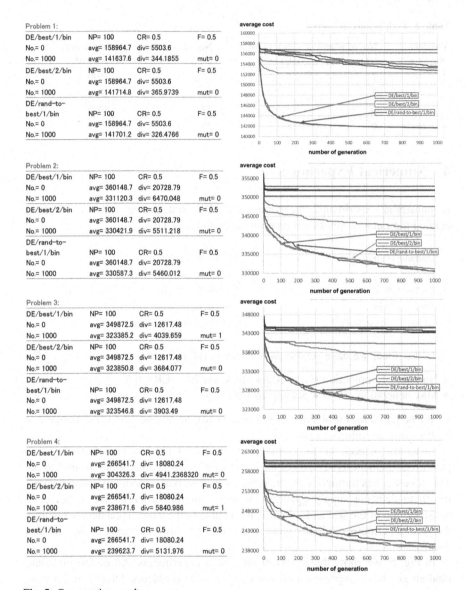

Fig. 5 Computation result

5 Conclusion

In this research, we propose multi-product two-stage transportation problem including opportunity loss and Inventory. This TP model designs delivery plan for multiple periods considering inventory cost and opportunity loss. To solve this problem, we prepared ten DEs that are included random key-based representation.

In numerical experiments, ten DEs with random key-based representation obtained the each solution. In particular, three types of DEs obtained good results in a stable. We are planning to consider more concrete inventory-control techniques and a shorter product life cycle.

Suggestion of the individual representation method that can investigate large solution space quickly and the experiment that used larger scale data sets or real data sets is a future problem.

References

1. Gen, M., Li, Y., Ida, K.: Spanning tree-based genetic algorithm for Bicriteria fixed charge transportation problem. J. Jpn Soc. Fuzzy Theor. Syst. **12**(2), 87–95 (2000). [in Japanese]
2. Yang, L.X., Liu, L.Z.: Fuzzy fixed charge solid transportation problem and algorithm. Appl. Soft Comput. **7**(3), 879–889 (2007)
3. Sun, M.: A tabu search heuristic procedure for solving the transportation problem with exclusionary side constraints. J. Heuristic **3**, 305–326 (1998)
4. Sun, M.: The transportation problem with exclusionary side constraints and two branch-and-bound algorithms. Eur. J. Oper. Res. **140**(3), 629–647 (2002)
5. Ataka, S., Gen, M.: Solution method for multi-product two-stage logistics network with constraints on delivery route. Electr. Eng. Jpn **92**(8), 18–24 (2009)
6. Ataka, S., Kim, B., Gen, M.: Optimal design of two-stage logistics network considered inventory by Boltzman random key-based GA. IEEJ Trans. Electr. Electron. Eng. **5**(2), 195–202 (2010)
7. Storn, R., Price, K.: Differential Evolution: A Simple and Efficient Adaptive Scheme for Global Optimization over Continuous Spaces, Technical Report TR-95-012. International Computer Science Institute, Berkeley (1995)
8. Storn, R., Price, K.: Differential evolution–a simple and efficient heuristic for global optimization over continuous spaces. J. Global Optim. **11**(4), 341–359 (1997)
9. Gen, M., Cheng, R.W., Lin, L.: Network Models and Optimization: Multiobjective Genetic Algorithm Approach. Springer, London (2008)

Diagnosis of ECG Data for Detecting Cardiac Disorder Using DP-Matching and Artificial Neural Network

Mohamad Sabri bin Sinal and Eiji Kamioka

Abstract Computational Intelligence has made a huge impact on solving many complicated problem particularly in the medical field. With the advancement of computational intelligence where the effectiveness of data analysis is at high stake, the process of classifying and interpreting data accurately based on logical reasoning in decision making is not a big issue. This study discusses the process of diagnosing cardiac disorder using computational intelligence with specific focus on the feature extraction where the attribute of identifying Normal Sinus and Atrial Fibrillation rhythms using Physionet.org database is examined. In this paper, an algorithm to diagnose the cardiac disorder based on DP-Matching will be proposed where the time and frequency domains of ECG signal segments are introduced. At the end of this paper, the performance evaluations of the proposed method will be shown with the analysis by ANN.

Keywords Electrocardiogram (ECG) · Dynamic programming (DP-matching) · Artificial neural network (ANN) · Atrial fibrillation rhythm · Normal sinus rhythm

1 Introduction

An electrocardiogram (ECG) signal is considered as one of the best alternatives available to learn the status of the heart condition's activities. There are many critical diseases which are interconnected with the heart condition and some of the diseases need special treatments or unexpected death may occur. Therefore, a special equipment is needed so that the useful information from the ECG data can

M.S.b. Sinal (✉) · E. Kamioka
Graduate School of Engineering and Science, Shibaura Institute of Technology, Tokyo, Japan
e-mail: ma14103@shibaura-it.ac.jp

E. Kamioka
e-mail: kamioka@shibaura-it.ac.jp

Y.-W. Chen et al. (eds.), *Innovation in Medicine and Healthcare 2015*,
Smart Innovation, Systems and Technologies 45,
DOI 10.1007/978-3-319-23024-5_15

be collected and interpreted. In addition to that, an expert is required to analyze the data in order to describe in detail the real situation of the heart to the patients. This can be a draw-back in situations where the experts are lacking in numbers and experience. Thus, an appropriate method is required to automatically analyze the ECG signal, as well as having the capability to interpret data without relying heavily on the experts and sophisticated equipment.

Dynamic Programming (DP) matching is one of the well-established techniques which have been used to extract certain patterns in a time series data or signal data. DP-Matching can be used to extract similar sub-pattern from two different sequential patterns and validate the similarity based on numerical result [1].

The main aim of this study is to straighten out an efficient and accurate method to discriminate the Atrial Fibrillation symptom from Normal Sinus symptom based on ECG data by using DP-Matching and Artificial Neural Network. Which pattern to be used as a reference for diagnosing ECG data and what kind of mechanism to measure the similarity based on the pattern will be highlighted in order to discriminate the two symptoms. It has been decided that the following methods are required; the first step is a feature pattern which is going to be used to represent the pattern to be referred to as a reference for comparison. The second step is the range of acceptance value for DP-matching to accept the similarity of two patterns and the mechanism to handle all patterns before making the interpretation.

In this paper, the pattern for Normal Sinus has been proposed as a main reference pattern since they can be the main indicator for a normal heart condition where it is able to differentiate two categories of symptoms in a row where either it is Normal Sinus or Atrial Fibrillation. By using DP-Matching algorithm, this technique will be used as a mechanism to validate the similarity between the two patterns for certain duration.

The remainder of this paper is organized as follows; Sect. 2 will discuss some related works towards this research area. Section 3 will introduce the abnormal pattern of Atrial Fibrillation and Normal Sinus Rhythm. Section 4 will describe the detail working custom DP-Matching algorithm. In Sect. 5, the analysis of experimental result will be discussed based on two technique which is DP-Matching and Artificial Neural Network. In Sect. 6, conclusions will be made with discussions on possible future research.

2 Related Works

Suzuki et al. [2], has proposed a method to diagnose cardiac arrhythmia by measuring ECG, blood oxygen, and blood pressure data by using Ant colony System. Her method resulted in high heart diseases classification accuracy.

Likewise, Kumar et al. [3], constructed an algorithm to identify heart disease based on certain characteristic points (CPs), the Q and S points in an ECG. In the proposed method, 3 main components are used which are a preprocessor, a DP-Matching and a detection algorithm. The detection algorithm was used to find

CPs from selected template pattern. MIT/BIH arrhythmia database was used to evaluate his proposed technique.

Lippincott Williams [4], have reviewed several techniques for detecting Atrial Fibrillation from Non-Episodic ECG Data. Several features extraction have been defined to diagnose the Atrial Fibrillation by focusing on segments P wave, QRS wave and R to R interval. In this paper, several methods were investigated to classify the feature extraction of ECG wave. Some of the discovered techniques are K-nearest neighbor (KNN), Bayer Optimal Classifier, Artificial Neural Network (ANN), Linear Discrimination Analysis and Empirical Detector. Even though these several techniques have some drawbacks, it is believed that this is a good start for diagnosing the Atrial Fibrillation through computerizing approach.

3 Time Series Features from ECG

In traditional medical diagnostic proceeding, cardiologists diagnose heart condition based on ECG rhythm visually where any kind of arrhythmia in the heart can be detected. Previously, arrhythmia used to be portrayed linguistically in a fashion which was difficult to understand. With the use of automated DP-Matching detection algorithm, feature extraction from several raw ECG signals will be translated where certain criteria and standard will be applied in order to diagnose the symptoms. At the end of the process, the result will be presented in numerical value. Hence, the description is visualized with numerical representative and can be easily be described.

3.1 Overview of Cardiac Disorder

3.1.1 Normal Sinus Rhythm

Sinus rhythm is reflective of a normally functioning conduction system in the body. The electrical current is following the normal conduction pathway without interference from other bodily system or disease processes [5].

3.1.2 Atrial Fibrillation

Atrial fibrillation (A fib.) occurs when electrical impulses come from areas of reentry pathways of multiple ectopic foci. Each electrical impulse results in depolarization of only a small group of atrial cells rather than the whole atria. Multiple atrial activities are recorded as chaotic waves, often with the appearance of fine scribbles [5].

3.2 Feature Extraction

3.2.1 P, Q, R, S, T Wave Morphology

As a Normal rhythm routine for a healthy heart condition, certain characteristics from the heart rhythm will consistently appear in every wave and in certain duration. By comparing Normal Sinus Rhythm with Atrial Fibrillation symptom as shown in the Fig. 1 for Normal Sinus and Fig. 2 for Atrial Fibrillation, both symptoms show a huge difference in many ways. This region is one of the best segments to differentiate the disease symptom from the normal healthy rhythm. Therefore, by referring to P, Q, R, S, T peak consistently and comparing them with other user patterns, DP-Matching will be able to give significant results.

3.2.2 R to R Interval

The most visible signal to detect in our hearts cycle is R peak especially for Normal Sinus Rhythm. R peak is considered the center of each beat rhythm cycle as shown in Fig. 3. In addition to that, R to R intervals for Normal Sinus Rhythm are very regular with only small variation between beats. Contrastively, the R to R interval during Atrial Fibrillation has a greater variation than P, Q, R, S, T interval variations [5].

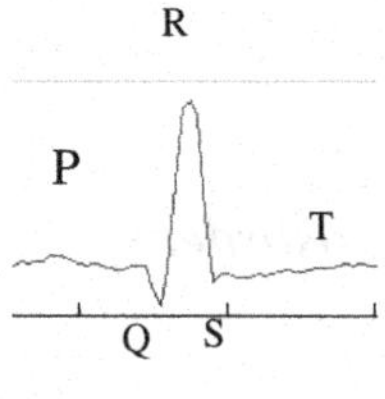

Fig. 1 Normal sinus rhythm pattern for P, Q, R, S, T

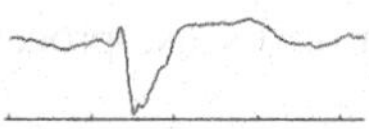

Fig. 2 Atrial fibrillation rhythm pattern for P, Q, R, S, T

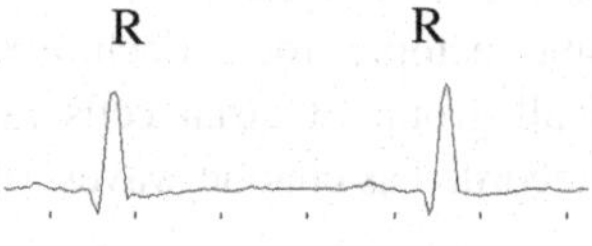

Fig. 3 Sample of R to R interval for normal sinus rhythm

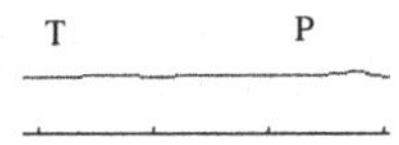

Fig. 4 Sample of T to P for normal sinus rhythm

3.2.3 T to P Interval

T peak to another P peak beat signal region is a location where many uncertain signals may appear due to certain reasons. A significant difference can be seen for Normal Sinus Rhythm and Atrial fibrillation where many fluctuation waves may appear in this region in various ways. Normal Sinus rhythms usually have only linear waves where there are no fluctuations except for some interference due to external factors as shown in Fig. 4.

4 Proposed Method

In this study, Physionet.org [6], has been selected as the main database resource where MIT-BIH Normal Sinus has been selected as the main reference for data analysis of the proposed DP Matching algorithm. In this database, several hundreds of patterns are available for diagnosis of the ECG signal.

Two types of symptoms are introduced as the main symptoms to be covered in this research. They are Normal Sinus rhythm and Atrial Fibrillation rhythm. The proposed DP-Matching algorithm will be used to identify the similarities of characteristic point of ECG and the result will be evaluated through a certain condition as proposed in this paper.

4.1 Overview of DP Matching

Dynamic programming (DP) matching is a method for comparing two sequential patterns which has been extracted from a time series data. The capabilities of DP-matching include the extraction of all similar sub patterns simultaneously while compensating the nonlinear fluctuation. Each comparison will be represented in numerical value [5].

The proposed algorithm by applying two criteria to distinguish the two symptoms is composed in the following stages:

- Data configuration: create several hundreds of patterns based on P, Q, R, S, T wave, R to R interval and T to P interval in each beat for Atrial Fibrillation and Normal Sinus Rhythm for pattern matching.
- Feature Extraction and comparison pattern: Extract feature from ECG signals and compare the similarities by using Euclidean metric in DP-Matching after

segmentation. All the numerical values of comparison in DP-Matching will be stored and measured through average values of each group to see the trend of the data.

- Disease Classification: Disease classification will be done after the average value of each pattern is analyzed using DP-Matching where two criteria will be used to distinguish both categories. The main criteria to classify the normal and abnormalities of heart condition are the average value and the standard deviation. If each value is larger than 20, it is considered as a sign of abnormalities. The second criteria is that the number of average range value and standard deviation above 20 which are tested with 10 reference data should be at least 7 over 10 reference data. This will be the best indicator in classifying the categories of diseases; be it atrial fibrillation or Normal Sinus Rhythm.

4.2 *Overview of Artificial Neural Network*

An Artificial Neural Network is inspired by the concept of biological neurons in the human brain. With the capability to duplicate sheer number of biological neurons with their high interconnectivity, the scaled down models of the artificial neural networks show similar capacity of learning and generalizing instinct characteristic of the information presented to it. In this paper, this method will be used for the performance comparison to the proposed DP-Matching algorithm using ECG data.

5 Evaluation

Physionet is one of the most popular free open source resources which provides a large collection of recorded physiologic signals and open-source software. In this website, a lot of data related to biomedical research and development which have been used by many researcher for data analysis and research are provided.

In this experiment, MIT-BIH Normal Sinus and MIT-BIH Atrial Fibrillation from Physionet.org has been selected to validate the performance of the proposed algorithm. 25 patients' data are used for this experiment where 13 data are taken from MIT-BIH Normal Sinus and the other 12 data are taken from MIT-BIH Atrial Fibrillation Database. It has been decided that 19 patient data are used for proposed DP-Matching and another 6 data are used for ANN experiment. Each data duration is 60 s per analysis.

After all the 3 segments are done in the experiments, All the DP scores and the average DP scores are distributed inconsistently in each segments for P, Q, R, S, T, R to R interval and T to P for both symptoms. It is difficult to divide both symptoms by just relying on all DP score, average DP score and standard deviation DP score. Therefore, by applying some criteria toward the result data, the possibilities to distinguish both symptoms are higher. One of the biggest issues in dealing with ECG signal data is the variability of individuals among the patients' heart cycle activities. In every comparison of pattern and shapes using DP-Matching technique with the reference data, the value of comparison might not get as small in value as 0 because each pattern is totally different in some ways thus making it almost impossible to have the same shape which is the reason why the 2 criteria range of value are introduced in the first place.

As seen in the result of the average DP score above 20 shows that the detection of Atrial Fibrillation for 9 patients data is at 55 % of accuracy for 3 segments as shown in Figs. 5, 6 and 7. This shows that the proposed algorithm based on the two criteria has some significance to the study. The proposed second criteria where the minimum detection data in segment P, Q, R, S, T has shown the detection of atrial fibrillation at 88 % while segment R to R interval and T to P segments are at 66 %. These three segments have demonstrated that this proposed method can detect over 50 % of the atrial fibrillation. In these experiments, the average DP score and the standard deviation DP score are two parameters that will be taken into consideration for discriminating two symptoms. Figures 5, 6, 7, 8, 9 and 10 show the result of accuracy over 9 Atrial Fibrillation patient data for average DP score and standard deviation DP score for segment P, Q, R, S, T, R to R and T to P where they have been tested with 10 Normal Sinus reference data.

Several issues are identified with some reference pattern which cannot be distinguished by both symptoms due to the lack of capabilities in DP-Matching technique itself. Therefore, the criteria which have been applied in DP-Matching will work to utilize the value of each matching pattern in order to discriminate the symptoms in some ways such as using the average DP score and the standard deviation DP score compared to each DP score itself. It is significant to use the average value of DP score as the main reference value to measure the symptom because this value is considered as the best approach to obtain cleaner data in order to discriminate existing noises in the data. Standard deviation DP score will be the secondary parameter to consider after average DP score due to its performance on

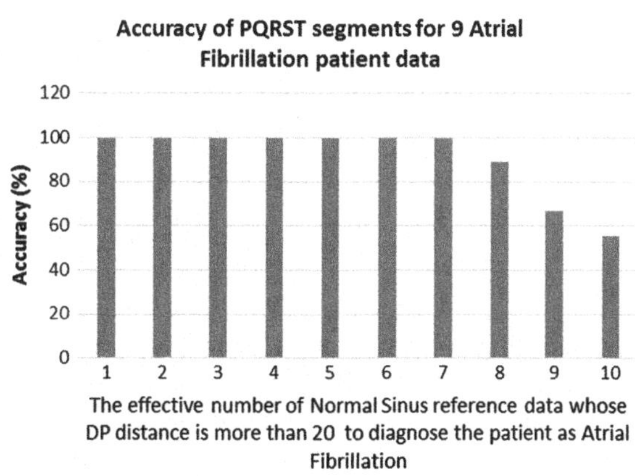

Fig. 5 Result of P, Q, R, S, T segment (average DP score)

Fig. 6 Result of R to R interval segment (average DP score)

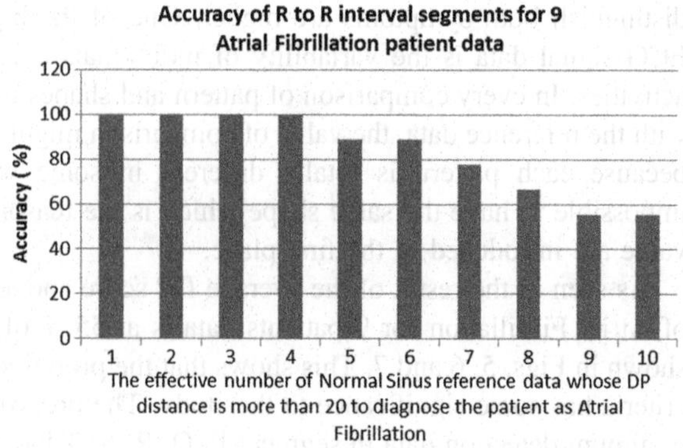

Fig. 7 Result of T to P segment (average DP score)

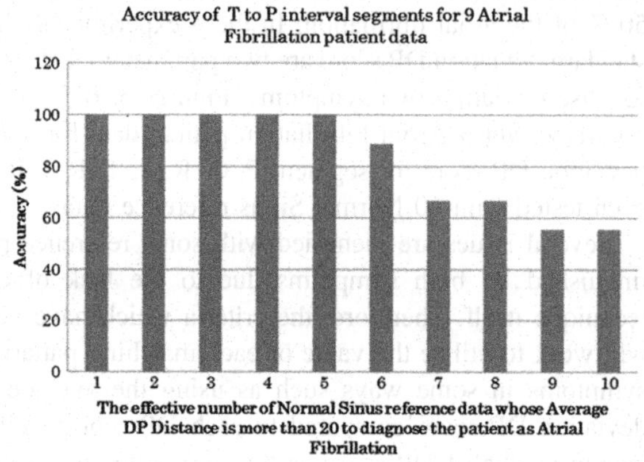

Fig. 8 Result of P, Q, R, S, T segment (standard deviation DP score)

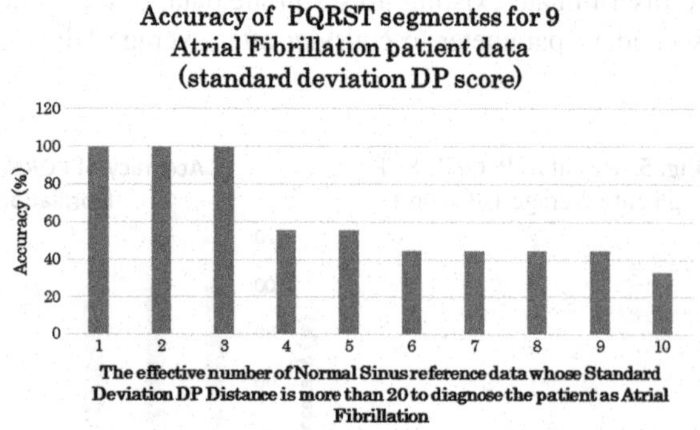

discriminating both symptoms in some ways. This is one of the main concerns as to why using the average DP scores and the standard deviation DP score is seen as one of the alternatives for analyzing and interpreting the data itself.

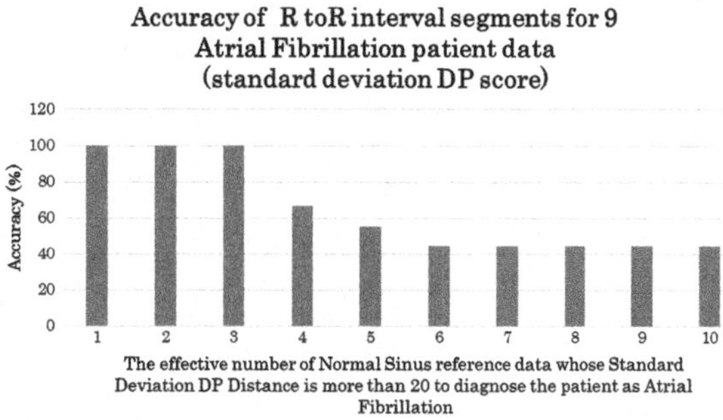

Fig. 9 Result of R to R interval segment (standard deviation DP score)

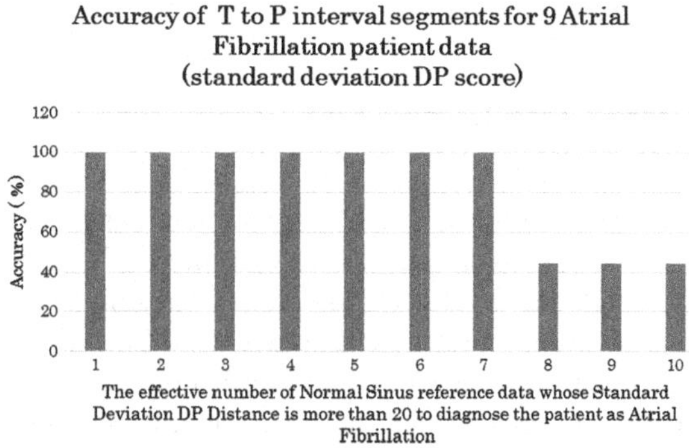

Fig. 10 Result of T to P segment (standard deviation DP score)

In this section, the performance of the proposed DP-Matching algorithm is compared with the Artificial Neural Network (ANN) while analyzing ECG data in order to diagnose and discriminate both symptoms in a row. 6 data are selected where 3 data are from MIT-BIH Normal Sinus and another 3 data are from MIT-BIH Atrial Fibrillation. In this ANN experiment procedure, these 6 data are prepared for train data and test data in order to see the performance of ANN in discriminating both symptoms. It has been decided in this procedure that the categorization for atrial fibrillation symptom must fall in value 1 and the categorization for Normal Sinus symptom should fall in value 0.

As shown in the Fig. 11, it is evident that the result for ANN in analyzing and discriminating Normal Sinus patient data and Atrial Fibrillation patient data are good. By comparing with DP-Matching performance in discriminating both symptoms, the proposed DP-Matching algorithm only have the capabilities to discriminate both symptoms in a certain segment linearly in ECG data. Even though, there are some data which are inconsistently distributed in ANN experiment for both symptoms, the number of noise data are very small compared to the average DP score or even DP score by using the proposed DP-Matching algorithm. However, there are some issues in using ANN as a tool to analyze ECG data such as the issue of overtraining and excessive computational overhead. Overtraining may affects the accuracy adversely while speed and required resources for ANN may become the main constraint that trigger on how to use ANN efficiently [7].

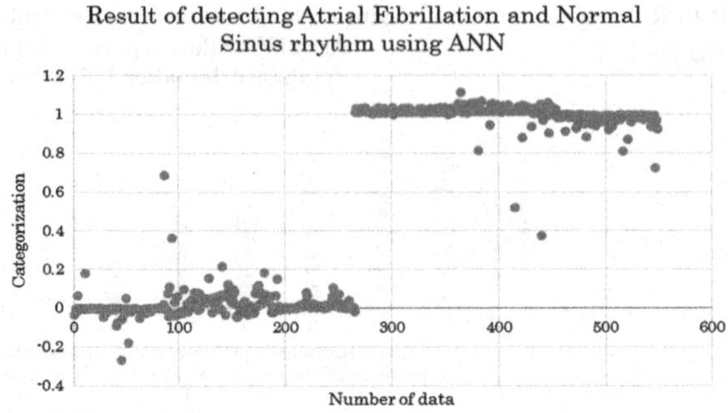

Fig. 11 Result of detecting normal sinus symptom and atrial fibrillation symptom for 6 patient in P, Q, R, S, T segments

6 Conclusion

In this research, a Dynamic Programming matching technique has been proposed. From the result obtained by the experiments of 3 segments in ECG data, it is proven that a high degree of detection rate in discriminating atrial fibrillation from normal sinus rhythm by using the proposed DP-Matching are over 50 % rate of accuracy over 9 patients data with Atrial Fibrillation symptoms. From the experiment result, it can be concluded that, the most significant parameter to use as a reference to determine the disorder is from average DP score. Meanwhile, standard deviation DP Score can be used as the secondary parameter to measure the heart condition for each segment as the performance of both parameter shows a huge relationship in distinguishing both symptoms.

As a conclusion, the best reference to be utilized in detecting Atrial Fibrillation from Normal Sinus by using DP matching tools is segment P, Q, R, S, T and T to P. Both segments are the best segments as they are involved with X axis comparison where DP-Matching is good at it. R to R interval segments were often dealing with Y axis pattern where it is difficult for DP matching to distinguish both symptoms based on some characteristics.

On the other hand, the best segment to describe Atrial Fibrillation is P, Q, R, S, T segments and T to P Segments. T to P is one of the segment which has not as yet been done before by many papers. In addition to this, it is a good segment to detect fluctuation of Atrial Fibrillation while P, Q, R, S, T segment is well known as a good segment to identify Atrial Fibrillation as referred to the characteristic of Atrial Fibrillation.

Comparing the performance of the proposed DP-Matching method and ANN shows that there is some huge potential to increase the rate of accuracy in detecting Atrial Fibrillation symptom from Normal Sinus symptom. The effectiveness of detecting Atrial Fibrillation and Normal Sinus symptoms by using both techniques rely on how data are been collected and from which segments of ECG data are being focused for diagnosis. Few number of patient data used in this experiment for

ANN are due to difficulty to collect all the peak value of P, Q, R, S, T automatically. However, the number of data point used in this experiment for ANN are 2745 which is good enough to measure the performance of ANN in detecting 6 patients data with sign of Normal Sinus and Atrial Fibrillation symptom. The result of ANN and DP-Matching shows that the idea of diagnosing ECG data for detecting cardiac disorder is possible to be established by utilizing computational intelligence way.

References

1. Fawziya, M.R.: Diagnosis of heart disease based on ant colony algorithm. In: International Journal of Computer Science and Information Security, USA (2013)
2. Suzuki, Y., Yukihisa, K., Sajjad, M., Junji, M.: A Method for extracting a QRS wave in an ECG based on DP matching. In:T.IEE, Japan (2001)
3. Kumar, S., Lu, W., Sitiani, D.T., Kim, D., Feng, M.: Detection of atrial fibrillation from non-episodic ECG data: a review of method. In: 33rd Annual International Conference of the IEEE EMBS, Massachusetts (2011)
4. Lippincott Williams, W.: ECG interpretation made Incredibly Easy! 5th edn. Wolters Kluwer Health, pp. 1–99 (2011)
5. Seiichi, U., Akihiro, M., Ryo, K., Rin-ichiro, T., Tsutomu, H.: Logical DP matching for detecting similar subsequence. In: 8th Asian Conference on Computer Vision, pp. 628–637. Springer, Heidelberg (2007)
6. The Research Resource For Complex Physiologic Signal. http://physionet.org/
7. Rajesh, G., Dr. Ghatol, A.A.: A brief performance evaluation of ECG feature extraction techniques for artificial neural network based classification. In: TENCON 2007–2007 IEEE Region 10 Conference, Taipei (2007)

Smart Technology for a Smarter Patient: Sketching the Patient 2.0 Profile

Luca Buccoliero, Elena Bellio, Maria Mazzola and Elisa Solinas

Abstract Patients' behaviors are changing over time as effect of the Health 2.0 phenomenon that entails the integration of information and communication technologies (ICTs) in healthcare. A new patient profile with growing expectations is emerging in today's healthcare world. In this scenario patient satisfaction has to be pursued through disruptive marketing strategies: healthcare providers are required to establish closer relationships with patients by leveraging both physical, experiential and technological service elements. Both qualitative and quantitative analysis were performed on a random sample of 2808 people divided into three groups: 737 outpatients and 861 inpatients of Niguarda Ca' Granda Hospital (Milan, Italy) and 1210 citizens reached through an online survey while browsing the hospital webpage between January and April 2014. Descriptive statistics and bivariate analysis were carried out. Beta coefficients were calculated to investigate the emerging patient satisfaction drivers. New healthcare guidelines were depicted in order to match patient 2.0 requirements.

Keywords Healthcare · Icts · Empowerment · Patient 2.0 · Italy

---

L. Buccoliero (✉) · E. Bellio
Department of Marketing, Bocconi University, CERMES
(Centre for Research on Marketing and Services), Milan, Italy
e-mail: luca.buccoliero@unibocconi.it

E. Bellio
e-mail: elena.bellio@unibocconi.it

M. Mazzola · E. Solinas
Bocconi University CERMES (Centre for Research on Marketing
and Services), Milan, Italy
e-mail: maria.mazzola@unibocconi.it

E. Solinas
e-mail: elisa.solinas@unibocconi.it

Y.-W. Chen et al. (eds.), *Innovation in Medicine and Healthcare 2015*,
Smart Innovation, Systems and Technologies 45,
DOI 10.1007/978-3-319-23024-5_16

1 Introduction

The development of information and communication technologies (ICTs) in the health sector has generated the so-called Health 2.0, enabling patient empowerment and education. Health 2.0 refers to personal and participatory healthcare where patients are invited to assume an active role in their own care and in the healthcare system in general [1, 2]. We refer in the present study to the new patient profile with the name of "patient 2.0" because of his/her behavioral and socio-demographic characteristics retrieved from international literature on the topic and derived from results of this study.

A shared understanding of the issue has brought to the identification of new patient's health habits and to the awareness that health service providers need to be prepared, starting from their academic education, in order to face those new requests [3].

Some authors try to identify the characteristics and attitudes of the new patient profile that is differently named depending on the study considered. Moreover, whereas Health 2.0 has been widely discussed in previous studies, there is a lack of specific knowledge about the characteristics of the users. The greatest attention has been paid to health informatics advances and the economic benefits deriving from the ICT implementation in the healthcare market [4], while less focus has been addressed to patient's behaviors and compliance to those new technologies in the health sector. Below the main findings in the available current literature regarding the emerging patient's characteristics are presented.

Profiling the "Patient 2.0". Gender, age and education appear to differentiate the way patients manage their health conditions [5, 6].

The search for health-related information online appears to be more widespread among women, younger and more-educated people [5–7]. Female internet users are the main health virtual community participants [8, 9]. They use the above-described tool to share personal experiences and to give encouragement rather to only gather or give information as man do [9].

Younger people are more willing to access medical records online [6] and at increasing education level potentially correspond higher innovation adoptions [3].

Emerging Patients' Requirements and Expectations. To better understand the patient's changing behaviors phenomenon and its implications for the healthcare sector, this section provides an overview on what this emerging profile refers to. As shown in Fig. 1, the "patient 2.0" is characterized by distinctive needs that can be categorized in three main areas.

"Patient 2.0" Need to Participate in the Decision-Making Process. The decision-making process about health and treatment choices of the detected profile differs from the one traditionally adopted by patients. Today's patients want to be involved in the healthcare process.

Physician are required to provide patients with more detailed information about their health conditions enabling a conscious decision-making about treatment choices. This increased need of engagement is achieved also through the use of

Fig. 1 The "patient 2.0" emerging needs

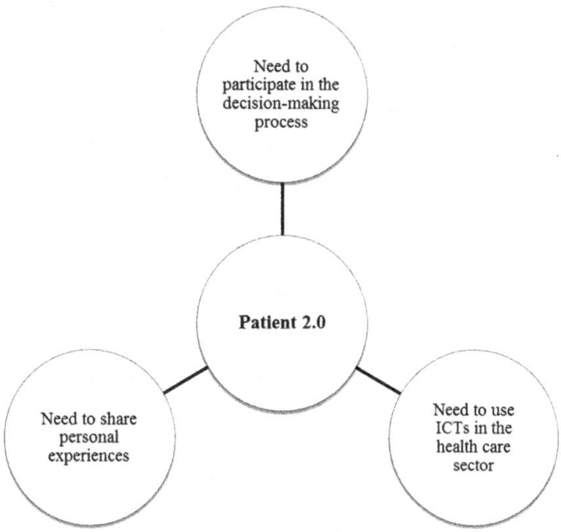

internet that acts as alternative source of information [10, 11]. This phenomenon is commonly defined by many authors as the "empowerment process" [12, 13] and can be considered as one of the key emerging characteristics of "patient 2.0" [4, 13, 14].

As confirmed by the American Medical Association, an increasing number of people seek medical information online rather than actually visiting health professionals [15]. Besides the learning experience, those patients tend to trust the internet tool and use the information gathered for making important decisions regarding their illness or condition, whether to consult or not a doctor and, eventually, to get a second opinion [5, 6]. Patients are increasingly using websites to retrieve and provide information about doctors [3, 6].

"Patient 2.0" Need to Use ICTs in the Health Care Sector. ICTs have the potential to streamline the communication process between patients and doctors.

Todays' patients are used to email care providers to carry out general health-related issues (e.g. the cancellation of an appointment) and to make contact with their physicians in a more informal and direct way [16].

Moreover, patients seem to recognize the advantages of getting clinical health care at a distance and are increasingly comfortable with telemedicine devices and applications [3]. Finally, the new patient wants to actively monitor his health conditions by accessing to online medical records, such as personal health records (PHR) [3].

"Patient 2.0" Need to Share Personal Experiences. New dynamics of social interactions among patients are arising. Patients use social media tool to communicate with each other in order to get online support and share personal stories.

These community participants use the social channel to get health-related information [9, 17], whether they are acting as patients or caregivers [5, 6]. The research drivers are wide-ranging: deepening the knowledge about one's own health conditions and illness in a cost-effective way, getting a second opinion especially when the information provided by the physician is not satisfactory, becoming more conscious about treatment options when talking to doctors [5].

2 Research Objectives

The aim of this research is to deepen and develop "patient 2.0" theme in the light of the ICTs adoption in the healthcare sector. The study focuses on the state of diffusion and use, satisfaction and acceptability of ICTs in support of patients in the current context of the Italian National Health Service (INHS).

What this study adds, comparing to the available literature on the topic, is an overview of the main items of value propositions that Italian healthcare providers should implement in order to adopt a "patient 2.0-centered" approach.

Research Questions. The following two research questions were used:

RQ1: Are there any distinguishable segments of patients within the study that are consistent with the "patient 2.0" definitions provided by scientific literature?
RQ2: Is it possible to identify in the target population different segments of "patient 2.0" whose satisfaction has to be achieved through different strategies?

3 Methods

The research methodology entailed three steps of analysis: a literature review, a qualitative and a quantitative investigation (see Fig. 2).

First, a qualitative study was carried out through semi-structured interviews to ICT and healthcare experts, then three focus groups were conducted involving from 6 to 8 citizens-patients to better understand the phenomenon of todays' patients' changing behaviors from both health providers and patients sides.

The quantitative research was conducted on a sample of 2808 citizens-patients of the Niguarda Ca' Granda Hospital (Milan-Italy) between January and April 2014 by administering a paper-based questionnaire to 737 outpatients and 861 inpatients and an online survey to 1210 users of the institutional hospital website. The health care center is acknowledged in Italy as one of the main transplant organizations with 26 specialized national referral centers. The hospital offers all clinical and surgical specialties and since its foundation in 1939 seeks the excellence by continuous improvements through investment in latest healthcare technologies and applications and health cooperation with various international organizations [18].

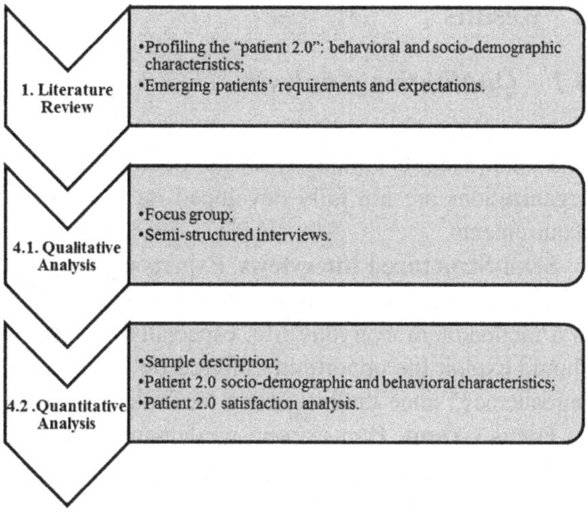

Fig. 2 Research methodology

The questionnaires were administered in Italian and gathered socio-demographics, the extent of use of ICT applications and social media as sources of health-related information. We collected opinions regarding three types of services: general web services (payments, appointment booking and cancellation, medical exam check-in, and so on), Personal Health Record and mobile health applications.

A specific section assessed patients' satisfaction with the "overall" service.

Responses were based on a Likert scale ranging from 1 to 7 (where the successive Likert category represents a "better" response than the preceding value), dichotomous and checklist items.

Statistical Package for the Social Sciences Program (SPSS) version 21 was used for the data analysis. Descriptive statistics were performed to investigate the sample composition. A Chi-squared test was used to assess the association between different categorical variables. Pearson correlation coefficients were calculated to measure the degree of linear dependence between satisfaction variables. The analysis of variance (ANOVA) was used to infer whether there are real differences between the means of independent groups in the sample data. Eta-squared values from ANOVA were reported as a measure of effect size for group mean differences [19]. Linear regressions were performed to assess the impact of each elements of the health service (independent variables) on the overall patient satisfaction (dependent variable). Regression analysis were then used again in the light of various socio-demographic variables to determine the differences in satisfaction drivers for various population subsets. The statistical significance was defined as p-value lower than 0.05 and all the β coefficients reported in this study were statistically significant.

4 Results

4.1 Qualitative Analysis

The main insights coming from the qualitative analysis underlined that healthcare organizations are not fully developed on the basis of today's patients' needs and requirements.

Semi-Structured Interviews. Experts claimed that information on webpages are usually not updated, resulting useless for patients. They highlighted that technology is a facilitator in everyday life, especially for younger people, and care providers should exploit the opportunity offered by IT applications to simplify processes and bureaucracy, since the increasing technology acceptance.

Focus Group. Focus group participants stated that many of their questions to doctors go unanswered. The need of more detailed information arose. Patients affirm that they usually rely on IT tools in order to fill their information needs.

Qualitative findings from both experts and patients confirm that the doctor-patient relationship is changing over time and that Health 2.0 is becoming more and more important for patients who are increasingly recognizing the benefits of using ICTs to carry out health-related activities.

4.2 Quantitative Analysis

4.2.1 Sample Description

Univariate Analysis (Descriptive Statistics). The average age of the sample is 49 years (youngest respondent 16 y.o and oldest 98 y.o) and respectively for outpatients 55.16 years, inpatients 55.85 years and online respondents 42.65 years. Females represent 52 % of the sample. The 97 % of respondents declare to have an education and to be Italian citizens.

Data show high prevalence of tablet and mobile devices owners (57 % of the sample have a smartphone and the average age of those respondents is 39.64 y.o). Mobile health applications (mHealth) are of undoubted importance for patients. Mean values of mHealth importance higher than 5 (out of 7) are detected for the following services: in first place, patient wish they could "make reservations via mobile", in second place they wish to "check-in" via mobile, then "to pay the ticket", in the fourth place to "download and view the reports", and lastly to "be oriented within the hospital" through a georeferentiation app.

42.9 % of outpatients and 39.4 % of hospitalized patients use social networks and both groups perceive as useful (respectively 4.58 out of 7 and 4.52 out of 7) the hospital presence on social media. The percentage of social network users increases (58 %) in the group of the online respondents, and only 9 % of cases declare to have used this channel to interact with the care provider.

Respondents' main reasons to access the hospital website are the search for health and administrative information. There is a great extent of use of ICTs to carry out health-related issues: 63 % of outpatients and inpatients use the health insurance card to access medical records.

The total sample claimed to be satisfied with its overall experience at the Niguarda hospital. The overall level of satisfaction is on average high for the three groups in the following order: in-patients (6.04 out of 7), on line respondents (6.00 out of 7) and outpatients (5.65 out of 7). Patients using online health services express an overall degree of satisfaction that is higher than the overall satisfaction of the sample (5.96 against 5.65 in the case of outpatients; 6.11 against 6.04 in the case of in-patients).

4.2.2 "Patient 2.0" Socio-Demographic and Behavioral Characteristics.

Chi-squared Test. According to the findings in the available literature, the usage of the "Niguarda online" (PHR) and the hospital's website appear to be more widespread, regarding both frequency and intensity of usage, among younger people and respondents with university or higher level of education, in comparison to those with high school or lower education. There is strong association between variables confirmed by Phi and Cramer's V values higher than 0.2.

ANOVA. Mobile health applications are clearly more important for younger people than for people belonging to the over 65 segment. Importance mean scores for mhealth apps equal or higher than 6 for the youngest people against mean values lower than 5 out of 7 for the oldest segment. Eta-squared values of 0.03 show that variables are strongly associated. For inpatients the education variable plays a significant role too in differentiating the importance related to mhealth apps (mean values higher than 5 out of 7 for people with a higher education).

4.2.3 "Patient 2.0" Satisfaction Analysis

Correlation Analysis. Pearson correlation coefficients show significant positive correlations between the amount of information received and overall satisfaction (0.682 significant at the 0.01 level) and between the amount of information received and the perceived quality of cure (0.675 significant at the 0.01 level). It is interesting to note that patients are more satisfied with their medical experience when care providers give them more information about their conditions.

ANOVA. The one-way ANOVA returned interesting results. Women, younger respondents and those with higher education (high school or undergraduate) are more demanding regarding the service received.

Younger patients show lower levels of overall satisfaction in comparison with older people ($\mu = 4.86/7$ for people aged 18–25 against $\mu = 5.78$ for over 65 respondents). Eta-squared value is equal to 0.34, indicating a strong association between variables. This phenomenon repeats in the satisfaction scores related to the following items of the experience: the access options to clinical data, clarity of information and the attention paid to patients by healthcare providers, timing of the services and, eventually, web services such as emailing and hospital website.

Gender and education differentiate the degree of satisfaction between population groups. Graduated patients are less satisfied of the overall experience ($\mu = 5.76$ against $\mu = 6.15$ of those with lower education). As regards the information received, women are harder to please compared to man ($\mu = 5.60/7$ against $\mu = 5.91/7$ of the male sample and Eta-squared equal to 0.20). In addition, females evaluate as more relevant the presence of a virtual community on the hospital's webpage contrary to males; getting online health support from care providers or other patients is also more important for women than for men ($\mu = 5.51/7$ against $\mu = 4.80/7$ of the male sample and Eta-squared equal to 0.16).

Regression Analysis. Patient satisfaction determinants were detected by analyzing the impact of different satisfaction drivers (independent variables) on overall patient satisfaction (dependent variable) through linear regression analysis. Four are the crucial elements in determining patient satisfaction, named in this study as "value drivers": *Patient Empowerment* (i.e. involvement of the patient in the care process), *Privacy and Dignity* (i.e. respectful attitude of healthcare providers towards patients), *Atmosphere and Comfort* (i.e. environmental aspects of the hospital) and *Technology* (i.e. ICTs integration in the health care service delivery). Value drivers are made up of different items related to the patient experience of care, and are derived through an aggregation of various questionnaire items intended to measure the corresponding construct presented above. Cronbach's alpha coefficients were performed to test the reliability of aggregated items and test scores show a good internal consistency reliability—alpha values higher than 0.6 [20].

All β coefficients were statistically significant since values were always lower than 0.05. The results testify that different patient's profiles exist whose satisfaction has to be pursued through different strategies. Results also show that *Patient Empowerment* plays a significant role in determining satisfaction in female patient and in patients which use technology (see Table 1). With regard to the youngest

Table 1 β standardized coefficients for the population subsets: female versus males, technology users versus non users, people aged 18–25 versus over 65

		β standardized coefficients		
Discriminating factors		Patient empowerment	Privacy and dignity	Atmosphere and comfort
Gender	Female	0.524	0.145	0.242
	Male	0.162	0.224	0.354
Technology usage	Health IT application users	0.531		0.354
	Health IT application non users	0.451		0.563
Age	18–25		0.879	
	65+	0.211	0.286	0.446

Table 2 β standardized coefficients for outpatients and inpatients

	β standardized coefficients	
Value drivers	Outpatients	Inpatients
Patient empowerment	0.358	0.249
Privacy and dignity	0.223	0.279
Atmosphere and Comfort	0.255	0.437
Technology	–	0.056

segment of patients, *Privacy and Dignity* proved to be the sole relevant value driver. Finally, while *Technology* appears to be irrelevant for the above population subsets, a regression analysis performed for the outpatients and inpatients groups (see Table 2) shows that *Technology* value driver was able to affect the overall patients' satisfaction and experience, meaning an increased attention to technological aspects of the healthcare service.

5 Conclusions

The main strength of this study was looking at Niguarda Ca' Granda Hospital performance from patients' perspective rather than from the organization's point of view.

Questionnaires allowed to measure patients levels of overall satisfaction and to understand how strong the impact of each value driver is in determining the overall patient satisfaction.

Results show the effective existence of a new patient profile, definable as "patient 2.0" since his/her new healthcare habits. Findings of this study are confirmed by the available literature: the "patient 2.0" mainly deals with a young and well-educated person, increasingly confident with the use of technology to carry out health-related activities, willing to accept IT health applications and to switch to unconventional service delivery solutions.

Finally, nontraditional communication channels as emails or virtual communities are perceived by the "patient 2.0" as an effective way to get health support and information.

In conclusion, investments in ICTs are a necessity to delight the new patient's perspective. Matching patient 2.0 requirements means health organizations must change the way they operate: it implies providing patients with more clear and detailed information through a dedicated social platform. More attention to patient data management and empowerment appears to be fundamental and must become the main objective that every innovation strategy in healthcare should achieve.

References

1. Yamout, Sani Z., et al.: Using social media to enhance surgeon and patient education and communication. Bull. Am. Coll. Surg. **96**(7), 7–15 (2011)
2. Normann, Andersen Kim, Rony, Medaglia, Zinner, H.H.: Social media in public health care: Impact domain proposition. Gov. Inf. Quart. **29**, 462–469 (2012)
3. Masters, Ken, Ng'ambi, Dick, Gail, T.: I found it on the internet. Preparing for the e-patient in oman. Sultan Qaboos Univ Med J. **10**(2), 169–179 (2010)
4. Stump, Terra, Alberto Coustasse, S.Z.: The emergence and potential impact of medicine 2.0 in the healthcare industry. Hosp. Top. **90**(2), 33–38 (2012)
5. Susannah, Fox, et al.: The Online Health Care Revolution: How the Web Helps Americans Take Better care of Themselves. The Pew Internet & American Life Project, Washington (2000)
6. Fox, S.: Health Information Online. Pew Internet & American Life Project, Washington (2006)
7. Tu, Ha T., R, C.G.: Striking Jump in Consumers Seeking Health Care Information. Health System Change, Washington (2008)
8. Mo Phoenix, K.H., Malik Sumaira, H., S, C.N.: Gender differences in computer-mediated communication: a systematic literature review of online health-related support groups. Patient Educ. Couns. **75**, 16–24 (2009)
9. White, M., Dorman, SM.: Receiving social support online: implications for health education. Health Educ. Res. **16**(6), 693–707 (2001)
10. Charles, C.A., et al.: Shared treatment decision making: what does it mean to physicians? J. Clin. Oncol. **21**, 932–936 (2003)
11. Godolphin, W.: The role of risk communication in shared decision making: first, let's get to choices. BMJ **327**, 692–693 (2003)
12. Lau, D.H.: Patient empowerment—a patient-centred approach to improve care. Hong Kong Med J. **8**(5), 372–374 (2002)
13. Bos, L., et al.: Patient 2.0 empowerment. In: Proceedings of International Conference on Semantic Web and Web Services, pp. 164–168 (2008)
14. Hawn, C.: Take two aspirin and tweet me in themorning: how twitter, facebook and other social media are reshaping healthcare. Health Aff. **28**, 361–368 (2009)
15. Forkner, D.J.: Internet-based patient self-care: the next generation of health care delivery. J. Med. Internet Res. **2**(5), e8 (2003)
16. Eysenbach, G., et al.: Health related virtual communities and electronic support groups: systematic review of the effects of online peer to peer interactions. BMJ **328**, 1166–1171 (2004)
17. AlGhamdi, K.M., Moussa, N.A.: Internet use by the public to search for health-related information. Int. J. Med. Informatics **6**(81), 363–373 (2012)
18. Azienda Ospedaliera Niguarda Ca' Granda. Niguarda Hospital. Health care and Culture: Regione Lombardia
19. Cohen, J.: Statistical power analysis for the behavioral sciences. New York University, New York (1988)
20. Cronbach, L.J.: Coefficient alpha and the internal structure of tests. Psychometrika **13**(3), 297–334 (1951)

Construction and Evaluation of Bayesian Networks Related to the Specific Health Checkup and Guidance on Metabolic Syndrome

Yoshiaki Miyauchi and Haruhiko Nishimura

Abstract Metabolic syndrome has become a significant problem worldwide, and health checkups and guidance aimed at preventing this condition were initiated in 2008 in Japan. Through this guidance, people considered at high risk of developing metabolic syndrome are expected to be made aware of their own problems in terms of their daily lifestyle choices and to improve their daily life behaviors by themselves. To this end, the instructors should be able to supply satisfactory and evidence-based information for these subjects. In order to support this large undertaking from the point of information technology, we here introduce our novel ideas based on data mining technology using Bayesian networks. The Bayesian network has emerged in recent years as a powerful technique for handling uncertainty in complex domains, and it is expected to represent an appropriate method for the health checkup domain, where medical knowledge is required for the analysis of the results. In this study, we constructed Bayesian networks connecting the findings from a physical examination and questionnaire on daily lifestyle choices, and evaluated the relationship between them. We applied these network models to the field data of 5423 subjects. The proposed method was found to provide good performance, and its usefulness was revealed by evaluating the level of change of the responses to the questionnaire.

Keywords Metabolic syndrome · Bayesian networks · Specific health checkup

---

Y. Miyauchi (✉)
College of Life and Health Sciences, Chubu University, 1200 Matsumoto-cho, Kasugai, Aichi 487-8501, Japan
e-mail: yomiyauchi@isc.chubu.ac.jp

H. Nishimura
Graduate School of Applied Informatics, University of Hyogo, 7-1-28 Minatojima-minami, Chuo-ku, Kobe 650-0047, Japan
e-mail: haru@ai.u-hyogo.ac.jp

Y.-W. Chen et al. (eds.), *Innovation in Medicine and Healthcare 2015*,
Smart Innovation, Systems and Technologies 45,
DOI 10.1007/978-3-319-23024-5_17

1 Introduction

Metabolic syndrome has become a major problem worldwide. In Japan, a health diagnostics and guidance program, known as "specific health checkups," was initiated in 2008 [1]. This health guidance, which targets subjects deemed at high risk of lifestyle-related diseases such as metabolic syndrome, aims to prevent the transition to such lifestyle-related diseases. It is necessary that the examinees themselves recognize the changes, both mental and physical, by understanding the medical examination results, and that they reflect on their lifestyle. Moreover, under the support of this health guidance, it is hoped that the examinees will be able to improve their health on their own. In other words, we believe that, in order to function effectively, it is important for the specific health checkup program to promote behavioral changes of the examinees in a manner that emphasizes individuality and to reduce their risks of lifestyle-related diseases by considering the circumstances of the individual examinees. To achieve this goal, we believe that further development and enhancement of the interface environment between the examinees and their health guidance providers are important.

From the perspective of data management, in the near future, interannual data from tens of millions of people across the country will be accumulated, and the development of a national health database is expected. However, this effort should not be stopped at only reference and statistical analyses by mere data accumulation. To help effectively utilize the research results in individual health guidance for supporting metabolic syndrome management in the clinical setting, it is insufficient to only perform research at the typical database level. To support such a large project from the point of information technology, we here introduce our novel idea based on Bayesian network data mining techniques [2]. Bayesian networks have emerged in recent years as a powerful technique for handling uncertainties in complex domains, and are an appropriate method for differentially analyzing a framework of a particular medical examination based on medical knowledge [3–6].

In this study, we constructed a Bayesian network that connects information obtained from a questionnaire regarding everyday lifestyle patterns and from physical examination findings, and examined its usefulness for providing health guidance information. We aimed to develop an information-providing tool that can be individualized for each health guidance examinee in order to provide health care solutions specifically designed for that person.

2 Preparation and Construction

2.1 Study Subjects

In this study, we studied the medical examination findings and results of a lifestyle-related questionnaire of 5423 anonymous male participants who underwent a health examination in certain establishments for two consecutive years. The following specific health checkup items were evaluated: waist circumference (cm), systolic blood pressure (mmHg), diastolic blood pressure (mmHg), neutral fat (mg/dl), high-density lipoprotein (HDL) cholesterol (mg/dl), fasting blood glucose level (mg/dl), glycated hemoglobin (HbA1c; %), and body mass index (BMI; kg/m2). The questionnaire included 36 multiple-choice questions (4-5 possible answers each), with 12 questions each related to the exercise, nutrition, and lifestyle habits of the subject. One question about smoking habits had only two possible answers. We allocated a numerical value of 1–5 points to the interview data based on the appropriate degree of choice. The potential sum of all 36 questions ranged from 36 to 180 points.

2.2 Layered Method Based on the Medical Examination Data

The health guidance of the specific health checkup consists of four layers, namely the positive and motivational support levels, the information provision level, and the excluded health guidance level, based on the medical examination results. Table 1 shows the concrete method used. The results of applying this hierarchical method (called stratification) to the data from the 5423 male participants described in the previous section are shown in Table 2.

2.3 Binary Representation of the Examination Data

As is clear from previous reports [7, 8] on the risk factors of metabolic syndrome, the following pairs of factors included in our inspection data are known to contribute to the risk of metabolic syndrome: (1) waist circumference and BMI, (2) fasting blood glucose and HbA1c, (3) neutral fat and HDL cholesterol, and (4) systolic and diastolic blood pressures. Therefore, as an expression of health according to the inspection data, these data (body shape, blood sugar, lipids, and blood pressure) can be represented by 4-bit representation of the 16 potential outcomes, ranging from the (0000) state to (1111) state, where 1 is defined as one or both of the two items of each factor being outside the reference value/range, and 0 is defined as both items being inside the reference (Fig. 1). In this study, we used these 16 states to determine the health condition of the examinees and for the classification of the learning data to the Bayesian network.

Table 1 Stratification of the health guidance into four levels

Step 1: Judge the risk of visceral fat accumulation by the waist circumference and BMI
I. Waist circumference ≥ 85 cm in male (90 cm in female)
II. Waist circumference < 85 cm in male (90 cm in female) and BMI ≥ 25
Step 2: Count additional risks from the results of physical tests and questionnaire
(1) Blood glucose: Fasting blood glucose ≥ 100 mg/dl or HbA1c ≥ 5.6 %, or Receiving drug treatment (<–checked from questionnaire)
(2) Lipid: Triglyceride ≥150 mg/dl or HDL cholesterol <40 mg/dl, or Receiving drug treatment
(3) Blood pressure: Systolic BP ≥130 mmHg or Diastolic BP ≥85 mmHg or Receiving drug treatment
(4) Smoking: Experienced (<–checked from questionnaire)
* (4) is included only if at least one risk exists throughout (1)–(3)
Step 3: Classify into four health guidance levels
For the examinees who correspond to the case I in Step 1,
According to the number of additional risks in (1)–(4) (– >abbreviate to #ARs):
If #ARs ≥ 2, then [Positive support] level
If #ARs = 1, then [Motivation support] level
If #ARs = 0, then [Information provision] level
For the examinees who correspond to the case II in Step 1,
If #ARs ≥ 3, then [Positive support] level
If #ARs = 1 or 2, then [Motivation support] level
If #ARs = 0, then [Information provision] level
And the others are classified into [Excluded health guidance] level.

Table 2 Results of applying the hierarchical method for the 5423 examinees

Case I in Step 1		
Positive support level	Motivation support level	Information provision
1328 people (24.5 %)	332 people (6.1 %)	552 people (10.2 %)
Case II in Step 1		
Positive support level	Motivation support level	Information provision
22 people (0.4 %)	59 people (1.1 %)	30 people (0.6 %)

2.4 Bayesian Network and Its Application

In the specific health checkup, the risk factors are quantified on the basis of the lifestyle questionnaire and the results of the physical examination, and the examinees are stratified into four levels (active support, motivational support, information provision, and excluded health guidance) according to the medical examination reference values (RV); subsequently, health guidance is offered. Thus, in this study, we constructed Bayesian networks with each node on a single network [9], where the

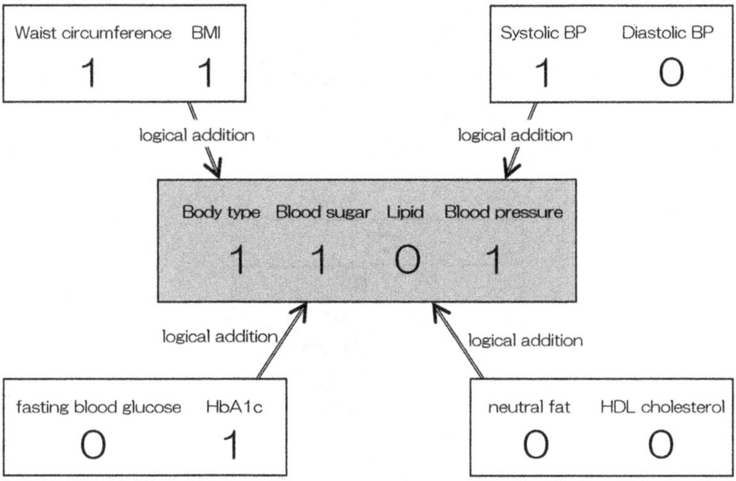

Fig. 1 Example of the binary representation of the examination data (BMI, body mass index; BP, blood pressure; HbA1c, glycated hemoglobin; HDL, high-density lipoprotein)

linked structures include the node of information from the lifestyle questionnaire, the node of the physical examination results indicating a health condition, the node representing the results of the hierarchical data described above, and the node representing the health status according to the 16 different states (Figs. 2, 3, 4, 5 and 6).

Figure 2 shows an example of a node for "waist circumference", and is represented by a two-state medical examination value: >85 cm (shown as "out of RV") and <85 cm ("in RV"). In this case, the probability of the state in RV (expressed as a percentage), indicates that 59.4 % of the examinees belonged to the state inside the RV.

Figure 3 shows an example of the interview node "Q1", and the 5 states, ranging from 1 to 5 points (Sect. 2.1), are represented. For example, the probability of 3 points of question Q1 was found to be 37.9 %. The average value (2.75 $\pm$ 1.1 points) is displayed at the bottom.

Figure 4 shows a hierarchical node ("Stratification"); the four support levels in the hierarchy of Sect. 2.2 are shown, namely the positive support level ("positive sup"), motivational support level ("motivation sup"), information provision level ("info prov"), and the level of excluded health guidance ("no need"). For example, the probability of a positive support level was 24.9 %, indicating that 24.9 % of the 5423 men had been layered to a positive support level.

Figure 5 shows the 16 health states-representation node ("16 conditions"); it is represented by the 16 states, ranging from the (0000) state to the (1111) state, according to the 4-bit representation described in Sect. 2.3. In the figure, the probability of the (0000) state, which represents the most healthy state, is 28.2 %, and the probability of the (1111) state, the least healthy state, is 3.53 %.

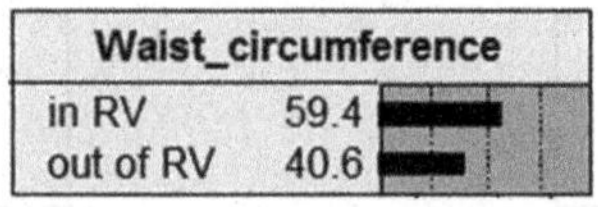

Fig. 2 Physical examination node: Waist circumference (RV, reference value)

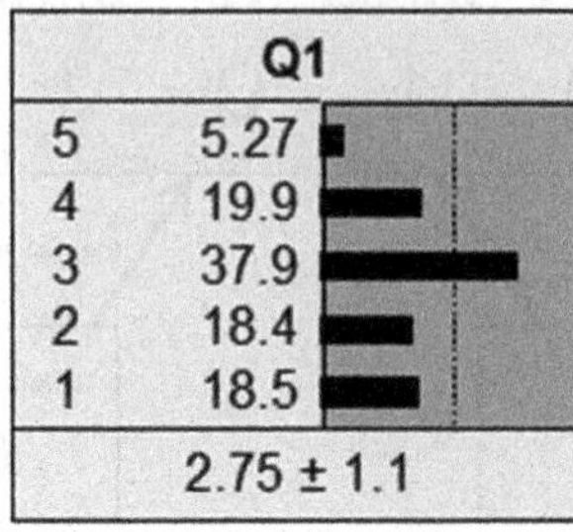

Fig. 3 Lifestyle questionnaire node: Q1

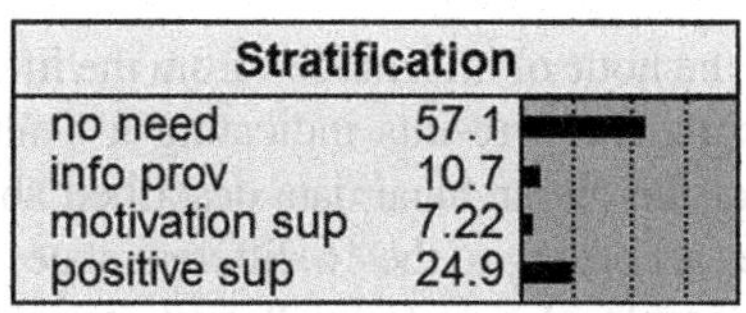

Fig. 4 Support level hierarchical node: Stratification

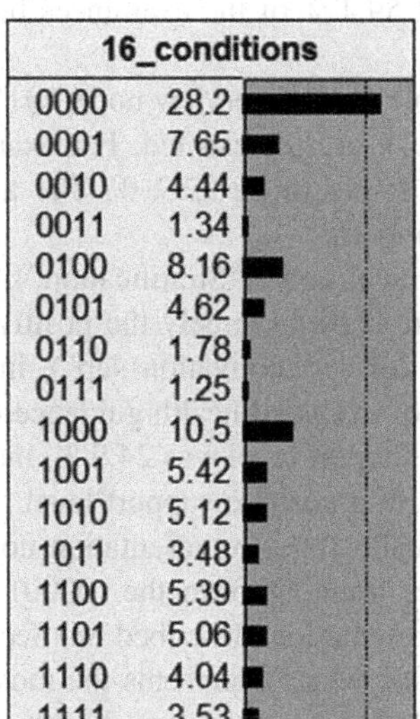

Fig. 5 The 16 health states representation node: 16 conditions

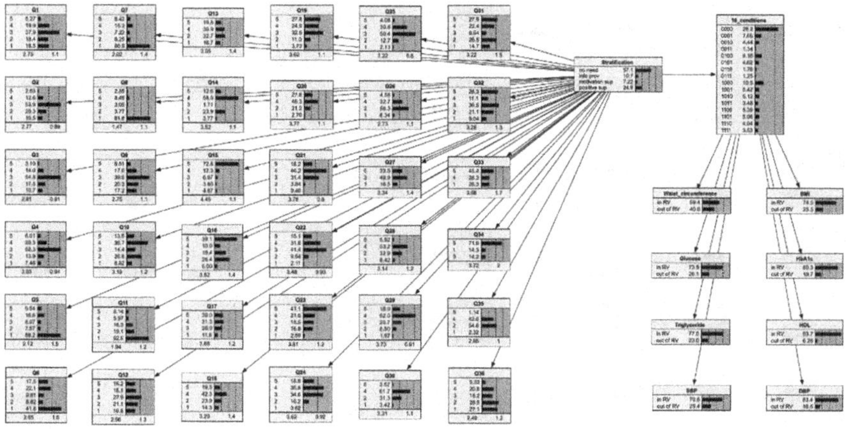

Fig. 6 Bayesian network for the specific health checkups on metabolic syndrome (BMI, body mass index; HbA1c, glycated hemoglobin; HDL, high-density lipoprotein; SBP, systolic blood pressure; DBP, diastolic blood pressure)

Figure 6 shows an overall picture of the Bayesian network constructed. We calculated the conditional probability using the health data of the 5423 examinees. All 36 question nodes (Q1-Q36) are shown on the left side. The lower right side shows the check node group with 8 nodes, namely the waist circumference, BMI, fasting blood glucose ("Glucose"), HbA1c, neutral fat ("Triglyceride"), HDL cholesterol ("HDL"), systolic blood pressure ("SBP"), and diastolic blood pressure ("DBP") nodes. The upper right indicates the 16 health states node ("16 conditions"), and the hierarchical node ("Stratification") is shown in the center of the figure.

3 Evaluation

Based on the results of the specific health checkup of examinee A, we evaluated our Bayesian network. Examinee A is a 56-year-old man (height, 165.9 cm) who had not received oral treatment for lifestyle-related diseases. All his inspection items, except for HbA1c and HDL cholesterol, were outside of the reference values, indicating a typical metabolic syndrome (1111) state according to the 16 health state-representation. He was a typical example of an individual belonging to the positive support level. Figure 7 shows a Bayesian network based on the questionnaire data of examinee A.

For evaluating our Bayesian network, we questioned what changes would occur in the health status of examinee A if he was able to change his behavior in terms of his lifestyle habits. In his questionnaire, he provided unsuitable answers to the question group about exercise. When the scores of the 6 questions relating to

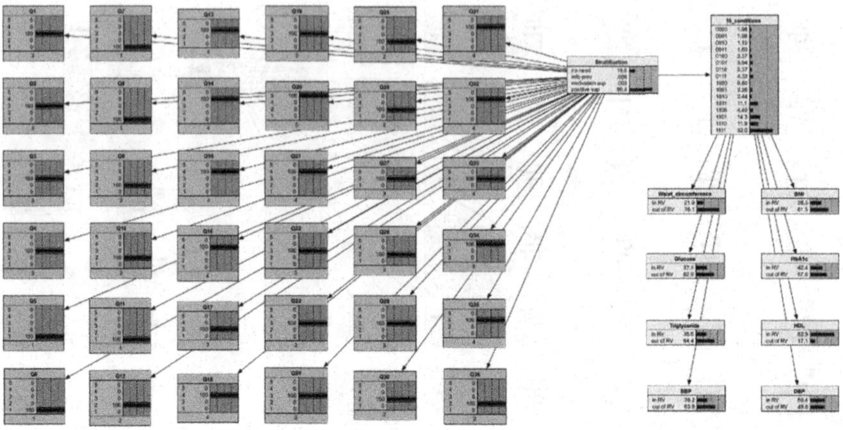

Fig. 7 Setting nodes based on the case of examinee A (BMI, body mass index; HbA1c, glycated hemoglobin; HDL, high-density lipoprotein; SBP, systolic blood pressure; DBP, diastolic blood pressure)

exercise were set as the highest scores, the probability that he would remain in the (1111) state decreased from 32.0 to 11.7 %, and the possibility of improvement to the (1000) state increased from 0.80 to 10.7 % (Fig. 8). That is, improving the lifestyle factors relating to exercise was expected to improve the health condition of the examinee.

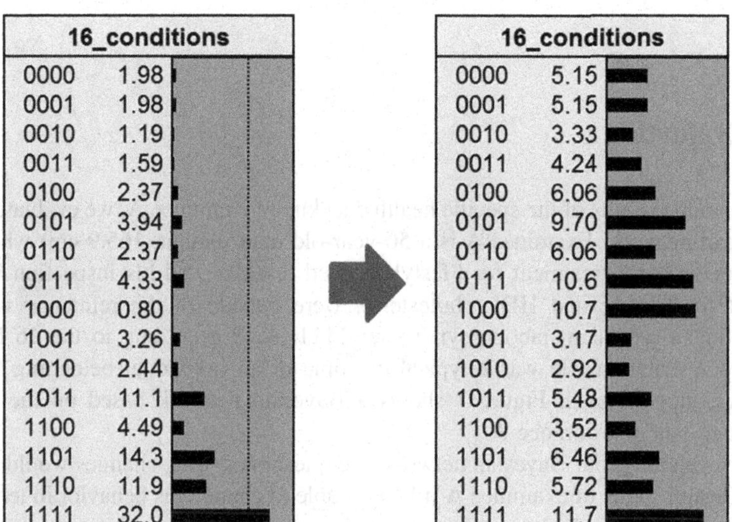

Fig. 8 Outcomes when the answers to the 6 questions relating to exercise were changed

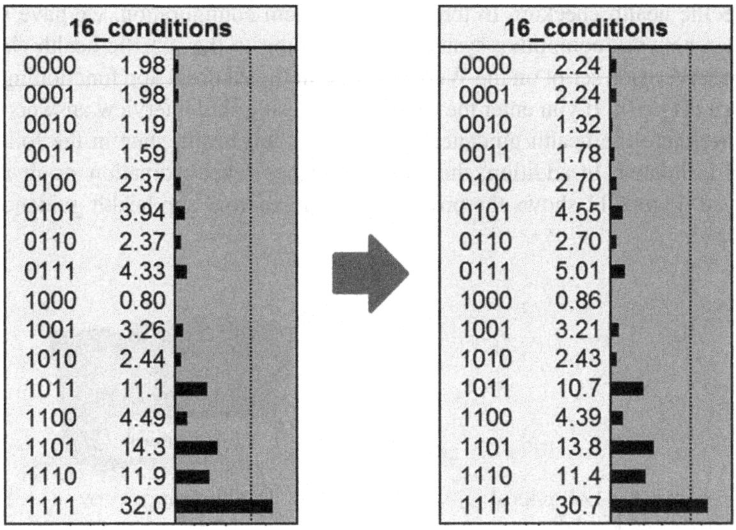

Fig. 9 Outcomes when the answers to the 6 questions relating to nutrition were changed

On the other hand, when we set the 6 questions relating to nutrition to the highest scores, the probability to stay in the (1111) state barely changed, decreasing from 32.0 to 30.7 % (Fig. 9). This indicates that, in the case of health guidance to examinee A, encouragement to exercise, rather than improving his diet, is expected to show positive effects on his health condition.

4 Conclusion and New Challenges

As described in the previous section, by showing the individual data directly to each examinee, the variations in the probability of disease according to the potential lifestyle changes are expected to provide the opportunity for the individual to initiate such lifestyle behavior changes. Based on our findings in this study, we consider our Bayesian network, which corresponds to the specific health checkup, to have the potential to become an effective tool for improving the chances of changing the lifestyle-related behavior of individual examinees. In this study, we were able to preliminary confirm the potential of this tool; however, it is desirable to simplify the use of Bayesian networks for the public health nurses actually performing the health guidance. Hence, as a new challenge, we are currently working on the development of Android apps, which are very common and are being increasingly used in recent years.

This Android health guidance tool will be simple to use and easy to understand, using a touch panel input. Internally, the system performs the probability estimation by the Bayesian network of outcome described in this study, which corresponds to the specific health checkup. In terms of the system configuration, we have built a Bayesian network computing system corresponding to the specific health checkup using a server-side script on the Web server, with the Android app functioning as an interface (Fig. 10). If you enter the examination results and interview answers of the examinees into the health guidance application, their health state in the following year is estimated. In addition, the health guidance level estimation result is also displayed. Figure 11 shows the prototype of the Android app health guidance tool developed.

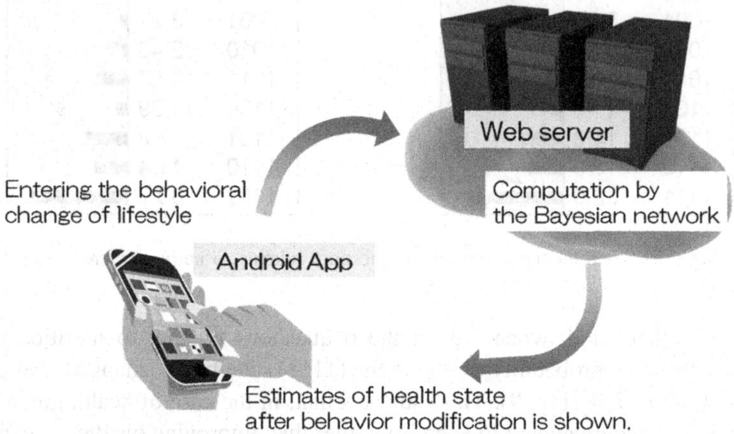

Fig. 10 Android health guidance application

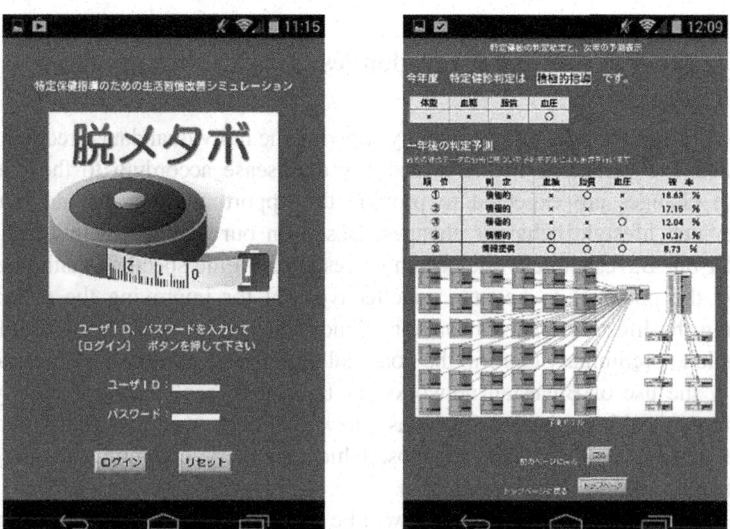

Fig. 11 Representative health guidance application screen shots

References

1. Specific Health Checkups and Specific Health Guidance. The Health Service Bureau of the Ministry of Health, Labour and Welfare (2007)
2. Miyauchi, Y., Nishimura, H.: Bayesian network for healthcare of metabolic syndrome. IEEE EMBC2013, Osaka, Short paper No. 3164 (2013)
3. Park, H.S., Cho, S.B.: An efficient attribute ordering optimization in Bayesian networks for prognostic modeling of the metabolic syndrome. ICIC2006, LNBI4115, pp. 381–391. Springer (2006)
4. Gamez, J., Moral, S., Salmeron, A. (eds.): Advances in Bayesian Networks. Springer, New York (2004)
5. Maglogiannis, I., Zafiropoulos, E., Platis, A., Lambrinoudakis, C.: Risk analysis of a patient monitoring system using Baysian network modeling. J. Biomed. Inform. **39**(6), 637–647 (2006)
6. Lee, S.M., Abbott, P.A.: Bayesian network for knowledge discovery in large datasets. J. Biomed. Inform. **36**, 389–399 (2003)
7. Shen, B., Todaro, J.F., Niaura, R., McCaffery, J.M., Zhang, J., Spiro III, A., Ward, K.D.: Are metabolic risk factors one unified syndrome? modeling the structure of the metabolic syndrome X. Am. J. Epidemiol. **157**, 701–711 (2003)
8. Shah, S., Novak, S., Stapleton, L.M.: Evaluation and comparison of models of metabolic syndrome using confirmatory factor analysis. Eur. J. Epidemiol. **21**, 343–349 (2006)
9. Netica User's Guide. http://www.norsys.com/. Application for Belief Network and Influence Diagrams

Medical Care Delivery at the XXVII World Summer Universiade Kazan 2013

Timur Mishakin, Elena Razumovskaya, Michael Popov and Olga Berdnikova

Abstract Medical care system is one of the important part in terms of the international sports events. It is clear that one of the key factors of success of international multi-sport competitions such as Olympic Games and Universiade is well established system of medical care delivery. The purpose of this paper was to analyze experience of the XXVII World Summer Universiade 2013 and to propose a practical framework methodology to assist construction of the health care system and medical service system in terms of mass international sporting events.

Keywords Health care system · Medical service · Mass gatherings · International sporting events

1 Introduction

Singularities of mass international sport events are: mass gatherings; the international level of the event; the probability of sports injuries among athletes, the need for athletes training and preparation, the doping control; the probability of emergency situations when a lot of people need medical assistance.

Accordingly to singularities such events are require a well-planned medical care system.

Physicians are increasingly called upon to provide medical support for mass gatherings such as concerts, sporting events, political conventions, and other special events. Until recently, individuals planning such support have had little reliable information to assist them in determining what specific personnel and equipment are necessary to optimally support a mass gathering [3].

T. Mishakin (✉) · E. Razumovskaya · M. Popov · O. Berdnikova
Kazan Federal University, 18 Kremlyovskaya Str., Kazan, Russia420008
e-mail: timur.mishakin@mail.ru

Y.-W. Chen et al. (eds.), *Innovation in Medicine and Healthcare 2015*,
Smart Innovation, Systems and Technologies 45,
DOI 10.1007/978-3-319-23024-5_18

The Universiade, often referred to as the World University Games, is an international multi-sport event, organized by the International University Sports Federation (FISU) for university athletes and is important second only to the Olympic Games.

XXVII World Summer Universiade 2013 was hosted in Kazan (Russia) during 6th to 17th July 2013. It was the most ambitious Universiade ever with the participation of 7980 athletes and 3798 officials from 160 countries [1]. For example, XXIV Summer Universiade 2005 in Bangkok had 6093 athletes from 152 countries [6]. The paper contains a comparison of some indicators between the two largest Universiade.

Experience of the XXVII World Summer Universiade 2013 in Kazan can be called the most successful and efficient. Preparation of medical service system played one of the main role in success of this event.

Kazan is the capital of the economically stable and dynamically developing subordinate entity of the Russian Federation—The Republic of Tatarstan. Kazan has 1.2 million citizens.

In 2005, the city celebrated the 1000th anniversary of its foundation. The city is inhabited by more than 100 nationalities, people of Christian, Muslim and other faiths, and is famous for it's good neighborliness and tolerance. Large-scale international competitions, which were held in Kazan, showed that the capital of Tatarstan has all the required resources, including human, for organizing such events on a high level.

All this determined the success of Kazan in bidding the right to hold the XXVII World Summer Universiade 2013. On May 31, 2008 The International University Sports Federation (FISU) in Brussels decided to hold the XXVII World Summer Universiade 2013 in Kazan.

Such large-scale events, on the one hand, need all resources to be concentrated, such as: material, organizational, intellectual, and on the other hand, provide a unique opportunity to develop the entire town infrastructure, economy, training, education, culture and student sport [4].

From this historical point of view, the highly symbolic dates associated with Student games 2013 in Kazan are being clarified: the 90th anniversary of the World Student Games in Paris and the 40th anniversary since the VII summer Student games in Moscow [2].

2 Main Activities and Indicators

Medical support of the Universiade 2013 was organized in accordance with the minimum requirements of the International University Sports Federation and the Concept of health, doping and sanitary-epidemiological security of the XXVII World Summer Universiade 2013 in Kazan.

Concept implementation plan included the following major sections:

1. Legal provision of medical care during the Universiade;
2. Construction and equipping of health facilities involved in medical support of the Universiade.
3. Staffing of the of health facilities involved in the medical and sanitary-epidemiological provision of the Universiade.
4. The organization of health care to participants and guests of the Universiade.
5. Health and sanitation activities in emergency situations during the Universiade.
6. Provision of sanitary and epidemiological welfare during the Universiade.
7. Anti-Doping providing of the Universiade.

The following measures have been implemented in preparing medical support for the Universiade 2013, Kazan:

- Specially created headquarters worked at the Ministry of Health.
- Universiade Village Medical Center was commissioned and equipped;
- The Emergency Hospital was constructed, commissioned and equipped;
- Health centers for athletes and visitors was opened and equipped;
- On-site medical centers for athletes and visitors was opened and equipped;
- 35 health medical posts for spectators and 55 for athletes were deployed on sports facilities
- Mobile medical teams was created;
- 28 ambulances class "B" and 39 class "C" was bought;
- Ambulance crews was provided in accordance with the schedule of events;
- Medical-evacuation plan, including air medical evacuation, was approved;
- Inspection exercises of medical facilities were held to prevent the proliferation of dangerous infections;
- Sanitary environment monitoring was carried out in Kazan;
- Laboratory monitoring of air quality, water and soil was carried out during the Universiade;
- Universiade staff and volunteers vaccination was carried out;
- Sanitary and quarantine epidemiology station was created;
- Anti-Doping supporting of the Universiade was carried out.

2.1 *Staffing*

An indispensable condition of perfect medical providing of the Games is the preparation and selection of medical personnel.

According to changes in Russian legislation, medical specialists of foreign teams had the right to carry out medical care of their teams in Russian Federation without passing the admission procedure for the implementation of medical and pharmaceutical activity.

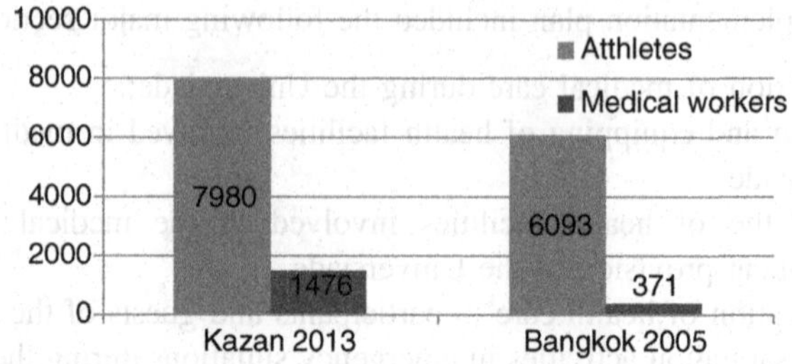

Fig. 1 The ratio of medical workers and athletes in Bangkok and Kazan

An important aspect of the preparations for the international sporting events is English language training courses for staff; 1100 medical workers were trained in English.

To work at the University Games were held in 1476 medical workers, including 167 specialists of Federal Medical and Biological Agency, 719 doctors and 757 nurses from hospitals in Tatarstan, 138 mobile teams, 1 aero-medical team worked at the University Games.

To compare with, XXIV Summer Universiade 2005 in Bangkok had only 371 medical workers [6].

Figure 1 indicates the ratio of medical workers and athletes on Universiade in Bangkok and Kazan.

587 medical volunteers worked at the Universiade in Kazan. The volunteers were members of the mobile teams, they assisted medical staff in health centers of sports facilities and ambulance crews. Also, volunteers worked in the Universiade Village Medical Center, hospitals of the Universiade, accompanied the athletes during hospitalization.

2.2 *Medical Facilities*

Seven Universiade Hospitals were provided a 24 h care system in order to keep medical support for all client groups of the Universiade 2013:

- The Republican Clinical Hospital;
- The Children's Republican Clinical Hospital;
- The Interregional Clinical Diagnostic Center;
- The Republican Clinical Hospital of Infectious Diseases;
- The Emergency Hospital (City Hospital # 7);
- The Republican Clinical Ophthalmological hospital;
- The Medical Center in the Universiade Village

For example, The Emergency Hospital (City Hospital # 7), was one of the main hospitals of the Universiade 2013, which provided medical support during opening and closing ceremonies at the Kazan Arena stadium. It included diagnostic department and 12-storey surgical building with a total area of 41.5 thousand meters.

It should be noted that during the Summer Universiade 2005 in Bangkok only two hospitals were involved: The Athletes Village Polyclinic and The Thammasat Hospital [6].

Medical center was built and equipped in the international zone of the Universiade Village. Medical care provided to the participants and guests of the Universiade In the medical center around the clock. The emergency unit with traumatologic point, infectious unit, functional and beam diagnostics rooms, department of rehabilitation treatment, outpatient monitoring was presented in the Medical Center of the Universiade Village. Doping control station, rooms for FISU Medical Commission was operated in the Medical Center. Before and after the Universiade Medical Center operates as a city student polyclinic provides medical care and the students of Kazan. Before and after the Universiade Medical Center worked as a city student polyclinic.

2.3 *Delivery of Health Care*

An important direction in organization of medical support of the Universiade in Kazan was simulation exercises.

A detailed contingency plan for mass casualty scenarios with the inclusion of other hospitals and level-A trauma centers should be present during planning and execution of a major sporting event [7]. Due to possible additional threats, emergent particularly during the last few years, an inclusion of emergency services and law enforcement in contingency planning should be considered to address the threat of terror attacks [5].

Interdepartmental training exercises in the practical preparedness of medical facilities of Kazan to provide medical care to patients and suspicious on especially dangerous infections was held on May, 2013. “The blasting of explosive device on Perron Hall subway station” and “Spraying toxic substance in the train” were simulated for the exercise. A special tactical exercise on liquidation of consequences of caving the ceiling in the Palace of Sports in Kazan was held in a framework of medical support preparedness.

Operational exercises “4 days of the Universiade”, which simulate actual game days of the Universiade was held in June 2013. More than 1400 medical workers participated in this action.

A special connection between all medical workers was introduced. Each medical worker had a radio that worked over a dedicated channel. Thus, all the actions were coordinated.

From June 24 to July 20, 2013 the headquarters of the medical support organization has worked round the clock. The system of organization of medical support of the Universiade included medical assistance in sports facilities, in places of arrival, accommodation of participants, in hospitals, medical support opening and closing ceremonies of the Games.

On sports facilities, medical assistance was provided by the mobile medical teams, which were located in competition and training areas. The mobile team includes doctor, nurse, and a medical volunteer. Medical stations for athletes and first aid rooms to spectators were organized on sport objects.

Depending on the sport, the number of active competition and training venues the total number of medical workers who were at the site at the same time, varied from 8 to 20 people.

According to procedure of hospitalization of client group, inpatient care to athletes, family members of FISU, judges, representatives of the media provided by 6 hospitals of the Universiade.

The medical service provided care for 12940 people that had accreditation for Universiade 2013 in Kazan, 3340 of cases were a result of sports injuries and 9600 of them were a result of common diseases, 158 people were hospitalized.

3 Conclusion

Providing medical care in the mass gathering sport events is a big challenge for the medical teams. Experience of the XXVII World Summer Universiade 2013 in Kazan can be called the most successful and efficient. Although the number of participants, medical assistance was provided on time and efficiently. This paper provides information on medical organization and overall medical care provided during the XXVII World Summer Universiade 2013.

This information might be useful for planning medical services in international multi-sport competitions in the future.

References

1. Burganov R.T.: Some results of XXVII world summer student games 2013 in Kazan. Teoriya i Praktika Fizicheskoy Kultury. No. 1 (2014)
2. Gafurov, I.R.: Historical traditions and development of university sport in Kazan university today. Teoriya i Praktika Fizicheskoy Kultury. No. 1 (2014)
3. Grange, J.T.: Planning for large events. Curr. Sports Med. Rep. **3**, 156–161 (2002)
4. Kadyrov A.R.: The effect from XXVII world summer students games on regional development. Teoriya i Praktika Fizicheskoy Kultury. No. 1 (2014)
5. Keim, M.E., Williams, D.: Hospital use by Olympic athletes during the 1996 Atlanta Olympic Games. Med. J. Aust. **167**, 603–605 (1997)

6. Lertwanich, P. et al.: Medical services during the 24th summer universiade. Siriraj Med. **63**, 8–11 (2011)
7. Milne, C., Shaw, M., Steinweg, J.: Medical issues relating to the Sydney Olympic Games. Sports Med. **28**, 287–298 (1999)

Part IV
Advanced ICT for Medical and Healthcare

Coccurrence Statistics of Local Ternary Patterns for HEp-2 Cell Classification

Xian-Hua Han, Yen-Wei Chen and Gang Xu

Abstract In this paper, we describe a novel image representation strategy for classifying HEp-2 cell patterns of fluorescence staining. Our proposed strategy extends local binary patterns (LBPs), which are state-of-the-art texture features, into local ternary patterns (LTPs) with data-driven thresholds according to Weber's law, a human perception principle; further, our approach incorporates the contexts of spatial and orientation co-occurrences among adjacent Weber-based local ternary patterns (WLTPs) for texture representation. The explored WLTP is formulated by adaptively quantizing differential values between neighborhood pixels and the focused pixel as negative or positive stimuli if the normalized differential values are large; otherwise the stimulus is set to 0. Our approach here is based on the fact that human perception of a distinguished pattern depends not only on the absolute intensity of the stimulus but also on the relative variance of the stimulus. By integrating spatial and orientation context information, we further propose a rotation invariant co-occurrence WLTP (RICWLTP) approach to be more discriminant for image representation. Through experiment on the open HEp-2 cell dataset used at the ICIP2013 contest, we confirmed that our proposed strategy can greatly improve recognition performance or achieve comparable performance as compared with state-of-the-art LBP-based descriptor, the conventional LTP, and adaptively codebook/model based methods.

1 Introduction

Indirect immunofluorescence (IIF) is a standard visualization technique for the determining autoantibodies and antibodies against infectious agents; this technique is widely used as a diagnostic tool via image analysis [1]. In IIF, the human larynx carcinoma (HEp-2) substrate is applied, and recognition of the HEp-2 cell pattern is

X.-H. Han (✉) · Y.-W. Chen · G. Xu
College of Information Science and Engineering, Ritsumeikan University,
Shiga 525-8577, Japan
e-mail: hanxhua@fc.ritsumei.ac.jp

Y.-W. Chen et al. (eds.), *Innovation in Medicine and Healthcare 2015*,
Smart Innovation, Systems and Technologies 45,
DOI 10.1007/978-3-319-23024-5_19

then used to identify antinuclear autoantibodies (ANA). The common ANA analysis using IIF is typically conducted by an expert who recognizes the staining patterns of HEp-2 cells through a fluorescence microscope; however, the practical procedure remains subjective, which not only needs highly specialized and experienced technicians or physicians to achieve acceptable diagnostic results but it is also time-consuming. Therefore, in this study, we focus on the automatic identification of Hep-2 staining patterns using progressive techniques developed in computer vision and machine learning. Previously, several attempts to construct automated system for HEp-2 staining pattern recognition have already been tried. Soda and Iannello [2] investigated a multiple expert system (MES) in which an ensemble of classifiers was combined using a fusion technique to label the patterns of single cells. Cataldo et al. [3] used both a grey level co-occurrence matrix (GLCM) and discrete cosine transform features to represent texture information of cell images. Williem et al. [4] explored a means to adaptively learn representative prototypes (i.e., codebooks) with a discrete cosine transform feature and scale-invariant feature transform (SIFT) descriptors; the coded vectors using the codebook were integrated for HEp-2 cell representation. Han et al. [5] proposed to model the micro-structure (local patch) using Gaussian mixture process instead of binary/uniformly quantization, and achieved promising performance compared with some state-of-the-art approaches. However, it is difficult to integrate context information of co-occurrences for the codebook- or model-based strategy because of the diversity of the learned codebook or models. Another state-of-the-art texture representation approach is to use local binary patterns (LBPs), formulated by a simple binarization of differential values between neighborhood pixels and a focus pixel [6]. LBP is robust against uniform changes and easy to extend because of the regularly decimated levels for all neighborhood pixels. Several HEp-2 cell classification systems using LBP-based descriptors that have shown acceptable performance levels [7] already exit; however, because of the lack of spatial relationships between local textures, these approaches have serious disadvantages in the original LBP representation. Therein, an extension of LBP called CoLBP [8] was proposed by considering the co-occurrence (spatial context) among adjacent LBPs [9]; this approach appeared promising performance for HEp-2 cell classification [7]. In addition, by integrating orientation context, Nosaka et al. explored a rotation invariant co-occurrence using LBP, which further improved recognition performances on HEp-2 cell classification as compared to CoLBP. Qi et al. [10] proposed a pairwise rotation invariant CoLBP for HEp-2 cell representation and achieved the best recognition performance combined with conventional BOF with SIFT descriptors on the second HEp-2 cell classification contest in ICIP2013.

Although LBP-based descriptors showed promising performances as compared to other feature representations, LBP only sets differential values between neighborhood pixels and the focus pixel to zero or one, which causes high sensitivity to noise existing in the processed image. Tan et al. extended LBP to a local ternary pattern (LTP) approach [11] that considers differential values between neighborhood pixels and the focused pixel as either a negative/positive stimulus or no stimulus whatsoever; they successfully applied their technique to facial recognition under difficult

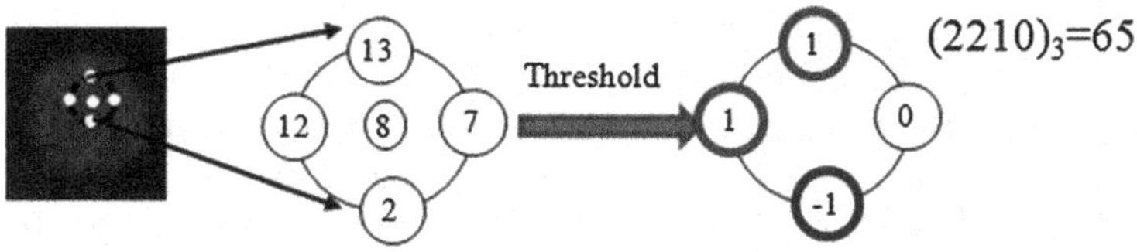

Fig. 1 The procedure of the proposed WLTP extraction

lighting conditions. Given a preset positive threshold η, LTP [11] was able to obtain a series of ternary values for local pattern representation; however, regardless of the magnitude of the focused pixel, the preset threshold η remained fixed, which violates the principle of human perception. Therefore, following the fact that human perception of a pattern depends not only on the absolute intensity of the stimulus but also on the relative variation of the stimulus, we propose quantizing the ratio between the neighborhood and center pixels, which is equivalent to adaptively deciding the quantization points according to the magnitude of the focused pixel (i.e., we take a data-driven approach). Our proposed quantization strategy is inspired by Weber's law, a psychological law, which states that the noticeable change of a stimulus such as sound or lighting by a human being forms a constant ratio with the original stimulus. When the stimulus has a small magnitude, a small change is noticeable. Thus, as illustrated in Fig. 1, we propose a Weber-based robust local ternary pattern (WLTP) approach that determines the activation status of neighborhood pixels by identifying data-driven thresholds for the noticeable change according to the stimulus of the focused pixel; more specifically, positive activation (i.e., a magnitude of 1) occurs if the ratio between the stimulus change and the focused pixel is larger than constant value η; further, negative activation (i.e., a magnitude of -1) occurs if the change ratio is less than η; finally, no activation (i.e., a magnitude of 0) occurs otherwise. By incorporating spatial and orientation contexts, we extend our proposed WLTP to a rotation invariant co-occurrence WLTP (RICWLTP) that handles image rotation and has high descriptive ability among WLTP co-occurrences. With extracted RICWLTP descriptors, we construct a support vector machine (SVM) classifier and automatically predict staining patterns of any input image. Experimental results on the open HEp-2 cell dataset used at the ICIP2013 contest show that the variability of recognition performance achieved by our proposed strategy was even significantly less than the observed intra-laboratory variability for both positive and intermediate intensity cell types.

2 Materials

The HEp-2 cell database used for our experimentation is made freely available for academic research from the second HEp-2 cell classification contest in ICIP2013. There are over 10,000 images in this dataset, each showing a single cell; images were obtained from 83 training IIF images by cropping in line with the bounding box of the cell. This HEp-2 dataset includes two intensity types of HEp-2 cells: intermediate and positive. The purpose of using this dataset for research is to recognize the staining pattern on the given intensity types. The studied staining patterns primarily include the following six classes, with available image numbers for positive and intermediate intensity types respectively shown in parentheses for each class: Homogeneous (1087, 1407); Speckled (1457, 1374); Nucleolar (934, 1664); Centromere (1387, 1364); NuMem (943, 1265); Golgi (347, 377). Please see the detailed explanation and example images in supplemental materials. Using the provided HEp-2 cell images and their corresponding patterns, we can extract features that are effective for image representation and train a classifier (i.e., a mapping function) using these extracted features of cell images and corresponding staining patterns. With the constructed classifier, the staining pattern can automatically be predicted given any HEp-2 cell image. In the next section, we describe our proposed methods for feature extraction from HEp-2 cell images.

3 Methods

Tan and Triggs [11] introduced local binary patterns (LBPs) as a means to summarize local gray-level structures. As noted above, LBP is a simple yet efficient texture operator that labels pixels of an image by establishing thresholds for the neighborhood of each pixel based on the value of the central pixel; the result is a binary number associated with each neighborhood pixel. Because LBP only sets differential values between neighborhood pixels and the focused pixel to zero or one, it has high sensitivity to noise in the processed image that in turn degrades discriminant image representation. Thus, as noted above, Tan et al. extended LBP to a local ternary pattern (LTP) approach [11], which considers differential values between neighborhood pixels and the focused pixel as either a negative/positive stimulus or no stimulus whatsoever. Next the series of ternary values are combined into an LTP index. Given intensities $[I(\mathbf{x}), I(\mathbf{x}+\triangle\mathbf{x}_1), \ldots, I(\mathbf{x}+\triangle\mathbf{x}_l), \ldots, I(\mathbf{x}+\triangle\mathbf{x}_{L-1})]$ of focused pixel $\mathbf{x}$ and its L neighbors $\mathbf{x} + \triangle\mathbf{x}_l$ (displacement vector), LTP thresholds differential values $[I(\mathbf{x}+\triangle\mathbf{x})_0 - I(\mathbf{x}), \ldots, I(\mathbf{x}+\triangle\mathbf{x}_l) - I(\mathbf{x}), \ldots, I(\mathbf{x}+\triangle\mathbf{x}_{L-1}) - I(\mathbf{x})]$ as

$$G(I(\mathbf{x}+\triangle\mathbf{x}_l) - I(\mathbf{x})) = \begin{cases} 1 & I(\mathbf{x}+\triangle\mathbf{x}_l) - I(\mathbf{x}) > \eta \\ -1 & I(\mathbf{x}+\triangle\mathbf{x}_l) - I(\mathbf{x}) < -\eta \\ 0 & otherwise \end{cases} \quad (1)$$

where η is the pre-set constant for thresholding the differential values. Regardless of the magnitude of the focused pixel, preset threshold η in LTP remains fixed, which violates the principle of human perception.

3.1 Weber LTP

Weber's law states that the just noticeable difference (JND) is a constant proportion of the original stimulus magnitude that corresponds to the perception excitation domain of humans. This observation exhibits that the JND between two stimuli is proportional to the magnitude of the stimuli, and can be formulated as

$$\frac{\triangle I}{I} = a \tag{2}$$

where $\triangle I$ denotes the increment threshold, I denotes the initial stimulus intensity, and a is the *weber fraction*, which indicates that the proportion on the left-hand side of the equation remains constant in spite of variances in I.

According to this law, the JND of a focused pixel in relation to its neighboring pixels is proportional to intensity $I(\mathbf{x})$ of the focused pixel. Thus, we quantize different values $[I(\mathbf{x} + \triangle\mathbf{x}_0) - I(\mathbf{x}), \ldots, I(\mathbf{x} + \triangle\mathbf{x}_l) - I(\mathbf{x}), \ldots, I(\mathbf{x} + \triangle\mathbf{x}_{L-1}) - I(\mathbf{x})]$ between a focused pixel $\mathbf{x}$ and its $L - 1$ neighbors $\{\mathbf{x} + \triangle\mathbf{x}_l\}(l = 0, 1, \ldots, L - 1)$ to form a ternary series as the follows:

$$G\left(\frac{I(\mathbf{x} + \triangle\mathbf{x}_l) - I(\mathbf{x})}{I(\mathbf{x}) + \alpha}\right) = \begin{cases} 1 & \frac{I(\mathbf{x}+\triangle\mathbf{x}_l) - I(\mathbf{x})}{I(\mathbf{x})+\alpha} > \eta \\ -1 & \frac{I(\mathbf{x}+\triangle\mathbf{x}_l) - I(\mathbf{x})}{I(\mathbf{x})+\alpha} < -\eta \\ 0 & otherwise \end{cases} \tag{3}$$

where η is a predefined constant, and α is a constant that avoids the case in which there is zero intensity (i.e., no stimulus); we always set α to one in our experimentation. Equation (3) adaptively quantizes differential values between the focus pixel and its neighboring pixels into a series of ternary codes; the WLTP index at $\mathbf{x}$ is defined as

$$WLTP(\mathbf{x}) = \sum_{l=0}^{L-1} \left[G\left(\frac{I(\mathbf{x} + \triangle\mathbf{x}_l) - I(\mathbf{x})}{I(\mathbf{x}) + \alpha}\right) + 1\right] 3^l \tag{4}$$

In general LBP, neighborhood pixel number L is usually set to 8. Due to the detailed quantization (i.e., the ternary representation instead of binary), L is set to 4 to reduce computational cost. The lth displacement vector $\triangle\mathbf{x}_l$ is formulated as $\triangle\mathbf{x}_l = (\mathbf{r}\cos(\theta_l), \mathbf{r}\sin(\theta_l))$, where $\theta_l = \frac{360°}{L} l$ and $\mathbf{r}$ is the scale parameter (i.e., the distance from the neighboring pixels to the focused pixel) of WLTP. As a result, as shown in Fig. 1, WLTPs have $N_P = 81$ ($=3^L$) possible patterns.

3.2 Integration of Spatial and Orientation Contexts

WLTP discards information regarding spatial relationships between adjacent patterns; such information would be crucial to describing texture information for images. In this study, we first integrate the spatial context between the adjacent WLTPs via co-occurrence information (CoWLTP). To obtain statistics of the co-occurrence (i.e., the spatial context) between two adjacent WLTPs, we consider the $N_P \times N_P$ auto-correlation matrix defined as:

$$H^{\varphi}_{p,q} = \sum_{\mathbf{x} \subset \mathbf{I}} \delta_{p,q}(WLTP(\mathbf{x}), WLTP(\mathbf{x} + \triangle\mathbf{x}_{\varphi}))$$
$$\delta_{p,q}(z_1, z_2) = \begin{cases} 1 \text{ if } z_1 = p \text{ and } z_2 = q \\ 0 \text{ otherwise} \end{cases} \tag{5}$$

where p, q (=[0, 1, ..., $N_P - 1$]) are possible pattern indexes for the two adjacent WLTPs and φ is the angle that determines the positional relations between the two WLTPs, which formulates displacement vector $\triangle\mathbf{x}_{\varphi} = (d \cos\varphi, d \sin\varphi)$ with interval d. Then auto-correlation matrix dimension 6561 (=$N_P \times N_P$).

Further, because of the possible different imaging viewpoints, rotation invariant (i.e., orientation context) is generally an indispensable characteristic for texture image representation. Thus, we also integrate orientation context among adjacent WLTPs and propose a rotation invariant co-occurrence WLTPs that would contribute much higher descriptive capabilites for HEp-2 cell image representation. We first denote two pairs of WLTP patterns, $P^{WLTP}_{\varphi=0} = [WLTP(\mathbf{x}), WLTP(\mathbf{x} + \triangle\mathbf{x}_{\varphi=0})]$ and $P^{WLTP}_{\varphi} = [WLTP^{\varphi}(\mathbf{x}), WLTP^{\varphi}(\mathbf{x} + \triangle\mathbf{x}_{\varphi})]$, where $WLTP(\mathbf{x})$ gives the 4-bit clockwise ternary digits with the first digit in the right-horizontal direction ($\varphi = 0$), and $WLTP(\mathbf{x} + \triangle\mathbf{x}_{\varphi=0})$ is the co-occurrence WLTP in the $\varphi = 0$ direction; $WLTP^{\varphi}(\mathbf{x})$ and $WLTP^{\varphi}(\mathbf{x} + \triangle\mathbf{x}_{\varphi})$ indicate the rotated entire WLTP pair with rotation angle φ. Thus, the rotation invariant statistics can be formulated if we assign the same index to P^{WLTP}_{φ} regardless of the different rotations designated by φ. Because we only used 4 neighbors of the focused pixel, only 4 rotation angles (i.e., $\varphi = 0°, 90°, 180°, 270°$) are available for computing rotation invariant statistics as shown in Fig. 2 (i.e., 4 equivalent WLTP pairs). According to the assigned labels for rotation invariant WLTP, the valid co-occurrence patterns can be reduced from 6561 to 2222. To efficiently calculate the rotation invariant co-occurrence of WLTP, we use mapping table $\mathbf{M}$ according to the algorithm shown in Table 1; the algorithm is to generate mapping table that converts a WLTP pair to an equivalent rotation index. In Table 1, *shift*($(p)_3, l$) means circle-shift l bits of the transformed ternary digits of p. With the calculated mapping table, statistics of the rotation invariant co-occurrence WLTP can be formulated as

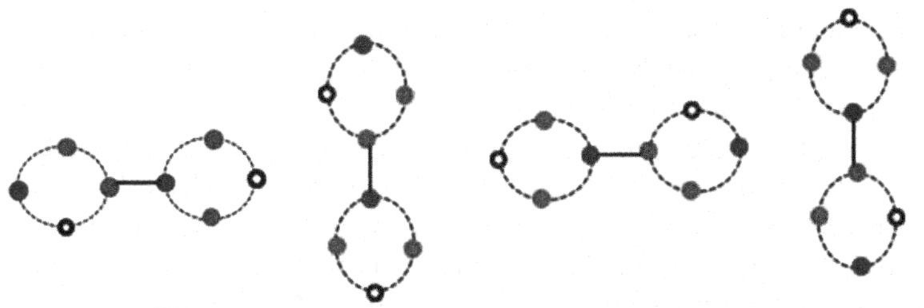

Fig. 2 The four equivalent WLTP pairs

Table 1 Calculation of mapping table between the WLTP pair and the rotation equivalent index

Mapping table generation algorithm
Input: Number of neighbor pixel L
Output: Mapping table $\mathbf{M}$ ($N_P \times N_P$ matrix)
Initialization: $Index$=1, $N_P = 3^L$, $\mathbf{M} \Leftarrow \{null\}^{N_P \times N_P}$
for: $p = 0, \ldots, N_P - 1$ and $q = 0, \ldots, N_P - 1$
if $M(p, q) = null$, **then**
$M(p, q) \Leftarrow Index, p' \Leftarrow shift((p)_3, 2), q' \Leftarrow shift((q)_3, 2), M(q', p') \Leftarrow Index$
$p' \Leftarrow shift((p)_3, 1), q' \Leftarrow shift((q)_3, 1), M(p', q') \Leftarrow Index$
$p' \Leftarrow shift((p)_3, 3), q' \Leftarrow shift((q)_3, 3), M(q', p') \Leftarrow Index$
$Index \Leftarrow Index + 1$
end if
end for

$$H^{RI}_{M(Index)} = \sum_{\mathbf{x} \subset \mathbf{I}} \bigcup_{\varphi} \delta^{index}[M(WLTP^{\varphi}(\mathbf{x}), WLTP^{\varphi}(\mathbf{x} + \triangle\mathbf{x}_{\varphi}))]$$
$$\delta^{index}(z) = \begin{cases} 1 \text{ if } z = index \\ 0 \text{ otherwise} \end{cases} \tag{6}$$

where $M(WLTP^{\varphi}(\mathbf{x}), WLTP^{\varphi}(\mathbf{x} + \triangle\mathbf{x}_{\varphi}))$ are the index of the rotation invariant co-occurrence between two WLTP pairs (RICWLTP). Finally, the statistics (i.e., histogram) of the RICWLTP can be used for discriminant representation of HEp-2 cell images.

4 Experimental Results

Given the HEp-2 cell dataset, we validate recognition performance for two types of intensities (i.e., intermediate and positive) using the statistics of our proposed WLTP, as well as spatial and orientation context integration in WLTP. We focused on the corresponding versions without the use of Weber's law (denoted as LTP and RICLTP, respectively) and the conventional LBP [4, 6] alone with its extensions that also incorporate spatial and orientation contexts into LBP, denoted as LBP_ex1 [8] and LBP_ex2 [10]. We also compare our results with the recently published work by Han et al. [5] (data-driven modeling of 3*3 micro-structure), which show promising performance for cell staining pattern recognition compared with other state-of-the art methods. Through our experimentation, we successfully showed that promising recognition performance can be achieved for HEp-2 cell classification via our methods. In the released HEp-2 cell database, each pattern has a different number of available cell images as introduced in Sect. 2. We observed that the Golgi pattern has very few cell images than other patterns. Thus, in our experiment, for training data, we randomly selected 600 cell images from the 5 patterns excluding Golgi and 300 cell images from Golgi; the remaining cell images were used to test both positive and intermediate intensity types. A linear SVM was used as our classifier on the root-squared statistics for both the proposed (W)LTP and LBP-based descriptors; note that we decided to use a linear SVM because it was much more efficient than using a nonlinear SVM. The above procedure was repeated 20 times, the final results were calculated as an average recognition performance of these 20 runs; results showed the percentages of properly classified cell images for all test samples. Table 2 shows comparative recognition results for both positive and intermediate intensity types. We conclude that our proposed WLTP with integrated spatial and orientation context (i.e., RICWLTP) achieved the best performance. For reference, the accuracy-reject rate curve of all six staining patterns and the confusion matrix of both intensity types are available the supplemental materials.

Table 2 The comparative results of our proposed framework and the state-of-the art descriptors

Method	LBP	LBP_Ex1	LBP_Ex2	Han et al. [5]	LTP	WLTP	RICLTP	RICWLTP
Positive %	78.22	89.13	91.83	95.5	87.55	87.79	**95.02**	**96.55**
Intermediate %	60.24	75.42	78.07	80.95	71.59	73.39	**84.82**	**85.88**

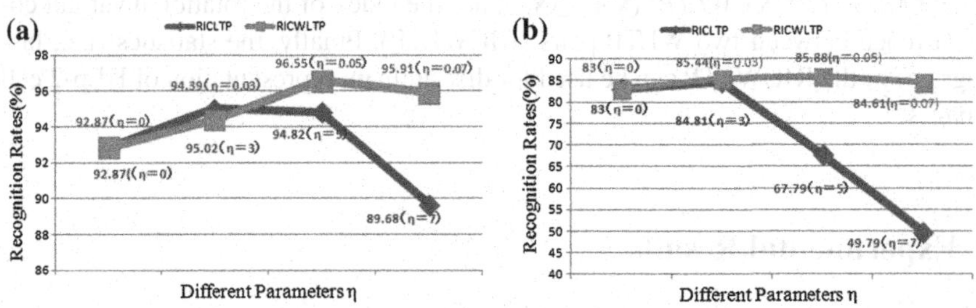

Fig. 3 Comparative results using rotation invariant co-occurrence WLTPs with and without Weber's law (data-driven thresholding), with η defined in Eq. (1) in Sect. 3. **a** Positive type. **b** intermediate type

As introduced in Sect. 3 above, the (W)LTP in our proposed framework is formulated by a quantization procedure with a pre-defined (data-driven) threshold η. Figure 3 shows the recognition performance using our proposed RICLTP and RICWLTP approaches with different values of η. From the Fig. 3, we observe that the RICWLTP with data-driven quantization results in a much more stable performance than that with an absolute threshold, regardless of the magnitude of the focused pixel.

5 Conclusions

In this paper, we described a robust representation strategy for classifying HEp-2 cell patterns of fluorescence staining. We proposed a local ternary pattern (LTP) with data-driven quantization according to Weber's law (called WLTP), and incorporated the spatial and orientation context into WLTP, called as rotation invariant co-occurrence among WLTP (RICWLTP). Our experiments on the open HEp-2 cell dataset used at the ICIP2013 contest confirmed that our proposed strategy greatly improved recognition performance as compared to state-of-the-art descriptor.

References

1. Conrad, K., Schoessler, W., Hiepe, F., Fritzler, M.J.: Autoantibodies in Systemic Autoimmune Diseases. Pabst Science Publishers, Lengerich (2002)
2. Soda, P., Iannello, G.: Aggregation of classifiers for staining pattern recognition in antinuclear autoantibodies analysis. IEEE Trans. Inf. Technol. Biomed. **13**(3), 322–329 (2009)
3. Cataldo, S.D., Bottino, A., Ficarra E., Macii, E.: Applying textural features to the classification of hep-2 cell patterns in IIF images. In: International Conference of Pattern Recognition (ICPR2012), pp. 28–43 (2012)
4. Wiliem, A., Wong, Y., Sanderson, C., Hobson, P., Chen S., Lovell, B.C.: Classification of human epithetial type 2 cell indirect immunofluorescence images via codebook based descriptors. In: Workshop on Application of Computer Vision, pp. 95–102 (2013)
5. Han, X.-H., Wang, J., Xu, G., Chen, Y.-W.: High-order statistics of microtexton for HEp-2 staining pattern classification. IEEE Trans. Biomed. Eng. **61**(8), 2223–2234 (2014)
6. Wang, X.Y., Han, T.X., Yan, S.C.: An HOG-LBP human detector with partial occlusion handling, ICCV (2009)
7. Foggia, P., Percannella, G., Soda, P., Vento, M.: Benchmarking HEp-2 cells classification methods. IEEE Trans. Med. Imag. **32**(10), 1878–1889 (2013)
8. Nosaka, R., Ohkawa, Y., Fukui, K.: Feature extraction based on co-occurrence of adjacent local binary patterns. In: The 5th Pacific-Rim Symposium on Image and Video Technology (PSIVT2011). Part II, LNCS, vol. 7088, pp. 82–91 (2011)
9. Nosaka, R., Fukui, K.: HEp-2 cell classification using rotation invariant co-occurrence among local binary patterns, Pattern Recognition (2013)
10. Qi, X.B., Xiao, R., Zhang, L., Guo, J.: Pairwise rotation invariant co-occurrence local binary pattern. In: 12th European Conference on Computer Vision (2012)
11. Tan, X.Y., Triggs, B.: Enhanced local texture feature sets for face recognition under difficult lighting conditions. IEEE Trans. Image Process. **19**(6), 1635–1650 (2010)

Combined Density, Texture and Shape Features of Multi-phase Contrast-Enhanced CT Images for CBIR of Focal Liver Lesions: A Preliminary Study

Yingying Xu, Lanfen Lin, Hongjie Hu, Huajun Yu, Chongwu Jin, Jian Wang, Xianhua Han and Yen-Wei Chen

Abstract Recently, content-based image retrieval (CBIR) in medical applications has attracted a lot of attentions. In this paper, we present a preliminary study on CBIR of focal liver lesions based on combined density, texture and shape features of multi-phase contrast-enhanced CT volumes. We improve the existing method from following two aspects: (1) in order to improve the retrieval accuracy, we propose a novel 3D shape feature for CBIR of liver lesions in addition to conventional density and texture features; (2) in order to reduce the computation time, we propose an improved local binary pattern, which is called imLBP, as the 3D texture feature. The effectiveness of our proposed method has been validated with real clinical datasets.

Keywords Content-based image retrieval · Multi-phase contrast-enhanced CT volumes · Focal liver lesions · Shape feature · Improved local binary pattern (imLBP) · Precision · Recall

Y. Xu · L. Lin (✉) · Y.-W. Chen
College of Computer Science and Technology, Zhejiang University, Hangzhou, China
e-mail: llf@zju.edu.cn

Y. Xu
e-mail: cs_ying@zju.edu.cn

H. Hu · H. Yu · C. Jin
Radiology Department, Medical School, Sir Run Run Shaw Hospital, Zhejiang University, Hangzhou, China
e-mail: hongjiehu@zju.edu.cn

J. Wang · X. Han · Y.-W. Chen
College of Information Science and Engineering, Ritsumeikan University, Shiga, Japan

Y.-W. Chen et al. (eds.), *Innovation in Medicine and Healthcare 2015*,
Smart Innovation, Systems and Technologies 45,
DOI 10.1007/978-3-319-23024-5_20

1 Introduction

With the development of digital imaging technology, more and more information nowadays is conveyed in the form of digital images or video clips. Content-based image retrieval (CBIR) becomes a useful and powerful technique for digital image searching in large databases [1–4]. Recently, CBIR in medical applications has attracted much attention of researchers [5]. The aim of CBIR of medical images is to assist the interpretation of medical images for radiologists and to share experience of other experienced radiologists.

Though researches on CBIR in radiology are very few, several CBIR methods have been proposed for identifying different types of liver lesions [6–8]. Most of them used 2D image based features extracted from a few representative slices for CBIR, which is incomplete to represent a 3D lesion. Roy et al. [9] proposed a CBIR framework for liver lesions based on 3D spatiotemporal features derived from multi-phase CT volumes. Four 3D features (density feature, temporal density feature, texture feature, temporal texture feature) were used for CBIR. The 3D features performed better results than existing 2D features. In this paper, we improve the Roy's work from following two aspects: (1) in order to improve the retrieval accuracy, we propose a novel 3D shape feature for CBIR of liver lesions in addition to conventional density and texture features; (2) in order to reduce the computation time, we propose an improved local binary pattern, which is called imLBP, as the texture feature. In [9], Roy et al. use a 3D gray-level co-occurrence matrix (GLCM) to extract texture feature. On the other hand, LBP is another method for texture representation, which is considered as one of the best descriptors in analyzing texture because of its robustness under different illumination condition. Furthermore, LBP responds well in both macro-textures and micro-textures with high performance and is simple to implement. In $3 \times 3 \times 3$ texture patterns for 3D images, the LBP value ranges from 0 to $2^{26} - 1$., which results in a histogram of a quite wide range with plenty of frequency being zero. Therefore, a uniform pattern was adopted to play down the upper bound of the LBP value. While transformation from ordinary LBP code to uniform LBP code for 3D images costs a lot of time. So in our study, we make some improvement on the basis of the original LBP algorithm that three 8-bit LBP codes are exploited instead of a 26-bit code.

This paper is organized as follows. In Sect. 2 we describe our proposed method including our proposed features. Experimental results are presented in Sect. 3. The conclusion is given in Sect. 4.

2 Dataset and Methodology

3D multi-phase contrast-enhanced CT images of the liver from 38 cases are used in our research, including 15 Cyst images, 7 FNH images, 7 HCC images and 9 HEM images. Each case contains three phases, namely non-contrast enhanced

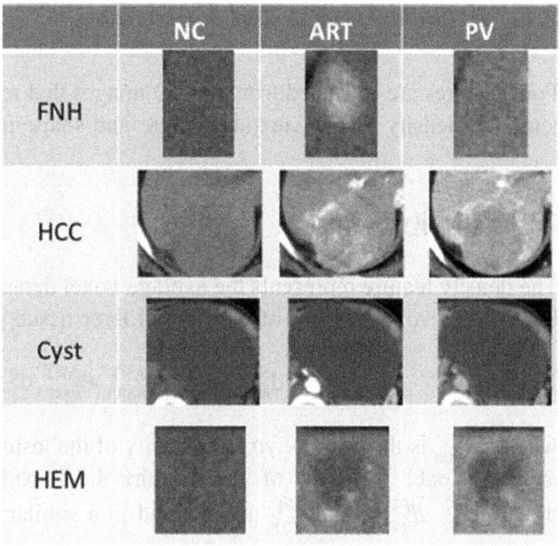

Fig. 1 Typical multi-phase CT images of focal liver lesions

(NC) phase, arterial (ART) phase and portal venous (PV) phase. Some typical images are shown in Fig. 1. In most cases, images of these three phases are enough for radiologists to identify the type of focal liver lesions and the delay (DL) phase is usually not used in order to reduce the radiation dose. The pathology type of the lesions were identified by diagnostic radiologists. We use a random walk based interactive segmentation algorithm proposed in [10] to segment both liver and lesions in a 3D image. Visual features are extracted from the segmented liver and lesions.

According to clinic observations, different kinds of lesions appear to have distinct enhancement patterns after contrast injection. The evolution pattern of the lesion plays a significant role in identification of hepatic lesions in clinical diagnosis. So we extract the temporal density feature from the multi-phase contrast-enhanced CT images as well as the density feature and the texture feature [9]. Another clinical observation is that different lesion may have a different shape, so we also extract the shape feature in addition to the density feature and the texture feature. Finally, we use four following features for CBIR of focal liver lesions: density feature, temporal density feature, texture feature and shape feature.

Features extracted from all these images are registered in a feature database for computation of similarity. For image retrieval, we first extract the designed features from the query lesion and then calculate the similarity between the query and each of cases registered in the database based on their features. Two similarity measures (L2 similarity measure and histogram intersection between the feature vectors) are used for retrieval. A shortest-distance based KNN algorithm is used for the identification of query.

2.1 Feature Design and Extraction

Four features are extracted from the 3D images that respectively are density feature, temporal density feature, texture feature and shape feature.

2.1.1 Density Feature

The density feature represents the average voxel density of the lesion normalized by the average voxel density of the normal liver tissue [9], which is defined as

$$F_1 = \{d^{NC}_{lesion}/d^{NC}_{liver}, d^{ART}_{lesion}/d^{ART}_{liver}, d^{PV}_{lesion}/d^{PV}_{liver}\} \tag{1}$$

where d^{NC}_{lesion} is the average voxel intensity of the lesion in NC phase and d^{NC}_{liver} *is* the average voxel intensity of the healthy liver parenchyma in the NC phase. d^{ART}_{lesion}, d^{ART}_{liver}, d^{PV}_{lesion}, and d^{PV}_{liver} are defined in a similar way.

2.1.2 Temporal Density Feature

The temporal density feature F_2 concerns about the enhancement of density over time after the injection compared with the density in the NC phase [9]. Thus, F_2 is a two-dimensional feature vector that consists of the enhancement of ART phase and PV phase. The expression of F_2 is shown as:

$$F_2 = \{TD^{ART}, TD^{PV}\} \tag{2}$$

here $TD^{ART} = (d^{ART}_{lesion} - d^{NC}_{lesion})/d^{NC}_{lesion}$., and $TD^{PV} = (d^{PV}_{lesion} - d^{NC}_{lesion})/d^{NC}_{lesion}$

2.1.3 Texture Feature

Texture features indicate spatial organization of voxel values in the ROI of each 3D image [4, 11]. We use an improved three-dimensional uniform local binary pattern (imLBP) to describe the local texture feature. Texture features of ART and PV phase form the feature vector F_3 of the lesion. F_3 is defined as:

$$F_3 = \{T^{ART}, T^{PV}\} \tag{3}$$

The term T^{ART} contains three histograms resulted from the uniform LBP images of ART phase. T^{PV} has a similar definition.

LBP is one of the best descriptors for texture representation because of its robustness under different illumination condition. Furthermore, LBP responds well in both macro-textures and micro-textures with high performance and is simple to implement. For a given voxel i, the conventional 3D LBP operator compares the voxel value with its 26 neighborhood voxels and gets a 26-bit binary number which yields a LBP value ranges from 0 to $2^{26} - 1$. The intensity of the given voxel is then replaced by the LBP value. The conventional 3D LBP will result in a histogram of a quite wide range (2^{26} bins) with plenty of frequency being zero. Even we adopt a uniform pattern [11] to reduce the length (number of bins) of histogram, the number of bins is still $26^2 - 26 + 3 = 653$. Furthermore, the transformation from ordinary LBP code to uniform LBP code for 3D images costs a lot of time.

In order to reduce the large computation time of 3D LBP, we propose an improved LBP (imLBP) for fast extraction of texture features. The imLBP only takes 24 neighborhood voxels to calculate the LBP value, excluding the voxels just above $(i, j, k - 1)$ and below $((i, j, k + 1))$ the given voxel in a $3 \times 3 \times 3$ cube. The conventional $3 \times 3 \times 3$ cube results in a descriptor of 26-bit size, whereas our imLBP codes are three 8-bit size descriptors (LBPs of three 2D slice images ($k - 1$, k, $k + 1$) with a central pixel of (i, j, k)). If we adopt a uniform pattern for our imLBP, the number of bins or the length of the histogram is $3 * (8^2 - 8 + 3) = 177$.

2.1.4 Shape Feature

Shape features are important for distinguishing different types of lesions. In this paper, the sphericity of a lesion extracted by Principle Component Analysis (PCA) is used as the shape feature of the lesion. Considering that the shape of lesions show no obvious change in different phases, we extract shape features from images of ART phase. The shape feature F_4 is denoted by three eigenvalues $\lambda_1, \lambda_2, \lambda_3$ $(\lambda_1 > \lambda_2 > \lambda_3)$ calculated via principle component analysis (PCA) as formulated below:

$$F_4 = \{\lambda_2/\lambda_1, \lambda_3/\lambda_1\} \quad (5)$$

2.2 *Similarity Assessment and Ranking*

The similarity between the query image and images in the database can be measured using four different distances for four respective feature vectors with corresponding weights. Distance between two images is defined as

$$\mathrm{D}(\text{query}, Image_D) = \sum_{i=1}^{4} w_i d_i \quad (6)$$

where d_i denotes the distance of i-th feature between the query lesion and the $Image_D$ in the database. w_i is its respective weight, whose selection will be discussed in Sect. 3.

As for density feature, temporal density feature and shape feature, we use Euclidean distance to calculate the distance.

$$d_1(F_{query}, F_D) = ||F_{query} - F_D||_{L^2} \tag{7}$$

where $d_1(F_{query}, F_D)$ is the Euclidean distance of density feature between the query image and images in the database. Similar definitions follow for distance of temporal density feature d_2 and distance of shape feature d_4.

Histogram intersection distance is an approach to measure the similarity between two LBP images based on histogram. Histogram intersection distance is formulated as

$$d_3(H_{query}, H_D) = \sum_{i=1}^{k} min[H_{query}(i), H_D(i)] \tag{8}$$

The images are sorted in decreasing order on the basis of their similarity to the query image. The first K images are retrieved as the nearest neighbors. The number of retrieved lesions K is experimentally chosen as 6 according the experiment described in experiment section. Basically, the query image is predicted to belong to the class c if C_i owns the maximal percentage among the K retrieved classes. While, if there exists another class C_j that has the same percentage, we should take mean distance of each class into account. Then the shortest-distance based KNN means is proposed to solve this problem. The prediction of the class of the query image is shown as follows:

$$\begin{aligned} &\text{query} \subseteq C_i \\ \text{if mean\_D}(C_i) &= \min_{i=1,\ldots n}(mean\_D(C_i)) \text{ where } C_i \subseteq \text{A}, \\ &\text{A} = \{C_k | \text{P}(C_k) = \max_{k=1,2,3,4}(\text{P}(C_k))\} \end{aligned} \tag{9}$$

Set A contains classes that have maximal percentage. mean_D(C_i) represents the mean distance to query image of class C_i. P(C_k) is defined as the percentage of the number of retrieved images belong to class C_k with respect to the top k results. n is the size of set A. We will chose the class C_i from set A and C_i has the minimal mean distance to the query image compared to other classes in the set A.

2.3 Evaluation

The leave-one-out method is employed to evaluate the performance of the retrieval system. One case is selected as a query case (unlabeled case) and the remaining 37 cases are used as labeled datasets in database for retrieving. The retrieval experiment is repeated on all cases. A total of 38 experiments with a different query are performed. Precision and recall are used to assess the retrieval performance. Precision represents the ratio of retrieved images relevant to the class of the query case with respect to the total number of images retrieved. Recall means the number of retrieved images relevant to the class of the query case divided by the total number of relevant images in the database. In order to manifest the overall performance of the retrieval and decision, another assessment parameter called correct decision rate (CDR) is proposed in the evaluation. For the 38 experiments, CDR indicates the percentage of how many lesions are correctly decided for each type of lesions in the database. CDR is defined as:

$$CDR_i = \#(lesions_i\_correct\_decided)/\#(lesions_i\_in\_database) \quad (10)$$

CDR_i where i ranges from 1 to 4 corresponds to the correct decided rate of different types of lesions. When one of the i-th type of lesions is selected as a query, and the prediction of its class matches its real class, the numerator should plus one.

3 Experimental Results and Discussion

As we use a KNN algorithm for deciding the class of the query lesion, the retrieval performance is dependent on the value of *K*. To investigate the function of *K*, we tested the performance with different *K*. Figure 2 exhibits the precision and recall versus different value of *K*. We observed from the experiments that when K equals to 6, precision and recall achieve a relatively ideal value.

The retrieval performance is also dependent on feature weights ($\mathbf{w} = [w_1, w_2, w_3, w_4]$). Before determining the weights, we first use F_1, F_2, and F_4 alone to obtain the contribution of the various features to the system performance. We conclude from the experiments that the features sorted by contribution in descending order are density feature, shape feature, temporal feature and texture feature. We set the initial value of the weight vector as [0.25, 0.25, 0.25, 0.25] with equal weight of

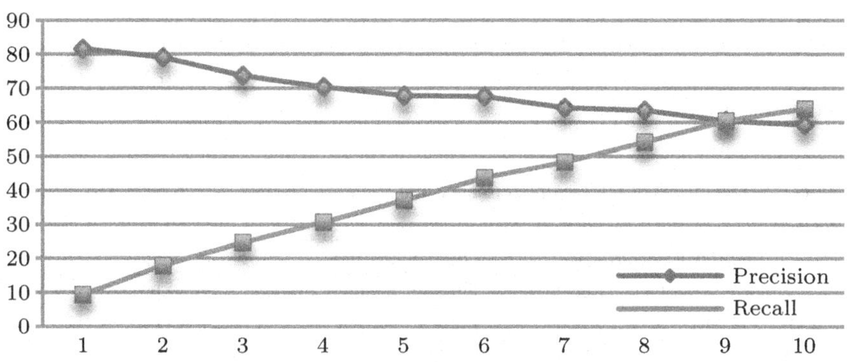

Fig. 2 Precision and recall versus different value of K

Table 1 Dependence of retrieval performance on weights (K = 6)

w	[0.3, 0.3, 0.2, 0.2]	[0.25, 0.25, 0.25, 0.25]	[0.3, 0.2, 0.2, 0.3]	[0.35, 0.2, 0.15, 0.3]	[0.4, 0.2, 0.1, 0.3]
Precision	61.84 %	61.84 %	64.91 %	65.79 %	67.54 %
Recall	40.29 %	40.15 %	41.56 %	41.93 %	43.69 %

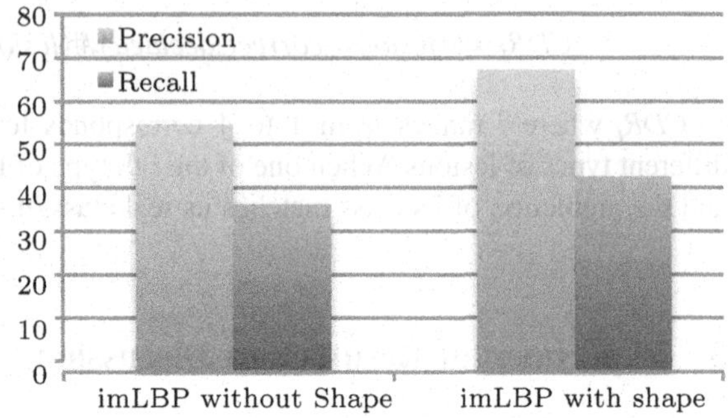

Fig. 3 Comparison of retrieval results with and without shape feature (K = 6, w = [0.4, 0.2, 0.1, 0.3])

each feature. Then we adjust the weights in steps of 0.05 increasing or decreasing the corresponding weight according to our previous practice. We choose several representative weights and show their precision and recall in Table 1. We can see that the best performance was achieved with the weights of [0.4, 0.2, 0.1, 0.3].

In order to demonstrate the positive effect of shape feature, we conducted two groups of experiments with and without the shape feature for comparison. The results are shown in Fig. 3. As shown in Fig. 3, the retrieval results (both precision and recall) with shape feature are much better than those without shape feature.

Next, we compared our proposed imLBP with conventional LBP and GLCM [9]. The comparisons of retrieval performance and computation time are shown in Table 2. The computation time is on a PC with a 3.40 GHz CPU. Feature extraction using imLBP performs 10 times faster than extraction with GLCM and more than 60 times faster than extraction with conventional LBP algorithm, while the retrieval performance using our proposed imLBP is better than GLCM and is the same as conventional LBP.

Table 2 Comparisons of retrieval performance and computation time (K = 6, w = [0.4, 0.2, 0.1, 0.3])

	Retrieval performance		Computation time	
	Precision (%)	Recall (%)	Time for texture extraction	Total processing time
imLBP	67.54	43.69	9.003 s	52.132 s
GLCM	62.28	42.24	116.986 s	163.707 s
LBP	67.54	43.69	>10 min	>10 min

The CDR reflects the detection degree of each class of lesion. The examination results show that with an approximate feature weight and K-value, the detection rate for Cyst and FNH can reach at 100 %. While the maximum rate for HCC and HEM can only run up to 85.71 and 77.78 %. The small validation of data set and complexity of some classes of lesions may be the potential reason accounting for the phenomenon. In our next-step work, we will enlarge our database to construct a more precise retrieval system based on a large training sets. This deficiency indicates that features adopted in this study may be not powerful enough to achieve an ideal result. Other symptoms like the degree of cirrhosis may help to identify the lesion class. We are supposed to design more effectual features for retrieving.

4 Conclusions

In this paper, we proposed a CBIR system based on combined density, texture and shape features of three-phase contrast-enhanced CT volumes. These features are meticulously designed according to clinic experts' clinical experience. The system performance was significantly improved by using shape features in addition to density and texture features. We also proposed an improved LBP operator for fast extraction of texture feature. Feature extraction using our improved 8-bit LBP operator (imLBP) performs 10 times faster than extraction with GLCM and more 60 times faster than extraction with conventional LBP algorithm, while the retrieval performance using our proposed imLBP is better than GLCM and is same as conventional LBP.

Preliminary results validated the potential of our method. However, there are still several issues we want to address in the future. The first issue is to increase the number of samples, especially the number of METS, which is not involved in this research because of limited number of samples. The second issue is to extract more distinct features to improve the system performance.

Acknowledgments This research was supported in part by National Science and Technology Support Program of China under the Grant No.2013BAF02B10, in part by the Recruitment Program of Global Experts (HAIOU Program) from Zhejiang Province, China, in part by the Grant-in Aid for Scientific Research from the Japanese Ministry for Education, Science, Culture and Sports (MEXT) under the Grant No. 2430076 and No. 15H01130, in part by the MEXT Support Program for the Strategic Research Foundation at Private Universities (2013–2017), and in part by the R-GIRO Research Fund from Ritsumeikan University.

References

1. Lew, M., et al.: Content-based multimedia information retrieval: state of the art and challanges. ACM Trans. Multimedia Comput. Commun. Appl. **2**, 1–19 (2006)
2. Niblack, W., et al.: The QIBC project: querying images by content using color, texture and shape. In: Proceedings SPIE Storage and Retrieval for Image and Video Database (1993)

3. Pentland, A., et al.: Photobook: Cont-based manipulation of image database. Int. J. Comput. Vis. **18**, 233–254 (1996)
4. Zeng, X.Y., et al.: A new texture feature based on PCA pattern maps and its application to image retrieval. IEICE Trans. Inf. Syst. E86-D, 929–936 (2003)
5. Akgul, C.B., et al.: Content-based image retrieval in radiology: current status and future directions. J. Digit. Imag. (2010). doi:10.1007/s10278-010-9290-9
6. Yang, W., et al.: Content-based retrieval of focal liver lesions using bag-of-visual-words representations of single- and multiphase contrast-enhanced CT images. J. Digit. Imag. **25**, 708–719 (2012)
7. Chi, Y., et al.: Content-based image retrieval of multiphase CT images or focal liver lesion characterization. Med. Phys. 40, no. 10, art. 103502 (2013)
8. Napel, S.A., et al.: Automated retrieval of CT images of liver lesions on the basis of image similarity: method and preliminary results. Radiology **256**, 243–252 (2010)
9. Roy, S., et al.: Three-dimensional spatiotemporal features for fast content-based retrieval of focal liver lesions. IEEE Trans. Biomed. Eng. **61**, 2768–2778 (2014)
10. Dong, C., et al.: A knowledge-based interactive liver segmentation framework using random walks, to be published. In: Proceedings of ICNC-FSKD2015 (2015)
11. Maenpaa, T., et al.: Robust texture classification by subsets of local binary patterns. In: Proceedings of the 15th International Conference on Pattern Recognition, vol. 3, pp. 947–950. Barcelona, Spain (2000)

Supporting Nurses' Work and Improving Medical Safety Using a Sensor Network System in Hospitals

Misa Esashi, Haruo Noma and Tomohiro Kuroda

Abstract New electrical medical instruments can report their status, which will improve the accuracy of electronic medical records (EMR) and reduce nurses' workload. Processing the data collected and providing feedback to nurses in real-time will reduce medical errors. We designed a sensor network system that uses Bluetooth to communicate with medical instruments to collect information on where, how, and by whom an instrument is being used. This should detect errors in instrument settings by comparing the data collected with the physician's order, and alerting nurses to any errors. This paper discusses our system, which was evaluated by interviewing nurses.

Keywords Hospital information system · Sensor network · Syringe driver · Bluetooth

1 Introduction

Hospital information systems (HIS) are used widely in large hospitals to improve the efficiency and safety of medical treatment. For example, an order entry system can alert physicians to medication errors, and a medicine authentication system can be used to determine whether a medicine matches the patient and to record who prescribed it. However, an HIS is incapable of preventing all human errors in

M. Esashi (✉) · T. Kuroda
Graduate School of Informatics, Kyoto University, Kyoto, Japan
e-mail: mesashi@kuhp.kyoto-u.ac.jp

M. Esashi · H. Noma
Department of Information and Communication Science, Ritsumeikan University, Shiga, Japan

T. Kuroda
Division of Medical Information Technology and Administration Planning, Kyoto University Hospital, Kyoto, Japan

Y.-W. Chen et al. (eds.), *Innovation in Medicine and Healthcare 2015*,
Smart Innovation, Systems and Technologies 45,
DOI 10.1007/978-3-319-23024-5_21

hospitals because the data that the HIS handles need to have been input into the HIS. Inputting data relies heavily on manpower and is a source of human error. The development of digital medical instruments has increased the data output, increasing the burden of inputting data into electronic medical records (EMR). In comparison, inputting data, such as measurements, directly into the HIS is precise and efficient [1]. Nurses frequently use personal computers to input data, but these are unsuitable for all uses because nurses spend much time walking around the hospital.

Data input is not the only problem with an HIS. The number of medical instruments that have serial ports for communication is increasing. However, to make use of the data saved in EMR, we need a method of validating the data and presenting the result to the medical staff in real time. For example, to use data on an ongoing infusion, the HIS needs to decide whether the flow rate is appropriate and immediately inform the nurse who is in charge of the patient if an error is detected.

In hospitals, the process of inputting data to the HIS, processing the data, and outputting the result should be automated, seamless, and happen in real-time.

Nevertheless, if the HIS were to check the data in minute detail and warn nurses about every error, it would disrupt the nurses' work. In addition, nurses might miss or ignore important messages. The need for a warning depends on many factors, such as the nurses' schedules and patients' condition. To design a system that gives alerts, we must consider various cases.

This paper focuses on medication errors. When administering medication, human error can occur at several stages, such as when the physician orders the medication, when the medicine is prepared, and at the patient's bedside. The use of medical instruments such as infusion pumps and syringe drivers involves a risk of setting errors, and a slight difference in a setting such as the flow rate can have serious effects on a patient.

We designed a system to collect and store the state of syringe drivers and monitor the status of the syringe drivers in real time to avoid medication errors caused by setting the flow rate incorrectly. Storing the state of the syringe drivers in the HIS enables the recording of detailed infusion data, including for which patient and how the device is being used. The data are collected automatically, so the data input process does not require nurses. Simultaneously, the location of the syringe driver inside the hospital is monitored, and which patient is allocated to the bed where the syringe driver is located is recorded. The identification of patients based on location serves as a backup medicine authentication system to avoid treating the wrong patient. It also helps to determine where a patient is when the patient is out of the sickroom during the infusion, improving the efficiency and safety of medical treatment.

A syringe driver allows the infusion of a small amount of fluid at a constant rate. Medicine authentication systems can avoid giving the wrong medicine or medicine to the wrong patient by reading the barcodes on the medicine package and patient's wristband. However, the flow rate of a syringe driver is set and checked manually.

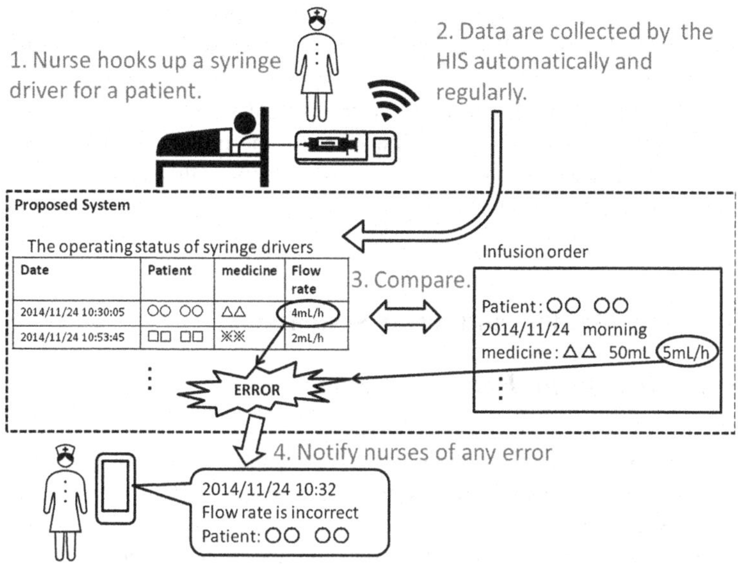

Fig. 1 The process by which the proposed system detects an infusion flow rate error

Flow rate errors can result from:

- Using two or more syringe drivers in a patient,
- Missing a change in the medication order, and
- Confusing the flow rate with the amount of medicine to administer.

Although syringe drivers have been designed to avoid flow rate errors and nurses double-check the flow rate after setting it, human error is not prevented completely.

Given these circumstances, we designed a system to check the flow rate of a syringe driver and alert staff if there are any errors. The system involves three steps: collecting data on the operating status of the syringe driver with a sensor network and recording it in the EMR, deciding whether the flow rate is appropriate and monitoring any alerts from the syringe driver, and informing the nurse looking after the patient of the error. In this paper, we discuss the system design used to put the first two steps into practice. Figure 1 shows the process by which the system identifies an infusion flow rate error.

2 Related Work

Emori et al. proposed a network system that detects the alarms generated by syringe drivers and infusion pumps at the University of Fukui Hospital [2]. The alerts include occlusion, the syringe being disconnected, a low battery charge, and forgetting to push the start button. In their system, small devices are connected to the syringe drivers and infusion pumps to communicate with a wireless network. Alerts are displayed on a screen at the nursing station and on the nurses' laptops. A trial of the system involving a small number of patients showed that it reduced the time taken for nurses to respond to an alarm. The system also helps nurses to recognize the reason for the alarm without going to the patient's bedside. Patients and their families are relieved that they do not have to use the nurse call button. Here, we discuss a method used to match medical instruments with physicians' orders to check the flow rate of syringe drivers.

3 Proposed Method and Trial System

3.1 Overview of the Proposed System

The proposed system involves three phases: collecting data from medical instruments, processing the data, and outputting the results. Here, we focus on data collection and processing.

The first phase involves collecting data on the state of the syringe drivers automatically and recording it in the EMR. At Kyoto University Hospital, medications are recorded by a medicine authentication system. The data stored in the EMR, the flow rate, and the amount of infusion administered do not always match. Recording the state of operation of a syringe driver directly to the EMR stores detailed medication information. Simultaneously, the location of the syringe driver is collected and input into the HIS.

The next phase is to monitor the state of the syringe driver to check the flow rate and raise an alert if it is incorrect. To compare the flow rate of the syringe driver with the order in the medical chart, the syringe driver must be paired with an order that includes information on the patient and medication. The method of linking them is described below.

When an error is detected, one or more nurses are notified via mobile terminals. Here, we will discuss to which nurse a message is sent and the content of the message, but we will not discuss the method used to send messages.

3.2 Data Collection

There are several requirements for data collection in a hospital: considering the movement of medical instruments inside the hospital, the electricity consumption of the communication device, and dealing with more than one medical instrument in one location. We developed a Bluetooth-based sensor network system to communicate with medical instruments and other Bluetooth-equipped devices and locate them within a hospital [3–5]. We selected Bluetooth (Class 2) for the proposed sensor network system because Bluetooth requires less energy than Wi-Fi. ZigBee

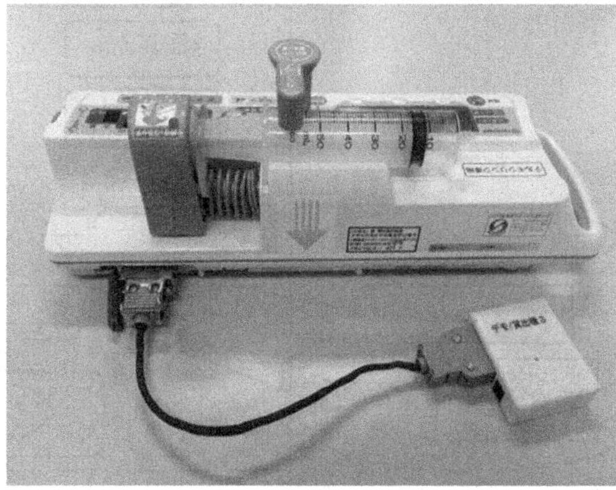

Fig. 2 A BT-SA connected to a syringe driver

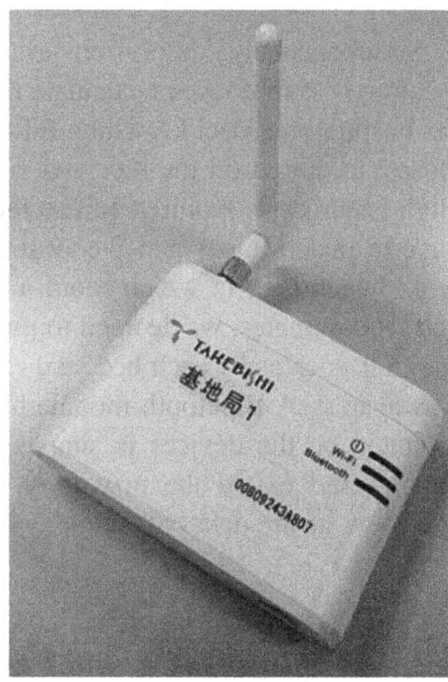

Fig. 3 A BT-AP/BT-ID base station

is another low-power wireless communication protocol, but Bluetooth is more reliable and more widely used. Radio frequency identification (RFID) is usually used for the transmission of small amounts of data over short distances.

To communicate with syringe drivers that are not equipped with a Bluetooth module, we developed the Bluetooth serial adapter (BT-SA) shown in Fig. 2. This is connected to a serial port in the syringe driver. In addition, Bluetooth access points (BT-AP) are installed in the patients' rooms (Fig. 3). The proposed system communicates with the syringe driver via BT-SA regularly and collects data on its state, including information on the syringe driver configuration. The system outputs the collected data to the EMR database.

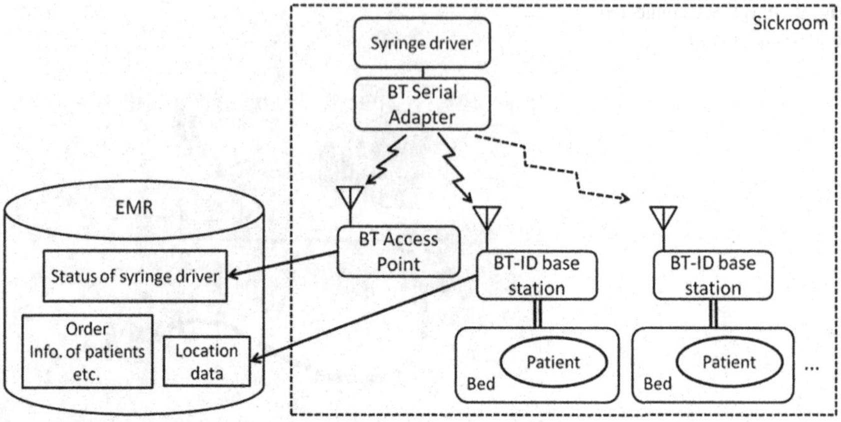

Fig. 4 Overview of the data collection system

Simultaneously, the system estimates the location of the syringe driver. The locating system does not calculate the *x*- and *y*-coordinates of syringe drivers inside the hospital, but decides which BT-ID base station (shown in Fig. 3) the BT-SA is closest to, based on the received signal strength of the Bluetooth inquiry process. High accuracy is required to use the *x*- and *y*-coordinates for positioning, and we have to match the *x*- and *y*-coordinates with a logical location inside the hospital (e.g., which bed, in which room, on which floor). Given the difficulty in using *x*- and *y*-coordinates, we decided to put BT-ID base stations at crucial spots inside the hospital, such as by each bed, and calculate to which BT-ID base station the BT-SA was nearest. A Bluetooth module has the ability to handle this process, so the unit mounted on the devices is simple. The output data contain the times the device entered and exited the proximity of a BT-ID base station. Figure 4 shows an overview of the data collection system.

3.3 Pairing the Syringe Driver and Medication Order

To decide whether the flow rate settings of the syringe drivers are appropriate, each syringe driver should be paired with the order regarding which patient and which medicine the syringe driver is being used for. We compared the three methods outlined below and chose method 2.

1. *Deciding from the position and time of medication*

From the information on the location of the syringe driver, the system identifies the patient by referring to the data on which patient is in which bed. Then, it determines the order by comparing the time at which data were output from the syringe driver with the time of the medication order. However there are two problems with this method. First, two or more medicines could be administered to one patient at the same time, making it difficult to decide for which medicine the syringe driver is being used. The second reason is that most medication orders do not include precise times. Rather, the timing of the medication is often described in the form "three times a day" and the time is adjusted to the nursing schedule.

2. *Put barcodes on syringe drivers*

Assign a unique barcode to each syringe driver to identify it when the system is introduced to the hospital. The barcodes are printed on labels, which are stuck on syringe drivers. Nurses scan the barcode at the time of medicine authentication to match the syringe driver with the order. Although this method increases the number of barcodes that must be scanned, the syringe driver is matched with the order precisely and inexpensively.

3. *Introduction of barcode pumps*

Syringe drivers with embedded barcode scanners are being adopted widely in Europe and America [6]. These syringe drivers are known as barcode pumps and they contain a medicine library that allows them to refer to the amount limit and flow rate of each medicine. Scanning the barcode printed on a medicine automatically matches the syringe driver with the order. However, replacing existing syringe drivers with barcode pumps is expensive and nurses have to be trained in the use of the new devices.

4 Evaluation of the Method

4.1 Interviews

To evaluate the proposed system's usability, we obtained feedback from nurses, the intended users of the system.

First, we outlined the system to seven nurses employed at Kyoto University Hospital. We explained the functions of collecting the working status of syringe drivers and warning of any error; and the necessity of scanning the barcode on the syringe driver in addition to the current medicine authentication process. Then, we discussed the following questions:

- Would the system improve the efficiency and safety of medical treatment?
- Would the system have negative effects on the medical staff?
- In what situations are even unimportant warnings required?
- Can you think of other functions that would be helpful?
- Can you think of any problems involved in introducing the system at the hospital?

4.2 Discussion

4.2.1 Advantages

1. *Automation of data input into HIS*

By collecting data on the operating status of syringe drivers, detailed records of infusions are available, including start/end times, flow rate, and amount of medicine.

2. *Double-checking the patient and medicine prescribed*

Using the data on which bed the syringe driver is located, the system can double-check that the medicine paired with the syringe driver is prescribed for the patient in that bed. This helps to detect oversight errors in the medicine authentication system.

3. *Checking the medicine flow rate and warning errors*

The system checks for a mismatch between the flow rate setting of the syringe driver and that of the order in real-time and alerts the nurses in the event of an error. Nurses usually give medication based on a printed order and can miss an updated order in the HIS. The system checks that the infusion flow rate accords with the newest order providing an opportunity for nurses to confirm that the correct order is being used. However, an alert might confuse the nurse.

4.2.2 Disadvantages

1. *The work of nurses is increased*

Introducing the system increases the number of barcodes that nurses must scan for medicine authentication. Although this is a small task individually, it would add considerably to the total daily workload. In addition, when several syringe drivers are used for the same patient, the nurse must be conscious of which syringe driver to use for which medicine.

2. *The effective term for pairing the order and syringe driver is ambiguous*

After matching the syringe driver and order, how long this pairing should remain in effect is unclear. If the pairing is continued until being overwritten when the syringe driver is used for other medicine or different patients, errors could arise when a nurse forgets to scan the barcode on the syringe driver.

3. *Warnings could disrupt nurses' routines*

When a nurse's treatment is not required immediately or the nurse has already dealt with a warning, reading the message could disrupt the nurse's routine. The same message sent to several nurses could cause more than one nurse to deal with the warning. This is at least a waste of labor. If the patient used the nurse call button when the alarm on the syringe driver sounded, there might be duplication of the same message sent to the nurse.

4.2.3 System Problems

We analyzed the problems raised in the discussion and classified them into groups: problems introducing the system into the existing HIS, which are the shortcomings of the system explained previously; problems that could be solved by changing the system design; problems that could be solved by changing the medication flow; and problems beyond the capacity of the system.

4.2.4 Problems that Could Be Solved by Changing the System Design

1. *Deciding which message to send and to whom*

The designed system sends warning messages to the nurse responsible for that patient. However, in some cases, such as when infusing a potent medicine, it would be more appropriate to send a message to the nurse nearest to the patient's bed to deal with the warning swiftly. Conversely, some alerts can be dealt with by any nurse, such as the alarm indicating that the infusion has been completed.

Sometimes a nurse who was not originally responsible for the patient dispenses medication. An infusion using a syringe driver could be in operation all day, during which time the attending nurse would change frequently. As described, there are many possible patterns of which messages to send to which nurse(s), depending on the medicine and the nurses' work schedules.

To solve these problems, the system must have a function that sets the destination and contents of the message. However, setting this for each message requires time and results in situations such as improper settings causing a message not to be sent, or nurses receiving unrelated messages. Therefore, it is necessary to design a default setting or consider the context automatically. The system used to locate medical instruments can also be implemented for nurses, to determine the destination of a message.

To design a system that gives important warnings, but does not disrupt the nurses' work by sending too many messages, we must analyze the classification of medications and nurses' services in more detail.

2. *Checking the order of medications*

The order of medications is vital in some treatments, such as chemotherapy. The system can check for mistakes in the order of medications by referring to the record of medications completed for each patient.

3. *Interruption during the infusion*

Sometimes syringe drivers are turned off, such as while examining the patient or transfusing blood. During this period, the system cannot collect information on the state of the syringe driver, although the system can detect the interruption and send an alert when a nurse forgets to restart the infusion. However, the interruption could last for hours, making it difficult to decide whether it is intended. One solution is to send an alert when the interruption of medication might cause a medical problem, depending on the medicine.

4.2.5 Problems that Could Be Solved by Changing the Medication Flow

1. *Some data are not input into the HIS*

The proposed system monitors the state of syringe drivers based on information in the HIS. However, nurses are sometimes given verbal instructions to change the flow rate or stop an infusion depending on the patient's condition; these instructions are often not recorded in the EMR. To introduce the system, it would be necessary to input every medical treatment order.

However, medical staff would have to derive a benefit from inputting information that otherwise needs only to be communicated orally, otherwise the entry task would be skipped. There are often discrepancies between the EMR and actual medical treatment. However, medical accidents are often caused by misunderstanding a verbal instruction, and medical treatment based on the orders entered in the EMR is meaningful, as every medical treatment is recorded.

2. *Medical treatment provided based on printed orders*

Nursing care is usually based on printed orders; therefore nurses only have information for patients for whom they are responsible. If nurses could refer to the EMR of all patients, they would be able to deal with a warning message from the proposed system for any patient.

4.2.6 Problems Beyond the Capacity of the System

1. *Validity of the physician's order*

The proposed system makes judgments on the presupposition that the order entered into the HIS is correct. Therefore, the system cannot detect incorrect orders.

2. *Detecting a disconnected tube*

It would be useful to inform a nurse when the tube connected to the syringe used for an infusion is accidentally disconnected. However, this is beyond the capacity of the system because syringe drivers do not have the ability to detect this.

4.2.7 Summary

The analysis of the discussion of the proposed system with the nurses identified many problems that must be solved to introduce our system into a hospital. Further research on the workflow of nurses and medication is required to design the decision function of the system.

To introduce the system, the data in the HIS should be more complete to avoid miscommunication among the medical staff. The system could increase the work of medical staff and disrupt their duties by sending an excessive number of warnings. However, if the system's merits outweigh the demerits, the system would be acceptable.

5 Conclusions

We proposed a sensor network system that collects and stores the state of medical instruments in the EMR. The system also monitors the state of medical instruments by referring to the order entered in the HIS. The system would help to improve the efficiency and safety of medical care. This study focused on checking the flow rate of syringe drivers.

The proposed system involves three steps: data collection, data processing, and outputting a result. First, the state and location of the syringe driver are collected automatically by a sensor network using Bluetooth, and the data are stored in the EMR. Each syringe driver is matched with an order by scanning the barcode on the syringe driver during medicine authentication by the nurses. The system processes the collected data and detects improper flow rate settings and alarms regarding the syringe driver. Any errors would be sent to the nurses when necessary.

To evaluate the system, we interviewed seven nurses and analyzed the problems raised, and considered methods to solve them to facilitate the system's introduction into hospitals.

As further work, we plan to apply the sensor network system to other medical instruments, nurses, and patients, and make effective use of the collected data. As a result, the efficiency and safety of medical care would be improved.

Acknowledgements This research was funded by Grant-in-Aid for Scientific Research 25280106 from the Japan Society for the Promotion of Science.

References

1. Kuroda, T., Noma, H., Naito, C., Tada, M., Yamanaka, H., Takemura, T., Nin Yoshihara, K.H.: Prototyping sensor network system for automatic vital signs collection. Methods Inf. Med. **52** (3), 239–249 (2013)
2. Emori, N., Ito, S., Ohkita, M., Kasamatsu, S., Yoshino, T., Yamashita, Y., Ihaya, A.: A trial of infusion monitoring system using ubiquitous sensor network (in Japanese). Japn. Soc. Qual. Saf. Healthc. **5**(1), 58–63 (2010)
3. Naya, F., Noma, H., Ohmura, R., Kogure, K.: Bluetooth-based indoor proximity sensing for nursing context awareness. Proceedings of IEEE, International Symposium on Wearable Computers, pp. 212–231 (2005)
4. Sato, K., Kuroda, T., Takemura, T., Seiyama, A.: Feasibility assessment of Bluetooth based location system for workflow analysis of nursing staff, IEEE EMBC Short Papers, no. 3316 (2013)
5. Kuroda, T., Noma, H., Takase, K., Sasaki, S., Takemura, T.: Bluetooth roaming for sensor network system in clinical environment. Proceedings of MEDINFO (2015) (In print)
6. Kasamatsu, S., Yoshino, T., Okita, M., Emori, N., Ogaito, T., Yamashita, Y., Ihaya, A.: A study of the dose error reduction system using ubiquitous networks (in Japanese). In: 30th Joint Conference on Medical Informatics, pp. 236–241 (2010)

Eye-Hand Coordination Analysis According to Surgical Process in Laparoscopic Surgery Training

Takafumi Marutani, Hiromi T. Tanaka, Nobutaka Shimada, Masaru Komori, Yoshimasa Kurumi and Shigehiro Morikawa

Abstract Laparoscopic surgery is a recent common surgical technique as one of minimally invasive surgery. This surgery is performed under the situation, such as the limited field of view egocentric video from a laparoscope, and poor force sensation from surgical instruments. Especially, the techniques called "Eye-hand coordination", which represents the collaboration of gazing action and hand action (instrument manipulation), is very important technique in the surgery. In this paper, we analyze gazing actions and instruments manipulation for evaluating the "Eye-hand coordination" technique in order to support the training of Laparoscopic surgery.

1 Introduction

Recently, laparoscopic surgery has become a common surgical technique as one of minimally invasive surgery. There are a number of advantages (e.g. smaller incision, less pain, less hemorrhage, and shorter recovery time) to the patient with Laparoscopic surgery comparing to an open procedure. However, advanced surgical techniques are required in the surgery, because doctors must perform the surgery according to the limited field of view from an endoscope with poor force sensation from surgical instruments. Therefore, it is important to support the training of the laparoscopic surgical techniques.

Generally, the trainings of the surgical techniques are mainly supported by experts' one-by-one coaching. Through the training, trainee learn the techniques about collabotration of gazing action and hand action, which is called Eye-hand coordination. To support the learning of the techinuque, various VR Laparoscopic surgery simulators have been developed. Almost of all VR-based Laparoscopic surgery simulator has the function to assess the surgical techniques of trainees from various

T. Marutani (✉) · H.T. Tanaka · N. Shimada
Ritsumeikan University, Kyoto, Japan
e-mail: marutani@cv.ci.ritsumei.ac.jp

M. Komori · Y. Kurumi · S. Morikawa
Shiga University of Medical Science, Otsu, Japan

Y.-W. Chen et al. (eds.), *Innovation in Medicine and Healthcare 2015*,
Smart Innovation, Systems and Technologies 45,
DOI 10.1007/978-3-319-23024-5_22

measurements (e.g. operating time, path length, and so on). These measurements can evaluate instrument manipulation technique. However the gazing action cannnot be evaluated in spite of its importance. Therefore, we aim to analyze the Eye-hand coordination technique of experts in order to evaluate the trainee's Eye-hand coordination technique.

2 Related Works

There are various researches to support the training of laparoscopic surgery. Ahmmad et al. investigate various assessment methods about surgical techniques [1]. In that research, they support trainees by assessing trainees' surgical techniques manually. Tagawa et al. developed a VR-based Laparoscopic surgery simulator, which can display visual, and force information in order to achieve laparoscopic surgical training of basic tasks [2]. They support trainees by developing training environment. However, it is not sufficient to substitute experts' coaching task by using the environments.

Neumuth et al. proposed Surgical Process Model, which represent operational steps and actions in surgical operation for various reasons: the evaluation of surgical assistant system, the control of surgical robots, and so on [3]. Surgical process represents a part of the operational step of surgery. However, the surgical process cannot suggest how trainees do in each operational step. Then it is not sufficient to describe the detail of Eye-hand coordination techniques.

Thijssen et al. reported various measurements in commercial VR simulators [4]. From their reports, almost of all VR-based Laparoscopic surgery simulator has the function to assess the surgical techniques of trainees from various measurements (e.g. operating time, path length, and so on). These measurements can evaluate the result of trainee's operation. However the measurements cannot evaluate the Eye-hand coordination techniques, because these measurements do not focus on gaze actions.

About detailed technical assessment research using electronic devices, Datta et al. analyzed technical differences between novice and expert according to operating time, path length of instruments, and number of movements in Vein patch insertion [5]. Egi et al. analyzed technical differences between novice and expert according to the trajectories of forceps [6]. These researches focused on how "instruments" are operated. Then, their systems also cannot evaluate the Eye-hand coordination techniques, because these measurements do not focus on gaze actions.

As for the research about gaze action analysis in Laparoscopic surgery, Ibbotson et al. [7] investigate when the doctor, who is performing the laparoscopic operation, look at object during the surgery. Tien et al. [8] analyze the difference of gaze action among in performing the surgery and watching the surgery video. They report some specific tendency of gaze actions about laparoscopic sergery, but focus on only the gaze movements. Then the relationship between gaze action and hand movements is not consider in their research. Therefore, to support the training of Eye-hand coordination, the framework for analyzing both of gaze and hand movements are necessary.

In this paper, at the first step of realizing the framework, we try to analyze the Eye-hand coordination technique of experts in order to reveal the important points about Eye-hand coordination technique.

3 Eye-Hand Coordination Analysis

3.1 Overview of Our Training Support Framework

In our research, we try to analyze trainee's techniques according to surgical processes. Figure 1 shows an overview of our laparoscopic surgical training support framework.

At first, we archive the expert's operation according to surgical process. In concrete, we record expert's operations of instruments and movements, gazing actions, and transformations of organs through surgical simulator. Then, we can describe a surgical process as time-sequential data of expert's actions about gaze and instruments, and transformations of organs. At the next time, by analyzing the trainee's action according to expert's surgical process, and by displaying visual and force information of expert's surgical techniques, trainees can train their techniques without expert's assistances. In this paper, we analyze the Eye-hand coordination techniques according to surgical processes, as the first step of our framework.

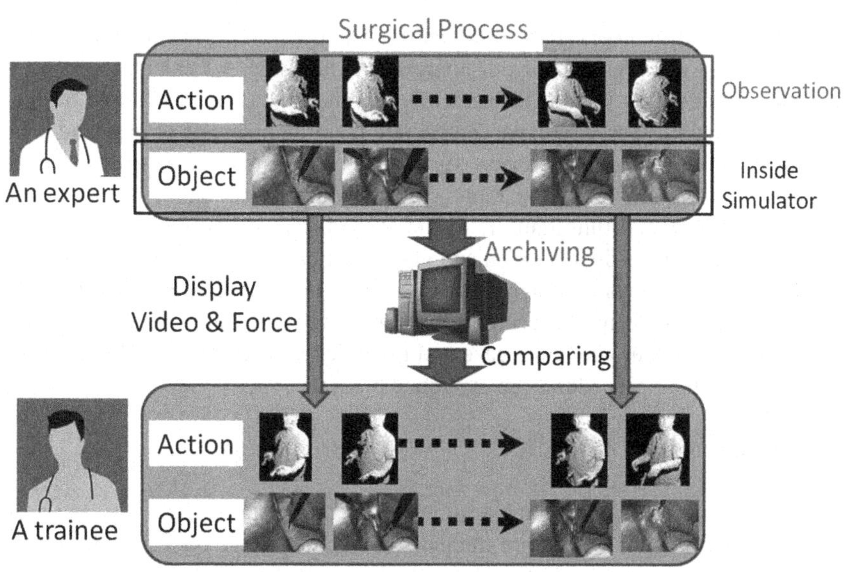

Fig. 1 Framework of our surgical techniques training support

3.2 Surgical Process Model

In our research, we represent surgical process by using Neumuth's Surgical Process Model [9]. Neumuth's Surgical Process Model represents surgical steps as computational representation in order to record and analyze surgical procedures. Neumuth's surgical process consists from following elements.

- *functional:*
  What is done in the work step (e.g. dissect, position).
- *organizational:*
  Who is performing the work (e.g. surgeon, right hand).
- *operational:*
  Which instruments, devices, or resources are used (e.g. forceps, scalpel).
- *spatial:*
  Where the step is performed (e.g. dura, cranial nerve).
- *behavioral:*
  When the step is performed (e.g. start, end).

In this paper, we focus on "*spatial*" element, because the element represent the target object in the process, and the position of the target object becomes the basis of position analysis.

3.3 Analysis Procedures

In order to analyze Eye-hand coordination, we perform following procedures. Figure 2 shows the overview of our analysis. At first step, we calculate the positions of feature points (target, instrument's tip, and target) in each frame of egocetric video. By this procedure, we can acquire many sample data of gaze and hand movement through a surgical process. A sample data consists of followings features acquired from a frame; target position $(x_t(t), y_t(t))$, tip's position $(x_f(t), y_f(t))$, gaze point $(x_g(t), y_g(t))$, and timestamp t. At the second step, we normalize the sample data by translating the tip's position and gaze point based on the position of target, and transforming the value range of tips and gaze in [−0.5;0.5] and t in [0;1]. At the last step, we perform clustering to the normalized sample points. Through the clustering, the data, in which the gaze and tip are closely related, may be revealed. The details of these procedures are explained below.

Position detection

In order to start analysis, we must acquire the position data of target, tip, and gaze point. In this research, we acquire the gaze point data by eye tracking device, and target position by manual operation, because the target changes drastically about it's position and shape, and is hard to extract by computational method. In opposite, the

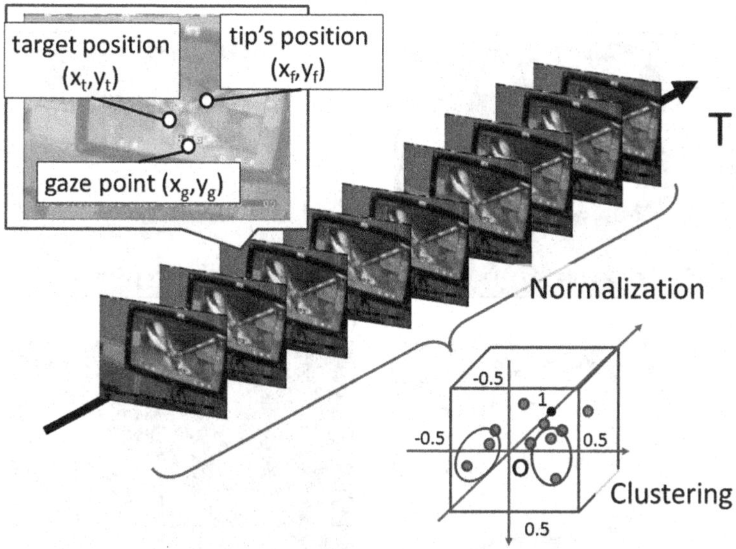

Fig. 2 Overview of Eye-hand coordination analysis

tip's position is relatively easy to detect, because the instruments are rigid objects. To detect the tip's position, we apply Fathi's method [10]. Figure 3 shows the position detection process. At first, we construct superpixel based on simila llity among neighboring pixels. After that, we segment the instrument area based on harmonic solution by selecting some superpixels as instruments, and some other superpixels as background. At last, we detect a position as tip's position based on the segmented region and instrument constraint (its' long and narrow shape and it's direction in the working area).

Normalization

In surgical process, the target position and the operating time differ by various reasons (manipulation, camera angle, skill level, and so on). Therefore, we analyze gaze position and tip's position by relative position from target position and reduce the scale differences among positon data and time data. Then, we suppose that there are sample points $\{\mathbf{P}(t) = (x_g(t), y_g(t), x_f(t), y_f(t), x_t(t), y_t(t), t)\}$ $(0 \leq x_g(t), x_f(t), x_t(t) \leq X_{max}, 0 \leq y_g(t), y_f(t), y_t(t) \leq Y_{max}, t_s \leq t \leq t_e)$, we calculate normalized sample point $\hat{\mathbf{P}}(t) = (\hat{x}_g(t), \hat{y}_g(t), \hat{x}_f(t), \hat{y}_f(t), \hat{t})$ by followings;

$$\hat{x}_{\{g,f\}}(t) = \frac{x_{\{g,f\}}(t) - x_t(t)}{X_{max}}$$

$$\hat{y}_{\{g,f\}}(t) = \frac{y_{\{g,f\}}(t) - y_t(t)}{X_{max}}$$

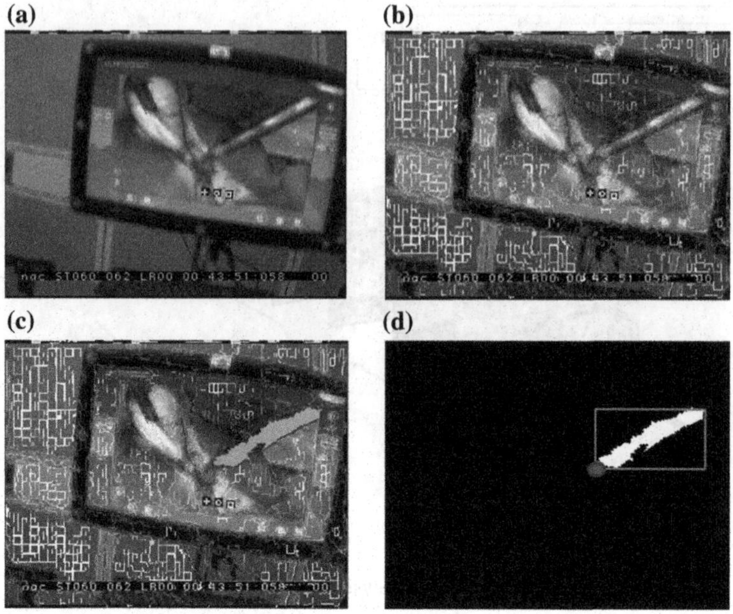

Fig. 3 Forceps' tip detection process (**a**) Original data (**b**) Superpixel (**c**) Segmentation based on manual labeling (**d**) Tip detection based on instrument's constraint

$$\hat{t} = \frac{t - t_s}{t_e - t_s}$$

Clustering

By clustering the data points $\{\hat{\mathbf{P}}(t)\}$, we aim to concentrate some specific combination of gaze movements and tip's movements. In this paper, we choose k-means algorithm as the clustering algorithm. After the clustering, we analyze each cluster by comparing the datapoints in the cluster and the egocantric video of corresponding duration.

4 Experiment

To analize Eye-hand coordination by our method, We measured the 3 experts' eye movement under VR laparoscopic cholecystectomy surgery training. We use commercial VR surgical simulator (Lap-Mentor [11]) and eye-tracking device (EMR-9 [12]) for the measurement. Figure 4 shows the experimental settings. The subjects demonstrate a series of surgical processes about laparoscopic cholecystectomy surgery by VR simulator. The details of the training surgical

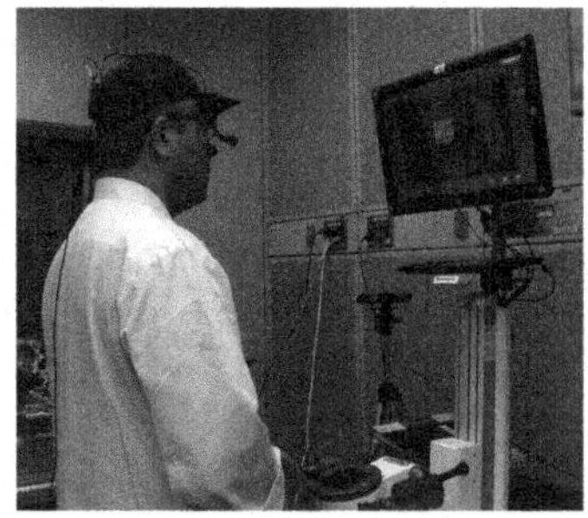

Fig. 4 Experimental settings (the case of expert clinician)

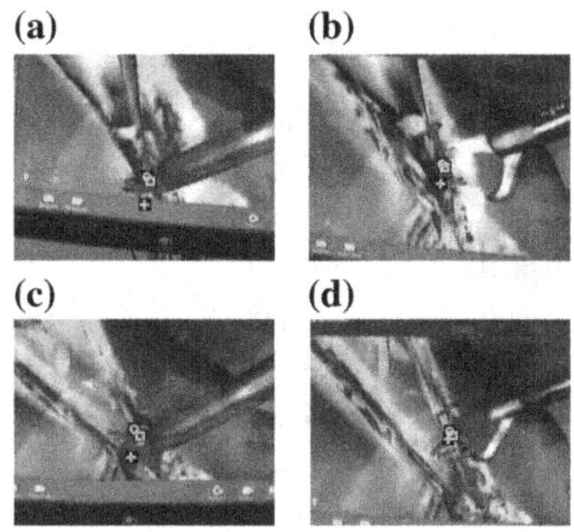

Fig. 5 Example of screenshot about surgical processes. **a** Clipping Cystic Duct. **b** Cutting Cystic Duct. **c** Clipping Cystic Artery. **d** Cutting Cystic Artery

processes are as follows; ablating fats, clipping cystic duct, cutting cystic duct, clipping cystic artery and cutting cystic artery. In these processes, we select 4 process for analysis, because there are clear target position in these processes. (The screenshots of the selected processes are shown in Fig. 5.) All subjects demonstrate through operation by 7–15 min. The sampling rate for eye movements is 60[Hz]. The effective number of pixels of head mounted camera view is 640[H] by 480[w], and the horizontal angle of view is 62°. We divided the eye movement data into each process manually. And the target position in each surgical process are attached manually.

Tables 1, 2 and 3 are the details of acquired data. In each table, "ClipCD", "CutCD", "ClipCA" and "CutCA" represent the surgical processes "clipping cystic duct", "cutting cystic duct", "clipping cystic artery" and "cutting cystic artery". Table 1 shows the elapsed time of subjects for completing each surgical process ([sec]). In addition, we measure the distance of eye movements and instrument's movement, because these measurement are used for technical assessment [4]. Table 2 shows the total eye movement distance in egocentric video of subjects for completing each surgical process([pixel]). Table 1 shows the total instrument movement distance in egocentric video of subjects for completing each surgical process([pixel]).

From the Table 1, novices spent less time to complete surgical processes than experts in many cases. The reasons for this may be as follows; All subjects in this experiment use the simulator for the first time. Therefore, novices can be familiar with the simulator soon. On the other hand, experts have trouble with controlling

Table 1 Elapsed time for completing surgical processes ([sec])

	Process			
subject	ClipCD	CutCD	ClipCA	CutCA
expertA	0:21	0:15	0:45	0:09
expertB	0:30	0:25	0:26	0:15
expertC	0:31	0:10	0:27	0:07
noviceA	0:28	0:15	0:13	0:13
noviceB	0:19	0:07	0:46	0:06
noviceC	0:17	0:03	0:17	0:02

Table 2 Total eye movement distances in surgical processes ([pixels])

	Process			
subject	ClipCD	CutCD	ClipCA	CutCA
expertA	7,706	5,748	8,987	1,539
expertB	4,013	2,137	1,887	1,402
expertC	3,488	800	2,053	460
noviceA	5,397	2,567	2,821	2,165
noviceB	4,265	3,362	10,858	816
noviceC	2,245	314	2,390	175

Table 3 Total instrument movement distances in Surgical Processes ([pixels])

	Process			
subject	ClipCD	CutCD	ClipCA	CutCA
expertA	3,735	2,465	4,919	433
expertB	2,316	1,879	1,420	1,096
expertC	2,518	682	1,761	404
noviceA	2,590	1,012	1,895	2,145
noviceB	1,784	1,121	3,106	498
noviceC	1,500	243	1,863	102

the simulator by feeling gap of real surgery. Especially, expertA failed in holding gallbladder many times. It is also be revealed that all subjects spent more time in clipping process than that in cutting process. This is because the clipped positions in clipping process affects the difficulty of cutting process. Therefore subjects tend to spend much time for deciding clipping positions.

From the Tables 2 and 3, expertA moved his eye and hand more than other subjects. However, as mentioned in Table 1, he had trouble to control the simulator. Therefore, we exclude his data for analysis. Comparing movement distances among experts and novices, the distances of experts are relatively shorter than that of novices

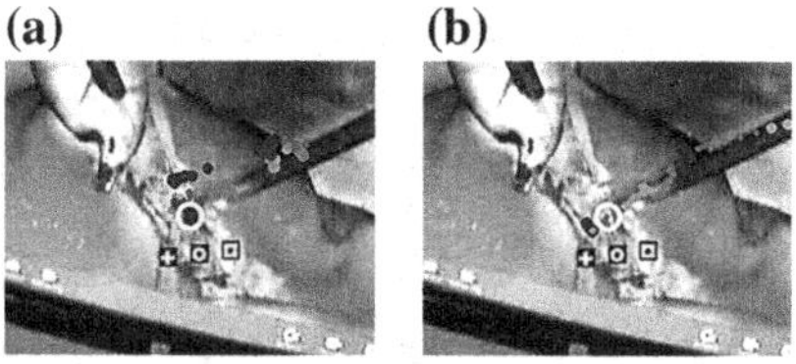

Fig. 6 Point distributions of gaze and forcep's tip about one subject in a surgical process (cutting cystic artery). **a** Gaze points distribution. **b** Tip's positions distribution

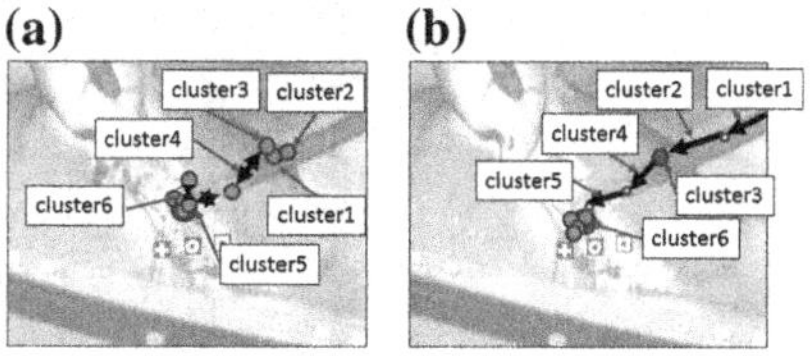

Fig. 7 Movements of gaze and forcep's tip about one subject in a surgical process (cutting cystic artery) **a** Gaze points movement. **b** Tip's positions movement

when we take into account of elapsed times. Especially, the eye movement distances of experts are obviously less than that of novices. This is because the experts can fix their gaze in particular points. Experts understood where to watch based on their surgical experiences.

Figure 6 shows the clustering result ($k = 10$) in cutting cystic artery process of a subject. In this figure, the left figure shows the position distribution of gaze point (relative position to target position.) And the right figure shows the position distribution of forceps' tip (relative position to target position.) The points of same color in both figures are belonging to same cluster. From this result, there are some cases that the tips' position approach to the gaze fixation points. This means that experts fix their attention to particular point, and then approach the instruments towards the point in a straight line.

Figure 7 shows the detailed movements of gaze and instruments in cluster 1–6. (In this experiments, we choose $k = 10$ for clustering. However the movements of gaze and instrument are very small in cluster 7–10. Then we omit their data in Fig. 7). In this figure, arrows show the movement and large circle represent the fixation of gaze and instrument. At first, expert look at the halfway position to the target and bring the instruments to the position in cluster 1 and 2. After he checked the condition of instrument tip in cluster 3, he checked the next position (around target) and move the instruments to the position in cluster 4. Then, he repeat checking the condition of the instrument tip and target position, and move the instrument to the target position in cluster 5. At last, he checked the condition around the target. This means that he did not move the instrument to the target position in one breath. This is because he avoided puncturing other organs. In Laparoscopic surgery, the workspace is very narrow and the distance among target and other organs is very short. Therefore, large movement of instrument may be dangerous.

For more detailed analysis, we make a graph, that shows the velocity transitions of gaze and instruments of same data, as shown in Fig. 8. In this graph, the vertical axis represents the velocity of gaze point and tip of instrument ([pix/frame]), and the horizontal axis represents the time ([frame]) from start time. The vertical lines

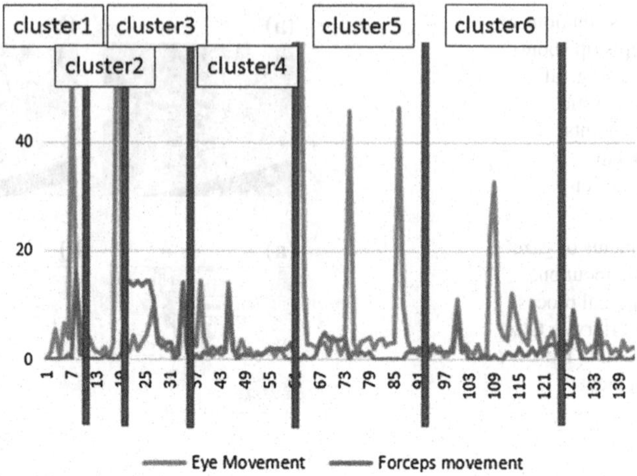

Fig. 8 Velocity transitions of gaze and forceps (closeup) [*pix*/*frame*]

in the graph show the borderline among clusters. From this graph, the clusters are mainly divided according to time sequences, and the width of cluster depends on the value of variances. In the graphs of cluster 1, the velocity of gaze make a peak before the border. This timing is that the expert looks at the target position. After that, the expert operate the instrument with stable speed (at the first half of cluster 2.) This means that the expert can control the instrument smoothly, and move it to appropriate position courteously. In addition, in the graph of cluster 4 and 5, there are some peaks about velocity of gaze. These timing are that the expert checks the state of instrument's tip or checks the state around the target position. During the timing, the velocity of tip's position are almost 0. This means that the expert can fix the instrument while checking surgical situation by their eyes. These tendency are also found in other processes and other experts.

5 Conclusions

In this paper, we analyze Eye-hand coordination based on egocentric video during laparoscopic surgery training according to surgical process. In order to analyze eye-hand coordination, we calculate the positions of feature points (target, instrument's tip, and target), normalize them based on the target position and value range, and perform clustering by using conventional clustering algorithm. After that, we compare the distance of eye movement and instrument among 3 experts and 3 novices, and analyze the cooperative movements of gaze and instrument in experts' training.

From the result of analysis, we could find some relationship between gaze movements and instrument movements. However, this analysis is based on only limited surgical processes. Therefore, we will apply our method to other surgical processes and check the differences among the experts and the novices for further analysis.

References

1. Ahmmad, S.N.Z., Ming, E.S.L., Fai, Y.C., Harun, F.K.C.: Assessment Methods for Surgical Skill, World Academy of Science, Engineering and Technology, vol. 58, pp. 752–758 (2011)
2. Tagawa, K., Tanaka, H.T., Kurumi, Y., Komori, M., Morikawa, S.: Laparoscopic Surgery Simulator Using First Person View and Guidance Force. Medicine Meets Virtual Reality, vol. 20, pp. 431–435 (2013)
3. Neumuth, D., Loebe, F., Herre, H., Neumuth, T.: Modeling surgical processes: a four-level translational approach. Artif. Intell. Med. **51**, 147–161 (2011)
4. Thijssen, A.S., Schijven, M.P.: Contemporary virtual reality laparoscopy simulators: quicksand or solid grounds for assessing surgical trainees? Am. J. Surg. **199**, 529–541 (2010)
5. Datta, V., Mackay, S., Mandalia, M., Darzi, A.: The use of electromagnetic motion tracking analysis to objectively measure open surgical skill in the laboratory-based model. Am. Coll. Surg. **193**, 479–485 (2001)
6. Egi, H., Okajima, M., Yoshimitsu, M., Ikeda, S., Miyata, Y., Masugami, H., Kawahara, T., Kurita, Y., Kaneko, M., Asahara, T.: Obejctive assessment of endoscopic surgical skills by analyzing direction-dependent dexterity using the hiroshima university endoscopic surgical assessment device (HUESAD). Surg. Today **38**, 705–710 (2008)
7. Ibbotson, J.A., MacKenzie, C.L., Cao, C.G.L., Lomax, A.J.: Gaze patterns in laparoscopic surgery. In: Medicine Meets, Virtual Reality, pp. 154–160 (1999)
8. Tien, G., Atkins, M.S., Jiang, X., Khan, R.S.A., Zheng, B.: Identifying eye gaze mismatch during laparoscopic surgery. In: Medical Meets, Virtual Reality, pp. 453–457 (2013)
9. Neumuth, T., Loebe, F., Jannin, P.: Similarity metrics for surgical process models. Artif. Intell. Med. **54**, 15–27 (2012)
10. Fathi, A., Balcan, M.F., Ren, X., Rehg, J.M.: Combining self training and active learning for video segmentation. Proc. BMVC 78.1–78.11 (2011)
11. Lap-Mentor. http://simbionix.com/simulators/lap-mentor/
12. EMR-9. http://www.eyemark.jp/product/emr_9/index.html

An Improvement of Surgical Phase Detection Using Latent Dirichlet Allocation and Hidden Markov Model

Dinh Tuan Tran, Ryuhei Sakurai and Joo-Ho Lee

Abstract In this paper, we present two methods to utilize Latent Dirichlet Allocation and Hidden Markov Model to automatically detect surgical workflow phases based on codebook which is built by quantizing the extracted optical flow vectors from the recorded videos of surgical processes. To detect the current phase at a given time point of an operation, some recorded training data with correct phase label need to be learned by a topic model. All documents which are actually short clips divided from the recorded videos are presented as mixtures over learned latent topics. These presentations are then quantized as observed values of a Hidden Markov Model (HMM). The major difference between two proposed methods is that while the first method quantizes all topic-based presentations based on k-means, the second method does this based on multivariate Gaussian mixture model. A Left to Right HMM is appropriate for this work because there is no switching the order between surgical phases.

Keywords Surgical phase detection · Latent Dirichlet allocation · Hidden Markov model

1 Introduction

In recent years, with the advancements in technology and medicine, the operating room (OR) in particular, has evolved into a highly complex and technologically rich environment. Error in medical became one of the most serious issues in daily practices. Although numerous research projects have been established to reduce the medical errors and a certain result was achieved, there is no radical solution to stop medical errors [1]. In OR, concepts such as context-aware ORs appeared. A key research field which is growing interest in context-aware concept is the analysis of

D.T. Tran (✉) · R. Sakurai · J.-H. Lee
Graduate of Science and Engineering, Ritsumeikan University, Kyoto, Japan
e-mail: is0050pi@ed.ritsumei.ac.jp

Y.-W. Chen et al. (eds.), *Innovation in Medicine and Healthcare 2015*,
Smart Innovation, Systems and Technologies 45,
DOI 10.1007/978-3-319-23024-5_23

the surgical workflow (SW) [2]. Surgical process models (SPMs) were first introduced to be a powerful tool to help surgeons by using a model of surgical progress. The model is able to identify meaningful information such as activities, steps, or even adverse events in a surgical intervention. By using SPMs, main purposes such as the surgical decision-making process as well as surgical teaching will be facilitated an assessment, thereby impact directly on patient safety. Also, SPMs could help in anticipating patient positioning, optimizing operating time or analyzing technical requirements.

Some methods have been developed to identify intra-operative activities, detect common phases in the surgical workflow and combine all gained knowledge into a SPM [3]. In surgical phase detection work, the signals that can be used are manyfold, varying from manual annotations by observers [4], to sensor data such as surgical tool tracking based on images from recorded videos [5].

In light of the growing interest in this field, we propose in this paper two methods to utilize Latent Dirichlet Allocation (LDA) and Hidden Markov Model (HMM) to automatically detect surgical workflow phases based on codebook which is built by quantizing the extracted optical flow vectors from the recorded videos of surgical processes.

This paper is organized as follows: In the next section, we describe the problem statement and the overview of our previous published method [6]. The disadvantage of our previous method is explained in Sect. 3. The detail of two proposed methods is described in Sect. 4. To this end, we conduct some experiments to compare two proposed methods with our previous one in Sect. 5.

2 Overview of Our Previous Method

The goal of this work is to output an appropriate phase for each given time point in a surgical operation. The phase concept mentioned here has the meaning of a specified work in a SW. Because each kind of surgery has its own order of works that needed to be done and there is no switching the order between these works, therefore our idea in this research is that by constructing a HMM based on this characteristic with the number of hidden states is corresponding to the number of phases in the SW, the observed value at a given time point will be calculated and the output likelihood will indicate the appropriate phase corresponding to that time point (Fig. 1).

2.1 Optical Flow Extraction

Optical flow (OF) is the pattern of apparent motion of objects, surfaces, and edges between two video frames that have a small time interval. In this work, from videos gained from multiple cameras, we extract OF in each pair of consecutive frames at

Fig. 1 Proposed method

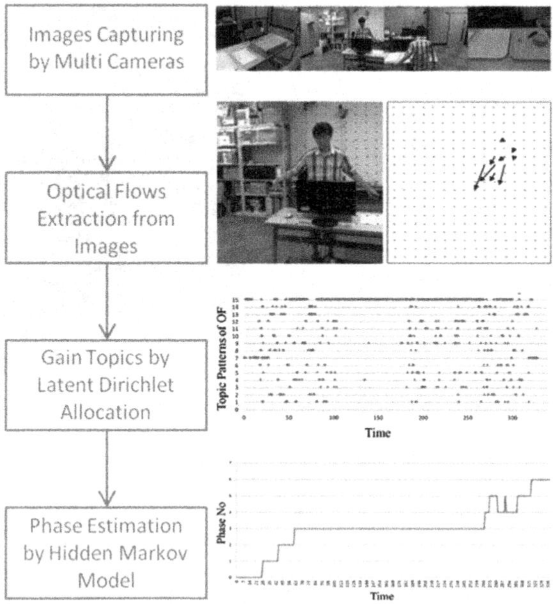

positions arranged on a grid with a spacing of fixed pixels using [7]. First, all extracted OFs are thresholded to remove noise. The remaining OF vectors are then quantized into 4 directions such as up, down, left, right using a codebook. After quantization is applied, all OF vectors have the same size. The final output of this step is a set of OFs at all time points and at all grid points (Fig. 2).

2.2 Topics Modeling Using Latent Dirichlet Allocation

Latent Dirichlet Allocation (LDA) [8] is a generative model that is widely used in natural language processing. LDA is an example of a topic model that is a statistical model to detect topics inside documents. In LDA, each document is actually a set of words and has a ratio of all topics that is assumed inside the document. The graphical model of LDA is showed in Fig. 3. In Fig. 3, M denotes the number of documents, N denotes the number of words in a document, K denotes the number of topics. Also, α is the parameter of the Dirichlet prior on the per-document topic distributions, β is the parameter of the Dirichlet prior on the per-topic word distributions, θ_i is the topic distribution for document i, φ_k is the word distribution for topic k, $z_{i,j}$ is the topic for the jth word in document i and $w_{i,j}$ is the specific word.

In this work, LDA is used for patterning the motions of surgeons represented by OFs in operating room and these gained patterns will be used as the observed values of a HMM in next step. The videos gained from multiple cameras are divided into a sequence of 1-second clips. Each clip corresponds to a document in LDA, each clip

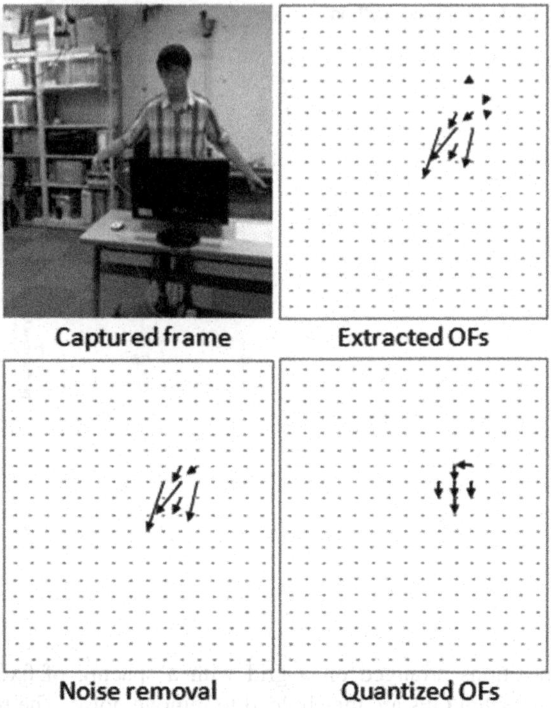

Fig. 2 OFs extraction

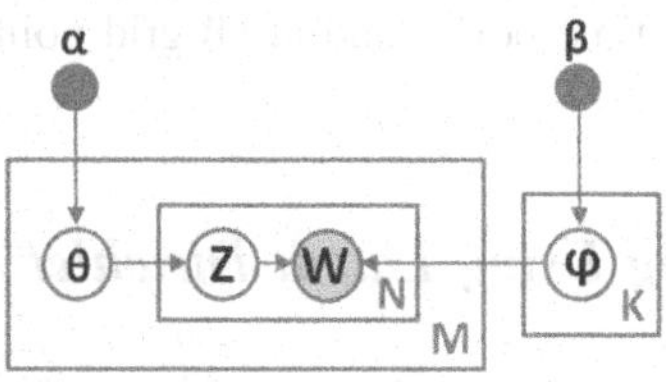

Fig. 3 The LDA graphical model

is represented by the words accumulated over its frames and each word indicates an OF vector at a rigid point. A word then corresponds to an OF vector and the position of the grid point where that vector occurred. The final output of this step is the distribution of all topics over each clip (1) and the distribution of all words over each topic (2).

$$\theta_i \sim \mathrm{Dir}(\alpha),\ i \in \{0, .., \mathrm{M}-1\} \tag{1}$$

$$\varphi_k \sim \mathrm{Dir}(\beta),\ k \in \{0, \ldots, \mathrm{K}-1\} \tag{2}$$

2.3 Hidden Markov Model Construction

Hidden Markov Model (HMM) [9] is a statistical Markov model in which the system being modeled is assumed to be a Markov process with unobserved (hidden) states. Each state has a state transition probability distribution that defines the transition probabilities from itself to other states, an emission probability distribution that defines the output probabilities for all observed values in the state, and an initial state probability distribution that represents the probability that this state is the starting state in HMM. Because each kind of surgery has its own order of works that needed to be done and there is no switching the order between these works, therefore a Left to Right HMM is appropriate in this work. The Left to Right HMM is limited in the transition probability distribution that all states are able to transit only to itself or the next state, and aren't able to return to the past ones (Fig. 4).

The transition probability from state q to state q' is calculated by using the following equation:

$$\mathrm{T}_{q,q'} = \frac{\sum(q \to q')}{\sum(q \to -)} \tag{3}$$

where, $\sum(q \to q')$ is number of transitions from state q to state q' and—means all states.

The estimation probability distribution is calculated as follows: First, from the distribution of all topics over each document θ_i which is the output of previous step (1), a quantization process is applied to transform the distribution to a binary-based one (4). Second, the observation value of each document is calculated using (5). The variance of the observed value becomes K power of 2. Finally, the emission probability distribution of the state q is calculated using (6).

$$\theta_{i,k} = \begin{bmatrix} 1 & \text{if } \theta_{i,k} \geq \frac{1}{\mathrm{K}} \times \sum_{k'=0}^{\mathrm{K}-1} \theta_{i,k'} \\ 0 & \text{otherwise} \end{bmatrix} \tag{4}$$

$$\mathrm{O}_i = \sum_{k=0}^{\mathrm{K}-1} (\theta_{i,k} \times 2^k),\ \mathrm{O}_i \in [2^0, 2^{\mathrm{K}}] \tag{5}$$

$$\mathrm{E}_{q,o} = \frac{\sum(i \in q | \mathrm{O}_i = o)}{\sum(i \in q)} + \epsilon \tag{6}$$

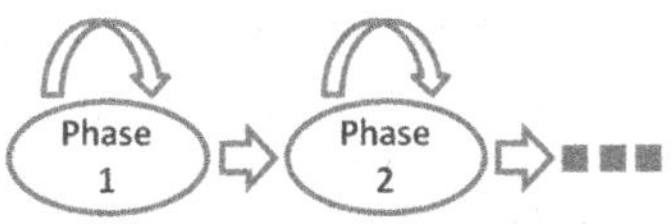

Fig. 4 *Left* to *Right* hidden Markov model

where, $\theta_{i,k}$ is the probability that the topic k appears in document i, $\sum(i \in q | O_i = o)$ is number of documents in state q that has the observation value o and $\sum(i \in q)$ is number of documents in state q. ϵ is a smoothing term that enable to estimate when an observed value is impossible to appear from constructed model.

The initial state probability distribution that represents the probability that a state is the starting state in the HMM is defined as follows:

$$\pi_q = \begin{cases} 1 & \text{if } q = 0 \\ 0 & \text{otherwise} \end{cases} \tag{7}$$

The HMM is initialized with all parameters calculated above. These parameters of the model are then estimated with the goal to maximize the likelihood of the data given the model. This is done for HMM with the Baum-Welch algorithm [10] which is actually an instance of the well-known Expectation-Maximization algorithm [11] for missing data problems in statistics. The process is iterative and hence we can call re-estimation.

2.4 *Phase Determination*

With each input clip at a given time point in surgical workflow of the same surgery type, OFs are extracted and removed noise as describled in Sect. 2.1. The distribution of all topics over this clip is then calculated based on the extracted OFs using topic model gained in Sect. 2.2. After that, the observation value of the clip is calculated by using (4) and (5). Finally, the appropriate state is estimated by the trained HMM.

3 Disadvantages of Our Previous Method

Although the method introduced above has been implemented and gotten a promising result, some disadvantages of the method have caused its decrease in reliability. The most significant problem is memory usage. In the method implementation, a double-type array needs to be used to implement the estimation probability distribution for a HMM state in (6). As shown in (5), the variance of observation value is K power of 2. Therefore, if a double-type variable has a size of 8 bytes, the required size S in bytes of the array is calculated using (8).

$$S = 8 * 2^K \tag{8}$$

where, K is the number of topics in the LDA, S is the size in bytes of the array required to implement the estimation probability distribution for a state in the HMM.

Table 1 Memory usage S in three methods

Number of topics (K)	S in our previous method	S in the method using k-means (c = 50) (KB)	S in the method using MGM (m = 5) (KB)
10	8 KB	0.4	4.4
20	8 MB	0.4	16.8
30	8 GB	0.4	37.2
40	8 TB	0.4	65.6
50	8 PB	0.4	102
60	8 EB	0.4	146.4
70	8 ZB	0.4	198.8

The second column of Table 1 shows some values of required size S when the number K of topics in the LDA is from 10 to 70. Because of these requirements, with computer hardware nowadays, the method is available only when the value of K is smaller than 40. Because a real surgical workflow often has a sequence of very large number of activities which each activity corresponds to a topic in the LDA, the limitation of small number of topics in the LDA therefore cause its decrease in reliability.

4 Proposed Methods

In this section, we propose two methods to resolve the significant problem described in Sect. 3. While the first method uses k-means clustering method to calculate the observation value for each document, the second method do this based on Multivariate Gaussian Mixture model.

4.1 Calculating Observation Value Using K-Means

K-means clustering is a method of vector quantization that solves the well-known clustering problem in data mining. In unsupervised learning, k-means is one of the simplest algorithms that its procedure follows a simple and easy way to classify a given n observations through a certain number of clusters (c clusters) in which each observation belongs to the cluster with the nearest mean.

Given a set of observations θ_i, $i = 1 \ldots n$, where each observation is a d-dimensional real vector, k-means classify the n observations into c ($\leq n$) clusters $S = \{S_1, S_2, \cdots, S_c\}$ by finding the positions μ_i, $i = 1 \ldots c$ of the clusters centers that minimize the within-cluster sum of squares which are distances from observations to the clusters centers:

$$\operatorname{argmin}_S \sum_{i=1}^{c} \sum_{\theta \in S_i} \|\theta - \mu_i\|^2 \tag{9}$$

In this method, after quantization process is done to transform the distribution of all topics over each document to a binary-based one in (4), instead of using (5) to calculate the observation value for each document, we use k-means to classify all documents which each document has a distribution of all topics θ_i, $i = 1 \ldots n$ where each distribution θ is a K-dimensional vector (K is the number of topics in the LDA) into c clusters (10). The result of classifying by k-means is used as observation values for documents to calculate the emission probability distribution for the state q in (6).

$$O_i = \operatorname{argmin}_a \|\theta_i - \mu_a\|, \ O_i \in [1, c] \tag{10}$$

In the method implementation, a double-type array needs to be used to implement the estimation probability distribution for a HMM state in (6). As shown in (10), the variance of observation value in this method is equal to the number c of clusters in the k-means. Therefore, if a double-type variable has a size of 8 bytes, the required size S in bytes of the array is calculated using (11).

$$S = 8 * c \tag{11}$$

The third column of the Table 1 shows the value of required size S when the number K of topics in the LDA is from 10 to 70 and the number c of clusters in the k-means is 50. The Eq. (11) and the third column of the Table 1 indicate that the value of S depends only on the value of c, does not depend on the value of K. Also, because the number of clusters in the k-means is often small, therefore the memory is needed to implement the estimation probability distribution is small and the significant disadvantage described in Sect. 3 is resolved perfectly.

4.2 Calculating Observation Value Using Multivariate Gaussian Mixture Model

In data mining, data clustering is a main task of exploratory that is the process of classifying observations into clusters so that observations in the same cluster are as similar as possible, and observations in different clusters are as dissimilar as possible. Data clustering has two types: hard clustering and soft clustering. In hard clustering, observations are assigned into distinct clusters, where each observation belongs to exactly one cluster. On the other hand, soft clustering assigns observations to clusters with certain probabilities. The first method described in Sect. 4.1 uses k-means that is a hard clustering. In this second method, we extend k-means to make a soft clustering. Given a set of clusters centers μ_i, $i = 1 \ldots c$, instead of directly assign all observations to their closest clusters, we assign them probabilistically based on the distances by using multivariate Gaussian mixture (MGM) distribution with a specified number of mixtures.

$$\mathrm{p}\left(x; a_j, S_j, \pi_j\right) = \sum_{j=1}^{m} \pi_j p_j(x) \tag{12}$$

$$\sum_{j=1}^{m} \pi_j = 1 \tag{13}$$

where m is the number of mixtures in MGM distribution, p_j is the normal distribution density with the mean a_j and covariance matrix S_j, π_j is the weight of the jth mixture.

In this method, after quantization process is done to transform the distribution of all topics over each document to a binary-based one in (4), instead of using (5) and (6) to calculate the emission probability distribution for the state q, we use a multivariate Gaussian mixture distribution with a specified number of mixtures which is estimated from binary-based distribution of all topics over each document in the same state q as the emission probability distribution for the state q (14).

In the method implementation, the double-type array is used to implement E_q in (14). If the number of topics in the LDA is K, the size of means in MGM is K and the size of covariance matrix is K^2. Therefore, if a double-type variable has a size of 8 bytes, the required size S in bytes of the array is calculated using (15).

$$\mathrm{E}_q \sim \mathrm{MGM}\left(\theta_{q1}, \theta_{q2}, \cdots, \theta_{qn}\right) \tag{14}$$

$$\mathrm{S} = 8 * \left(m + \left(\mathrm{K} + \mathrm{K}^2\right) * m\right) \tag{15}$$

where θ_{qi} is binary-based distribution of all topics over ith document in the state q. m is the number of mixtures in MGM distribution.

The fourth column of the Table 1 shows some values of required size S when the number K of topics in the LDA is from 10 to 70 and the number m of mixtures in MGM distribution is 5. Although the memory usage S increases when the number of topics increases, the biggest value of S (19,8840 bytes) is very small, much smaller than 8 Zettabytes in our previous method. Therefore, we can conclude that the method that uses multivariate Gaussian mixture distribution has resolved the significant disadvantage described in Sect. 3.

5 Experiments

In this section, some experiments are conducted to compare performance of two proposed methods described in Sect. 4 and our previous method summarized in Sect. 2.

5.1 Settings

The type of surgery used in our experiments is cholecystectomy, which is a typical laparoscopic surgery. This surgery has a basic flow and assumed to consist of following 7 phases: Entrance, preparation, dissection, operation, suturation, cleanup, exit.

Figure 5 shows the surgical room, the surgical instruments and the positions of 5 cameras used in the experiments. 4 of 5 cameras are used to capture the surgical room, the rack, the trays and operation field. The remaining one is laparoscope. All cameras have the resolution of 640 × 480. Figure 6 shows the images captured from multiple cameras. The number on the top-left of each image in Fig. 6 corresponds to the position in Fig. 5. We recorded the surgical workflow 5 times, 4 times are for learning the parameters of the HMM and the remaining time is for testing the

Fig. 5 Environment setting

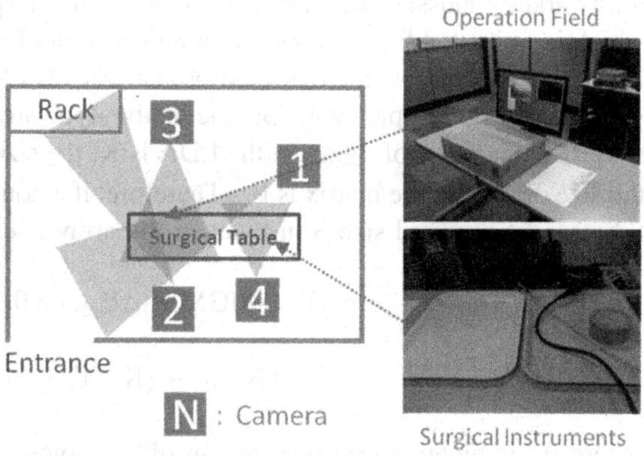

Fig. 6 Images captured from multiple cameras

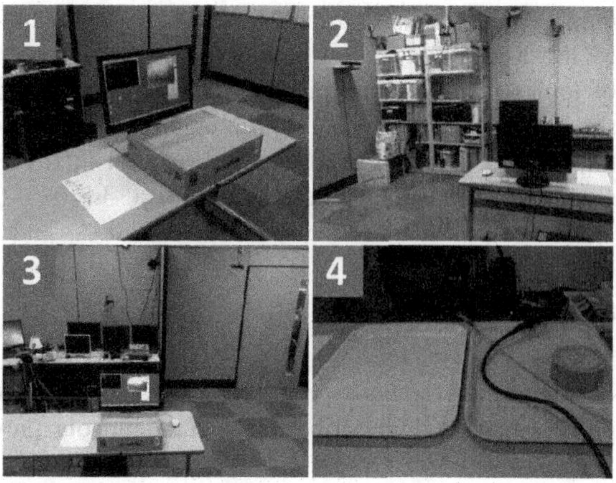

accuracy of the phase detection of 3 methods. We did this so that every set of images was used for testing once in leave-one-out-fashion.

The grid points mentioned in Sect. 2.1 have a spacing of 20 × 20 pixels. The number K of topics is 10, α and β in the LDA are set to 1.0 and 0.1. The smoothing term ϵ in (6) is set to 0.0001. The number c of clusters in the k-means in Sect. 4.1 is 50 and the number m of mixtures in MGM distribution in Sect. 4.2 is 5.

5.2 Experimental Results

Figure 7 shows the comparisons between the detection results of our previous method summarized in Sect. 2 and the correct labels of phases. Figures 8 and 9

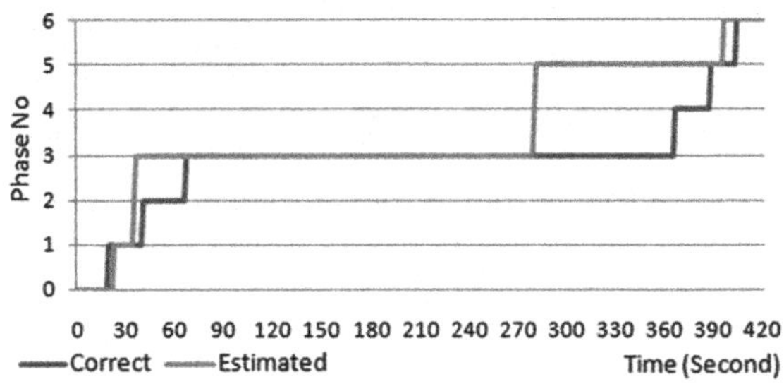

Fig. 7 Detection results of our previous method (Sect. 2). The *blue line* is the correct phase label and the *red line* shows estimation results

Fig. 8 Detection results of the proposed method using k-means (Sect. 4.1)

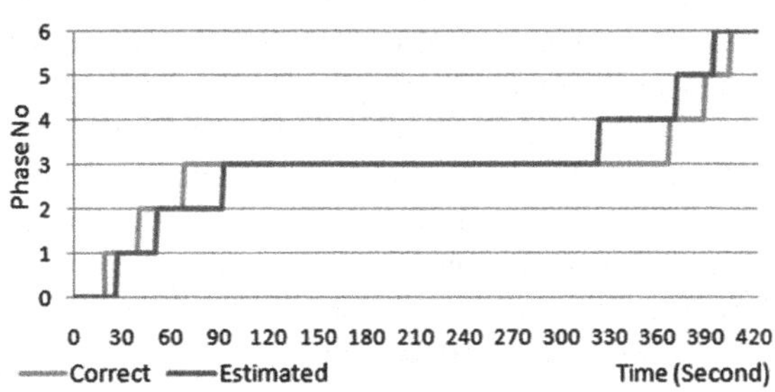

Fig. 9 Detection results of the proposed method using MGM (Sect. 4.2)

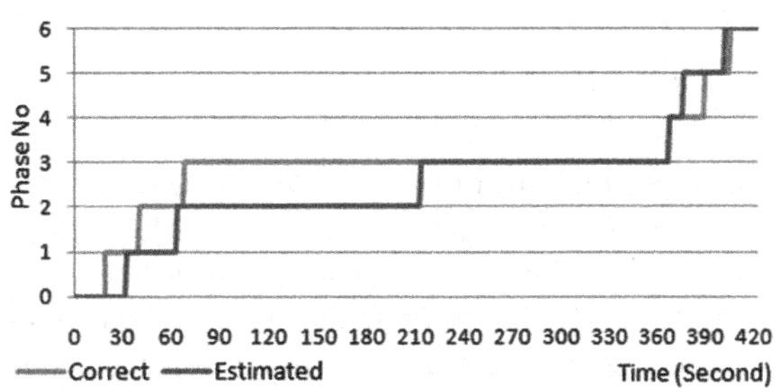

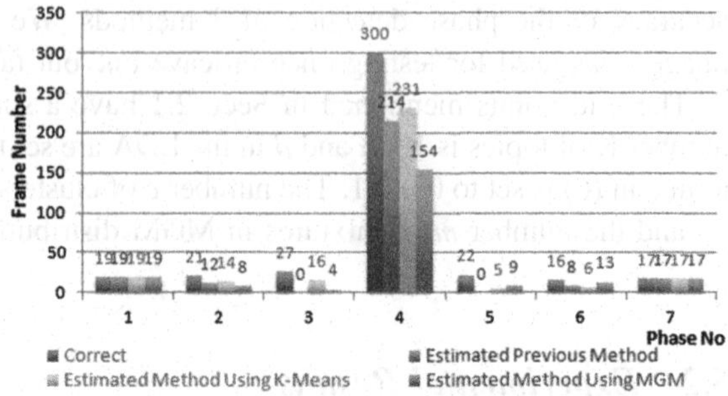

Fig. 10 Detection results in each phase of all 3 methods

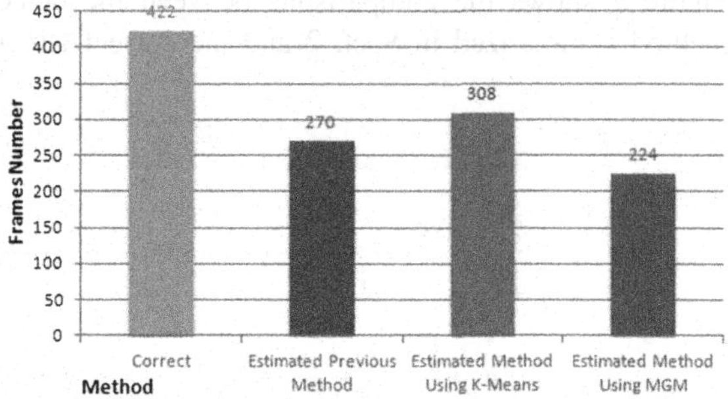

Fig. 11 Detection results of all 3 methods

shows the same comparisons for the proposed methods described in Sect. 4. Figure 10 shows the comparisons of the number of correct detection results in each phase between all 3 methods. Figure 11 shows the same comparisons but is average in all phases. Although 3 methods detected correctly all documents in phase 1 and phase 7, the numbers of correct detection results of 3 methods in the remaining phases are different. The proposed method using k-means detected better than other methods in phases 2, 3 and 4. In phases 5 and 6, the best method is the proposed method using multivariate Gaussian mixture distribution. Figure 11 indicates that the method using k-means has the best performance (73 %). Although the method using multivariate Gaussian mixture distribution (53 %) has worse average performance than our previous method (64 %) in all phases, our previous method was not able to detect phases 3 and 5.

6 Conclusions

This paper described two methods inherited our previous method that uses Latent Dirichlet Allocation and Hidden Markov Model to automatically estimate phases in a surgical workflow. The input of the methods is multiple videos gained from multiple cameras. After all processes including optical flow extraction, topics modeling using Latent Dirichlet Allocation and Hidden Markov Model construction are done, the appropriate phase at a given time point of a workflow is estimated. The paper also proved that the two proposed methods resolved perfectly the significant disadvantage of memory usage in our previous method. Through conducted experiments, while our previous method was not able to detect some phases, the two proposed methods were able to detect all phases and had promising results.

For future work, the usage of the surgical instruments should be recognized and the phase detection algorithm should be improved to get higher performance.

Acknowledgement MEXT-Supported Program for the Strategic Research Foundation at Private Universities, 2013-2017.

References

1. McCannon, J., Berwick, D.M.: A new frontier in patient safety. JAMA **305**(21), 2221–2222 (2011)
2. Lemke, H.U., Ratib, O.M., Horii, S.C.: Workflow in the operating room: a summary review of the arrowhead 2004 seminar on imaging and informatics. Int. Congr. Ser. **1281**, 862–867 (2005)
3. Neumuth, T., Strauß, G., Meixensberger, J., Lemke, H.U., Burgert, O.: Acquisition of process descriptions from surgical interventions. In: Database and Expert Systems Applications Lecture Notes in Computer Science, vol. 4080, pp. 602-611 (2006)
4. Neumuth, T., Jannin, P., Schlomberg, J., Meixensberger, J., Wiedemann, P., Burgert, O.: Analysis of surgical intervention populations using generic surgical process models. Int. J. Comput. Assist. Radiol. Surg. **6**(1), 59–71 (2011)
5. Padoy, N., Blum, T., Ahmadi, S.A., Feussner, H., Berger, M.O., Navab, N.: Statistical modeling and recognition of surgical workflow. Med. Image Anal. **16**(3), 632–641 (2012)
6. Yoshimura, A., Lee, J.H.: A phase estimation method for workflow based on optical flow and Hidden Markov Model. In: IEEE/SICE International Symposium on System Integration (SII), pp. 919–924 (2013)
7. Zach, C., Pock, T., Bischof, H.: A duality based approach for realtime tv-l1 optical flow. In: The 29th DAGM conference on Pattern recognition, pp. 214–223 (2007)
8. Blei, D.M., Ng, A.Y., Jordan, M.I., Lafferty, J.: Latent dirichlet allocation. J. Mach. Learn. Res. **3**, 993–1022 (2003)
9. Kuettel, D., Breitenstein, M.D., Gool, L.V., Ferrari, V.: What's going on? Discovering spatio-temporal dependencies in dynamic scenes. In: IEEE Conference on Computer Vision and Pattern Recognition, pp. 1951–1958 (2010)
10. Welch, L.R.: Hidden Markov Models and the Baum-Welch Algorithm. IEEE Inf. Theor Soc. Newsl. **53**(4), 1–24 (2003)
11. Hartley, H.O.: Maximum likelihood estimation from incomplete data. Biometrics **14**(2), 174–194 (1958)

Implementing a Human-Behavior-Process Archive and Search Database System Using Simulated Surgery Processes

Zhang Zuo, Kenta Oku and Kyoji Kawagoe

Abstract Recently, the development of motion data detection, as well as of behavior information management, has become very rapid. However, no appropriate database system exists for comprehensively archiving and searching of human behavior processes. In this paper, we present the implementation of a human-behavior-processes database system which can archive and search for surgery processes. The database system can be applicable to find the similar human processes to a given process and distinguish the differences between them, which can be used for supporting medical skill training. The whole development of our system is based on simulated surgery processes. In this paper, we describe the surgery data processing, the architectural framework and the development phases of database system.

Keywords Human behavior process archive · Database system · Surgery support

1 Introduction

With the development of science and technology, various kinds of sensor devices, such as motion and location sensors, have been widely used. The sensor devices such as Kinect and LeapMotion, are currently used primarily for analyzing object movements, as well as for visualizing them. As a result of this rapid popularization, huge amounts of monitored data has been obtained and analyzed for application-oriented purposes by using advanced sensor devices. However, although a large amount of data has been detected, the efficient reuse of human behavior data is still a hard

Z. Zuo (✉) · K. Oku · K. Kawagoe
Graduate School of Information Science and Engineering, Ritsumeikan University, Kusatsu Shiga, Japan
e-mail: gr0186rk@ed.ritsumei.ac.jp

K. Oku
e-mail: oku@fc.ritsumei.ac.jp

K.Kawagoe
e-mail: kawagoe@is.ritsumei.ac.jp

Y.-W. Chen et al. (eds.), *Innovation in Medicine and Healthcare 2015*, Smart Innovation, Systems and Technologies 45,
DOI 10.1007/978-3-319-23024-5_24

task because of the complexity of human behavior data. Especially, when a certain behavior is sensed, searching behaviors similar to it is important. Therefore, it is necessary to develop a human behavior-based service such as e-learning and human task support services. However, there is no appropriate database system exists for comprehensive archiving and efficiently managing human behavior data.

In this paper, we developed a novel human-behavior-process database system to obtain behaviors that are similar to a given behavior and distinguish the differences between the processes. In addition, our system is designed to be used for supporting medical skill training by presenting users the proper surgery processes and the differences need to be noticed. In our system, the human behavior can be archived from many aspects comprehensively, from the low level such as individual motions related entities, to the abstract level such as surgery processes.

Our developed human-behavior-process database system includes some special functions for management and a Human Behavior Processes (HBP) database. The functions for management provide us with a comprehensive storage and efficient query processing. The human behavior can be archived in the HBP database with those functions.

In order to realize a useful human behavior-based service or application, the first question is to represent the complex human behaviors and archive them into a database. It is very important whether a good method for archiving is employed. In our HBP database system, we realize the archive function of system by using a process meta model for describing people's activities (MLPM) [1]. Therefore, it is possible to ensure the completeness of information stored in the system and ensure the efficiency of querying it.

On the other hand, another key question of the system is the search method. In our proposed system, we use the similarity calculation method which is called Extended LDSD [2] to realize the query function. Because the objects of Extended LDSD method are human behaviors, this method ensures the efficient query of our system which has the same objects.

In this paper we focus on the development process of our system. The process of our system development contains several stages. In order to make the system development to be reasonable and to demonstrate the effectiveness of surgery support at the same time, the whole development of our system is based on simulated surgery processes, which simulates the process of Laparoscopic Cholecystectomy operation. Therefore, the first step of our system includes data collection and data modeling.

In our development, we firstly set up the architectural framework of the system including the functions, the database design and the information interchange between them. We focus on the introduction of architectural framework. Because there are some function modules in our framework, we describe the development of search function in details.

The rest of our paper is organized as follows: The surgery data collection is described in Sect. 2. Section 3 describes whole structure of system as well as the architectural framework. This paper also contains brief introduction of the similarity search method. Finally, the conclusion and the future work are described.

2 Simulated Surgery Processes

In our system development, we used human behavior data which is taken from Laparoscopic Cholecystectomy simulation operation and we made a series of data processing.

2.1 Data Source

The laparoscopic cholecystectomy simulation is conducted using a virtual reality training system (Fig. 1). The equipment can simulate the entire surgical phase, including air injection, clipping and cutting, etc. The user can operate the equipment based on the manual. The equipment includes a trunk, which simulates the patient, and related operating tools. A complete operation takes about ten minutes. The operation process is recorded by four cameras inside and outside the patient's body. The camera data are stored in the form of videos and text.

2.2 Data Modeling

As stated above, we used human behavior process MLPM to represent complex humandata to a data which can be saved in the database efficiently. In MLPM, behaviors are decomposed into three layers: process/task layer, activity layer, and action layer. And further, the three layers model can be decomposed into seven layers, such as entity and motion. Based on MLPM, the human behavior process can be represented by behavioral components and the links between them. According to this theory, we decomposed all the experimental data into nodes which are added by tag to

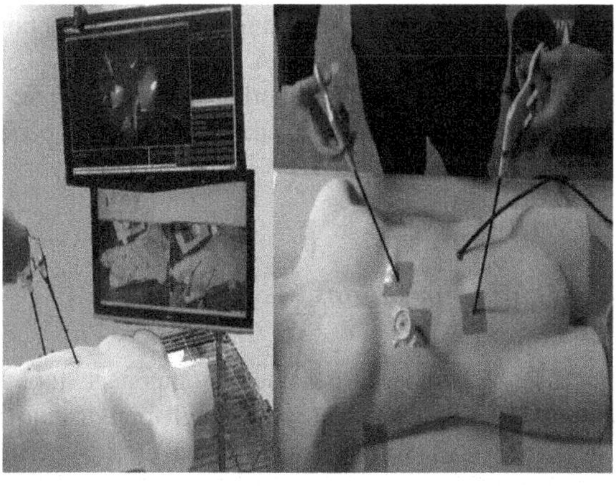

Fig. 1 Surgery simulation. [3]

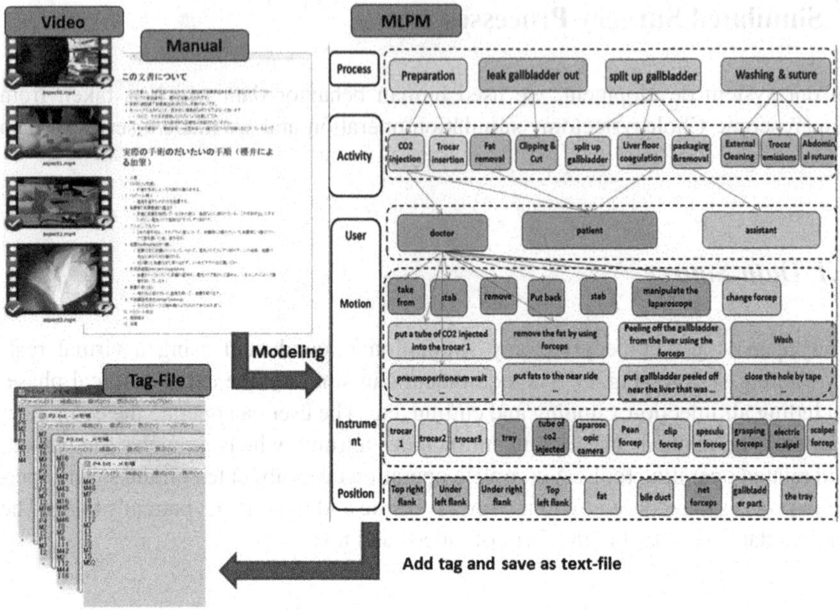

Fig. 2 Modeling of surgery processes

indicate their properties. In this data modeling process, simulated surgery processes are decomposed into 6 kind of nodes{process, activity, user, instrument, position and motion}. And all of the nodes are divided into three layers {process, activity, and content}. Beside, we took four processes from the whole surgery as four different processes because that a complete procedure generally has four stages. The result of data modeling is shown in Fig. 2. You can find the four processes in the figure easily by recognizing the color.

In the modeling of surgery processes data, there are some entities, which are used to perform a process. They are divided into either user or instrument classes, in our example, such as a doctor or a trocar. An action is an abstract movement related to one entity. One entity is related to a sequence of actions used to perform an activity associated with other entities. A motion is an actual entity's movement used to represent a specific action. The motion data are aggregated and integrated from various kinds of motion expressions, such as video. The position is stated as motion status information.

2.3 Data Generation

Because the number of behavioral components took from the simulated surgery is around 200. Those nodes are not enough for us to construct the system reasonably, we generated lots of artificial data from real data using an automated test data generator.

Our data generator inputs a collection of manually constructed processes. The outputs are a series of varying data. In the deformation, some predefined variation functions, such as add nodes, cut nodes, and change nodes, are used. During the data collection, we got lots of processes which can be divided into four categories.

3 Architectural Framework of Our HBP Database System

3.1 Motivations

In the medical filed, it is a difficult problem to improve young doctors' skills. For example, suppose that a skilled doctor is fostering junior doctors in order to impart to them better skills for the task of giving intravenous or subcutaneous injections. It is difficult for junior doctors to understand and to perform the task without any practical experience of it. Even if they have some experience of giving the injections, appropriate real-time comments from experienced doctors are very necessary and helpful. However, when they use a subcutaneous-injection simulator, such useful comments are not available to them. There is thus no opportunity to improve their skills in such situations.

In order to improve this situation, we propose a human behavior processes database system to support medical treatment education by archiving a huge amount of surgery processes for reference and presenting young doctors the differences between the activity as executed by a skilled doctor and by a junior doctor with specific details. Using our system, skilled doctor can review their executed surgery processes or share them with other persons. Moreover, the junior doctors can access the database system to learn by themselves in any time.

3.2 Architectural Framework

As is states in the design of the prototype system [4], our system is generally divided into two parts, which are archiving management component and HBP database component. And there are some functions in the archiving management component. In management component, given data can be recorded into the database, a record can be updated, or a query can be conducted. The contents of basic function are shown in Table 1.

In HBP database component, a relational database is built and store nodes and edges. This determines the characteristics of the table. Beside, because nodes and edges each have their own type which should be reflected in their attributes. Besides nodes and edges, there are also some tables like process and data source in the HBP database.

Figure 3 shows the architectural framework of the system.

Table 1 System basic function

Function name	Content
Aggregation	Human behavior will be represented by MLPM, decomposed into behavioral components
Registration	Human behavior components and associations will be inserted in to DB
Similarity calculation	Similarities between query and other processes be calculated by Extended LDSD
Detailed output	Details of results presented in last step can be checked
Process visualization	Original data can be visualized

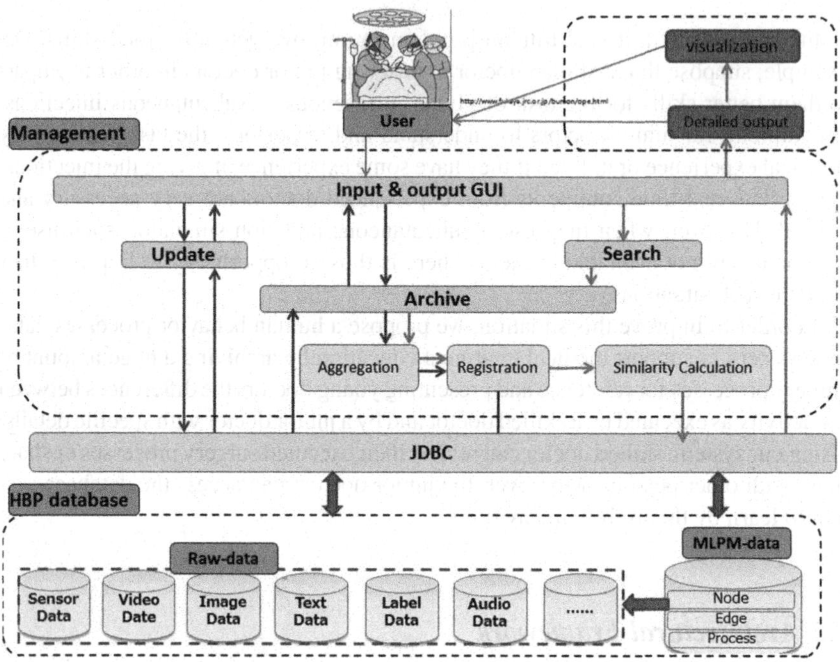

Fig. 3 Architectural framework

3.3 Development Phase

The development of the whole system is divided into several phases. According to the development phases, we imagine several versions of our system as a guideline of the next development.

Version1: a HBP archive and search system based on file system. All the processes are stored and searched in the format of file (video or image) in a normal OS in this vision.

Version2: a HBP archive and search system based on SQL Database. In this version, all the processes are archived in a relationship database in the format of records.

Version3: a HBP database management system. This version will be a combination of version1 and version2, which will keep all the processes in the records in DB and also offer the visualization function, using which the users can check the original data.

4 Searching HBP Data

In this section, a brief introduction of the similarity search method Extended LDSD [2] will be made. The Extended LDSD is a method that extends the semantic distance calculation method Linked Data Semantic Distance (LDSD) and applies it to human behavior distance calculations.

4.1 Original LDSD [5]

Before introducing our proposed method called Extended LDSD, we describe here the original LDSD. The objective of LDSD (Linked Data Semantic Distance) is to define a semantic distance between two nodes in Linked Data. As is well-known, Linked Data network can be abstracted into a graph, which consists of nodes and directed edges. Therefore, the LDSD actually calculates the semantic distance between nodes in a digraph.

Calculation of the linked data from LDSD is carried out as follows. A dataset is a graph G such as $G = (N, E, L)$, in which $N = \{N_1, N_2, \ldots, N_n\}$ is a set of nodes, $E = \{E_1, E_2, \ldots, E_m\}$ is a set of typed links, and $L = \{L_1, L_2, \ldots, L_p\}$ is a set of instances of these links between data nodes, such as $E_i = < L_j, N_a, N_b >$. In this case, the semantic distance between nodes N_a and N_b, $LDSD(N_a, N_b)$ is defined as follows.

$$LDSD(N_a, N_b) = \frac{1}{1 + \alpha + \beta + \gamma + \delta} \tag{1}$$

$$\begin{cases} \alpha = \sum_i \frac{C_d(L_i, N_a, N_b)}{1+\log(C_d(L_i, N_a, N_n))} \\ \beta = \sum_i \frac{C_d(L_i, N_b, N_a)}{1+\log(C_d(L_i, N_b, N_n))} \\ \gamma = \sum_i \frac{C_{ii(L_i, N_a, N_b)}}{1+\log(C_{ii(L_i, N_a, N_n)})} \\ \delta = \sum_i \frac{C_{io(L_i, N_a, N_b)}}{1+\log(C_{io(L_i, N_a, N_n)})} \end{cases}$$

C_d is a function that computes the number of direct and distinct links between nodes in a graph G. $C_d(L_i, N_a, N_b)$ is equal to one if there is an instance of L_i

from a node N_a to a node N_b, otherwise, it is zero. C_d can be used to compute the total number of direct and distinct links from N_a to N_b, which is defined as $C_d(L_n, N_a, N_b)$. Further, the total number of distinct instances of link L_i from N_a to any node ($C_d(L_i, N_a, N_n)$) can be defined and calculated.

C_{io} and C_{ii} are functions that compute the number of indirect and direct links, both outgoing and incoming, between nodes in a graph, respectively. $C_{io}(L_i, N_a, N_n)$ equals of 1 if there is a node N_n that satisfy both $< L_i, N_a, N_n >$ and $< L_i, N_b, N_n >$, 0 if not. $C_{ii}(L_i, N_a, N_b)$ equal 1 if there is a node N_n that satisfy both $< L_i, N_n, N_a >$ and $< L_i, N_n, N_b >$, 0 if not.

4.2 Extensions to LDSD

The purpose of our extensions is to find the similarity between entities such as processes, activities, actions. There are three types of extended distance definitions: temporal extension, granularity extension, and content extension, which all are extensions to the original LDSD. In original LDSD, whether there is a link between two specific nodes or not is concerned. But in our Extended LDSD, in each extension we are also concerned about the distance of each kind of links mentioned above.

ExtendedLDSD(N_a, N_b) is defined as follows.

$$ExtendedLDSD(N_a, N_b) = \frac{1}{1 + \alpha + \beta + \gamma + \delta + \tau + \chi + \psi} \tag{2}$$

1. Temporal extension to LDSD
   In this extension, the distances τ of temporal-link are calculated using the time interval assigned to nodes.
   $$\tau = \left|T_{N_a} - T_{N_b}\right|$$
2. Granularity extension to LDSD
   In this extension, the distances χ of granularity-link are calculated by comparing the number of hierarchical-link linked to nodes.
   $$\chi = \left|C_d(E_i, N_a, N_n) - C_d(E_j, N_b, N_m)\right|$$
   $C_d(E_i, N_a, N_n)$ is the total number of direct instances of all hierarchical-link from N_a to any node N_n.
3. Content extension to LDSD
   According to the hierarchical structure of the human behavior linked data network, we can build the virtual-content-link on the network. Firstly, We define a value ω to describe the tightness of this kind of association between N_c and N_d as follow.
   $$\omega = C_{io}(E_i, N_c, N_d)/C_{io}(E_i, N_c, N_n)$$

Secondly, we set a threshold value Θ to check whether a virtual-content-link can be constructed or not. That is, if the ω of two nodes is greater than Θ which means the indirect association between them is strong , then, a virtual-content-link will be constructed.

Finally, due to the increase of virtual-content-link, the human behavior network can be rebuilt. The virtual content distance between two upper lever nodes N_e and N_f in this situation is defined as follow:

$$\psi = \sum_i \frac{C_{io}(E_i, N_e, N_f)}{1 + log(C_{io}(E_i, N_e, N_n))}$$

5 Discussion

In our study so far, we had proposed the MLPM model to completely describe human behavior. And we also proposed the similarity method Extended LDSD to search for a similar behavior to a given a particular behavior. Some experiments were conducted by our automated test data generator and shown the superiority of our method in terms of similarity precision [6]. Based on all the theory, we designed a human behavior processes database prototype. Finally, we presented the architectural framework of system and the development phases in implementing the system we proposed in previous study. Although we finished some part of the HBP archive and search system, there are still a lot of work need to be finished, such as the search in a database rather than in a file system and visualization. As the ultimate goal of our study, we will build a complete medical treatment system process archive database management system to support the medical treatment or nursing activity.

On the other hand, there are some problems which need to be solved in the future. Firstly, in order to achieve higher precision of storage, we need to build an efficient data collection system which can turn multidimensional real surgery processes to database data. Because of the diversity in the medical process and recording equipments, the human behavior processes raw data may be video data, audio data or sensor data. Based on this situation, we need mature data processing technology, such as video analytic technology to process the raw data. Secondly, in our HBP search method, we compare human behavior from aspect of temporal similarity, granularity similarity and content similarity. consider the complexity of human activity, especially medical activities, the contrast of more aspects need to be considered.

6 Related Work

There are some research studies on retrieval of the medical data, mainly medical image data. The work in [7], Data Grid for Large-Scale medical image archive and analysis has been studied. They also implemented computational services in the Data Grid for image analysis and data mining. In work [8], a completely new approach has been developed to enrich the existing information in clinical information systems with additional meta-data, such as the actual treatment phase from which the information entity originates.

On the other hand, there have been many research studies on motion index storage and retrieval. In work [9] parameterizes motions by recomputing match webs. Neighbor graphs are proposed in [10] for storage and indexing. However, the quadratic memory requirement in these methods makes it impractical for large databases. Content-based retrieval methods [11] compute a small set of geometric properties which are used to find logically similar motions. Following the pioneering work of [12], different techniques have been used for spatial indexing of motion data.

7 Conclusion

In this paper, we presented the implementation of a human-behavior-process database system which can archive and search surgery processes. As a data collection, we made use of some real human behavior processes and we have shown the content of data processing. As the main content of this paper, we focused on architectural framework of system and the development phases. A search method is a key to a search system, which we made a brief introduction. At the end of this paper, we presented a comprehensive summary of our research so far. On the other hand, we made in-depth discussion about the tasks need to be completed in next step and the problem we should solve in the future. We will implement all the functions in the system and improve the system in next step.

Acknowledgments This work was partially supported by MEXT-Supported Program for the Strategic Research Foundation at Private Universities, 2013-2017. I thank Professor Joo-Ho Lee and Mr. Ryohei Sakurai for permitting us to use their simulated surgery data [3].

References

1. Zuo, Z., Huang, H.H., Kawagoe, K.: MLPM: A Multi-Layered Process Model Toward Complete Descriptions of People's Behaviors. eKNOW 2014. The Sixth International Conference on Information, Process, and Knowledge Management, pp. 167–172 (2014)
2. Zuo, Z., Huang, H.H., Kawagoe, K.: Similarity Search of Human Behavior Processes Using Extended Linked Data Semantic Distance. ISSASiM2014. Proceedings of the 4th DEXA

Workshop on Information Systems for Situation Awareness and Situation Management, pp. 178–182 (2014)
3. Haptic Vision Lab.: http://www.cv.ci.ritsumei.ac.jp/haptic/works.html. Accessed May 2015
4. Zuo, Z., Huang, H.H., Kawagoe, K.: A human behavior processes database prototype system for surgery support. The 14th IEEE/ACIS International Conference on Computer and Information Science, pp.241–246 (2015)
5. Alexandre, P. Measuring Semantic Distance on Linking Data and Using it for Resources Recommendations. AAAI Spring Symposium: Linked Data Meets Artificial Intelligence, pp. 93–98 (2010)
6. Zuo, Z., Huang, H.H., Kawagoe, K.: Evaluation of a similarity search method for human behavior (Extended LDSD). The International MultiConference of Engineers and Computer Scientists, pp. 96–101 (2015)
7. Huang, H.K., Zhang, A., Liu, B. J., Zhou, Z., Documet, J., King, N., Chan, L.W.: Data Grid for Large-Scale Medical Image Archive and Analysis. Proceedings of the 13th ACM International Conference on Multimedia, pp. 1005–1013 (2005)
8. Meier, J., Dietz, A., Boehm, A., Neumuth, T.: Predicting treatment process steps from events. J. Biomed. Inform. **53**, 308–319 (2015)
9. Kovarr, L., Gleicher, M., Pighin, F.: Motion graphs. ACM Trans. Graph **21**, 473–482 (2002)
10. Chai, J., Hodgins, K.: Performance animation from low-dimensional control signals. SIGGRAPH, pp. 686–696 (2005)
11. Muller, M., Roder, T.: Motion templates for automatic classification and retrieval of motion capture data. SCA, pp. 137–146 (2006)
12. Faloutsos, C., Ranganathan, M., Manolopoulos, Y.: Fast Subsequence Matching in Time-series Databases, pp. 419–429. ACM SIGMOD, New York (1994)

Unobtrusive Sensing of Human Vital Functions by a Sensory Unit in the Refrigerator Door Handle

D. Zazula, S. Srkoč and B. Cigale

Abstract This paper opens new insights into short-duration photoplethysmography (PPG) in dynamic condition when opening a refrigerator. Light-emitting diodes illuminate fingers in the door handle and 512 PPG signals are recorded in parallel with the acceleration information, which indicates the moment of the door opening. Eight healthy volunteers participated in the experiments with opening the refrigerator's door. A Critikon Dinamap Pro 300 was used to record a referential level of their blood oxygen simultaneously. We derived novel algorithms for assessing blood oxygenation based on a very short transient segment of PPGs in the very moment of the refrigerator opening. The approach does not need either heartbeat detection or calibration. A comparison between our estimates and referential data yields the mean absolute error of 1.23 %.

Keywords Unobtrusive sensors • Photoplethysmography • Contact pressure on fingers • Blood oxygenation • Blood pressure

1 Introduction

New paradigms and more efficient healthcare and medical services will have to ameliorate the burden loaded on the national budgets by fast growing population of elderly and chronical diseases. By 2050, 11 % of world population is expected of age over 80, national healthcare expenses will double. Current trends, for example,

---

D. Zazula (✉) · S. Srkoč · B. Cigale
System Software Laboratory, Faculty of Electrical Engineering and Computer Science, University of Maribor, Smetanova 17, 2000 Maribor, Slovenia
e-mail: damjan.zazula@um.si

S. Srkoč
e-mail: sandi.srkoc@student.um.si

B. Cigale
e-mail: boris.cigale@um.s

Y.-W. Chen et al. (eds.), *Innovation in Medicine and Healthcare 2015*, Smart Innovation, Systems and Technologies 45,
DOI 10.1007/978-3-319-23024-5_25

predict 35 % of gross domestic product spent by 2025 on health and social care in Slovenia.

Home and continuous care for the elderly and people with disabilities can facilitate and prolong their independent living. It has been shown this could loosen mentioned bottleneck problems. However, home services must be automated and widely accepted, which haven't happened yet in spite of high-tech solutions feasible. A major drawback lies in observations that are obtrusive (users must take care of measurements, devices' operation, data collection and forwarding, etc.).

Unobtrusiveness depends on the ability of measuring the effects of human vital signs when a person, during his or her daily activity, unconsciously establishes a direct or indirect contact with sensors built in the appliances and elements of the living environment. A variety of suitable sensors are available today, such as the accelerometers, fibre-optic interferometers, capacitive electrodes, optic and thermal cameras, radar, sonar, etc. Their sensitivity and efficiency is a key to detect tiny stimuli of human vital signs, but this also causes superimpositions and many unwanted disturbances. Sophisticated signal and image processing algorithms are, therefore, of paramount importance to extract and assess the physiological parameters looked for.

Photoplethysmography (PPG) has been known a convenient means for blood oxymetry since 1930s [1, 2]. Two light sources of red (R) and infrared (IR) wavelengths illuminate a thin body part, usually a finger, and an optical sensor recollects the transmitted or reflected light. A significant breakthrough was achieved in 1970s when the modern pulse oximetry was born with the realization that pulsatile changes in light transmission through living tissues are due to alteration of the arterial blood volume in the tissue. This requires a detection of heartbeats in the PPG signals prior to the estimation of oxygenation.

We have developed a robust method to detect heartbeats in PPG signals [3] and applied it to extract the information about heart rate, its variability, and blood oxygen saturation. It has also been shown the blood pressure can be assessed from the PPG signals [4]. The most known approach is based on pulse transit times measured as a time difference between the electrocardiogram (ECG) R-peak and a characteristic point of the PPG-based heartbeat detections [5, 6].

To apply PPG measurements unobtrusively and to avoid often unreliable heartbeat detections, we developed and patented a novel construction of a photoplethysmograph outfitted to be installed in human living environment [7]. This paper focuses on new insights obtained by this invention on short-time PPG analysis in dynamic condition, when no heartbeat detection and device calibration are required. Section 2 reveals a construction of novel sensory device, experimental setup, and signal analysis methods. Section 3 explains briefly the experimental findings, whereas Sect. 4 discusses obtained results and concludes the paper.

2 Materials and Methods

2.1 Experimental Setup

When people open a refrigerator, they grasp the door handle and pull until the door opens. Due to the sealant rubber along the door edges, the door does not open easy, but must be pulled by using a certain force. If the door handle is of an ergonomic shape, fingers slip behind it and when pulling the external force oppresses the fingers. At the same time, the artery, arteriolas, and veins in the fingers are oppressed too. Then, at the moment when the door suddenly slackens, the external oppression releases instantaneously.

We took advantage of this phenomenon and decided to observe a transition period immediately after the door opening. When pulling the door handle, the blood is part squeezed out of the fingers. The door opening releases the external contact force and the blood inflow begins. To observe this change, we built a special sensory unit that consists of a two-wavelength photoplethysmograph and an accelerometer. Our photoplethysmograph works in transmission mode with optical sensors at the one side of the fingers and the light sources on the other. The optical sensor is fixed to the inner side of the door handle and the light comes from the light emitting diodes (LEDs) inserted in the door frame behind the handle. Thus, fingers touch the optical sensor when a person opens the refrigerator and the light illuminates the transparent parts of fingers. The moment of the door opening is registered by the accelerometer.

In the experiments we wanted to study the transients that appear in the PPG signals in the instant when the door pressure releases. In this paper, we particularly focused on a relationship among the parameters that we extracted from the transitional parts of PPGs and the person's blood oxygenation. Referential data were measured by a Critikon Dinamap Pro 300, a professional oximeter and sphygmomanometric blood pressure measuring device. Oxygenation was recorded during the entire experimental trials. Time alignment of all the signals was achieved on the microcontroller level in our sensory unit.

2.2 The Sensory Unit Construction

The construction of our sensory unit is adapted to a special L-shaped type of the refrigerator door handle. This type is most convenient for the placement that warrantees stable PPG measurements. The unit's embodiment has been revealed [8] and will be merely recapitulated here.

As mentioned, the PPG sensor operates in transmission mode, so that optoelectronic sensors are placed opposite to the light sources. The door handle construction anticipates sensors and the electronic circuits encapsulated in a plastic

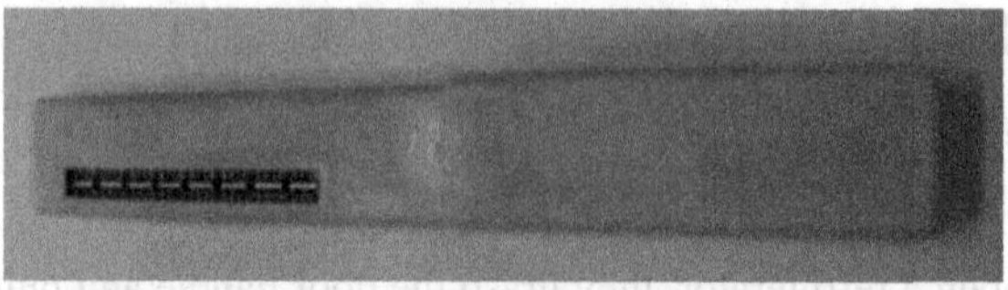

Fig. 1 The plethysmograph's plastic housing: optical sensors are visible on the left-hand side, while the controlling and computing electronic circuits are encapsulated in the right-hand side of the housing

housing (Fig. 1) and attached to an L-shaped handle, while the light sources in the form of LEDs reside vis-à-vis in the door frame.

Figure 1 shows 8 analogue optical plethysmographic sensors TSL1401CL (amc AG company) in a row. Each sensor incorporates 128 in-line photodiodes with controllable exposition, i.e. integration time. We deployed every second channel only, which totals in 512 simultaneous PPG signals (samples in a vector) equally distributed across an 80 mm distance. The sampling frequency was set equal to 225 Hz.

Four pairs of LEDs illuminate fingers along the whole length of the optical sensor array. Each pair consists of diodes with two different wavelengths: one in the red spectrum at 660 nm, the other one in the infrared spectrum at 940 nm. The duty cycle of light switching is divided into three thirds and is in a synchrony with optical-sensor sampling frequency: in the first interval, the red LEDs are turned on, in the second the infrared LEDs, and in the third all LEDs are turned off, so that in this interval the ambient light is the only illumination. In this way, the influence of the ambient light can be eliminated from the measurements with R and IR lights.

Figure 2, left, depicts a montage of the handle with sensors to the refrigerator's door. The sensors are placed vertically and a unit with LEDs and their drivers is inserted into the door frame vis-à-vis. IR illumination is turned on all the time at a slower test rate. Whenever the optical sensors detect the light was interrupted for a predefined time and number of PPG channels, all the sensors begin data acquisition with full sampling rates of both the R and IR illumination (Fig. 2, right).

The printed circuit with LEDs carries a three-axial accelerometer as well. The acceleration signals are sampled and synchronised with the PPG signals. Whenever the refrigerator's door moves, the acceleration signals detect the movement. In the instant of the door opening, an abrupt acceleration change points out this even.

2.3 *Data Processing and Analysis Methods*

In every experimental trial, 512 PPG signals are acquired along with the acceleration and referential oxygenation signals. To avoid high-frequency disturbances, we apply low-pass filtering to all obtained signals.

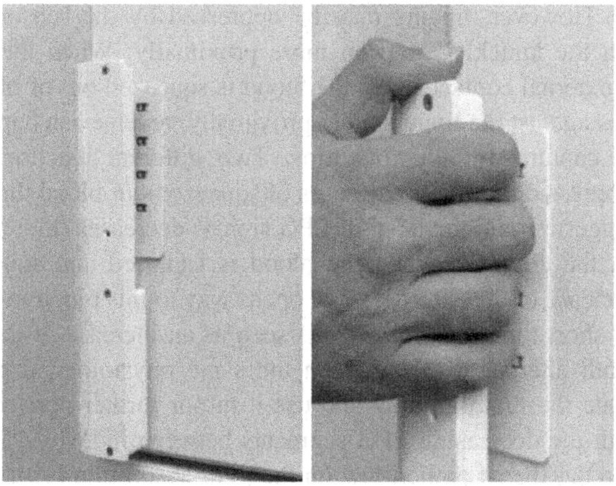

Fig. 2 The unit with optical sensors and controlling electronics is vertically affixed to the door handle. Opposite to the optical sensors, a subunit with LEDs and electronic drivers is inserted in the door frame (*left* subfigure). Fingers when opening the door are forced to a position where the light passes through to the sensors that acquire the PPG signals (*right* subfigure)

Suppose the signals are of length N. Second norm, $a(n)$, of a directional vector of the three acceleration signals is composed at sample n. Then the first maximum is found in $a(n)$:

$$N_a = \mathrm{argmax}_n a(n);\; n = 0, \ldots, N-1 \tag{1}$$

Index N_a indicates the time interval of the most accelerated door movement, which happens immediately after the door opening. This is then the point where transient changes must be looked for in the PPG signals.

Some of the PPG signals are saturated, because they belong to the spaces where no finger touched the optical sensors. Only those signals that do not saturate in any time are kept for further processing. Suppose N_j signals qualify and form the initial analysis set of filtered PPG signals, $\mathbf{s}(n) = [s_1(n), \ldots, s_{Nj}(n)]^T$; $n = 0, \ldots, N\text{-}1$.

It is typical for a transient period when the blood inflow fills up fingertips with blood again after the door opening that the PPG signals change rapidly. This PPG segment begins with a local maximum and ends up with a local minimum. Thus, our search continues as follows:

$$\begin{aligned} N_b &= \mathrm{argmax}_n s_m(n);\; n < N_a; m = 0, \ldots, N_j \\ N_e &= \mathrm{argmin}_n s_m(n);\; n > N_a; m = 0, \ldots, N_j \end{aligned} \tag{2}$$

where N_b and N_e denote the initial and termination indexes of the PPG segment that corresponds to observed transient phenomenon in the PPG signals.

There is no unique way of how people grasp the handle when they open a door. Our embodiment of the refrigerator handle forces person's fingers to touch the optical sensors. However, fingers may be oppressed by the sensors right on the fingertips or on the knuckles or even more proximally. When the fingertips are exposed to the external contact force, the blood is squeezed out of blood vessels. If the force presses against the fingers more proximally, reverse can happen: the blood is pushed and captured in the fingertips. Two different reactions follow after releasing the oppression force. In the cases of squeezed-out blood the inflow begins filling up the fingertips and the level of PPG signals decreases (more blood absorbs more light). In the contrary, when the blood is captured and squeezed into the fingertips, the release of the external force opens way to this blood to flow out of the fingertips for a short time interval. This is seen as an increase of the PPG level.

Although both alternatives depend on the same physiological parameters, we decided to isolate the first one only and use it in our further derivation. Thus, we dealt solely with the decreasing PPG segments between indexes N_b and N_e.

According to the Beer-Lambert law on the light absorption [10], an exponential relationship exists between the intensity of the light passing a medium and the properties of this medium, i.e. its extinction coefficient, concentration, and depths. Talking about a finger, the transparent parts belong to the finger soft tissues, in particular blood vessels and the blood. Suppose the finger artery diameter, d, changes with time: $d(n)$; n stands for discrete time moments. All other tissues remain unchanged within the observation interval. Beer-Lambert law can be applied with this assumption as follows:

$$s_l^{(k)}(n) = I_{0,k} e^{-\varepsilon_k \bar{d}} e^{-\varepsilon_k d(n)} \tag{3}$$

where $I_{0,k}$ stands for the kth light source intensity, $s_l^{(k)}$ for the intensity of the kth light as acquired by the lth sensor, ε_k the generalised extinction coefficient for the kth light, and $\bar{d}$ adapted thickness of the finger tissue surrounding the artery. The generalised extinction coefficient is defined as:

$$\varepsilon_k = c_0 \varepsilon_{o,k} + (1 - c_0)\varepsilon_{d,k} \tag{4}$$

where c_0 stands for the blood oxygen concentration (oxygen saturation level or oxygenation), $\varepsilon_{o,k}$ for the oxyhemoglobin extinction coefficient, and $\varepsilon_{d,k}$ for the deoxyhemoglobin extinction coefficient.

On the other hand, we are interested in dynamic circumstances when the blood volume increases and inflates the vessels whose diameter, therefore, increases. This happens in the observed time interval between N_b and N_e. Blood volume can be described by the following model [9]:

$$V = \begin{cases} V_0 e^{\frac{C_m}{V_0} P_t}; P_t \leq 0 \\ V_m - (V_m - V_0) e^{-\frac{C_m}{V_m - V_0} P_t}; P_t \geq 0 \end{cases} \tag{5}$$

where P_t stands for the transmural pressure on blood vessels, C_m for the vessels' compliance, V_0 for their volume at zero transmural pressure, and V_m for their maximum volume. The transmural pressure is computed as:

$$P_t = P_i - P_e \tag{6}$$

with P_i denoting the internal, distending blood pressure and P_e the external pressure.

The only time-dependent parameter in Eq. (5) is transmural pressure, all others are constant in short term. Indeed, in the observations of blood inflow after the release of external contact pressure on the fingertips, $P_e = 0$ and the transmural pressure changes from P_i-P_e to P_i. This does not happen instantaneously but lasts for an interval, say t. If we further consider the oppressed blood vessel is circular and of length L, a relationship between dynamic volume and blood vessel diameter yields:

$$d(n) = \sqrt{\frac{4}{\pi L} V(n)} \tag{7}$$

Now, we only need to draw a conclusion about the dynamic volume changes in the two conditions related to P_t in Eq. (5).

Suppose the external pressure P_e is high enough to surpass the point $P_t = 0$. In this case, the abovementioned interval t of blood inflow must be divided into two parts: one before $P_t = 0$ and the other after that point. But what about the cases when the external contact force does not overwhelms the internal blood pressure? In this case, we only see the consequences of the second model of volume change, as depicted in the lower part of Eq. (5). Logically, this model of volume changes is always applied, regardless the external contact forces, and it fades out with the transition interval after the door opening. This means that we have to go first to the end of observed PPG segment, i.e. to index N_e, and then take into account the samples backwards.

At this point we can combine the Beer-Lambert law, Eq. (3), with the dynamic volume change as derived from Eq. (5):

$$s_l^{(k)}(n) = I_{0,k} e^{-\varepsilon_k \bar{d}} e^{-\varepsilon_k \sqrt{\frac{4}{\pi L} V(n)}}; N_b < n < N_e \tag{8}$$

A logarithm of Eq. (8) yields:

$$\log s_l^{(k)}(n) = \log I_{0,k} - \varepsilon_k \bar{d} - \varepsilon_k \sqrt{\frac{4}{\pi L} V(n)} \tag{9}$$

If we move the first two terms from the right-hand side of Eq. (9) to the left-hand side, square the equation, and then rearrange the terms with respect to Eq. (5), a new result is obtained:

$$\log^2 s_l^{(k)}(n) = 2\log s_l^{(k)}(n)(\log I_{0,k} - \varepsilon_k \bar{d}) - (\log I_{0,k} - \varepsilon_k \bar{d})^2 + \varepsilon_k^2 \frac{4}{\pi L} V_m - \varepsilon_k^2 \frac{4}{\pi L}(V_m - V_0)e^{-\frac{C_m}{V_m - V_0}P_t(n)}; n < N_e \tag{10}$$

This outcome shows that a squared logarithm of the PPG segment related to the door opening comprises three constant terms and the fourth, exponential one. The equation holds for the samples near the end of the signal segment where index n is close to N_e.

The final step in our derivation is fitting $\log^2 s_l^{(k)}(n)$ from Eq. (10) by an exponential curve model:

$$\log^2 s_l^{(k)}(n) = p_l^{(k)} - q_l^{(k)} e^{r_l^{(k)}} \tag{11}$$

where $p_l^{(k)}$, $q_l^{(k)}$, and $r_l^{(k)}$ stand for the parameters of this curve fitting of the lth PPG signal taken at the kth illumination.

2.4 *Estimation of Blood Oxygen Saturation*

Recall Eq. (4) with the generalised extinction coefficient ε_k. If two coefficients are known at two different light wavelength, their ratio and the corresponding extinction coefficients for oxyhemoglobin and deoxyhemoglobin extract blood oxygen saturation c_O. This well-known fact is used in all pulse oxymeters that depend on reliable heartbeat detection from the PPG signals. To collect a few heartbeats reliably, the acquired signals must be at least 5 to 10 s long. If all the time we have is limited to a short interval during the refrigerator door opening, we have no chance to catch more than one or two heartbeats, and these will be very unreliable due to high dynamics that accompanies the door opening. Hence, the conventional approaches to assess the blood oxygen saturation in this way fail.

Equations (11) and (10) show that if we estimate two parameters $q_l^{(k)}$ at two different illuminations, their ratio equals the ratio of the generalised extinction coefficients at those two lights. This is all we need to compute blood oxygen saturation.

3 Experimental Results

Seven young healthy volunteers aged 19–24 years, 2 of them females, and a male at 64 signed informed consents before the experimental trials they participated in. Throughout all trials their referential oxygenation was monitored by a Critikon Dinamap Pro 300 and automatically stored to a computer file. They were instructed

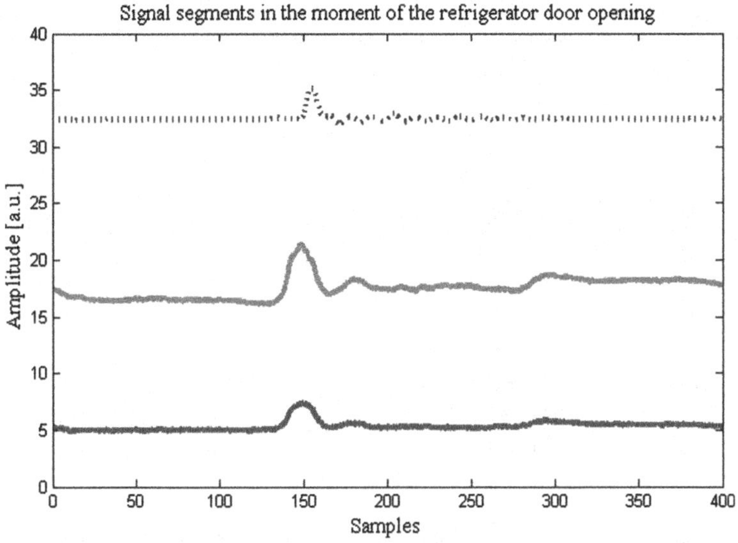

Fig. 3 Signal segments in the moment of the refrigerator door opening: acceleration (*blue dotted, top*), IR PPG (*magenta solid, middle*), R PPG (*red solid, bottom*)

to approach the refrigerator, grasp the door handle and, in most natural way, open and, after a while, again close the door.

The acquired PPG and acceleration signals were low-pass filtered at 15-Hz cut-off frequency. The moment of maximum acceleration was found and the PPG segment located for the interval of the door opening. We applied the algorithms described in Sect. 2.3. Figure 3 depicts part of acceleration signal and two PPG signals in parallel. A typical transient is seen at the moment of the door opening.

Then we selected the relevant PPG channels for the R and IR illuminations. The segments were modelled according to Eq. (11). Thus we obtained a number of parameters $q_l^{(R)}$ and $q_l^{(IR)}$. A well-known fact again is that the R light may not take the same way as the IR one. This is even more probable in our experimental set-up as the R and IR LEDs do not share the same housing and between them there is a small distance.

Therefore, the ratios of the generalised extinction coefficients, $\frac{\varepsilon_R}{\varepsilon_{IR}}$, vary slightly across the signal channels and the two illuminations. To improve robustness, we computed the ratios between all possible pairs of $q_l^{(R)}$ and $q_l^{(IR)}$. If, for example, we extracted Q acceptable R and IR PPG signal segments, we computed Q^2 possible ratios $\frac{q_l^{(R)}}{q_l^{(IR)}}$ and, subsequently, the same number of oxygen saturations, c_0. The results are depicted in Table 1 with their means and standard deviation. Referential oxygen saturation is added for comparison reasons.

Table 1 Instantaneously assessed blood oxygen saturation at the refrigerator door opening and its referential oxygenation measured by a Critikon Dinamap Pro 300

Person ID	Referential oxygenation [%]	Estimated oxygenation [%]	Absolute error for mean estimated oxygenation [%]	Absolute error for mean oxygenation –STD [%]	Absolute error for mean oxygenation +STD [%]
1	96	96.9 ± 2.1	0.94	3.13	1.25
2	97	98.0 ± 1.6	1.03	2.68	0.62
3	95	93.8 ± 2.2	1.26	1.05	3.58
4	96	98.1 ± 1.4	2.19	3.65	0.73
5	97	98.4 ± 0.8	1.44	2.27	0.62
6	99	99.0 ± 0.5	0.00	0.51	0.51
7	97	94.5 ± 2.5	2.58	0.00	5.15
8	98	97.6 ± 1.9	0.41	1.53	2.35

Statistical comparison of our estimates with the referential measurements totals in an overall absolute error of 1.23 % if the estimated mean oxygenations are taken into account. The figure changes to 1.85 % at one standard deviation lower limit, and the same at one standard deviation higher limit.

4 Discussion and Conclusions

We developed a novel approach to short-time estimation of blood oxygen saturation. A special sensory device measures it instantaneously at the refrigerator's door opening. No conventional approach based on a detection of heartbeats in the PPG signals under the illumination with two different wavelengths is applicable in such a case. The fact is that during a 1 to 2-second-long interval of the door opening no heartbeat detection is practically possible.

We derived an innovative algorithm that analyses the dynamical changes in the PPG segments during the refrigerator door opening. Equations (11) and (10) link the parameters of an exponential fitting of the PPG segments to the blood and vascular parameters. Most evident is the relationship with oxygenation, as we explained in previous sections. The exact oxygen saturation depends on the assumption that the blood volume causes the same changes in R and IR light on the optical sensors. This is not quite true in the reality, which necessitates a calibration of pulse oxymeters [10].

We made advantage of several PPG channels that we measure at the same time. The illumination paths traverse fingers at various places and under different angles. Due to slightly displaced R and IR light sources to each other, also the R and its neighbouring IR paths differ. Assuming that a statistically relevant set of the PPG segments is available, and that the variations causing inaccuracies are zero-mean, averaging of all possible outcomes must improve their accuracy and robustness. The results in Table 1 confirm the expectations. Estimation errors are small, though the number of different oxygenation levels met in our preliminary experiments is low. Actually, healthy subjects have their blood oxygen saturation always above 95 % and close to 100 %, unless they hold their breath for a while. In such a population variations are not significant. Our further research will have to introduce more statistically relevant variability.

It is worthwhile mentioning that if a heartbeat falls within the transient interval after the door handle release, this disturbs the expected PPG segment considerably. Appropriate solutions will have to be looked for in such cases.

Equations (11) and (10) lead up to a conclusion that all other vascular parameters, and also the distending blood pressure may be estimated from the transient PPG segments that we observed and modelled. This is going to be our future research focus. Relationships among blood pressure, blood inflow times after an instantaneous release of finger oppression, and their impact on the light transmission through fingers will have to be investigated in more detail on their physical background.

Acknowledgement Authors acknowledge a financial support of the Slovenian Ministry of Education, Science, and Sport and the European Regional Development Funds for the Biomedical Engineering Competence Centre. We are grateful to partners from Gorenje Group, Velenje, Slovenia, who designed the photoplethysmograph housing and placement in the refrigerator's door frame.

References

1. Kamat, V.: Pulse oximetry. Indian J. Anaesth. **46**(4), 261–268 (2002)
2. Zislin, B.D., Chistyako, A.V.: The history of oximetry. Biomed. Eng. **40**(1), 53–56 (2006)
3. Pirš, C., Cigale, B., Zazula, D.: A feasibility study of heartbeat detections from photoplethysmograms with fingers compressed. In: Proceeding of the 5th WSEAS International Conference on Sensors and Signals, pp. 47–52 (2012)
4. Spigulis, J., Erts, R., Rubins, U.: Micro-circulation of skin blood: optical monitoring by advanced photoplethysmography techniques. In: Proceeding of the SPIE, vol. 5119, pp. 219–225 (2003)
5. Choi, Y., Zhang, Q., Ko, S.: Noninvasive cuffless blood pressure estimation using pulse transit time and Hilbert-Huang transform. Comput. Electr. Eng. **39**, 103–111 (2013)
6. McCombine, D.B., Reisner, A.T., Asada, H.H.: Motion based adaptive calibration of pulse transit time measurements to arterial blood pressure for an autonomous, wearable blood pressure monitor. In: Proc. of the 30th Annual International IEEE EMBS Conference, pp. 989–992 (2008)
7. Cigale, B., Zazula, D., Đonlagić, D., Pirš, C., Benkič, K.: Računalniška naprava in postopek za nemoteče merjenje parametrov funkcionalnega zdravja. SI 24037 (A), 2013–10-30, Ljubljana, Urad Republike Slovenije za intelektualno lastnino (2013)
8. Zazula, D., Pirš, C., Benkič, K., Đonlagić, D., Cigale, B.: Short-term photoplethysmography embedded in household appliances. In: The 6th European Conference of the International Federation for Medical and Biological Engineering, MBEC 2014, pp. 922–925. Springer, Berlin (2014)

9. Teng, X.-F., Zhang, T.: Theoretical study on the effect of sensor contact force on pulse transit time. IEEE Trans. Biomed. Eng. **54**(8), 1490–1498 (2007)
10. Rhee, S.: Design and analysis of artifact-resistive finger photoplethysmographic sensors for vital sign monitoring. Ph.D. Thesis, MIT, Boston (2000)

Measurement of 3-D Workspace of Thumb Tip with RGB-D Sensor for Quantitative Rehabilitation

Tadashi Matsuo and Nobutaka Shimada

Abstract The three dimensional workspace of the thumb tip, where a thumb tip can reach, is closely related to functions that can be performed by the thumb. However, on the hand and finger rehabilitation, one dimensional range of motion for each joint is manually measured for evaluating the current state of the hand. It requires a therapist to measure the ranges. In addition, it is difficult to evaluate the three dimensional workspace from the one dimensional ranges. We propose a method to automatically estimate three dimensional position of the thumb tip with a contactless depth sensor. To evaluate the relative position to the palm, we also propose a method to estimate three dimensional configuration of the palm. With experiments, we show the effectiveness of the proposed method.

1 Introduction

The functions by a hand such as grasping, picking or moving an object, are achieved by the complex structure consisting of tendons, muscles and bones. When one's hand or finger is injured, rehabilitation is required for restoring the functions in addition to a surgical operation for restoring the complex structure. Since the rehabilitation should be adapted to the states of the injury and restoration, it is very important to measure the functional state of the hand. On the medical front, muscular strength, tactile sensation and movable range are used as indices of the functional state of the hand [3]. Currently, the movable range is represented as a set of one dimensional ranges of possible angles of each joint. In addition, each one dimensional range is manually measured with a protractor by a therapist [9].

The thumb tip can move in a wide three dimensional extent, which is called "workspace", and the workspace is closely related to the functional state of the hand [7]. However, it is difficult to evaluate the workspace from the set of one dimensional ranges. In addition, manual measurement for each finger is a work load of a therapist.

T. Matsuo (✉) · N. Shimada
Ritsumeikan University, Shiga, Japan
e-mail: matsuo@i.ci.ritsumei.ac.jp

Y.-W. Chen et al. (eds.), *Innovation in Medicine and Healthcare 2015*,
Smart Innovation, Systems and Technologies 45,
DOI 10.1007/978-3-319-23024-5_26

Automatic measurement of the three dimensional workspace of the thumb tip will enable a therapist to numerically evaluate the functional state of the hand with a lighter work load.

Such a three dimensional workspace can be measured by equipping a patient with a data glove or markers [4]. However, it is not desirable because it may be a heavy load for a patient with an injured hand and the patient may require a helper for the equipment. As a contactless measurement, there are methods by using X-ray, but it is not desirable because a patient and a therapist will be exposed to radiation. As a contactless measurement without radiation, Leap Motion Controller [5] has been sold on the market. It is said that the device can measure the three dimensional positions of finger tips. Although we have tried it, it seems not to measure correctly the positions when the palm and the tips are overlapped in view of the sensor. To evaluate the functional state of the hand, the position of the thumb tip, which often moves against the palm, is important. Therefore, a method should work even if the palm and the thumb tip are overlapped.

In this paper, we propose a method to estimate the position of the thumb tip by learning the shape of the tip on an output of a depth sensor. And also, we propose a method to estimate standard positions (the wrist, the root of the little finger and the root of the forefinger). By using the proposed methods, we can calculate the thumb tip position relative to the hand with a depth sensor. The numerically estimated three dimensional workspace will bring more accurate evaluation of the functional state of the hand. In addition, it will reduce a work load of therapists.

2 Proposed System

As a contactless depth sensor, we use Microsoft Kinect [8]. By placing a hand in front of the sensor as shown in Fig. 1, we can obtain a depth image (Fig. 2), which contains depths from the sensor to a position corresponding to each pixel. In Fig. 2, nearer pixel is rendered as blacker and further pixel is rendered as whiter. In this paper, we suppose that the depth from the hand to the sensor is within 700 $\sim$ 800 [mm] and there are no other objects in the range.

Fig. 1 Environment

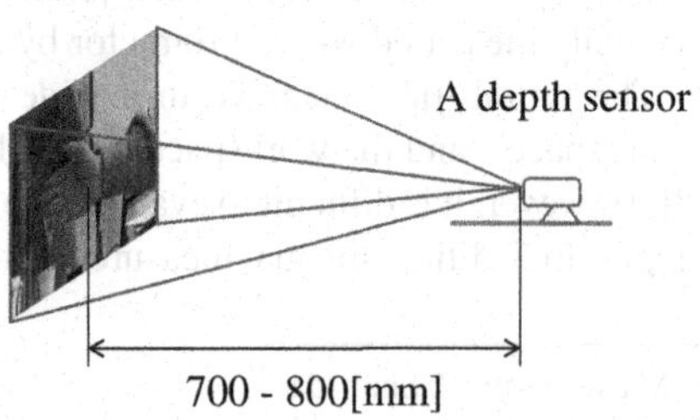

Fig. 2 Depth image

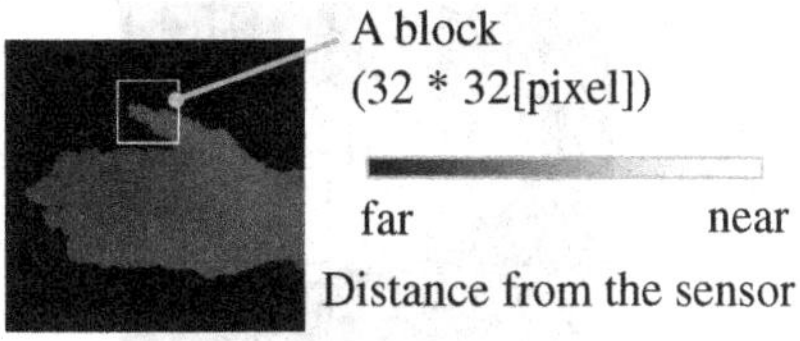

The proposed method estimates the thumb tip position by using the distribution of depths in a block including the thumb tip (Fig. 2). The size of the window is 32×32[pixel], which corresponds to a region $40 \sim 45$ [mm] square at a distance of $700 \sim 800$ [mm] from the sensor.

The estimation of the thumb tip position consists of the following steps.

1. Collect overlapping blocks from a depth image, and then discriminate blocks including the thumb tip from those excluding the thumb tip (Fig. 3a). This is described in Sect. 4.
2. Estimate the relative position of the thumb tip in each block including the thumb tip (Fig. 3b), and then collect the corresponding positions in the depth image as candidate positions. This is described in Sect. 5.
3. Find the candidate position supported by the most blocks and consider it as the estimated thumb tip position.

By the above steps, we can estimate the position represented by the coordinate system based on the sensor.

To evaluate the functional state of the hand, the spatial relation between the hand and the three dimensional reachable extent is important. By constructing a relative coordinate system based on the palm, we estimate the spatial relation. We derive the relative coordinate system from the three standard positions (the wrist, the root of the little finger and the root of the forefinger). Since it is difficult to find the standard positions by the local shape, each standard position is estimated from the distribution of depths of the whole hand. This is described in Sect. 6.

3 Feature Vector of a Block

Since the thumb tip has a characteristic shape, we find the tip by learning the local shape of the tip. To represent a local shape of the thumb tip, we use a feature vector derived from a relative depth distribution of a block because local shapes of the thumb tip are characterized by relative depth to neighbourhood. A feature vector of a block is constructed as follows:

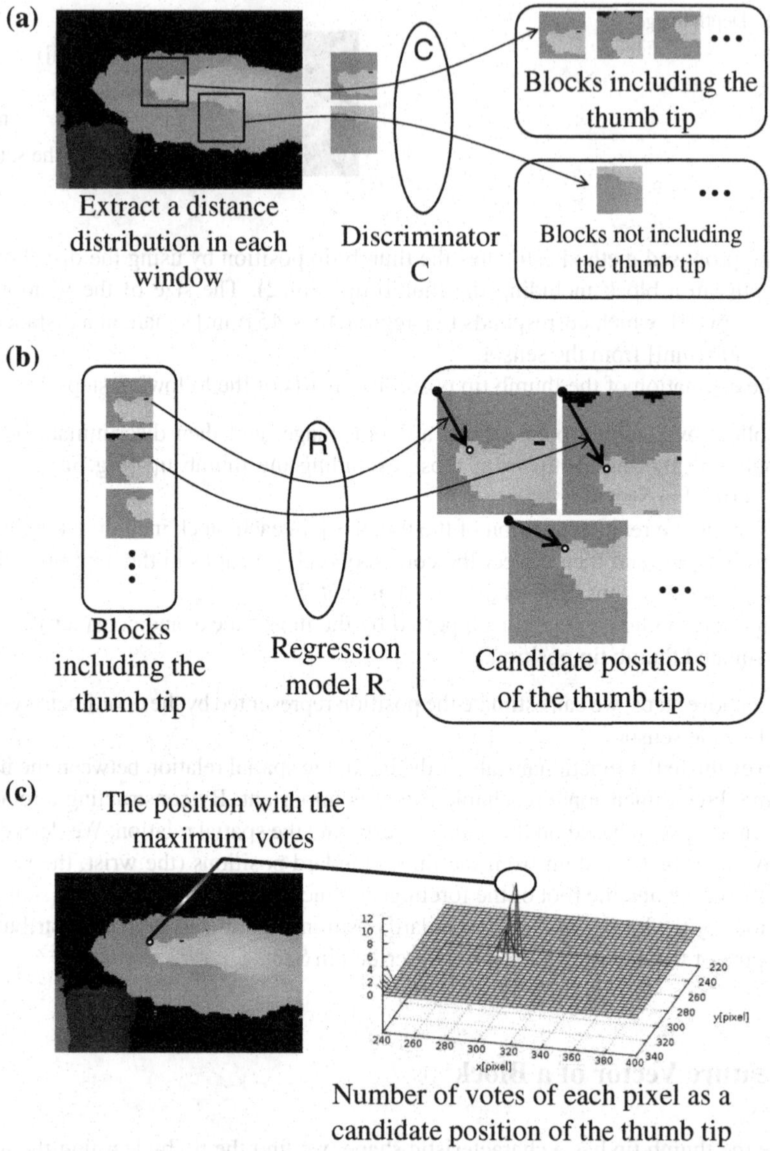

Fig. 3 Flow of estimation. **a** Block-wise discrimination. **b** Candidates of the thumb tip position. **c** Estimation by voting

1. Calculate normalized depth distribution of the block.
   (a) Separate the block into the hand region and the other region by depth.
   (b) Calculate the median of depths on the hand region.
   (c) Generate a normalized distribution $\hat{d}(x, y)$ as follows:

$$\hat{d}(x, y) = \begin{cases} d(x, y) - d_{\text{median}} & ((x, y) \text{ in the hand region}), \\ 100\,[\text{mm}] & (\text{otherwise}), \end{cases} \tag{1}$$

   where $d(x, y)$ denotes the original depth [mm] in the block and d_{median} denotes the median. On the background, we define $\hat{d}(x, y)$ as 100 [mm] since depths on the hand region will be within 100 [mm] from the median when the palm is nearly parallel to the sensor screen.

2. Calculate low resolution components (256 elements) and relative components (120 elements) and generate 376 dimensional vector by joining the components.

Low resolution components 256 elements sub-sampled with 2×2[pixel] interval from $\hat{d}(x, y)$ smoothed by the 4×4 constant filter.

Relative components Divide the 32×32[pixel] block into 16 sub-blocks (8×8[pixel]) and then calculate differences of the average depths in the sub-blocks for all combinations of two sub-blocks (${}_{1}6C_2 = 120$).

4 Block-Wise Discrimination

We discriminate blocks including the thumb tip from those not including the thumb tip by Random Forest Classifier [2]. We use the forest including 100 trees and we evaluate weak learners by Gini impurity [1] when training the forest.

We collect teacher labels from color images and depth images including a hand equipped with a blue thumbstall (Fig. 4). If a block includes the gravity center of the thumbstall region, it is labeled as a block including a thumb tip. We train the random forest classifier by pairs of the label and the corresponding feature vector.

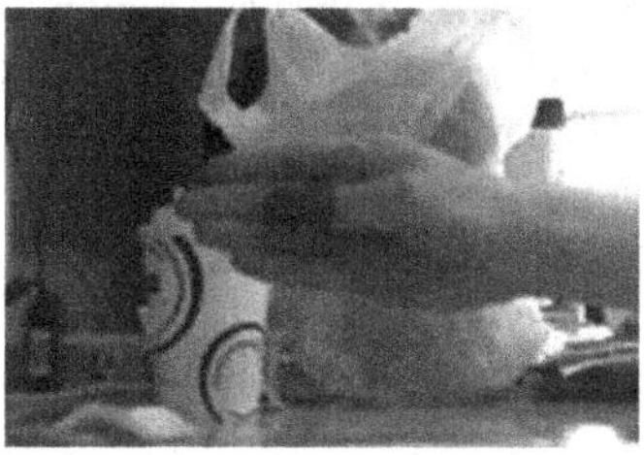

Fig. 4 Teacher of block-wise discrimination

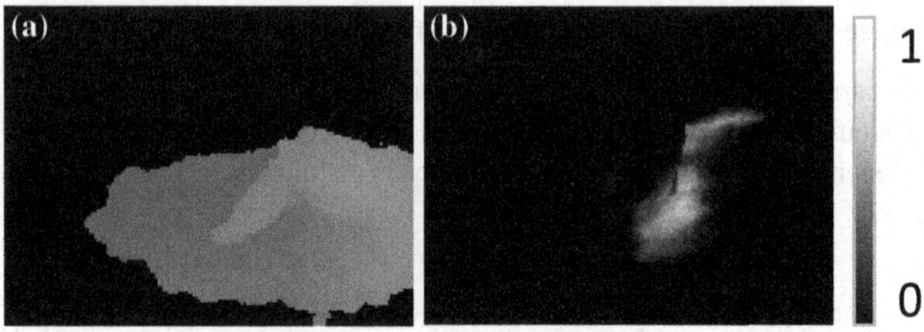

Fig. 5 Probability of a block including the thumb tip. **a** An input depth image. **b** Estimated probability

In this experiment, we took 85 scenes where the thumb tip moved and the fingers were naturally stretched. And then, we trained the classifier by 408,000 pairs of a teacher label and a feature vector, which were collected from 4800 blocks near to the hand region for each scene.

In Fig. 5, we show the estimated probability of a block including the thumb tip. The classifier outputs high probability on neighbour hood of the true thumb tip even though the thumb tip touches the palm.

5 Estimation of the Thumb Tip Position

We estimate the thumb tip position in a block including the tip by Random Forest Regression [2]. We use the forest including 100 trees and weak learners are evaluated by the mean squared error. The input of the regression model is a feature vector of a block and the output is the relative position of the thumb tip in the block.

We trained the regression model by the teachers extracted from the scenes use in Sect. 4. We manually determined the true position of the thumb tip for each scene and we trained the model by 21,760 pairs of a relative position of the thumb tip and a feature vector.

If a block really includes the thumb tip, the regression model outputs the near position for the overlapping blocks. Each discrimination and regression may be incorrect, but the influence of incorrect results can be reduced by voting. We collect overlapping blocks on the hand region, and then obtain candidate positions by the regression model. Finally, we find the candidate position supported by the most blocks and consider it as the estimated thumb tip position. An example of the voting is shown in Fig. 3c.

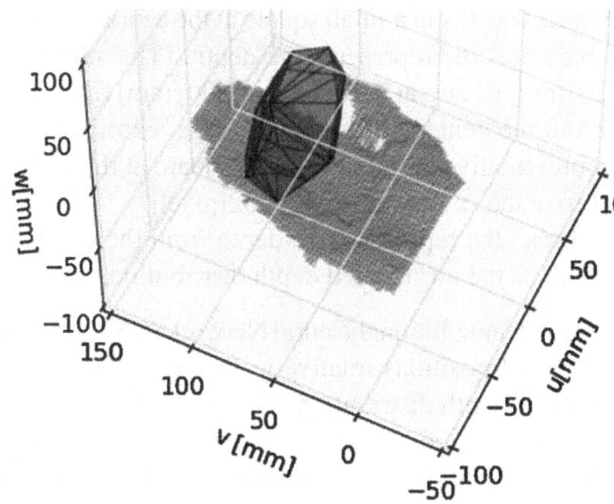

Fig. 6 A convex hull of possible positions of the thumb tip

In Fig. 6, we show the convex hull of positions of the moving thumb tip when the hand stands still and the thumb tip moves as widely as possible. The hull agrees with the reachable workspace.

6 Relative Coordinate System

We construct a relative coordinate system based on the following three position; the wrist, the root of the little finger and the root of the forefinger (Fig. 7), which we call the standard positions. Since it is difficult to find the standard positions by the local shape, each standard position is estimated from the distribution of depths of the whole hand.

The hand is nearer to the sensor, the hand region in the depth image is larger. To extract the whole shape of the hand without depending on its position, we estimate the standard positions by the depth distribution normalized as follows;

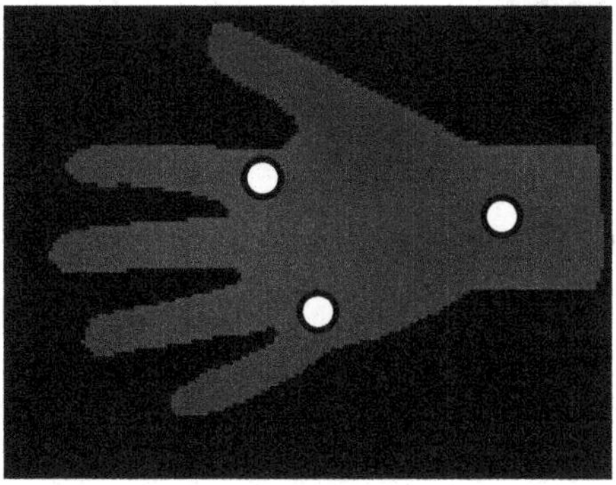

Fig. 7 The three standard positions of the palm

1. Collect depths in a small square at the center of the depth image and consider their median as the representative depth. (The small square corresponds to a region 20 [mm] square at a distance of 800 [mm] from the sensor.)
2. From the center of the depth image, extract a sub-image corresponding to the representative region 200 [mm] square at the representative depth.
3. Resize the sub-image to 32×32[pixel].
4. Subtract the representative depth from the depth of each pixel and consider the result as the normalized depth distribution.

We train a Convolutional Neural Network (CNN) [6] shown in Fig. 8 so that it outputs the standard positions relative to the center of the representative region from the normalized depth distribution.

To collect training samples, we use three dimensional computer graphics (CG) hand model because the true standard positions can be calculated easily. In this experiment, we manually specify the three points on the CG hand model as the standard points, and we generate 1000 training samples of the normalized depth distributions by moving the CG model within ± 20 [mm] and changing a joint angle within $0 \sim 5°$ randomly and independently.

In Fig. 9, we show the standard positions estimated from a real human hand. The standard positions are accurately estimated.

In Fig. 10, we show the convex hull of estimated positions when the hand moves without changing joint angles. In the figures, the hand at the initial positions is also drawn. In Fig. 10a, we show the positions represented by the absolute coordinate system based on the sensor. In Fig. 10b, we show the positions represented by the relative coordinate system based on the estimated standard positions. In the latter, the convex hull is small. This agrees with the fact that the relative position of the thumb tip does not change.

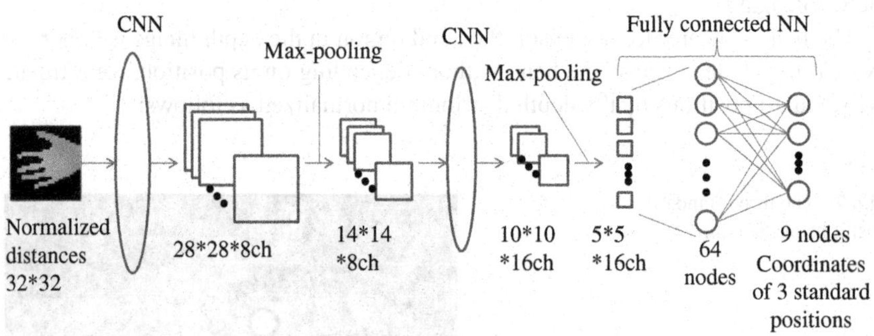

Fig. 8 Convolutional Neural Network

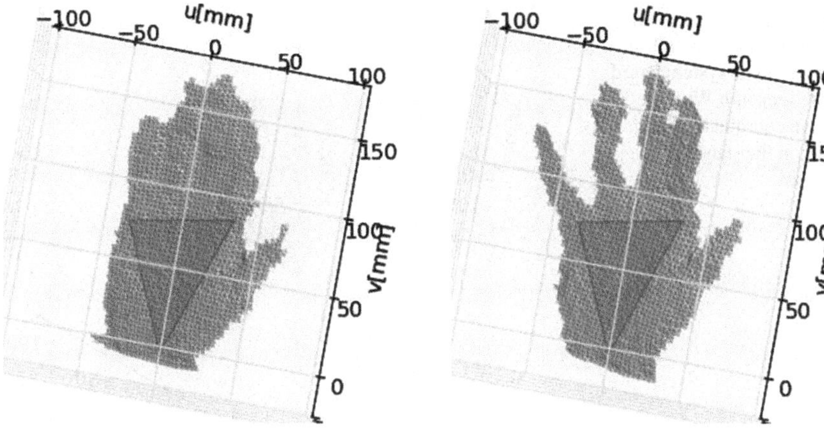

Fig. 9 Estimated standard positions

(a) **(b)**

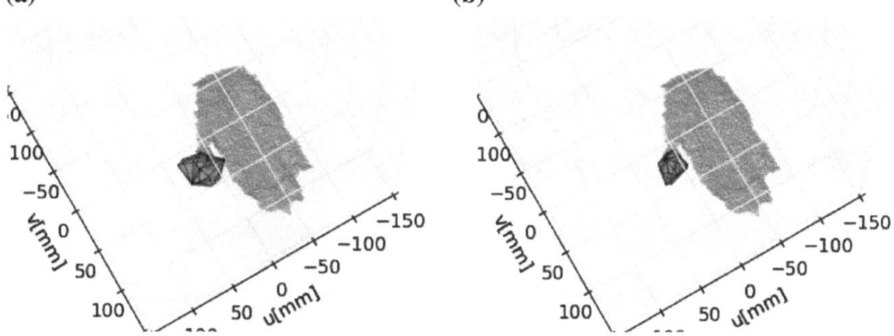

Fig. 10 The extent of thumb tip positions when bending only the wrist. **a** With the absolute coordinate system. **b** With the relative coordinate system

In Fig. 11, we show the convex hull of the estimated positions when the thumb tip moves circularly and the hand is not fixed. In the figures, the hand at the initial positions is also drawn. In Fig. 11a, the estimated position includes the motion of the whole hand and the convex hull is longer than the real three dimensional extent. In Fig. 11b, the convex hull is more similar to the real three dimensional extent because the motion of the whole hand is reduced.

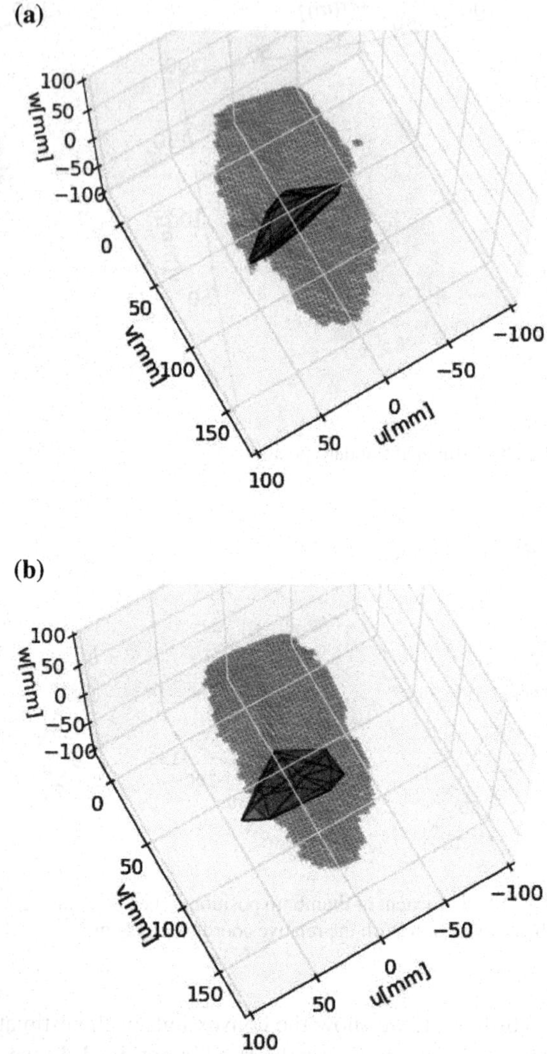

Fig. 11 The extent of the thumb tip positions. **a** With the coordinate system based on the sensor. **b** With the relative coordinate system based on the standard positions

7 Conclusion

We proposed a method to automatically estimate three dimensional position of the thumb tip with a contactless depth sensor and a method to estimate three dimensional configuration of the palm. We demonstrate the estimation of the workspace where the thumb tip can reach. But we have not analyzed the accuracy yet. We will evaluate the accuracy of the proposed methods by a high precision three dimensional sensor.

Acknowledgments This work was supported by JSPS KAKENHI Grant Number 24500224, 15H02764 and MEXT-Supported Program for the Strategic Research Foundation at Private Universities, S1311039, 2013–2016.

References

1. Breiman, L.: Technical note: Some properties of splitting criteria. Mach. Learn. **24**(1), 41–47 (1996). http://dx.doi.org/10.1023/A3A1018094028462
2. Breiman, L.: Random forests. Mach. Learn. **45**(1), 5–32 (2001). http://dx.doi.org/10.1023/A3A1010933404324
3. Health, J.L., Organization, W.: External injury: hand rehabilitation. http://www.research12.jp/gaisho/08.html, Accessed 29 May 2015
4. Kuo, L.C., Chiu, H.Y., Chang, C.W., Hsu, H.Y., Sun, Y.N.: Functional workspace for precision manipulation between thumb and fingers in normal hands. J. Electromyogr. Kinesiol. **19**(5), 829–839 (2009). http://www.sciencedirect.com/science/article/pii/S1050641108001193
5. Leap Motion, I.: Leap motion controller. https://www.leapmotion.com/product. Accessed 29 May 2015
6. Lecun, Y., Bottou, L., Bengio, Y., Haffner, P.: Gradient-based learning applied to document recognition. Proceedings of the IEEE **86**(11), 2278–2324 (1998)
7. Marzke, M.W.: Precision grips, hand morphology, and tools. Am. J. Phys. Anthr. **102**(1), 91–110 (1997)
8. Microsoft: Kinect for windows. http://www.microsoft.com/en-us/kinectforwindows/. Accessed 29 May 2015
9. Yonemoto, K., Ishigami, S., Toru, K.: Display and measurement of movable range of joints. The Japanese Journal of Rehabilitation Medicine **32**(4), 207–217 (1995)

Automatic Segmentation Method for Kidney Using Dual Direction Adaptive Diffusion Flow

Xu Qiao, Wujing Lu, Xuantao Su and Yen-Wei Chen

Abstract In this paper, we mainly focus on automatic segmentation method of sequence kidney images from CT based on adaptive diffusion flow (ADF) method and morphological analysis. We modified the energy function by focusing on tangent direction diffusion which considered that the shapes of kidney mainly are convex. We design to evolve the dynamic curve with dual direction to improve the precision of segmentation and to deal with the local optimization problems. Experiments applied on kidney volumes show good property of segmentation using the proposed method.

Keywords Kidney · Segmentation · Adaptive diffusion flow · Energy function

1 Introduction

Image segmentation is the fundamental and key approach of image processing and pattern recognition, which has been extensively used in many aspects including medical imaging, video tracking, remote-sensing and so on. The segmentation aims to divide the image into several meaningful objects so that it is easier to analyze or extract the regions of interest.

Active contour model (ACM), which was proposed by Kass et al. [1], has been proven to be an efficient and interactive method in the domain of image segmentation in the past decades. The principal idea of ACM is to evolve a dynamic curve under some constraints to extract the exact objective boundary. There are two main categories of active contour: the region-based models and the edge-based models.

X. Qiao (✉) · W. Lu · X. Su
Department of Biomedical Engineering, Shandong University, Jinan, China
e-mail: qiaoxu@sdu.edu.cn

Y.-W. Chen
Intelligent Image Processing Lab, Ritsumeikan University, Kyoto, Japan

Y.-W. Chen et al. (eds.), *Innovation in Medicine and Healthcare 2015*,
Smart Innovation, Systems and Technologies 45,
DOI 10.1007/978-3-319-23024-5_27

The region-based model segment the region of interest based on the image statistical information, especially applied to the homogeneous image with similar intensity distributions. Compared with the region-based models, the edge-based models utilize the image gradient information as a driven force to attract dynamic curve towards to the objective boundary. This kind of method can deal with the inhomogeneous regions or complicated circumstance for the reason that it just needs an appropriate initialization, especially for extracting the single target surrounded by complicated backgrounds. Considering the complexity of image we are going to cope with, this paper mainly focuses on the edge-based models.

Parametric active contours models have obtained a great development since original method was proposed. This kind of method is modeled by an energy function that the dynamic curve is moved towards to the desired boundary by minimizing the energy functions. The energy functions usually contain two terms: internal energy and external energy. The internal energy serves to make the dynamic curve smooth in the process of curve evolution, which is usually represented by the first and second derivatives on the boundary. Meanwhile, the external energy obtained according to the image property could serve to attract the curve to close the boundary, and act as a leading role to drive the contours has been extensively studied.

The original method also suffers from several shortcomings: initialization sensitivity, poor convergence rate, topology adaptive and detecting high curvature boundaries. To deal with these issues, plenty of efforts have been made to provide feasible solutions, such as balloons [2], distance potential force [3], gradient vector flow(GVF) [4], and the variant of GVF [5, 6]. GVF has proven to be the most successful algorithm among these methods. The method produces a kind of external force field, which generated from image by diffusing the gradient vector calculated from image edge map. The field could control the initial contour to evolve toward the object edge, which has successfully improved the drawback of traditional snakes: initialization sensitivity. Ning et al. [6] decomposed the diffusion term into normal direction diffusion and tangent direction diffusion, and updated the GVF by choosing normal gradient vector flow(NGVF) as the external force. The updated method could fix the drawback of concavity convergence while at the cost of losing the weak edge. Bing Li et al. [7] put forward an idea of modifying the external force by convolving a vector field with the edge map derived from image, which called VFC. It can obtain a larger capture range than GVF method, especially for the robustness and flexibility of tailoring the force field, and for the reduction in computational cost. But the method cannot preserve the weak edges, which might be overwhelmed by the strong edges along with the noise. Mishra et al. [8] addresses the limitations of capturing regions of very high curvature by applying internal and external image forces independently. The method employs a Hidden Markov Model and Viterbi search, and then a separate prior step, which modifies the updated curve based on the relative strengths of the measurement uncertainty and non-stationary prior. Kovacs et al. [9] utilized a modified function of Harris corner detector based on active contour external force to detect high curvature and noisy object boundaries.

The typical drawbacks of kidney CT images usually include: weak edge that easily leak into adjacent strong ones, blurring edge, lower-contrast, and inhomogeneous interior intensity distribution. In such a situation, the traditional methods cannot get the better kidney boundaries. Some academics proposed segmentation method by combining prior shape knowledge with special segmentation algorithms [10–13]. These methods usually construct a mathematical model and aims to designated segmentation object.

Recently, a novel method called adaptive diffusion flow (ADF) [14, 15] has been proposed. The method redefine the external force based on GVF by putting forward a rigorous mathematical framework according image characteristics, which could converge to narrow and deep concavity, adjust the diffusion process adaptively, and preserve the weak edge, especially neighbored by strong ones. In our work, this paper focus on automatic segmentation method of sequence kidney images from CT based on ADF method and morphological analysis. Simultaneously, this paper modified the energy functional by focusing on tangent direction diffusion which considered that the shapes of kidney mainly are convex. On the other hand, the dynamic curve easily falls into local optimization rather than global optimization due to the fact that lower-contrast in different regions and inhomogeneous interior and exterior intensity distribution. Therefore, this paper designs to evolve the dynamic curve with dual direction to improve the precision of segmentation. We divide the image into two different groups according the object boundary, and evolve the initial curves separately from inside of object boundary and outside of object boundary. Afterwards, this paper calculates the segmentation curve according to the final curve evolution result. Finally, we can obtain the dual initial values of adjacent images by incorporating the previous image segmentation result and morphological method. The creativities of our method are as follows: (a) automation initialization, (b) evolve dynamic curve in dual direction, (c) no prior shape is needed, (d) detect blurring and low-contrast edges.

2 Background

The original method was first proposed by Kass et al. [1] evolve the dynamic x (s) = [x(s), y(s)], s ∈ [0, 1] toward the object boundary by minimizing the following energy functional:

$$E_{internal} = \frac{1}{2}\left[\alpha(s)|x'(s)|^2 + \beta(s)|x''(s)|^2\right] \tag{1}$$

$$E_{internal} = \frac{1}{2}\left[\alpha(s)|x'(s)|^2 + \beta(s)|x''(s)|^2\right] \tag{2}$$

$$E_{external} = E_{ext}(x(s)) \tag{3}$$

The first term and the second term of Eq. (1) are usually called the internal force and the external force, respectively. For $E_{internal}$, α(s) and β(s) usually are the positive constant weighting parameters that dominate the tension and rigidity components of internal energy. x′(s) and x″(s) are the first order derivative and the second order derivative with respect s, usually serves to keep initial contour smooth and control contour bending in the process of evolving, respectively. For $E_{external}$, usually act as the external force for attracting the evolution curve to the object boundary. The common functional forms of the external force expressed as follows [6]:

$$E_{ext}(x(s)) = -\nabla|I(x,y)|^2 \tag{4}$$

$$E_{ext}(x(s)) = -|\nabla(G_\sigma(x,y)*I(x,y))|^2 \tag{5}$$

where G_σ is the Gaussian function with standard deviation σ, I(x, y) is the image intensity at (x,y), ∇ is the gradient operator, and * means the convolution operation.

To minimize E_{snake}, according to the variational calculus technique [16], Eq. (1) need to satisfy the following Euler equation:

$$\frac{\partial}{\partial s}\left(\alpha(s)\frac{\partial x(s)}{\partial s}\right) - \frac{\partial^2}{\partial s^2}\left(\beta(s)\frac{\partial^2 x(s)}{\partial s^2}\right) - \nabla E_{ext}(x(s)) = 0 \tag{6}$$

3 Dual Direction Adaptive Diffusion Flow

Xu and Prince [5] replaced the external force of active contour methods with gradient vector flow for settling the drawbacks of traditional method: initialization sensitivity, concavity convergence etc. We define the gradient vector flow field with the mathematical description $V(x,y) = [u(x,y), \nu(x,y)]$, and $V(x,y)$ obtained by the means of minimizing the energy functional:

$$E_{ext} = \iint \mu(u_x^2 + u_y^2 + \nu_x^2 + \upsilon_y^2)dxdy + \iint |\nabla f|^2 |V - \nabla f|^2 dxdy \tag{7}$$

where μ is a regularization parameter, u_x, u_y, ν_x, υ_y are the partial derivatives, f(x,y) is the edge map which derived from the original image I(x,y). The first integral in Eq. (7) is the smooth term, yielding a slowly varying field, which could increase the capture range of force field and robust to noise. For the second integral, it produced a desired effect of keeping force field nearly equal to the edge map when ∇f is large. Afterwards, Xu and Prince replaced the parameter μ and $|\nabla f|^2$ with new function forms for solving the opposite force field caused by proximity edge [6]. The mathematical model as follows:

$$E_{ext} = \iint g(|\nabla f|)(u_x^2 + u_y^2 + v_x^2 + v_y^2)dxdy + \iint h(|\nabla f|)|V - \nabla f|^2 dxdy \tag{8}$$

$$g(|\nabla f|) = e^{-(|\nabla f|/K)} \tag{9}$$

$$h(|\nabla f|) = 1 - g(|\nabla f|) \tag{10}$$

where $\boldsymbol{K}$ is a calibration parameter, determines to some extent the degree of tradeoff between field smoothness and gradient conformity.

To minimize the Eqs. (7) and (8), using the calculus of variations [17], we can obtain gradient vector flow field by solving the Euler equations:

$$\mu\nabla^2 u - (u - f_x)\left(f_x^2 + f_y^2\right) = 0 \tag{11}$$

$$\mu\nabla^2 v - (v - f_y)\left(f_x^2 + f_y^2\right) = 0 \tag{12}$$

for generalized gradient vector flow:

$$g(|\nabla f|)\nabla^2 u - (u - f_x)h(|\nabla f|) = 0 \tag{13}$$

$$g(|\nabla f|)\nabla^2 v - (v - f_y)h(|\nabla f|) = 0 \tag{14}$$

where ∇^2 is the laplacian operator.

Wu and Wang [14] improved the first integral in Eq. (7) for preserving the weak edge and entering into long and deep concavity by the following models:

$$\begin{aligned} \mathrm{E_{ext}} = &\iint \mathrm{g}(|\nabla \mathrm{f}|)(-\mathrm{m}\cdot \Theta_{\mathrm{L}^{\infty}(\Omega)})\mathrm{dxdy} + \iint \mathrm{g}(|\nabla \mathrm{f}|)(1-\mathrm{m}) \\ &\frac{1}{\mathrm{p}(|\nabla \mathrm{f}|)}\left(\sqrt{1+\Theta}\right)^{\mathrm{p}(|\nabla \mathrm{f}|)}\mathrm{dxdy} + \iint \mathrm{h}(|\nabla \mathrm{f}|)|\mathrm{V} - \nabla \mathrm{f}|^2\mathrm{dxdy} \end{aligned} \tag{15}$$

Here,

$$p(|\nabla f|) = 1 + 1/(1 + |\nabla G_\sigma * f(x,y)|).$$

$$\mathrm{m} = \begin{cases} \left[1 - f(x,y)^2/5K^2\right]^2 & if\, f(x,y)^2/5 \le K^2 \\ 0 & others \end{cases} \tag{16}$$

where $\Theta = |G_\sigma * \nabla V|^2$, L^∞ means the infinity Laplacian, K is a parameter computed by $K = 1.4826 \cdot E(||\nabla f(x,y)| - E(|\nabla f(x,y)|)|)$ [17] and E(·) denotes average value. The first integral of Eq. (13) produce the diffusion field along normal direction in image smoothing region rather than opposite direction, which could drive the dynamic curve entering into the concavity. The second integral of Eq. (13) serves to preserve weak edge and yield a smooth force field.

Using variation calculus, the minimizes of Eq. (13) can be solved by the following equations:

$$\frac{\partial V}{\partial t} = g\cdot\left[m\cdot\left(\frac{1}{|\nabla V|^2}\Delta_\infty V\right)+(1-m)\cdot\left((\sqrt{1+\Theta})^{p-2}\cdot V_{TT}\right.\right.$$
$$\left.\left.+\left((p-2)\cdot\Theta\cdot(\sqrt{1+\Theta})^{p-4}+(\sqrt{1+\Theta})^{p-2}\right)\cdot V_{NN}\right)\right]-h\cdot(V-\nabla f)$$
$$V_{TT} = \frac{1}{|\nabla V|^2}\left(V_x^2V_{yy}+V_y^2V_{xx}-2V_xV_yV_{xy}\right) \tag{17}$$

$$V_{NN} = \frac{1}{|\nabla V|^2}\left(V_x^2V_{xx}+V_y^2V_{yy}+2V_xV_yV_{xy}\right) \tag{18}$$

where $\Delta_\infty V$ is infinity Laplacian equation.

4 Experimental Results

In this section, we are going to report our results with two steps. The first step is to analyze the difference of dual direction with synthetic images from real kidney segmentation results. The second step is to show the segmentation results of kidney images and measures the segmentation quality using TPR and PPV indices compared with manually segmented by experts.

In order to demonstrate the difference of dual direction segmentation of kidney images, this paper compared the segmentation result with the ground truth using the indices of true-positive (TP), false-positive (FP), and false-negative (FN).They were counted to calculate the measurement of TPR and PPV. TPR can be defined as the probability that the ground truth objects are recognized. PPV is the probability that the segmentation results are recognized correctly. TPR and PPV are computed as follows:

$$\text{TPR} = \frac{Tp}{Tp+Fn} \tag{19}$$

$$\text{PPV} = \frac{Tp}{Tp+Fp} \tag{20}$$

We apply an OTSU method [17] to produce the binary image, which selects the global optimal threshold by maximizing the between-class variance based on image histogram. Afterwards, the initial contour is determined by dilating and eroding the

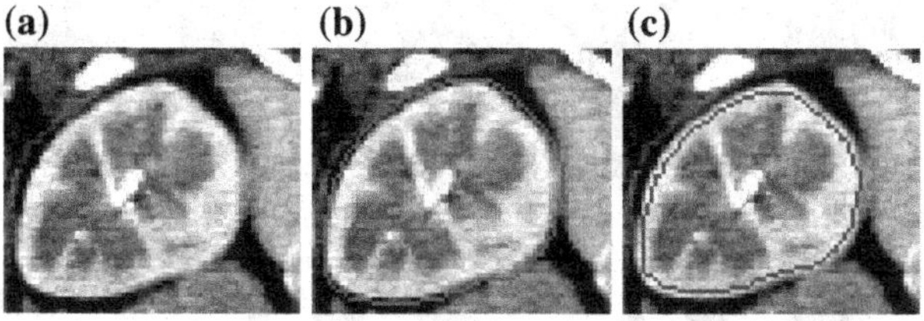

Fig. 1 **a** Original kidney image. **b** Initial outside of kidney image. **c** Initial inside of kidney image

binary image of kidney images two times respectively. Figure 1 listed three cases of segmentation result, where the blue and red lines represent the segmentation boundaries. It is obvious that the final segmentation results are different with evolving the initial contour in opposite direction. Two reasons are concluded here: (i): the first reason is the adjacent similar intensity regions. The kidney CT images are usually neighbored by some regions with strong gray value, which limits the choice of initial contour. However, the strong ones have no influence on the initial contour with inside unless the regions closely enough. (ii): the second reason is the fuzzy connectedness in different regions.

In detail, we evaluates the segmentation quality by specific data, as shown in Table 1. AVERAGE and SD means the average value and standard deviation of corresponding columns.

They are calculated according to the manual one and segmentation result with different initial contour. From the Table 1, we have the conclusion that the TPR is larger with initial contour outside of objects than initial inside, on the contrary, PPV are smaller. The results could be explained by the two reasons we have mentioned before. Because of the objects usually neighbored by strong ones and fuzzy connectedness, the dynamic curve usually converge to local minimum rather than global optimization in the process of evolving. Therefore, for the initial contour outside of objects, the dynamic curve usually is attracted by the strong ones, or converges to the external local minimum. Meanwhile, the dynamic curve with the initial contour inside of objects easily converges to internal local minimum, and almost has nothing to do with the strong ones. Therefore, the true-positive pixels inside of the red lines usually are larger than the blue lines when obtain the intersection with manual one respectively.

Table 1 Slices correspond to the image in Fig. 2

Image	Outside—Inside		Inside—Outside	
	TPR (%)	PPV	TPR (%)	PPV (%)
SLICE_1	99.285	96.525	99.229	97.504
SLICE_2	99.057	96.974	98.900	97.840
SLICE_3	99.329	98.453	98.985	98.693
AVERAGE	99.224	97.317	99.038	98.012
SD	0.146	1.009	0.171	0.613

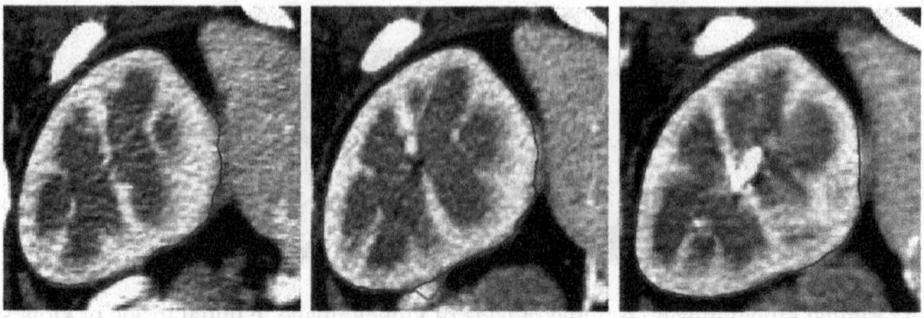

Fig. 2 Segmentation result of three kidney images. The *red line* represents the segmentation result with initial contour outside of object. The *blue line* represents the segmentation result with initial contour inside of object

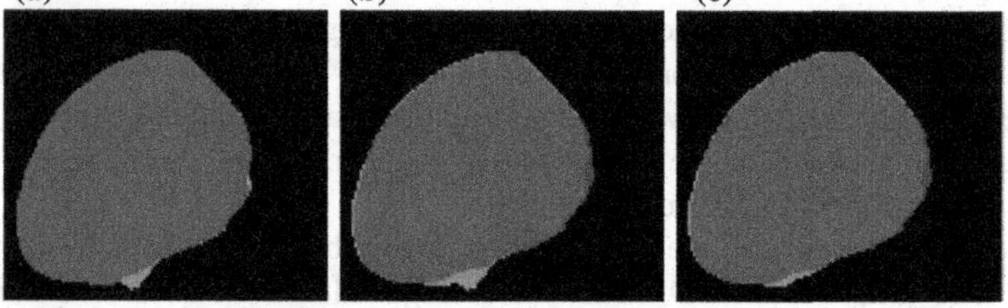

Fig. 3 **a** Segmentation result. **b** Segmentation result compared with manual one with initial contour outside of objects. **c** Segmentation result compared with manual one with initial contour inside of objects

We have listed other type of graph to display the segmentation result, as shown in Fig. 2. On Fig. 2, the three synthetic images are demonstrated according to the real segmentation data which come to the same kidney image. It is easy to observe the difference of initial inside and initial outside from the first image. Meanwhile, the second image and the third image demonstrate the difference between the segmentation result and manual one.

In Fig. 3, the red represented the common parts, green parts are the part of the segmentation result with initial contour outside and blue parts are the parts of the segmentation result with initial contour inside. In Fig. 3b, c, blues parts are the part of manual one, the green parts are the parts of the segmentation result with initial contour outside and inside respectively.

5 Conclusion

In this paper, we proposed an automatic segmentation method for medical volumes based on dual direction ADF. Experiments applied on kidney volumes show good property of segmentation using our method. In future, we will apply this method for other organs in medical images and try to combine the two contours obtained from different directions using a probability optimal function in order to get more accurate results.

Acknowledgement This work is supported by Natural Science Foundation of Shandong Province (ZR2014HQ054) and Doctoral Fund of Ministry of Education of China (20130131120035).

References

1. Kass, M., Witkin, A., Terzopulos, D.: Snakes: active contour models. Int. J. Comput. Vision **1**(4), 321–331 (1988)
2. Cohen, L.: On active contour models and balloons. CVGIP: Image Underst. **53**(2), 211–218 (1991)
3. Cohen, L., Cohen, I.: Finite element methods for active contour models and balloons for 2D and D images. IEEE Trans. Pattern Anal. Mach. Intell. **15**, 1131–1147 (1993)
4. Xu, C., Prince, J.: Snakes, shapes, and gradient vector flow. IEEE Trans. Image Process. **7**(3), 359–369 (1998)
5. Xu, C., Prince, J.: Generalized gradient vector flow external forces for active contours. Sig. Process. **71**(2), 131–139 (1998)
6. Jifeng, N., Chengke, W., Shigang, L., Shuqin, Y.: NGVF: an improved external force field for active contour model. Pattern Recogn. Lett. **28**(1), 58–63 (2007)
7. li, B., Acton, S.: Active contour external force using vector field convolution for image segmentation. IEEE Trans. Image Process. **16**(8), 2016–2096 (2007)
8. Mishra, A., Fieguth, P., Clausi, D.: Decoupled active contour(DAC) for boundary detection. IEEE Trans. Pattern Anal. Mach. Intell. **33**(2), 310–324 (2011)
9. Kovacs, A., Sziranyi, T.: Harris function based active contour external force for image segmentation. Pattern Recogn. Lett. **33**(9), 1180–1187 (2012)
10. Tsai, A., Yezzi, A., Wells, W.: Diffusion-snakes: combining statistical shape knowledge and image information in a variational framework. In: IEEE Workshop on Variational and Level Set Methods, IEEE, Vanconuver, pp.137–144 (2001)
11. Shen, D., Zhang, Y., Davatzikos, C.: Segmentation of prostate boundaries from ultrasound images using statistical shape model. IEEE Trans. Med. Imaging **22**(4), 539–551 (2003)
12. Chen, F., Hua, R., Yua, H.M., Wang, S.Y.: Reduced set density estimator for object segmentation based on shape probabilistic representation. J. Vis. Commun. Image Represent. **23**(7), 1085–1094 (2012)
13. Huang, J., Yang, X., Chen, Y., Tang, L.: Ultrasound kidney segmentation with a global prior shape. J. Vis. Commun. Image Represent. **24**, 937–943 (2013)
14. Wu, Y., Wang, Y., Jia, Y.: Adaptive diffusion flow active contours for image segmentation. Comput. Vis. Image Underst. **117**, 1421–1435 (2013)
15. Black, M., Sapiro, G., Marimont, D., Heeger, D.: Robust anisotropic diffusion. IEEE Trans. Image Process. **7**(3), 421–432 (2002)
16. Aubert, G., Kornprobst, P.: Mathematical Problems in Image Processing: Partial Differential Equations and the Calculus of Variations. Springer, New York (2006)
17. Otsu, N.: A threshold selection method form gray-level histograms. IEEE Trans. Syst. Man Cybern. **9**(1), 62–66 (1979)

Automatic Registration of Deformable Organs in Medical Volume Data by Exhaustive Search

Masahiro Isobe, Shota Niga, Kei Ito, Xian-Hua Han, Yen-Wei Chen and Gang Xu

Abstract This paper proposes a novel framework for fully automatic localization of deformable organs in medical volume data, which can obtain not only the position but also simultaneously the orientation and deformation of the organ to be searched, without the need to segment the organ first. The problem is defined as one of minimizing the sum of squared distances between the organ model's surface points and their closest surface points extracted from the input volume data. The geometric alignment, or so-called registration, of three-dimensional models by least square minimization always has the problem of initial states. We argue that the only way to solve this problem is by the exhaustive search. However, the exhaustive search takes much computational cost. In order to reduce the computational cost, we make efforts in the following three ways: (1) a uniform sampling over 3D rotation group; (2) Pyramidal search for all parameters; (3) Construction of a distance function for efficiently finding closest points. We have finished experiments for searching the six parameters for position and orientation, and the results show that the proposed framework can achieve correct localization of organs in the input data even with very large amounts of noise. We are currently expanding the system to localize organs with large deformation by adding and searching parameters representing scaling and deformation.

M. Isobe · S. Niga (✉) · K. Ito · X.-H. Han · Y.-W. Chen · G. Xu
College of Information Science and Engineering, Ritsumeikan University,
Shiga 525-8577, Japan
e-mail: is0081ef@ed.ritsumei.ac.jp

M. Isobe
e-mail: is0100px@ed.ritsumei.ac.jp

G. Xu
e-mail: xu@is.ritsumei.ac.jp

Y.-W. Chen et al. (eds.), *Innovation in Medicine and Healthcare 2015*,
Smart Innovation, Systems and Technologies 45,
DOI 10.1007/978-3-319-23024-5_28

1 Introduction

Medical volume analysis and understanding is a great challenge for the research and clinical communities. Organ registration plays an increasingly important role in clinical applications. In the conventional research, the first step is to segment the volume into different organs. Then the second step is to register these organs. And finally, these registered organs are used for specific applications.

The most intuitive way for organ segmentation is the manual implementation by medical doctors and researchers with medical knowledge, which takes a lot of time and imposes heavy burdens. Recently, some researchers were dedicated to explore automatic or semi-automatic organ segmentation approaches from the medical volumes, which mainly include intensity- and gradient-based approaches [1–5] and methods [6–10] combined with anatomical information. In the intensity- or gradient-based approaches, the prior knowledge has to be provided such as the manually labeled seeds of both the target organs and background for graph-cut [5], initial contour for level-set [3], and general parameters for intensity-based methods [2]. These approaches have achieved promising results both for organs having small intensity variation without human interaction, and for organs having large intensity variation with human interaction. On the other hand, the anatomical information such as organ's probabilistic atlas and distinguishable landmarks [6–10] has been combined into the intensity-based framework, which, to some extent, can give more precise organ region even for large variation of intensity. The organ segmentation needs firstly to align the distinguishable landmarks between the input volume data and the previously constructed model. However, it does not guarantee the alignment between the target organ and the organ model. Thus there is still much to be done in automatic organ localization from medical volumes.

This research devotes to explore a novel framework for fully automatic localization of deformable organs in medical volume data, which can obtain not only the correct position but also simultaneously the orientation and deformation of the organ to be searched, without the need to segment the organs first. Instead of the intensity itself that may vary widely, we prefer to use discontinuities in intensity that can be extracted more stably from medical volume [11]. The discontinuities in intensity, called surfaces, are then used to register to the surfaces of the previously constructed organ model.

The conventional way for obtaining registration parameters firstly assumes that desirable initial parameters can be obtained manually or according to some prior knowledge, and then these initial parameters are optimized by algorithms such as Gauss-Newton. However, in most real applications, it is difficult to obtain desirable initial parameters, and this leads to local minimums. To solve this local minimum problem, Genetic algorithm (GA) [12] was proposed. However, unfortunately it cannot guarantee reaching the global minimum.

We propose to use the exhaustive search, which is the only way to solve the problem of initial states. It has been considered to be impractical for high-dimensional parameter space. However, recently the computational power of computers has been exponentially increased, and promises the potential for the exhaustive search in high-dimensional parameter space.

In order to reduce the seemingly wasteful matching computations, we do the following three things: (1) a uniform sampling over 3D rotation group [13, 14] is explored; (2) Pyramidal search for all parameters is applied; (3) the distance function is constructed in advance to efficiently find the closest points.

This paper is organized as the following. We define the problem in a more formal way in Sect. 2, and describe how to solve this problem in Sect. 3. In Sect. 4, we describe preliminary experimental results of the proposed framework. Section 5 concludes the paper.

2 Problem Definition and General Framework

2.1 Unknown Parameters and Objective Function

What we want to do is, (1) to localize the organs in medical volume data, (2) to determine the position and orientation of the organs, and (3) to determine the deformed shape of the organs, all simultaneously.

Firstly, the model of an organ is defined as a set of model points, denoted by $\mathbf{X}_i (i = 1, \ldots, N)$. The model is deformable, and the deformed model is represented in the form of linear combination by

$$\mathbf{X}_i = s\left(\overline{\mathbf{X}}_i + \sum_{k=1}^{K} b_k \mathbf{v}_{ik}\right) \quad (1)$$

where s is the coefficient for scaling, $\overline{\mathbf{X}}_i$ is the coordinates of the ith point in the base shape, b_k is the coefficient for the kth principal deformation, $\mathbf{v}_{ik}$ represents the deformation for the i th point in the kth principal deformation. The base shape and the principal deformation are obtained by principal component analysis given a set of aligned organ models.

Secondly, the orientation and position are represented by $\mathbf{R} \in \mathrm{SO}_3, \mathbf{t} \in \mathrm{R}^3$, respectively. By $\mathbf{R}$ and $\mathbf{t}$, the model can be aligned to the input volume data by

$$\mathbf{R}\mathbf{X}_i + \mathbf{t} \quad (2)$$

Lastly, we need to evaluate the fitness between the input volume data and the unknown parameters $\mathbf{R}$, $\mathbf{t}$, s, $b_k (k = 1, \ldots, K)$. This fitness is defined here by the sum of the squared Euclidean distances between each model point and its closest surface point in the volume data, represented by

$$C = \sum_{i=1}^{N} \left\| \mathbf{Y}_i - \left(s\mathbf{R}\left(\bar{\mathbf{X}}_i + \sum_{k=1}^{K} b_k \mathbf{v}_{ik} \right) + \mathbf{t} \right) \right\|^2 \quad (3)$$

where $\mathbf{Y}_i$, in the surface point set extracted by Canny detector from the input volume data, is the closest extracted surface point to the ith surface point $\bar{\mathbf{X}}_i$ in the model.

By minimizing C, we can determine the unknown parameters $\mathbf{R}, \mathbf{t}, s, b_k$ $(k=1, \ldots, K)$, simultaneously. This means that the conventional segmentation, registration and deformation, which are treated separately in medical volume analysis and understanding, can now be done simultaneously in a single framework.

2.2 *Initial State Problem and Exhaustive Search*

However, optimization such as the least-squares minimization always has the problem of initial states. Since the optimization algorithms always converge monotonically to a local minimum from any given initial parameters of model data points, the desired global minimum cannot be guaranteed. Assuming a good initial guess, the distance metric in Eq. (3) can then be minimized, which means that the target points can be correctly localized and aligned well with the model points. In order to obtain a good initial state and to reach the desired global minimum with certainty, it is important to partition the registration state space into regions of sufficient resolution and optimize the objective function in Eq. (3) by selecting initial state in all regions for achieving global minimization point. The partition of the registration state space is equivalent to sampling all parameters to be searched such as rotation, translation, scaling and deformation parameters. The only certain solution to reaching the global minimum is the exhaustive search of the space of all parameters, which leads to a very high computational cost.

3 Algorithms to Reduce Computation

The disadvantage of the exhaustive search is that, in real applications, the number of parameter candidates for the solution becomes prohibitively large and it takes much computational cost. In our case, there are 3 parameters in rotation $\mathbf{R} \in SO_3$, 3 parameters in translation $\mathbf{t} \in R^3$, a scaling parameter s, and K deformation parameters. Assuming that each parameter is divided into 100 cells, the number of candidates to be searched is 100^{7+K}. This number is prohibitively large, and thus smart algorithms are required to reduce the search space and reduce computation. In this section, we present 3 such algorithms.

3.1 Distance Function(DF)

In order to evaluate the distance metric between the target point set and the model point set, it is necessary to know the correspondence between the target point set and model point set. However, it takes long to determine which point is the nearest neighbor. Assuming that both the target point set and model point set each have N points, the computation is in the order of N^2.

To solve the problem, we propose to use the distance function. A distance function is a three-dimensional lookup table, in which each voxel stores the index of its nearest neighbor point in the point set on a given volume, together with the Euclidean distance from that voxel to its nearest neighbor point. The distance function is created in advance, and its computational cost is in the order of N. Once the distance function is created, searching the corresponding points and evaluating the distances is straightforward (see Fig. 1).

When performing the exhaustive search, we do non minimum suppression, that is, those parameter candidates that do not have locally minimal SSD are deleted, and only those parameter candidates that have locally minimal SSD are retained for finer search in the next step.

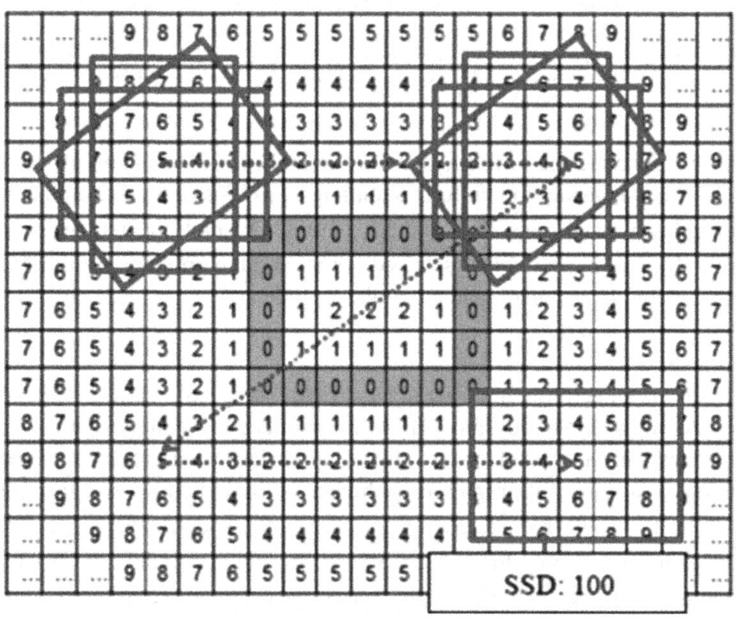

Fig. 1 The exhaustive search using distance function. This figure two-dimensionally illustrates the exhaustive search over the space of distance function. By constructing the distance function, we can efficiently access the measure metric of difference between the model and target surfaces extracted from the input volume data. When performing the exhaustive search, we evaluate the SSD for each parameter candidate

3.2 Uniform Sampling Over 3D Rotation Group

The exhaustive search requires the samples of searching parameters. In order to search these parameters efficiently, uniform sampling over all searching parameters is required. However, uniform sampling over 3D rotation group is very difficult because the three parameters of 3D rotation are not able to be partitioned by the ordinary uniform sampling, such as 3D translation.

In this paper, we generate uniform incremental grids over 3D rotation group using Hopf Fibration [13], an approach to the uniform sampling over 3D rotation group. In this approach, the 3D rotations are represented by Hopf coordinates. Hopf coordinates are unique for both the 3D rotation group and 3-sphere, $\mathbf{S}^3$. They naturally describe the intrinsic structure of both spaces and provide a natural tool for obtaining uniform distributions on these spaces. Hopf Fibration describes 3D rotation group in terms of the circle $\mathbf{S}^1$ and the ordinary 2-sphere $\mathbf{S}^2$. 3D rotation group is composed of non-intersecting fibers, such that each fiber is a circle $\mathbf{S}^1$ corresponding to a point on the 2-sphere $\mathbf{S}^2$. This fiber bundle structure is denoted as 3D rotation group , $SO_3 \cong \mathbf{S}^2 \otimes \mathbf{S}^1$. Each rotation in Hopf coordinates can be written as (θ, Φ, Ψ), in which $\Psi \in [0, 2\pi)$ parameterizes the circle $\mathbf{S}^1$, and $\theta \in [0, \pi]$ and $\Phi \in [0, 2\pi)$ represent spherical coordinates on $\mathbf{S}^2$. The transformation to a quaternion $\mathbf{q} = (x_1, x_2, x_3, x_4)$ can be expressed using the following formula:

$$\mathbf{q} = \left(\cos\frac{\theta}{2}\cos\frac{\Psi}{2},\ \cos\frac{\theta}{2}\sin\frac{\Psi}{2},\ \sin\frac{\theta}{2}\cos\left(\Phi + \frac{\Psi}{2}\right),\ \sin\frac{\theta}{2}\sin\left(\Phi + \frac{\Psi}{2}\right)\right) \tag{4}$$

Next, we generate the uniform sampling points over 3D rotation group. In the paper [13], they consider the uniform sampling of 3D rotation as a combination of the two uniform samplings in $\mathbf{S}^1$and $\mathbf{S}^2$. In order to partition the two rotations uniformly, HEALPix grid [14] is selected for $\mathbf{S}^2$, and the ordinary grid for $\mathbf{S}^1$. If $\mathbf{S}^2$ is partitioned by the ordinary grid along the latitude and longitude, it leads to large density differences of the grids on $\mathbf{S}^2$, and thus results in over sampling on and near the two poles.

HEALPix is an acronym for Hierarchical Equal Area isoLatitude Pixelization of a sphere. As suggested in the name, HEALPix produces a subdivision of a spherical surface in which each pixel covers the equal surface area. Figure 2 shows the partitioning of a sphere at progressively higher resolutions, from left to right.

Let Ψ be the angle parameterizing the circle, $\mathbf{S}^1$, and (θ, Φ) be the spherical coordinates parameterizing the sphere, $\mathbf{S}^2$. Let m_1 and m_2 be the numbers of sampling points at the base resolution of $\mathbf{S}^1$, and $\mathbf{S}^2$, respectively. Considering the space $\mathbf{S}^2 \otimes \mathbf{S}^1$, the multi- resolution grid sequence for 3D rotation group has $m_1 \cdot m_2 \cdot 2^{3l}$ points at the resolution of level $l (l \geq 0)$, in which every 2^3 points falling into a single grid cell comprise a cube in Hopf coordinates. Each element of the sequence is

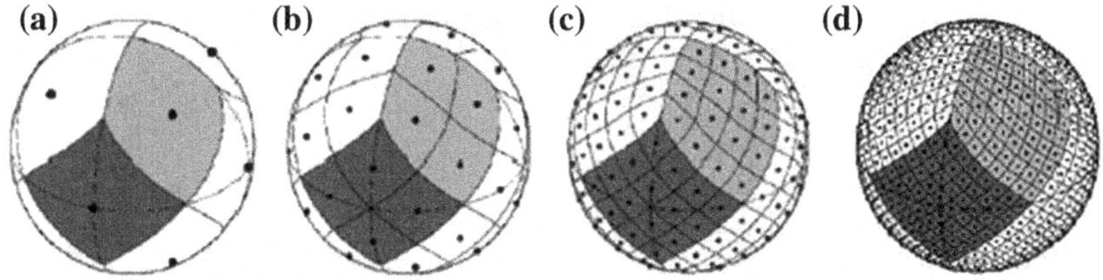

Fig. 2 HEALPix Multi-Resolution Grids: resolution of partitioning increases from (**a**) to (**d**). **a** Resolution Level 0: The base grid of the 2-sphere has 12 points. **b** Resolution Level 1: The 2-sphere has 48 points. **c** Resolution Level 2: The 2-sphere has 192 points. **d** Resolution Level 3: The 2-sphere has 768 points

obtained by combining the corresponding coordinates in the subspace, $\mathbf{S}^1$ and $\mathbf{S}^2$, using Eq. (4).

One of the issues raised by combining the two grids from $\mathbf{S}^1$and $\mathbf{S}^2$ is the length of a grid cell edge along each of the coordinates. In order to solve this problem, we have to match the number of cells in each base grid on both of the subspaces, so that they have cell sides of equal lengths. That is, the following equation should hold for natural numbers m_1 and m_2:

$$\frac{\mu(\mathbf{S}^1)}{m_1} \approx \sqrt{\frac{\mu(\mathbf{S}^2)}{m_2}}, \tag{5}$$

in which $\mu(\mathbf{S}^1)$ is the arc length of the circle $\mathbf{S}^1$ and $\mu(\mathbf{S}^2)$ is the surface area of $\mathbf{S}^2$. According to the paper [13], both $\mu(\mathbf{S}^1)$ and $\mu(\mathbf{S}^2)$ values are equal to π.

In our particular case, the base HEALPix grid consists of $m_2 = 12$ cells (see Fig. 2a). Therefore, the number of points in the base resolution of the grid on $\mathbf{S}^1$ is $m_1 = 6$. The base grid of the sequence for 3D rotation group then consists of $m_1 \cdot m_2 = 6 \cdot 12 = 72$ points.

In the ordinary partitioning case, when $\mathbf{S}^1$ is divided into 6 points, $\mathbf{S}^2$ is divided into 18 points (3 points along the latitude and 6 points along the longitude). The number of sampling points of HEALPix is roughly 2/3 = 12/18 of that in the ordinary partitioning on $\mathbf{S}^2$ (see Fig. 3).

3.3 Pyramidal Search

In order to reduce the parameter candidates to be searched when performing the exhaustive search, we create the pyramidal structure for all parameters and the volume data to be searched (see Fig. 4). By creating the pyramidal structure, we can implement the coarse-to-fine search of the parameters, such as rotation, translation, scaling and deformation, and then greatly fasten the exhaustive search.

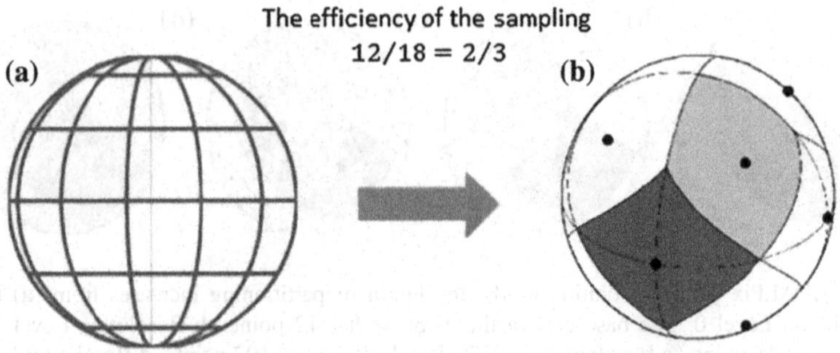

Fig. 3 The efficiency of sampling on $\mathbf{S}^2$. **a** The ordinary partitioning on $\mathbf{S}^2$ by the latitude and longitude divisions. The latitude and longitude are at 60 degree interval and thus it generates about 18 sampling points on $\mathbf{S}^2$. **b** The partitioning of HEALPix. Under the same condition as (**a**), it generates 12 sampling points on $\mathbf{S}^2$. The ratio of the samplings is about 12/18 = 2/3

4 Experimental Results

We ran our system on a standard desktop PC running 64-bit Windows 7 with an Intel Xeon 3.50 GHz CPU and 16 GHz RAM. Our proposed algorithm was implemented in C ++. The CT volume we used is from Osaka University (a resolution of $0.683 \times 0.683 \times 1\text{mm}^3$ with size of $512 \times 512 \times 159$) (see Fig. 5a). The model data of Liver was originally segmented manually by experienced experts or researchers (see Fig. 5d), and the original CT volume is used as the input target data. We visualize the CT volume and the experimental results using the 3DSlicer [15].

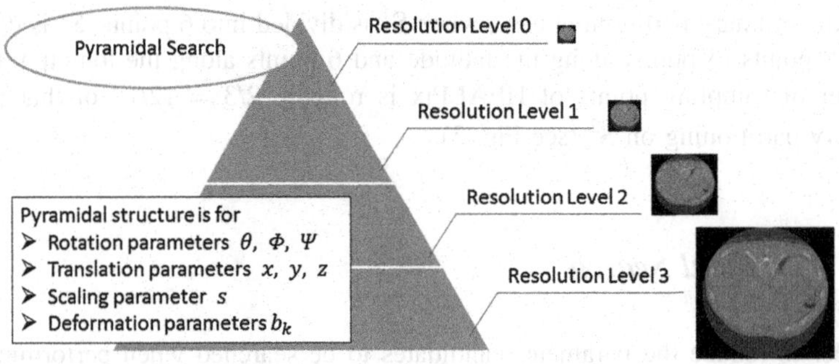

Fig. 4 Pyramidal structure. Pyramidal structure is created for all parameters, such as rotation, θ, Φ, Ψ, translation, x, y, z, scaling s and deformations b_k. We create a pyramidal structure of four stages for the input volume data to be searched. In the figure, the resolution of volume data is progressively higher resolutions, from level 0 to 4

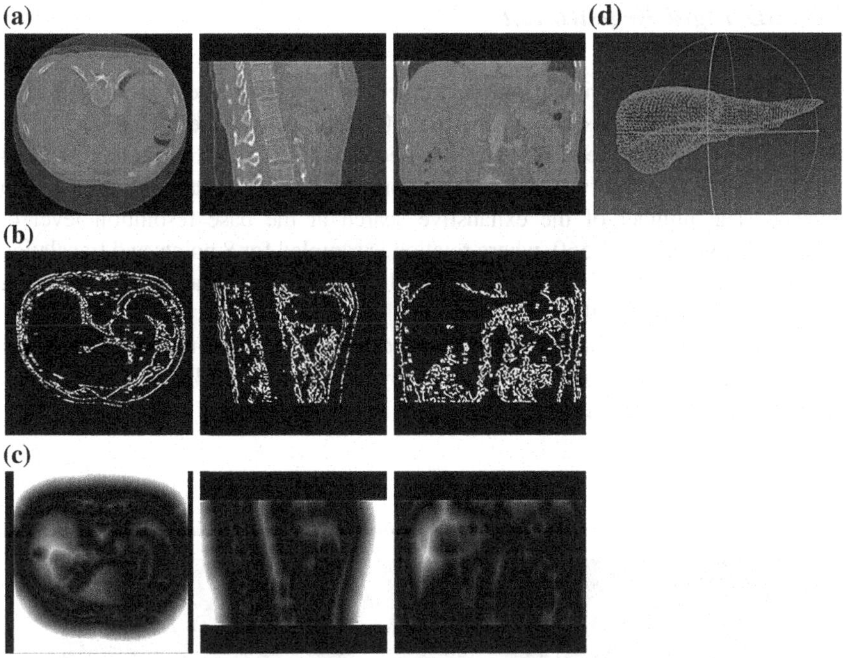

Fig. 5 Surface extraction from the segmented liver model. **a** shows the volume data, **b** shows the surfaces extracted by the 3D Canny surface detector, with the original intensities, and **c** shows the distance function created from the surfaces in the Fig. 5(**b**). **d** shows the model data of Liver, which consists of 1,000 points

4.1 Preprocessing

As a preprocessing step before the exhaustive search and registration, we extract the surfaces from the volume data, using Canny surface detector [11]. The basic formula in the 3D Canny surface detection is

$$\nabla[G(x,y,z)*V(x,y,z)], \tag{13}$$

where $V(x,y,z)$ is the intensity value at the voxel coordinate (x,y,z), $G(x,y,z)$ is a 3D Gaussian function and ∇ is the partial derivatives in x, y and z directions. Figure 5b shows the surfaces extracted from the original volume data.

Next, we create the distance function from the surfaces. Figure 5c shows the distance function created from the surfaces in the Fig. 5b.

4.2 3D Rigid Registration

As the preliminary experiment, we performed the exhaustive search of the 6 rigid transformation parameters only, using the 1,000 points of model (see Fig. 5d) and the input volume data (see Fig. 5a). The used model is fixed (rigid model without any deformation) which was segmented from the volume data to be searched in advance. The number of the exhaustive search at the base resolution level of pyramidal structure is 11,560, where rotation is sampled for 8 points and translation is sampled for $17 \times 17 \times 5$ points per 4 voxels. This means that we search $11,560 \times 64^3$ points at the finest resolution level.

The parameters obtained after exhaustive search serve as the initial state for optimization. After minimization of Eq. (3) by the Levenberg-Marquardt algorithm, we obtained the correct matching as shown in Fig. 6 (Tables 1 and 2).

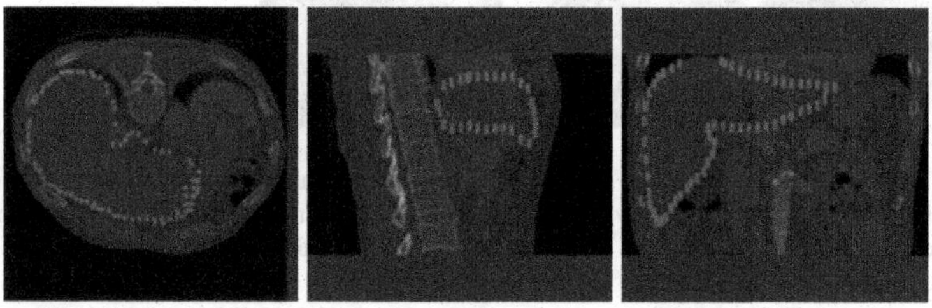

Fig. 6 The experimental result after optimization. The *red* points are the model of Liver. Optimization uses the registration result by the exhaustive search as the initial state

Table 1 The distance measure of the corresponding points with/without optimization

RMS Error between corresponding points [voxel]	
Before optimization	4.56
After optimization	0.97

Table 2 The computation time in each step

The computation time [s]	
Generating pyramidal data	0.11
Edge detection	0.73
Generating distance function	0.95
Exhaustive search	4.00
Optimization	0.96
Sum of the time of all steps	6.75

5 Conclusions and Future Work

In this paper, we proposed a novel framework of automatic organ localization by the exhaustive search of the previously constructed organ model in the input volume data. The exhaustive search in the whole parameter space ensures finding a good initial state required by most optimization algorithms. In order to search the 3D rotation parameters more efficiently, we applied "Generating Uniform Incremental Grids on SO(3) Using Hopf Fibration [13] " for uniform sampling over 3D rotation group, and combined the pyramidal search for sampling translation, scaling and deformation parameter spaces to reduce computational cost. Preliminary experiments show that localization of a rigid organ model can be achieved robustly and fully automatically.

We are currently extending the search from the 6 parameters of the rigid transformation to more parameters including scaling and deformation as well. We are also currently implementing parallel processing with GPU and exploring more efficient algorithms for sampling parameter spaces to reduce computational cost.

References

1. Adams, R., Bischof, L.: Seeded region growing. IEEE Trans. on Pattern Anal. Mach. Intell. **16** (6), 641–647 (1994)
2. Chen, Y.W., Tsubokawa, K., Foruzan, A.H.: Liver Segmentation from Low Contrast Open MR Scans Using K-Means Clustering and Graph-Cuts, Lecture Notes in Computer Science LNCS6064, pp.162–169. Springer, Berlin (2010)
3. Chen, Y.-T., Tseng, D.-C.: Medical Image Segmentation Based on the Bayesian Level Set Method, Medical Imaging and Informatics. Lecture Notes in Computer Science, vol. 4987, pp. 24–34 (2008)
4. Foruzan, A.H., Chen, Y.W., et al.: Segmentation of liver in low-contrast images using K-means clustering and geodesic active contour algorithms. IEICE Trans. **E96-D**, 798–807 (2013)
5. Boykov, Y.: Graph cuts and efficient N-D image segmentation. Int. J. Comput. Vision **70**(2), 109–131 (2006)
6. Rikxoort, van Y.A.E., Ginneken, van B.: Automatic segmentation of the liver in computed tomography scans with voxel classification and atlas matching. In: MICCAI Workshop 3-D Segmentat. Clínic: A Grand Challenge, pp. 101–108 (2007)
7. Park, H., Bland, P.H., Meyer, C.R.: Construction of an abdominal probabilistic atlas and its application in segmentation. IEEE Trans. Med. Imaging **22**, 483–492 (2003)
8. Zhou, X., Kitagawa, T., Hara, T., Fujita, H., Zhang, X., Yokoyama, R., et al.: Constructing a probabilistic model for automated liver region segmentation using non-contrast X-Ray torso CT images. In: IEEE International Conference on International Conference for Medical Image Computing and Computer-Assisted Intervention, MICCAI 2006, pp. 856–863 (2006)
9. Linguraru, M.G., Sandberg, J.K., Li, Z., Shah, F., Summers, R.M.: Automated segmentation and quantification of liver and spleen from CT images using normalized probabilistic atlases and enhancement estimation. Int. J. Med. Phys. **37**(2), 771–783 (2010)
10. Li, C.Y., Wang, X.Y., Eberl, S., Fulham, M., Yin, Y., Feng, D.G.: Fully automated liver segmentation for low—and high-contrast ct volumes based on probabilistic atlases In: IEEE International Conference on Image Processing, ICIP 2010, pp. 1522–1736 (2010)

11. Canny, J.: A computational approach to edge detection. IEEE Trans. Pattern Anal. Mach. Intell. **8**, 679–714 (1986)
12. Ziarati, A.: A multilevel evolutionary algorithm for optimizing numerical functions. IJIEC **2**, 419–430 (2010)
13. Yershova, A., Jain, S., LaValle, S.M., Julie C. Mitchell: Generating uniform incremental grids on SO(3) using Hopf fibration, In Int. J. Robot. Res. IJRR (2009)
14. Górski, K.M., Hivon, E., Banday, A. J., Wandelt, B. D., Hansen, F. K., Reinecke,M, Bartelmann,M. : HEALPix: a framework for high-resolution discretization and fast analysis of data distributed on the sphere. arXiv: astro-ph/0409513, **622**, 759–771 (2005)
15. 3DSlicer.: http://www.slicer.org/

Part V
Simulation and Visualisation/ VR for Medicine

GPU Acceleration of Monte Carlo Simulation at the Cellular and DNA Levels

Shogo Okada, Koichi Murakami, Katsuya Amako, Takashi Sasaki, Sébastien Incerti, Mathieu Karamitros, Nick Henderson, Margot Gerritsen, Makoto Asai and Andrea Dotti

Abstract Geant4-DNA is an extension of the general purpose Geant4 Monte Carlo simulation toolkit. It can simulate particle-matter physical interactions down to very low energies in liquid water. The simulation in that energy scale needs enormous computing time since it simulates all physical interactions following a discrete approach. This work presents the implementation of the physics processes/models of the Geant4-DNA extension in GPU architecture. We observed impressive performance gain with the same physics accuracy as existing methods.

1 Introduction

Simulating biological damage of ionizing radiation is a challenge of today's radiobiology research. A number of worldwide activities to develop simulation software are currently ongoing [1]. The application domain of such software covers

S. Okada (✉) · K. Murakami · K. Amako · T. Sasaki
High Energy Accelerator Research Organization, KEK, 1-1 Oho,
Tsukuba, Ibaraki 305-0801, Japan
e-mail: shogo@post.kek.jp

K. Murakami
e-mail: koichi.murakami@kek.jp

K. Amako
e-mail: katsuya.amako@kek.jp

T. Sasaki
e-mail: takashi.sakaki@kek.jp

S. Incerti · M. Karamitros
Centre D'Etudes Nucléaires de Bordeaux Gradignan, Université de Bordeaux,
CNRS/IN2P3, 33175 Cenbg, Gradignan, France
e-mail: incerti@cenbg.in2p3.fr

M. Karamitros
e-mail: matkara@gmail.com

Y.-W. Chen et al. (eds.), *Innovation in Medicine and Healthcare 2015*,
Smart Innovation, Systems and Technologies 45,
DOI 10.1007/978-3-319-23024-5_29

a wide range of effective dose. For example, chronic exposure to radiation during medical diagnosis or during frequent and long-duration flights correspond to doses under 100 mSv, while the estimation of deleterious effects for very high doses (>10 Sv) is required for long stays aboard the International Space Station and future manned missions to the Mars planet.

A possible simulation method is the Monte Carlo approach that computes all physical, chemical and biological interactions taking place when ionizing radiation penetrates into the biological medium [2]. Among the recently developed software codes, the Geant4-DNA extension [3] of the Geant4 general-purpose simulation toolkit [4, 5] provides a variety of physics, physico-chemistry, and chemistry processes and models. It can simulate particle-matter interactions in liquid water and the chemistry initiated by water radiolysis up to one microsecond after irradiation. The Geant4-DNA physics processes and models are described in detail in the work of Incerti et al. [6] and Francis et al. [7], and the new physico-chemistry and chemistry processes and models are described in the work of Karamitros et al. [8]. The physics processes in the Geant4-DNA cover dominant interactions of electrons, protons and neutral hydrogen atoms, alpha particles and their charged states and a few ions (Li, Be, B, C, N, O, Si, Fe). These interactions include: elastic scattering, electronic excitation, ionization, vibrational excitation, and dissociative attachment for electrons; electronic excitation, ionization, and charge transfer for protons, hydrogen, and alpha particles including their charged states; ionization for ions with $Z > 2$. An example of verification of the physics accuracy of Geant4-DNA is presented in Ref. [9].

All the processes are simulated as discrete processes in Geant4-DNA. They are described as step-by-step interactions without using condensed history approximation. This approach gives sufficient spatial accuracy for the track structure at sub-micrometer scale, dimensions similar to DNA fragments. On the other hand, enormous computation time is needed for the simulation of all particles interactions especially for the transport of high LET (Linear Energy Transfer) particles in larger volumes. The availability of GPU (Graphics Process Units) brings a new and promising opportunity to drastically improve the performance of Geant4-DNA

N. Henderson · M. Gerritsen
Institute for Computational and Mathematical Engineering,
Stanford University, 475 via Ortega, Stanford, CA 94306, USA
e-mail: nwh@stanford.edu

M. Gerritsen
e-mail: margot.gerritsen@stanford.edu

M. Asai · A. Dotti
SLAC National Accelerator Laboratory, 2575 Sand Hill Road, Menlo Park,
CA 94025, USA
e-mail: asai@slac.stanford.edu

A. Dotti
e-mail: adotti@slac.stanford.edu

physics as further shown in this paper. The work described in this paper focuses exclusively on the physics processes of Geant4-DNA.

2 Material and Method

2.1 *GPU Acceleration of Standard EM Physics for Electron and Gamma*

G4CU is a GPU implementation of the core Geant4 algorithm [10, 11]. Its implementation was done based on the original Geant4 codes. Many cores in GPU devices allow the processing of many particles in parallel. Geant4 standard EM physics processes for electrons, positrons, and gamma particles are available in G4CU. The current application of interest is the simulation of the absorbed dose calculation for photon and electron radiotherapy.

G4CU relies on CUDA, a GPU programming environment developed by NVIDIA. CUDA is an extension of the C and C++ languages. The programming model is called SIMT (Single-Instruction, Multiple-Thread) and is implemented in CUDA kernels that are executed in parallel in sets of thread blocks. The best performance is achieved when all threads in a block are executing the same instruction on different pieces of data. If the code contains branches, some threads may have to stall until the branches converge and all threads are issued the same instruction. Minimizing code branches is an important point to get better performance. GPU memory layout and access patterns also have large implications for overall application performance. NVIDIA GPUs have a large bank of "global" memory and a set of caches that reside "on-chip". The hardware is able to bundle requests by contiguous threads to contiguous memory locations. In CUDA these are known as coalesced memory reads/writes and are a crucial component for high performance. So far, we achieved up to 250 times faster than single CPU (Intel Xeon E5-2643V2) for electron and gamma simulation using Tesla K20 GPU.

2.2 *Implementation of Geant4-DNA Processes in CUDA*

The Geant4-DNA physics models available in the Geant4 version 10.0 for electrons, protons, neutral hydrogen atoms, alpha particles and their charged states were implemented in CUDA, called G4CU-DNA, as an extension of physics processes of the G4CU framework. Along with the porting of Geant4-DNA physics models to CUDA, we reformatted all total cross section data tables. The original data tables of total cross section for Geant4-DNA have interpolation tables of shell total cross sections per molecular electronic shell as a function of incident energy with non-uniform bin widths. The standard lookup method uses bisection, which has a particularly bad computation pattern for GPUs. We reformatted these tables to have uniform bin intervals. This allows for efficient computation of bin index. As for data interpolation between data points, G4CU-DNA adopts the same approach as Geant4-DNA that is one-/two-dimensional linear or logarithmic interpolations.

2.3 Physics Verification of G4CU-DNA

We verified the CUDA implementation of Geant4-DNA physics processes prior to testing computational performance. All related physics models are turned on, and we checked the validity of the dose calculation. Electrons, protons and doubly charged heliums (He^{++}) with specific kinetic energy were shot into a voxelized water phantom. Figure 1 shows the comparisons of depth dose distributions in the center voxels (2 um for electron and 0.5 um for proton and He^{++}) for different initial particles. G4CU-DNA can reproduce the simulation of Geant4-DNA reasonably well.

2.4 Dose Accumulation

Each GPU thread has access to a shared array to store accumulated dose. The array length is equal to the total number of voxel cells. A race condition exists if multiple threads attempt to add dose to the same voxel at the same time. We use the CUDA function atomicAdd for dose accumulation. With atomicAdd, simultaneous requests to add dose to the same cell are serialized. Thus, excessive calls to atomicAdd could limit performance. In G4CU-DNA, the physics processes update a thread local temporary variable for dose storage. The transport process is responsible for atomically updating the shared array only when a particle moves between voxels. This technique minimizes the number of calls to atomicAdd and results in a factor 2 × speedup compared to using atomicAdd in each step.

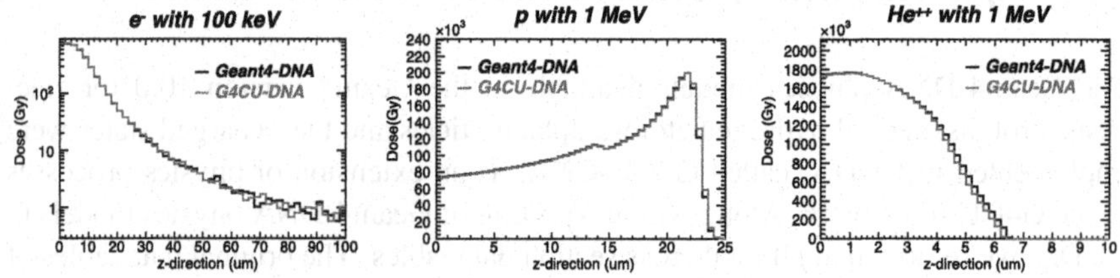

Fig. 1 Comparisons of Depth dose distributions between GPU and CPU

Table 1 Typical number of secondary particles generated from one primary particle and stack size allocated

Incident particle	Initial energy	# of secondary particles		Stack size per thread (memory size)
		Max.	Avg.	
e^-	100 keV	2,058	989	2,500 (0.11 MB)
p	1 MeV	17,784	17,064	21,000 (0.90 MB)
He^{++}	1 MeV	20,279	19,831	25,000 (1.1 MB)

2.5 Secondary Stack

Each CUDA thread in G4CU has a stack to store secondary particles generated in physical interactions (mainly ionization process). Each element in the stack has information about a secondary particle: position, kinetic energy, type of particle, etc. The memory size of a stack element is approximately 44 bytes. Table 1 shows typical number of secondary particles generated from a primary particle and stack size per thread needed. The large per-thread memory requirement limits the degree of parallelism at runtime. We will consider performance effects quantitatively in terms of thread occupancy in a following section.

3 Results

3.1 Thread Configurations

In CUDA, threads are organized into blocks. The number of threads per block ($N_{thd/blk}$) and the number of blocks (N_{blk}) are configurable parameters for each kernel launch. The total number of threads executed by a kernel is simply $N_{thd/blk}$ times $N_{thd/blk}$. The number of threads that can be executed concurrently in hardware depends on several parameters. The NVIDIA Tesla K20 GPU (Kepler architecture) has 13 streaming multiprocessors (SMX) with 192 CUDA cores each for a total of 2496 cores. In hardware, threads are executed in warps, which are groups of 32 threads. In the Kelper architecture, the maximum number of resident blocks per SMX is 16, resident warps is 64, and resident threads is 2048. It is best to maximize the number of resident warps so that the warp scheduler is able to keep the CUDA cores busy and hide instruction latency.

In G4CU-DNA, the maximum total number of running CUDA threads depends on the memory allocation of secondary stacks (see Table 1) in GPU global memory. NVIDA Tesla K20 GPU has the global memory of 5 GB. We can run 32,768 CUDA threads for electrons with 100 keV incident energy while 4,096 CUDA threads for protons and He^{++} with 1 MeV incident energy. The memory usage of the secondary stack is 3.4 GB for electrons with 100 keV, 3.6 GB for protons with 1 MeV, and 4.3 GB for He^{++} with 1 MeV, respectively. The CUDA thread

Table 2 Processing time among thread configurations for 100 keV electron. The unitis m sec/primary particle

	$N_{thd/blk}$				
N_{blk}	32	64	128	256	512
32	116.7	64.6	38.2	22.8	14.5
64	64.7	38.3	22.7	14.1	11.4
128	38.2	22.7	14.0	10.8	–
256	28.1	16.3	**10.5**	–	–
512	19.5	11.7	–	–	–

The unit is m sec/primary particle

configuration was optimized experimentally. For electrons with 100 keV, we tested 18 combinations of N_{blk} and $N_{thd/blk}$ with 32,768 CUDA threads. We measured simulation time for simulating 32,768 primary electrons and found the best pair giving the shortest processing time. Table 2 shows the processing time per electron for each configuration. The best CUDA thread configuration was determined to be $N_{block} = 256$ and $N_{thd/blk} = 128$.

For proton and He^{++} cases, we tested six configurations with 4,096 threads. 4,096 primary proton/He^{++} were simulated. The measured processing times per primary particle for each configuration are shown in Table 3. The best CUDA thread configuration is $N_{blk} = 64$, $N_{thd/blk} = 64$ for both cases. These configurations cannot use GPU hardware resources fully because large memory requirement of the secondary stack limits the number of running threads. We will improve the thread occupancy in future work.

3.2 Computational Performance

The comparison of computation time was made between Geant4-DNA (CPU) and G4CU-DNA (GPU). Geant4-DNA simulations ran in single-thread mode with Intel Xeon E5-2643V2 processor. The performance metric is the time for processing an incident particle. The GPU thread configuration used in performance measurement is 256 blocks with 128 threads per block for an electron, and 64 blocks with 64 threads per block for proton and He^{++}. Table 4 shows the computing performance in each case. G4CU-DNA achieves approximate 20–70 times speedup against Geant4-DNA simulation with single CPU core.

Table 3 Processing time comparisons among thread configurations for 1 MeV Proton (*left*) and 1 MeV He^{++} (*right*), respectively

Proton case				He^{++} case			
	$N_{thd/blk}$				$N_{thd/blk}$		
N_{blk}	32	64	128	N_{blocks}	32	64	128
32	2.216	1.139	0.619	32	2.403	1.241	0.665
64	1.141	**0.618**	–	64	1.243	**0.663**	–
128	0.619	–	–	128	0.666	–	–

Time unit is sec/primary particle

Table 4 Comparisons of computation time between GPU and CPU simulations

Incident particle	Initial energy	Geant4-DNA (CPU) (sec/particle)	G4CU-DNA (GPU) (sec/particle)	Speedup factor (=G4/G4CU)
e^-	100 keV	7.64×10^{-1}	1.05×10^{-2}	**72.9**
p	1 MeV	11.8	6.10×10^{-1}	**19.4**
He^{++}	1 MeV	12.3	6.63×10^{-1}	**18.6**

3.3 *Comparing GPU Performance Between Standard EM and DNA Physics*

Table 5 shows the comparison of GPU performance between the Standard EM physics for electrons with 20 MeV and DNA physics for different particle types. In the Standard EM physics, G4CU simulation with a typical thread configuration of 4,096 blocks with 128 threads per block (524,288 threads in total) achieves up to 250 times speedup against the CPU simulation. On the other hand, in DNA case for proton with 1 MeV using thread configuration of 64 blocks with 64 threads per block (4,096 threads in total), speed up factor is limited up to approximately 20. This large performance gap is due to the difference in number of active threads. As previously mentioned, active thread number in DNA process is limited by GPU memory usage storing secondary particles. For example, an electron with 20 MeV in Standard EM process generates less than 100 secondary particles because secondary particles are suppressed above a given production cut energy. On the other hand, a proton with 1 MeV in DNA process with no production threshold generates approximately 21,000 secondary particles. Most of the GPU threads are still vacant in the DNA simulation. We expect that performance of the DNA physics can be improved as comparable with the Standard EM physics if the low thread occupancy problem is fixed.

Table 5 Comparisons of speedup factors and thread occupancy for different simulations

	Incident particle	Initial energy	Stack size/thread	Total thread number ($N_{blk} \times N_{thd/blk}$)	Speedup factor
Standard EM process	e^-	20 MeV	100 (4.4 kB)	524,288 (4,096 × 128)	<250
DNA process	e^-	100 keV	2,500 (110 kB)	32,768 (256 × 128)	72.9
	p	1 MeV	21,000 (924 kB)	4,096 (64 × 64)	19.4
	He^{++}	1 MeV	25,000 (1100 kB)	4,096 (64 × 64)	18.6

3.4 Register Requirements of CUDA Kernels

The CUDA compiler allocates a certain number of registers for each CUDA kernel. Recall that a CUDA kernel is a function that is executed on the GPU in parallel in many threads. Registers are the memory storage locations with the fastest access time, followed by the on chip L1 and L2 caches, and then global memory (off-chip DRAM). NVIDIA Tesla K20 GPU has 65,536 registers per SMX. Each SMX can process 2,048 CUDA threads at the same time, thus 32 registers per thread is the maximum number to achieve 100 % thread occupancy. The situation where a CUDA kernel uses more than 32 registers causes the degradation of thread occupancy, because of the limit on number of registers. Therefore, the number of registers used in device functions is important information for performance profiling. CUDA provides a visual profiler (NVIDIA Visual Profiler) that displays various performance parameters including usage of registers, thread occupancy, etc. for each kernel (see Fig. 2). As an example, Table 6 shows the register requirement and thread occupancy for DNA simulation kernels. Most of the kernels for DNA models use more than 32 registers, so the thread occupancy is low. In future work, we plan to reduce the usage of registers by code refactoring and thus improve thread occupancy.

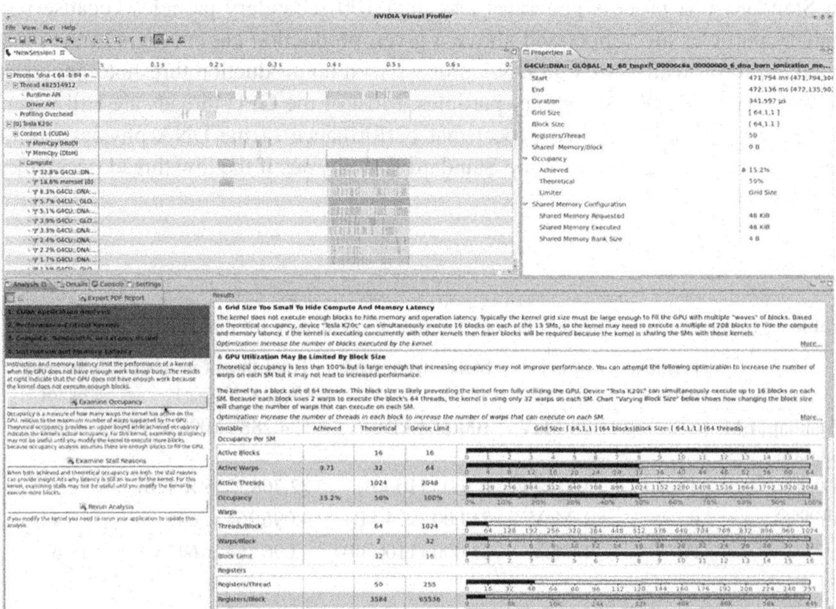

Fig. 2 NVIDIA Visual Profiler

Table 6 Usage of register memory and thread occupancy of device functions for several DNA models

Physics models in G4CU-DNA	# registers/thread	Thread occupancy (%)
Born excitation model	38	14.3
Rudd ionization extended model	71	2.5
Born ionization model	50	15.2
Dingfelder charge decrease model	42	15.1

4 Conclusion

We implemented the Geant4-DNA physics processes for electrons, protons, neutral hydrogen atoms, and helium atoms with charged states (He^0, He^+ and He^{++}) in the G4CU framework (A CUDA port of the core Geant4 simulation algorithm). G4CU-DNA gains a significant (20–70 times) speedup against CPU simulation with the same physics accuracy. We did some performance optimizations for the GPU code. However, there is still a large performance gap between Standard EM physics (G4CU) and DNA physics (G4CU-DNA) in the GPU speedup factors. This is because the number of active threads is limited by large GPU memory consumption of secondary stacks, and thread occupancy is not sufficient. In future work, we will improve the thread occupancy and expect that the GPU speedup factor of DNA physics will be comparable with the Standard EM physics. Further improvements on G4CU will enable scientific progress in various fields where quantitative simulation is necessary for the study of radiation effects at cellular and DNA levels.

Acknowledgments This work was supported by JSPS KAKENHI Grant 25246044, Japan-U.S. Cooperation in Research and Development in Science and Technology, and by the U.S. Department of Energy contract number DE-AC02-76SF00515. This work was partly supported by the Associated International Laboratory KEK (Japan)—CNRS (France)—CEA (France) "France-Japan Particle Physics Laboratory (FJPPL)". The authors would like to thank NVIDIA for their generous support of this project and the CUDA Center of Excellence at Stanford University.

References

1. Nikjoo, H., Uehara, S., Emfietzoglou, D., Cucinotta, F.A.: Track-structure codes in radiation research. Radiat. Meas. **41**, 1052–1074 (2006)
2. El Naqa, I., Pater, P., Seuntjens, J.: Monte Carlo role in radiobiological modelling of radiotherapy outcomes. Phys. Med. Biol. **57**, R75–R97 (2012)
3. "The Geant4-DNA project". http://geant4-dna.org (2014)
4. Agostinelli, S., Allison, J., Amako, K., Apostolakis, J., Araujo, H., Arce, P., et al.: Geant4—a simulation toolkit. Nucl. Instrum. Methods Phys. Res. A **506**, 250–303 (2003)
5. Allison, J., Amako, K., Apostolakis, J., Araujo, H., Dubois, P.Arce, Asai, M., et al.: Geant4 developments and applications. IEEE Trans. Nucl. Sci. **53**, 270–278 (2006)

6. Incerti, S., Ivanchenko, A., Karamitros, M., Mantero, A., Moretto, P., Tran, H.N., et al.: Comparison of GEANT4 very low energy cross section models with experimental data in water. Med. Phys. **37**, 4692–4708 (2010)
7. Francis, Z., Incerti, S., Capra, R., Mascialino, B., Montarou, G., Stepan, V., et al.: Molecular scale track structure simulations in liquid water using the Geant4-DNA Monte-Carlo processes. Appl. Radiat. Isot. **69**, 220–226 (2011)
8. Karamitros, M., Luan, S., Bernal, M.A., Allison, J., Baldacchino, G., Davídková, M., et al.: Diffusion-controlled reactions modeling in Geant4-DNA. J. Comput. Phys. **274**, 841–882 (2014)
9. Incerti, S., Psaltaki, M., Gillet, P., Barberet, P., Bardiès, M., Bernal, M.A., et al.: Simulating radial dose of ion tracks in liquid water simulated with Geant4-DNA: A comparative study. Nucl. Instrum. Methods Phys. Res. B **333**, 92–98 (2014)
10. Henderson, N., Murakami, K. et al.: A CUDA Monte Carlo simulator for radiation therapy dosimetry based on Geant4. In: SNA + MC 2013—joint international conference on supercomputing in nuclear applications + Monte Carlo. doi:http://dx.doi.org/10.1051/snamc/201404204 (2014)
11. Murakami, K., Henderson, N. et al.: Geant4 based simulation of radiation dosimetry in CUDA. In: Nuclear science symposium and medical imaging conference (NSS/MIC). doi:10.1109/NSSMIC.2013.6829452 (2013)

A Study on Corotated Nonlinear Deformation Model for Simulating Soft Tissue Under Large Deformation

Kazuyoshi Tagawa, Takahiro Yamada and Hiromi T. Tanaka

Abstract In surgery simulators, a computationally efficient and geometrically nonlinear deformation simulation approach is required for soft tissue simulation. Especially, in the case of presenting haptic sensation to users, computational cost becomes a large problem because a higher update rate is required in stable haptic feedback. In this paper, we propose an interactive nonlinear soft tissue simulation approach using an adaptive and corotated deformation model. In the approach, computation of nonlinearity consideration and deformation simulation are performed at different suitable resolution of tetrahedral adaptive mesh. We also propose the criterion for subdivision and simplification in the adaptive and corotated deformation simulation. In evaluation experiments, we implemented the proposed approach into our surgery simulator, and we confirmed the computation time, the accuracy of deformations and the stability of reaction forces. We believe that this approach is also useful for haptic interaction with other elastic materials (e.g. jelly and rubber) under large deformation.

Keywords Elastic objects · Deformation simulation · Geometric nonlinearity · Corotated deformation model · Tetrahedral adaptive mesh

K. Tagawa (✉) · T. Yamada · H.T. Tanaka
Ritsumeikan University, 1-1-1 Noji-higashi, Kusatsu, Shiga, Japan
e-mail: tagawa@cv.ci.ritsumei.ac.jp

T. Yamada
e-mail: tyamada@cv.ci.ritsumei.ac.jp

H.T. Tanaka
e-mail: hiromi@cv.ci.ritsumei.ac.jp

Y.-W. Chen et al. (eds.), *Innovation in Medicine and Healthcare 2015*,
Smart Innovation, Systems and Technologies 45,
DOI 10.1007/978-3-319-23024-5_30

1 Introduction

A fast soft tissue simulation is required of surgical simulators. In particular, in case presenting stable reaction force to users when grasping and touching organs, a higher update rate (about several hundred Hz) of the deformation simulation and the calculation of reaction force is required. In addition, in the surgery simulation, large object deformation that involves rotation often occurs [1]. Therefore, computationally efficient deformation simulation which can consider the geometric nonlinearity is required.

As a geometric nonlinear deformation model, there is Saint Venant Kirchhoff (StVK) Model [2]. Delingette [3] and Kikuuwe [4] have proposed efficient computation procedures for the StVK model by using the biquadratic and quadratic springs. However, it is difficult to reduce computation time due to discontinuous memory accesses in the computation.

Recently, in the field of computer graphics, corotated deformation models have been proposed [5]. In the corotated deformation model, the local coordinate system of each tetrahedral element is defined, and shape matching between the tetrahedral element at initial state and that at deformed state is performed. The component of rotational motion is then removed, and the deformation simulation using a linear finite element model is performed on the local coordinate system thus consideration of geometric nonlinearity becomes possible. However, there is a problem that a large amount of computation is required for this shape matching (extraction of the component of the rotational motion) [6].

As for the other acceleration approaches, (a) online re-mesh (multi-resolution model) [7, 8, 9] and (b) parallel computation [10] have been proposed. By applying these approaches to the corotated deformation model, further acceleration can be expected.

In this paper, a novel interactive nonlinear deformation simulation approach is proposed. In our approach, corotated deformation model and online re-mesh are used together. The elastic object is represented by a multi-resolution hierarchy of tetrahedral adaptive volume mesh. The tetrahedral adaptive volume mesh is locally refined by online re-mesh to concentrate the computational load into the regions that deform the most. To get a reduction in the number of times of shape matching, we used two different mesh resolutions. One is used for shape matching and the other is for linear finite element deformation simulation. Reduction of shape matching is realized by substituting the rotation of tetrahedra at deep depth for rotation of tetrahedra at shallow depth [11]. In addition, we propose the criterion for subdivision and simplification in the adaptive corotated deformation simulation.

In an evaluation experiment, we compare computation time, the accuracy of deformation and reaction force among (1) proposed approach, (2) linear finite element model (L-FEM), and (3) nonlinear finite element model in which StVK model is used (NL-FEM). Through these experiments, we show the effectiveness of our proposed approach.

2 Related Works

In this section, overviews of the online re-mesh deformation simulation and the corotated deformation model are stated.

2.1 Online Re-Mesh Using Tetrahedral Adaptive Mesh

In our past research, we proposed an online re-mesh approach [9] using tetrahedral adaptive mesh [12].

Our tetrahedral adaptive mesh is generated by the following procedure. Initially, the object model is enclosed with six root tetrahedral (Fig. 1). Then, as shown in Fig. 2, the root tetrahedra are recursively bisected by adding new nodes to the midpoints of the longest edges according to local features (e.g. non-uniformity of material properties, curvature of the isosurface). This subdivision process is repeated until the approximation accuracy of the whole model is satisfied.

The online re-mesh approach uses this tetrahedral adaptive multi-resolution mesh, and recursively refines (bisects) or simplifies each tetrahedron according to the rate of elongation σ of the longest edge of the tetrahedron.

The advantages of our online re-mesh approach using the tetrahedral adaptive mesh are as follows.

(1) Low computational cost: Computational complexity of this online re-mesh process is $O(\log n)$, where n is the division number of a side of an initial cube in Fig. 1. This is because of neighboring regions considered in the subdivision is limited.
(2) High quality mesh: In our approach, only three types (TYPE0, 1 and 2) of tetrahedra are used. The lower limit of aspect ratio of these tetrahedra is 0.64. The upper limit of the radius-shortest edge ratio of these tetrahedra is 1.11.

Fig. 1 Six root tetrahedra

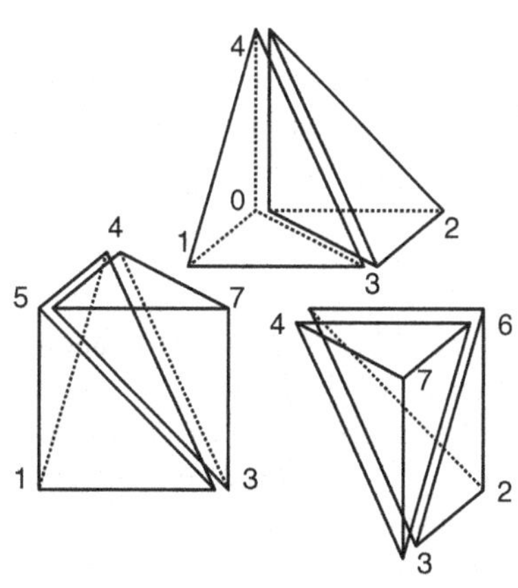

Fig. 2 Binary refinement and simplification

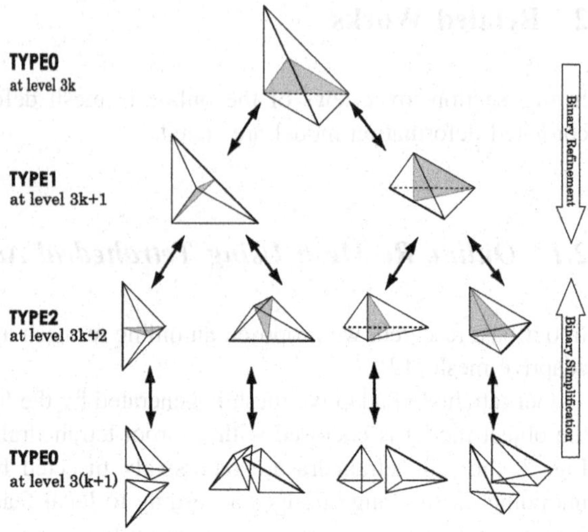

(3) Mesh isotropy: In our approach, mirror symmetric tetrahedra are recurrently generated, thus cancellation of affections of artifacts in the computation is possible.

2.2 Corotated Deformation Model

In the linear finite element model, the relationship between force vector $\mathbf{f}_T$ of four nodes of tetrahedron T and displacement vector $\mathbf{u}_T$ is described using the following equation,

$$\mathbf{K}_T\mathbf{u}_T = \mathbf{f}_T, \tag{1}$$

where $\mathbf{K}_T$ is an element stiffness matrix of tetrahedron T.

In contrast, in the corotated deformation model, the relationship between force vector $\mathbf{f}_T^c$ of four nodes of tetrahedron T and position vector $\mathbf{x}_T$ is described using the following equation,

$$\mathbf{R}_T\mathbf{K}_T\left(\mathbf{R}_T^{-1}\mathbf{x}_T - \mathbf{x}_T^0\right) = \mathbf{f}_T^c, \tag{2}$$

where $\mathbf{R}_T$ and $\mathbf{x}_T^0$ are the rotation matrix and the initial position vector of tetrahedron T, respectively.

In this model, large deformation which involves rotation (geometrical nonlinearity) can be considered, however, the computational cost of the extraction of $\mathbf{R}_T$ becomes a problem.

3 Adaptive and Corotated Deformation Model

In this section, approaches to reduce shape matching which is realized by substituting the rotation of tetrahedra at deep depth for rotation of tetrahedra at shallow depth are proposed.

3.1 *Reducing Shape Matching Computation Using Hierarchical Structure*

As stated in the previous section, the six root tetrahedra are recursively bisected and then the binary tree is constructed in the tetrahedral adaptive mesh generation. In this process, two child tetrahedra are generated from one parent tetrahedron and four grandchild tetrahedra are generated from one parent tetrahedron and so on. Therefore rotation matrices of these child or grandchild or descendant terahedra are nearly equal to that of their ancestor tetrahedra.

In this paper, we propose an approach to reduce the shape matching computation. This is realized by substituting the rotation matrices of descendant tetrahedra for rotation matrices of ancestor tetrahedra. In our previous online re-mesh approach, suitable resolutions of tetrahedra which can approximate when given accurate criterion are selected online and are used for the deformation simulation. In contrast, in this approach, as shown in Fig. 3, suitable resolutions of tetrahedra for the rotation extraction are separately selected online. If the difference of rotation between neighboring tetrahedra is large, in other words, the curvature of the object is large, high resolution tetrahedra should be used for rotation extraction. In other parts, low resolution tetrahedra should be used for rotation extraction and substitute the rotation matrices of descendant tetrahedra for rotation matrices of these selected tetrahedra. By using this approach, we can reduce the number of times of shape matching computation.

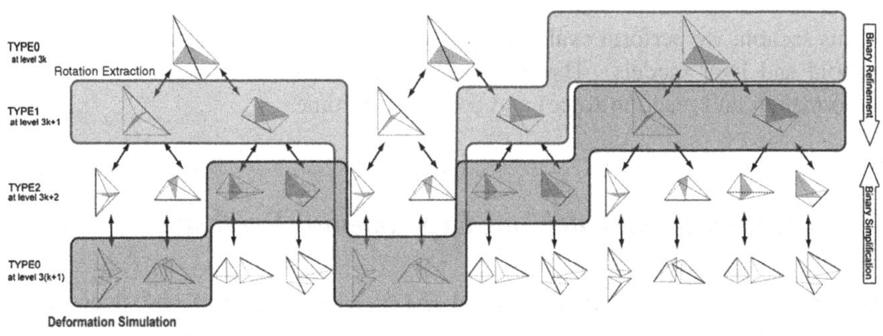

Fig. 3 Tetrahedra for rotation extraction and deformation simulation

3.2 Criterion for Subdivision and Simplification in the Adaptive Corotated Deformation Simulation

In this paper, we also propose a criterion for subdivision and simplification in the adaptive corotated deformation simulation. As an index of difference of rotation of neighboring tetrahedron, we propose the square of the Frobenius norm of difference of rotation matrices of neighboring tetrahedron. The relationship between the square of the Frobenius norm of difference matrix between rotation matrix $\mathbf{R}^{T_n}$ of tetrahedron T_n and rotation matrix $\mathbf{R}^{T_m}$ of neighboring tetrahedron T_m and difference of rotation θ between of tetrahedron T_n and neighboring tetrahedron T_m is described as follows.

$$\|\mathbf{R}^{T_m} - \mathbf{R}^{T_n}\|_F^2 = 4(1 - \cos\theta). \tag{3}$$

If rotation matrix $\mathbf{R}^{T_n}$ of tetrahedron T_n and rotation matrix $\mathbf{R}^{T_m}$ of whose neighboring tetrahedron T_m satisfy Eq. (4), these tetrahedra should be subdivided, where θ_{max} and F_{max} are subdivision threshold of the rotation matrix and the Frobenius norm, respectively. Otherwise, if they satisfy Eq. (5), these tetrahedra should be simplified, where θ_{min} and F_{min} are simplification threshold of the rotation matrix and the Frobenius norm, respectively.

$$\|\mathbf{R}^{T_m} - \mathbf{R}^{T_n}\|_F^2 >= 4(1 - \cos\theta_{max}) = F_{max} \tag{4}$$

$$\|\mathbf{R}^{T_m} - \mathbf{R}^{T_n}\|_F^2 <= 4(1 - \cos\theta_{min}) = F_{min} \tag{5}$$

Computation of the Frobenius norm is easy, thus fast computation of Eq. (4) and (5) is possible.

4 Evaluation Experiments

In this section, we perform evaluation experiments using two experimental models (cuboid and liver models). Through these experiments, we confirm the accuracy (deformation and reaction force) and computation time.

4.1 Experimental Model and Experimental Equipment

As experimental models, cuboid model (64 × 64 × 192 mm) and liver model were used. Figure 4 shows a cuboid model (all tetrahedra are TYPE0, subdivision

Fig. 4 Experimentl model (cuboid model)

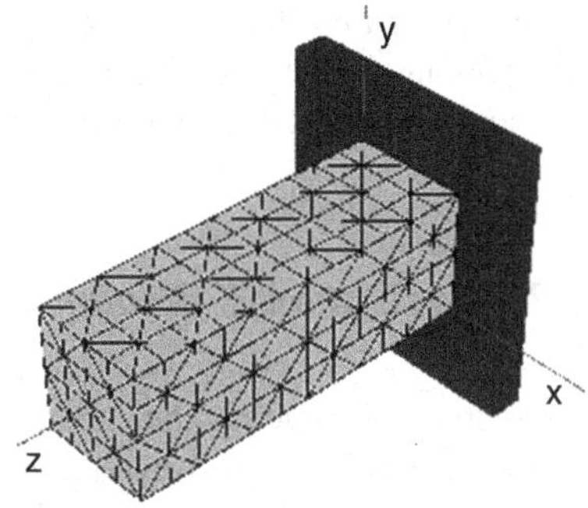

Fig. 5 Experimental equipment

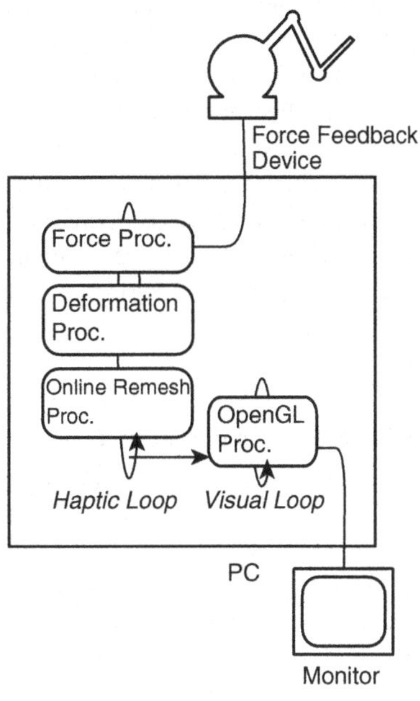

level was 6, the number of nodes was 325, the number of tetrahedra was 1152.) We used Young's modulus $E = 0.5$ [kPa], Poisson ratio $\nu = 0.49$, density $\rho = 10$ [Kg/m^3].

Figure 5 shows our experimental equipment. For whole computation, we used a PC (CPU: Intel Core i7-2760QM 2.4 GHz, Memory: 8 GB, OS: Scientific Linux 6.1). A haptic loop (which included processes of deformation simulation, online re-mesh and presentation of reaction force) run at 1 [kHz]. A visual loop run at 30 [Hz] asynchronously. Reaction force was presented by a force feedback device (Sensable PHANToM omni).

We compared the accuracy (deformation and reaction force) and computation time among (1) proposed approach, (2) linear finite element model (L-FEM), and (3) nonlinear finite element model in which StVK model was used (NL-FEM).

4.2 Evaluation 1 (Evaluation of Deformation)

Simulation of bending the cuboid (curvature of the cuboid model was almost constant) was performed by applying displacement boundary conditions to nodes on both ends of the cuboid model. We compared the deformation and computation time among (1) proposed approach, (2) linear finite element model (L-FEM), and (3) nonlinear finite element model in which StVK model was used (NL-FEM).

Table 1 shows maximum, minimum and average error of displacement of all nodes at different threshold F_{max} which were used for rotation extraction. Figure 6a shows simulation results of deformation, and the bold (red) wireframe shows that these terahedra were used for rotation extraction. We can find that the error in volume increment was observed in the result of L-FEM. In contrast, results by using the proposed approach was similar to NL-FEM. In the proposed approach, except in case $\theta_{max} = 25.8$ [deg], maximum of the average of error of displacement was 0.4 [mm].

Table 1 Errors of displacement [mm]

	L-FEM	Threshold θ_{max} [deg.]						
		25.8	8.1	4.1	2.6	1.8	0.9	0.1
Num. of tetrahedra	1151	18	48	300	578	696	908	1072
Average	26.180	1.107	0.367	0.064	0.032	0.020	0.019	0.007
Maximum	49.763	4.395	1.474	0.224	0.174	0.138	0.153	0.053
Minimum	3.206	0.08	0.02	0.009	0.002	0.002	0.001	0.0002

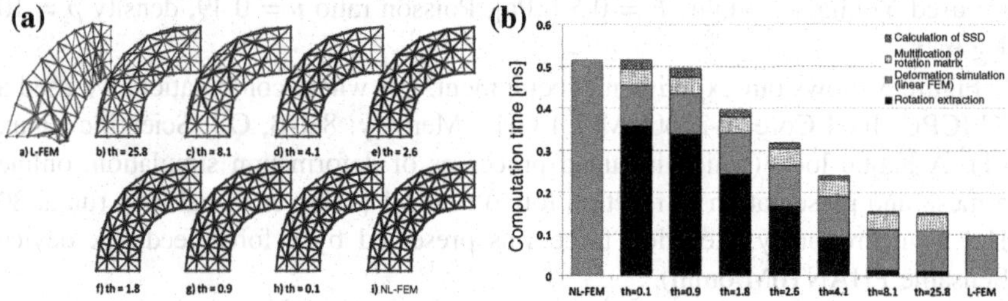

Fig. 6 Results (cuboid model was bended to almost constant curvature) **a** Deformation **b** Computation time [ms]

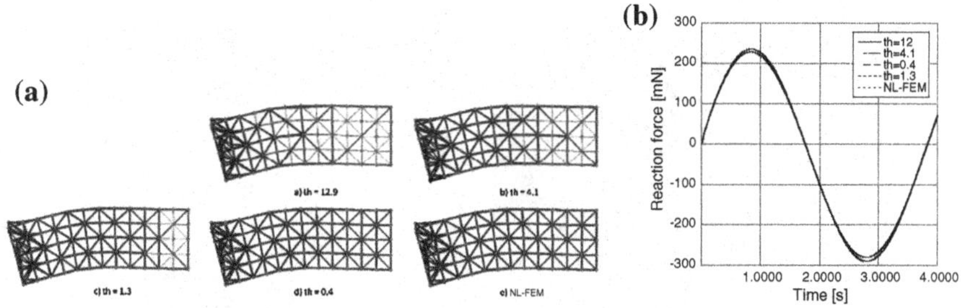

Fig. 7 Results (sinusoidal displacement boundary condition was applied to a node of the cuboid model) **a** Deformation **b** Reaction force

Figure 6b shows result of computation time. We can find that the computation time of rotation extraction was decreased in case that larger threshold θ_{max} was used. Computation time of each online re-mesh process was 0.015 [ms].

4.3 Evaluation 2 (Evaluation of Reaction Force)

We evaluated reaction force when the user was interacting with a deformable object (a cuboid model). The sinusoidal displacement boundary condition u was applied to a node of the cuboid model, as follows:

$$\mathrm{u} = \left(0.0, 50\sin 0.072k\frac{\pi}{180}, 0.0\right),$$

where k was a number of simulation cycle.

Figure 7a, b show result of deformation and intensity reaction force, respectively. We can find that the reaction force was very smooth, even if our approach was used.

4.4 Evaluation 3 (Surgery Simulation)

We are also developing an embedded deformation model in order to simulate inhomogeneous elastic objects like a liver with a vascular system [13]. It is possible to apply this proposed approach to the embedded deformation model.

Figure 8 shows results of linear FEM (L-FEM) and our proposed approach where a gallbladder was grasped and pulled. In both simulation, the embedded deformation model was also used. In L-FEM, volume increment of gallbladder was observed. In case of proposed approach, the users did not feel any unpleasant reaction force.

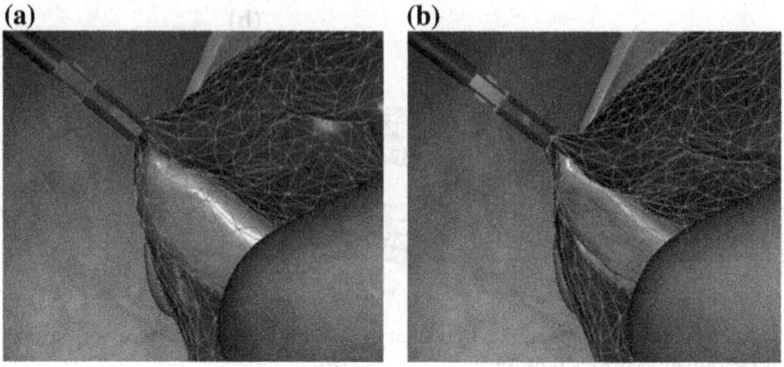

Fig. 8 Results of surgery simulation **a** L-FEM **b** Proposed approach

5 Conclusions

In this paper, we proposed a novel interactive nonlinear deformation simulation approach for surgery simulation. In our approach, corotated deformation model and online re-mesh are used in combination. To get a reduction in the number of times of shape matching, we used two different mesh resolutions. In addition, we proposed the criterion for subdivision and simplification in the adaptive corotated deformation simulation.

In current implementation, the tensor mass model approach [14] was used in the deformation simulation. This means that the forward difference method was used as a solver and the computational cost per one simulation cycle becomes low, however, a higher update rate is required to maintain stable simulation. In the future, we will apply proposed approach to another solver which uses backward difference method. Also, we are planning to investigate a GPU implementation of the proposed approach.

References

1. Fung, Y.C.: Foundations of Solid Mechanics. Prentice-Hall, Upper Saddle River (1965)
2. Fung, Y.C.: Biomechanics: Mechanical properties of living tissues. Springer, Berlin (1993)
3. Delingette, H.: Biquadratic and quadratic springs for modeling St Venant Kirchhoff materials. In: Proceeding of ISBMS, pp. 40–48, 2008
4. Kikuuwe, R., Tabuchi, H., Yamamoto, M.: An edge-based computationally efficient formulation of Saint Venant-Kirchhoff tetrahedral finite elements. ACM Trans. Graph. **28**, 1–13 (2009)
5. Muller, M., Dorsey, J., McMillan, L., Jagnow, R., Cutler, B.: Stable real-time deformations. In: Proceeding of ACM SCA, pp. 49–54 (2002)
6. McAdams, A., Zhu, Y., Selle, A., Empey, M., Tamstorf, R., Teran, J., Sifakiss, E.: Efficient elasticity for character skinning with contact and collisions. ACM Trans. Graph. **30**, 1–37 (2011)

7. Paloc, C., Faraci, A., Bello, F.: Online remeshing for soft tissue simulation in surgical training. IEEE Comput. Graphics Appl. **26**, 24–34 (2006)
8. Debunne, G., Desbrun, M., Cani, M.-P., Barr, A. H.: Dynamic real-time deformations using space and time adaptive sampling. In: Proceeding of SIGGRAPH, pp. 31–36 (2001)
9. Tanaka, H. T., Tsujino, Y., Kamada, T., Viet, H. Q. H.: Bisection refinement-based real-time adaptive mesh model for deformation and cutting of soft objects. In: Proceeding of ICARCV, pp. 1–8 (2006)
10. Courtecuisse, H., Jung, H., Allard, J., Duriez, C.: GPU- based real-time soft tissue deformation with cutting and haptic feedback. J. Progress Biophys. Mol Biol. **103**, 159–168 (2010)
11. Tagawa, K., Xu, C., Prince, J., Yamada, T., Tanaka H. T.: A rectangular tetrahedral adaptive mesh based corotated deformation model for interactive soft tissue simulation. In: Proceeding of IEEE EMBC, pp. 7164–7167 (2013)
12. Tanaka, H. T., Takama, Y., Wakabayashi, H.: Accuracy-based sampling and reconstruction with adaptive grid for parallel hierarchical tetrahedrization. In: Proceeding of VG, pp. 79–86 (2003)
13. Tagawa, K., Oishi, T., Tanaka, H. T.: Adaptive and embedded Deformation Model: an approach to haptic interaction with complex inhomogeneous elastic objects. In: Proceeding of IEEE WHC, pp. 169–174 (2013)
14. Delingette, H., Cotin, S., Ayache, N.: A hybrid elastic model allowing real-time cutting, deformations and force-feedback for surgery training and simulation. In: Proceeding of Computer Animation, pp. 70–81 (1999)

Remote Transparent Visualization of Surface-Volume Fused Data to Support Network-Based Laparoscopic Surgery Simulation

Rui Xu, Asuka Sugiyama, Kyoko Hasegawa, Kazuyoshi Tagawa, Satoshi Tanaka and Hiromi T. Tanaka

Abstract To assist a network-based laparoscopic surgery simulation, we developed a remote and fused 3D transparent visualization method. Our method enables us to create precise 3D see-through images of internal human organs at multiple distant places simultaneously. Besides, the method supports flexible fused visualization of surface data and volume data. Traditional transparent visualization methods require the time-consuming depth sort of rendering primitives. Therefore, it has been difficult to execute quick and precise fused visualization, which must treat both polygon data for surfaces and voxel data for volumes at one time. Our fused visualization is realized by applying the stochastic point based rendering that we recently proposed. We applied this rendering technique to remote fused visualization of surgery simulation, combining the technique with network-based distributed computing of visualization.

Keywords Visualization · Fusion · Point-based rendering · Network-based surgery simulator

1 Introduction

Minimally invasive surgery has gradually been paid a lot of attention because of its remarkable benefit compared to the conventional cut-open surgery, especially for abdominal organs. In such a surgery, surgeons firstly drill several holes on the patient's belly, and then insert laparoscopic tools into the abdominal cavity through these holes in order to operate surgery on inner organs. Since the wound that is made by

R. Xu (✉) · K. Tagawa
Ritsumeikan Global Innovation Research Organization,
Ritsumeikan University, Nojihigashi 1-1-1, Kusatsu, Shiga 5258577, Japan
e-mail: xurui@fc.ritsumei.ac.jp

A. Sugiyama · K. Hasegawa · S. Tanaka · H.T. Tanaka
College of Information Science and Engineering,
Ritsumeikan University, Nojihigashi 1-1-1, Kusatsu, Shiga 5258577, Japan

Y.-W. Chen et al. (eds.), *Innovation in Medicine and Healthcare 2015*,
Smart Innovation, Systems and Technologies 45,
DOI 10.1007/978-3-319-23024-5_31

this surgery is much less than that of the cut-open surgery, the patients usually can recover in less time.

Although minimally invasive surgery has the benefit for the recovery of patients, its operation is very difficult for surgeons who have to use tiny operation tools in a limited laparoscopic view field. A surgeon needs a lot of training in order to master the required skills, however the training cannot be operated directly on patients. Therefore, a simulator that is able to simulate vivid process of laparoscopic surgery is very useful to train inexperienced surgeons. Such a simulator is traditionally constructed on a single server, and both of the trainee and trainer should be at the same place. This makes the training very limited. In order to break the spatial limit, a network-based simulator of minimally invasive surgery has been under research [1, 2]. Since the network communication techniques are utilized, where the trainee and trainer can be at separate places.

Remote visualization is required to assist the network-based laparoscopic surgery simulator. The results that are generated by the simulator have to be visualized at a remote place where the trainer is. The simulator simulates how a liver is deformed in the surgery. It calculates the 3D deformable fields and the deformed surfaces of the liver. The deformable fields are 3D volume data, and the deformed surfaces are surface data. In order to render them simultaneously at a remote place, remote and fused visualization method should be developed by utilizing the network communication and visualization techniques. The network communication technology is quite advanced, however fast transparent visualization to fuse volume and surface data in a remote way is not a trivial work.

The conventional transparent visualization method is based on a ray-casting model [3–5] that simulates the refraction of light that rays through transparent materials. It has to sort the spatial relationship of all visualized primitives that a light goes through. This requires a high computational cost, especially for irregular grid based data. The simulator utilized finite element method (FEM) to calculate the deformation of the liver, and the 3D deformable fields are represented by tetrahedrons, which are the irregular grid based data. In order to render these data transparently with a fast speed, we have to develop a new transparent visualization method.

A novel framework that is called stochastic point based rendering (SPBR) has recently proposed [6–8] for transparent visualization. 3D opaque particles are utilized as the visualized primitives, and the stochastic based methods are used to calculate pixels intensities on the final visualized image in order to avoid the time-consuming depth sorting. In this paper, we present a fast transparent visualization method for the fusion of both volume and surface data by using the SPBR-based framework.

The main contribution is that we implemented a fast remote transparent visualization method that is able to fuse volume and surface data for a network-based laparoscopic surgery simulator, by using techniques of network communication and the SPBR based visualized framework. A previous study that utilized the same rendering framework for remote visualization was present in the paper [9], however it was proposed for visualization of volume data, not for the fusion of volume and surface data. The details of our contribution are presented in the following parts of this paper.

2 SPBR-Based Transparent Visualization to Fuse Volume and Surface Data

Stochastic point based rendering (SPBR) is a novel visualization framework for the transparent visualization of both volume and surface data [6–8]. Different from other methods, it adopts self-colored 3D points that are fully opaque as the visualized primitives. These points are called particles in this paper. No matter a rendered object is a volume or a surface, it is transparently rendered by the three-step procedure that is illustrated by Fig. 1.

STEP 1. Particle generation: At the first step, a large number of particles are generated for a rendered target. The particle number is related to the opacity of rendered target.

STEP 2. Particle projection with occlusion: At the second step, the particles are randomly separated into L subsets, and the particles of each subset are projected onto the image plane independently to create an intermediate image. Since the particles are fully opaque, the projection is operated with particle occlusion, by which only the nearest particles to the eye position remain on the image plane. As the results of this step, L intermediate images are created.

STEP 3. Averaging images: The final transparent image is generated by averaging the L intermediate images generated in the STEP 2.

The difference to render volume and surface data is in the step of particle generation. The STEP 2 and the STEP 3 are the same for both of them. It should be noticed that no sorting is required in this rendering procedure. Once the particles are generated, the STEP 2 and the STEP 3 can be operated very efficiently. In the following subsections, we firstly present how to generate particles for surface and volume data separately, and then introduce how to fuse the two kinds of data in the SPBR method.

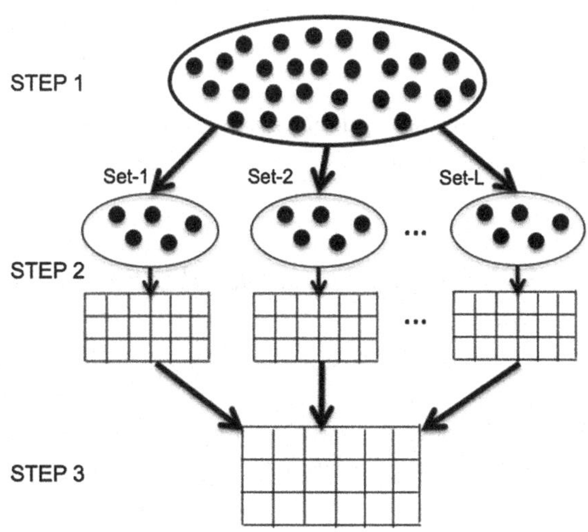

Fig. 1 The three-step procedure of stochastic point based rendering (SPBR) framework

2.1 Particle Generation for Surface Data

The particle generation for surface data is derived from a solid stochastic mechanism [8]. It is assumed that the generated particles uniformly spread on the target surface. During the particle projection, the probability of the number of particles projected onto a certain pixel is governed by the binomial distribution. Given s and S are the area of the cross-section of a particle and the area of the local surface segment respectively, the number of generated particles N can be controlled by a user specified opacity of the target surface α, according to the Eq. (1).

$$N = L\frac{\log(1-\alpha)}{\log(1-\frac{s}{S})} \tag{1}$$

For a polygon mesh, the necessary number of particles can be directly calculated by Eq. (1). Since it is assumed that particles uniformly spread on the surface, we place the particles along scan lines with constant intervals. It is easy to determine the value of intervals based on the above formula.

2.2 Particle Generation for Volume Data

Particles are generated in each cell for volume data. Since the volume data are 3D deformable fields that are represented by a tetrahedron mesh, particle generation is operated within each tetrahedron. The SPBR method utilizes the Metropolis algorithm [10], which is an efficient Monte Carlo technique widely used in chemistry and physics, during the particle generation for volume data [6, 7]. The number of particles for one tetrahedron can be determined by Eq. (2)

$$N \approx -\frac{L\log(1-\alpha)}{w_{pixel}^2 \Delta t}V \tag{2}$$

where w_{pixel} is the width of a pixel, V is the volume of the tetrahedron and Δt is 0.5 in the implementation.

2.3 SPBR-Based Fused Visualization of Volume and Surface Data

The fusion of volume and surface data is very straightforward by using the PBSR framework. After the particles are generated for both volume and surface data according to the descriptions in the Sects. 2.1 and 2.2, all particles are mixed together.

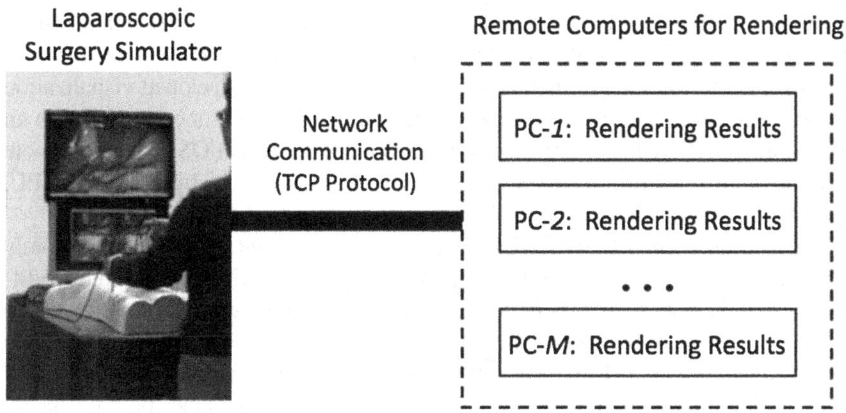

Fig. 2 The developed remote visualization for the laparoscopic surgery simulator

Then the STEP 2 and STEP 3 are operated for the unified particle set to realize the fused visualization for the volume and surface data. Since there is no sorting in the SPBR based method, the fusion can be rendered very efficiently.

3 Remote Visualization for Laparoscopic Surgery Simulator

The results of the laparoscopic surgery simulator are visualized at multiple places by making use of techniques of network communication. The developed remote visualization for the simulator can be illustrated by Fig. 2. The simulator simulates how a liver is deformed during the laparoscopic surgery, by calculating the 3D deformable fields and the deformed liver surface that are represented by tetrahedron meshes and triangular meshes respectively. The two meshes are warped into an ASCII datastream and sent to several computers that are located in multiple remote places via the internet. In order to ensure the data are correctly received by the remote computers, the transmission control protocol (TCP) is utilized for data transmission. Once a remote computer is received the ASCII datastream, it renders the fused results by using the SPBR-based method that is described in the Sect. 2. It should be noticed that all three steps of the SPBR method are performed at remote computers.

4 Experiments and Results

We evaluated the developed remote and fused visualization method in a local network environment. A trainer operates the laparoscopic surgery simulator. When he needs the help of a trainer, the results of the simulator will be sent and the fused results will be rendered on the computer that the trainee uses. We evaluated both of the data transmission and the fused visualization. Although our visualized system are designed for multiply remote computers, we tested the developed visualization on two remote computers in this paper. The simulator runs on a computer with an Intel Core i7-4771 CPU, 8 GB memory and Windows 7 64-bit OS. The two remote computers for rendering have the same specification that is an Intel Core i7 CPU, 8GB memory and Windows 7 64-bit OS.

We measured the data transmission speed by making the simulator to randomly send 35 frames during the training of laparoscopic surgery. Since we found little differences on the data transmission for the two remote computers, transmission speed for one computer were reported in this paper. The transmission speed of all frame are given by the Fig. 3. The average time of data transmission is 4.97 ms per frame. The speed is related to the transmitting data size. The data includes both of the 3D deformed fields (a tetrahedron mesh) and deformed liver surface (a triangular mesh). The triangular mesh that includes 2130 vertices and 4256 triangular facets is with a static data size, however the tetrahedron mesh is with a varied size. In order to make the deformation to be calculated efficiently, an adaptive-resolution based tetrahedron mesh is utilized to represent the 3D deformed fields [1, 2]. In the beginning of the surgery, there is less deformation and the deformed fields are represented by a tetrahedron mesh with a low resolution that has several hundred tetrahedrons. When the deformation becomes larger in the training, a finer tetrahedron mesh that has several thousand tetrahedrons is used. This is why the data transmission speed is increased as what is shown in the Fig. 3. However, the transmission speed is fast even when a tetrahedron mesh with higher resolution is used. In the experiments, the speed is always less than 7ms. This transmission speed is quite satisfactory for interactive visual analyses during the surgery simulation. Note that the particle generation (STEP 1 of PBSR) is made at remote computers after it receives the volume and/or surface data. Sending surface/volume data is faster than sending particle data. Once the

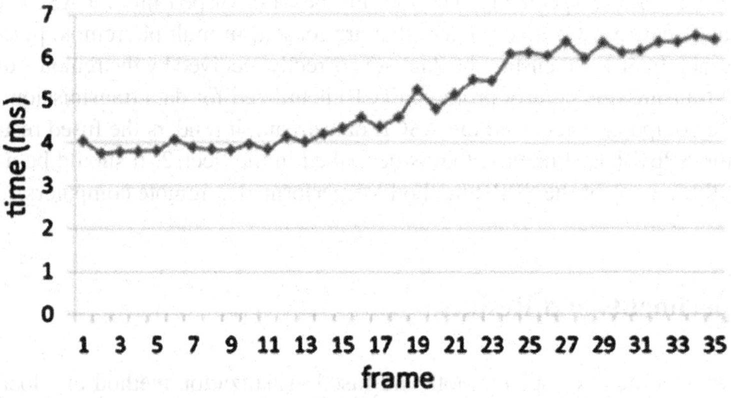

Fig. 3 Evaluation of data transmission. The average time of data transmission is 4.97 ms

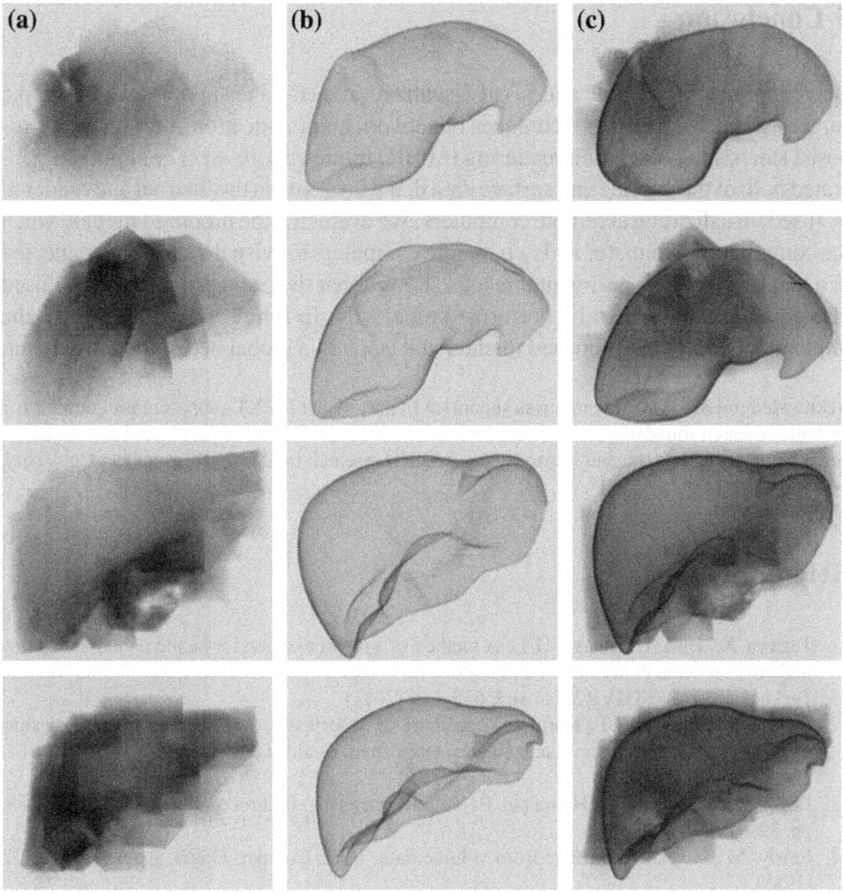

Fig. 4 The SPBR-based rendering results for the network-based laparoscopic surgery simulator. **a** Volume rendering results for the 3D deformable fields (volume). **b** Surface rendering results for the deformed liver surface. **c** Fused visualization of the 3D deformable fields and the deformed liver surface

surface/volume data are received, the remote computer can generate particles with any density, i.e., for any opacity.

The SPBR-based visualization results for randomly selected four frames are shown in Fig. 4. The volume visualization results of the stress field are shown in the left column of Fig. 4. This stress is caused by deformation of the liver in the surgery simulation. We adopted the standard rainbow color map, where high stress values are shown by red and low stress values by blue. This volume visualization is unsatisfactory, because we cannot see shape of the deformed liver. This problem is solved by fusing the surface visualization results in the middle column of Fig. 4. The result of the fusion is shown in the right column of Fig. 4, where we can understand relation between the liver shape and the stress field. The average rendering speed for this fused visualization is about 10.67 fps (frame per second).

5 Conclusion

We proposed a fast remote and fused visualization method to support a laparoscopic surgery simulator by using techniques of network communication and a recently proposed stochastic point based rendering (SPBR) framework [6–8]. The simulator generated both of the volume and surface data that were sent via the internet and rendered by fused visualization at remote computers. We evaluated the proposed method when the computer for simulator and two remote computers for visualization are connected in a local network. Experimental results showed that the proposed remote and fused visualization method can be performed efficiently. In future, we will optimize the implementation of the proposed method and test it in a global network environment.

Acknowledgments This research was supported in part by the MEXT-supported program for the strategic research foundation at private universities (2013-2017), and in part by JSPS KAKENHI Grant Numbers 25280044, and in part by the R-GIRO research fund from Ritsumeikan University.

References

1. Tagawa, K., Bito, T., Tanaka, H.T.: A method of synchronization for haptic collaborative virtual environments in multipoint and multi-level computer performance systems. Stud. Health. Technol. Inform. (MMVR2011) **163**, 638–644 (2011)
2. Tagawa, K., Tanaka, H.T., Kurumi, Y., Komori, M., Morikawa, S.: Laparoscopic surgery simulator using first person view and guidance force. Stud. Health Technol. Inform. (MMVR2013) **184**, 431–435 (2013)
3. Drebin, R., Carpenter, L., Hanrahan, P.: Volume rendering. In: Proceeding of SIGGRAPH'88, pp. 29–37 (1988)
4. Levoy, M.: Display of surface from volume data. IEEE Comput. Graph. Appl. **8**(3), 29–37 (1988)
5. Sabella, P.: A rendering algorithm for visualizing 3D scalar fields. Comput. Graph. **22**(4), 51–58 (1988)
6. Koyamada, K., Sakamoto, N., Tanaka, S.: A particle modeling for rendering irregular volumes. In: International Conference on Computer Modeling and Simulation (UKSIM 2008), pp. 372–377 (2008)
7. Sakamoto, N., Kawamura, T., Koyamada, K., Nozaki, K.: Improvement of particle-based volume rendering for visualizing irregular volume data sets. Comput. Graph. **34**, 34–42 (2010)
8. Tanaka, S., Shimokubo, Y., Kaneko, T., Kawamura, T., Nakata, S., Ojima, S., Sakamto, N., Tanaka, H.T., Koyamada, K.: Particle-based transparent rendering of implicit surfaces and its application to fused visualization. In: EuroVis 2012 (short paper), pp. 25–29 (2012)
9. Lorant, A., Ancel, A., Zhao, K., Sakamoto, N., Koyamada, K., Raffin, B.: Particle based Volume Rendering of Remote Volume Datasets Using FlowVR. In Proceedings of Asia Simulation Conference (AsiaSim2012), pp. 285–296 (Part 1) (2012)
10. Metroplis, N., Rosenbluth, A., Rosenbluth, M., Teller, A., Teller, E.: Equation of state calculations by fast computing machine. J. Chem. Phys. **21**(6), 1087–1092 (1953)

Study of Surgical Simulation of Flatfoot Using a Finite Element Model

Zhongkui Wang, Kan Imai, Masamitsu Kido, Kazuya Ikoma and Shinichi Hirai

Abstract A finite element (FE) model of flatfoot deformity was proposed in this paper for use in surgical simulations to improve individualized treatments. The external geometries of the flatfoot skeleton and encapsulated soft tissue were obtained by 3D reconstruction of CT images. A total of 63 major ligaments and the plantar fascia were manually created with wire parts to connect the corresponding attachment points on the bone surfaces. The bones, ligaments, and plantar fascia were defined as linearly elastic materials, while the encapsulated soft tissue was defined as nonlinearly hyperelastic material. The model was implemented in Abaqus®, and simulations of balanced standing were performed. The simulated plantar stress distribution was compared to actual measurements. Surgical simulations of medializing calcaneal osteotomy (MCO) and lateral column lengthening (LCL) were conducted, and we found that both surgeries alleviated the stress around the talo-navicular joint and shifted high stress from the medial area towards the center and lateral areas, but the improvement instilled by LCL was more obvious than that instilled by MCO.

Keywords Flatfoot · Finite element · Biomechanics · Surgical plan · Medializing calcaneal osteotomy · Lateral column lengthening

Z. Wang (✉) · S. Hirai
Department of Robotics, Ritsumeikan University, Shiga 525-8577, Japan
e-mail: wangzk@fc.ritsumei.ac.jp

S. Hirai
e-mail: hirai@se.ritsumei.ac.jp

K. Imai · M. Kido · K. Ikoma
Department of Orthopaedics, Kyoto Prefectural University of Medicine, Kyoto 602-8566, Japan
e-mail: kan-imai@koto.kpu-m.ac.jp

M. Kido
e-mail: masamits@koto.kpu-m.ac.jp

K. Ikoma
e-mail: kazuya@koto.kpu-m.ac.jp

Y.-W. Chen et al. (eds.), *Innovation in Medicine and Healthcare 2015*,
Smart Innovation, Systems and Technologies 45,
DOI 10.1007/978-3-319-23024-5_32

1 Introduction

Flatfoot is a very common foot deformity in which the foot arch collapses and the entire sole reaches complete or near-complete contact with the ground. Patients with flatfoot may develop lower extremity pain, swelling, abnormal gait, and difficulty walking [1]. In severe cases, surgery is required to correct the deformity. Despite its commonality, the biomechanics of flatfoot are not fully understood, and the optimal surgical methodology has not yet been established. Foot surgeons tend to have different opinions regarding optimal surgery for individual patients.

To study flatfoot biomechanics, cadaveric foot models have been frequently used by researchers. Due to the lack of donors, healthy foot samples have often been used to artificially generate a flatfoot deformity by releasing or sectioning specific ligaments and tendons [2, 3]. However, it is difficult to fully reproduce clinically accurate flatfoot functions with these artificially created flatfoot models. Moreover, the flatfoot deformity is patient-dependent and phase-dependent. A study of one cadaveric model does not provide sufficient information for instructing surgical planning.

On the other hand, computer-based models can be adjusted for individual differences in deformities and can easily simulate surgical treatments. The FE method has frequently been used to model human tissues due to its characteristic of continuum mechanics and its capability of modeling irregular geometries and complex material properties. One FE model of flatfoot described by [4] modeled 14 bones, 65 ligaments, and a portion of the plantar tissue, but the toes and dorsal tissue were omitted. A computational model of the foot skeleton was proposed by [5] to study the effects of surgical correction for the treatment of adult-acquired flatfoot deformity. The expected dynamic motions of the bones after different surgical procedures were simulated; however, the encapsulated soft tissue was not included in that model. In addition to flatfoot, FE models of healthy foot and other foot deformities have been developed for different purposes, such as improving footwear design [6, 7], studying clawed hallux deformity [8], and developing ankle prostheses [9].

In this paper, a complete flatfoot model is presented based on CT measurements and the FE package Abaqus®. The development of the FE model is described in Sect. 2. Balanced standing simulation results and validation, surgical simulations of MCO and LCL, and discussions are presented in Sect. 3. Finally, the paper is concluded in Sect. 4 with suggestions for future works.

2 FE Model of Flatfoot

2.1 Geometry Generation of Skeleton and Encapsulated Tissue

The geometries of the skeleton and encapsulated soft tissue of a flatfoot (right foot) were generated from a series of CT images obtained from a 38-years-old male subject of 168 cm in height and 62 kg in weight. During the CT scan, a custom-made

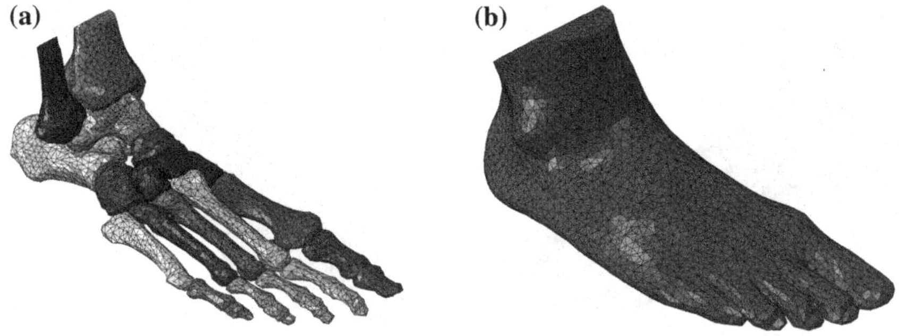

Fig. 1 Geometries of the flatfoot skeleton (**a**) and the encapsulated soft tissue (**b**)

foot loading device was used to fix the subject's lower limb [10]. The boundaries of the bones and encapsulated tissue were segmented from CT images using Mimics® (Materialise Inc., Leuven, Belgium). The resulting surface meshes were imported into the free mesh editor Meshlab to smooth the meshes and reduce the node densities to decrease the computation time of the FE simulation. Finally, the edited surface meshes were imported into the FE package Abaqus®. Figure 1a shows the foot skeleton consisting of 17 bone segments: tibia, fibula, talus, calcaneus, cuboid, navicular, cuneiform (3 merged into 1), 5 metatarsals, and 5 phalanxes (proximal, middle, and distal phalanxes were merged together). These bone segments were cut out from the tissue segment to generate an encapsulated tissue part surrounding the bone segments, as shown in Fig. 1b.

2.2 Creation of Ligaments and Plantar Fascia

From CT images, ligaments and plantar fascia cannot be discriminated from the surrounding soft tissue. Therefore, the geometries of the ligaments and plantar fascia were created manually by referring to an anatomy book [11] and also by following the suggestions of foot surgeons. These tissues were modeled as wire parts and were meshed with tension-only linear truss elements. The anatomical origins and insertions of the ligaments and plantar fascia were approximately located at the corresponding nodes on the bone surfaces. Wire parts were then defined to connect these corresponding nodes. A total of 63 ligaments (colored cyan in Fig. 2) and the plantar fascia (colored red) were modeled with 82 wire parts. The joint capsules connecting the metatarsals and phalanxes were modeled by 4 wire parts evenly surrounding the two bones. The cross-sectional areas of the wire parts were set to 18.4 and 58.6 mm^2 for the ligaments and plantar fascia respectively, according to [6].

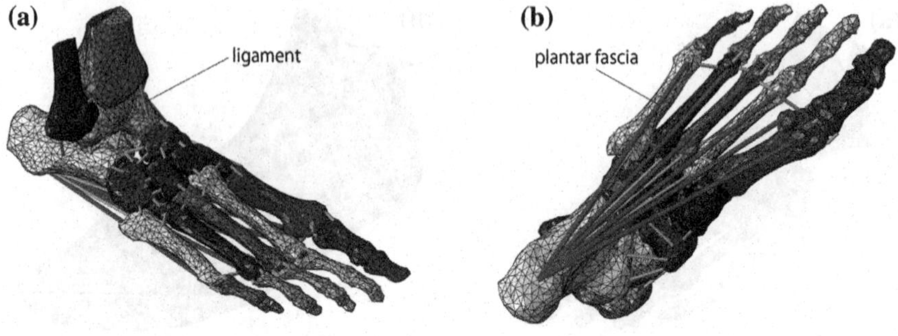

Fig. 2 Created ligaments and plantar fascia from a (**a**) dorsal and (**b**) plantar view

2.3 Material Properties, Contact Interactions, and Constraints

The material properties of the bones, ligaments, plantar fascia, and ground plate were considered linearly elastic, while the encapsulated soft tissue was considered nonlinearly hyperelastic (the second order polynomial model defined by the material constants C_{ij} and D_i). The mechanical parameters of these materials are listed in Tables 1 and 2 respectively, which are accompanied by the referenced literatures.

Contact interactions among neighboring bones and between the encapsulated tissue and the ground plate were defined by tangential and normal behaviors using the penalty method with a default stiffness value assigned automatically by Abaqus®. According to [6], the contact behavior between neighboring bones was considered frictionless because of the lubricating nature of the articulating surfaces. The friction coefficient between the foot and ground plate was set to 0.6 according to [8]. A total of 21 contact pairs were defined in the model. Tie constraints were defined to connect the ligaments and plantar fascia to corresponding bones and also to connect the bones to the encapsulated soft tissue. A total of 183 tie constraints were defined in the model.

Table 1 Mechanical parameters of linearly elastic material

Parts	Young's modulus (MPa)	Poisson's ratio
Bone	7,300 [6, 7]	0.3 [6, 7]
Ligament	260 [6, 7]	0.4 [7]
Plantar fascia	350 [6, 7]	0.4 [7]
Ground plate	17,000 [6, 7]	0.1 [6, 7]

Table 2 Mechanical parameters of nonlinearly hyperelastic material

C_{10} (MPa)	C_{01} (MPa)	C_{20} (MPa)	C_{11} (MPa)	C_{02} (MPa)	D_1 (MPa^{-1})	D_2 (MPa^{-1})
0.08556	−0.05841	0.03900	−0.02319	0.00851	3.65273	0.00000

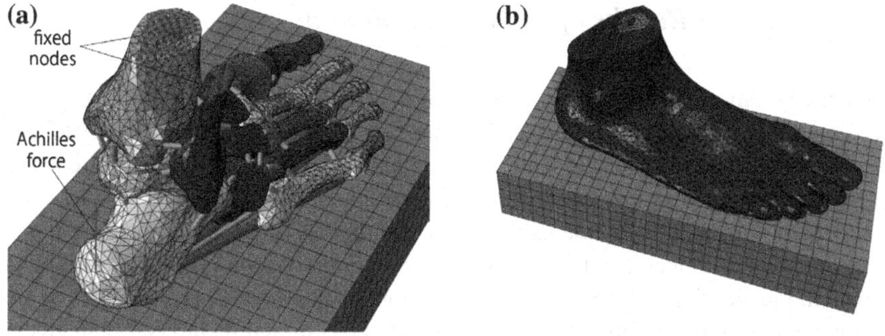

Fig. 3 **a** Boundary conditions for the tibia and fibula, and **b** the complete FE model

2.4 Loading and Boundary Conditions

During the balanced standing simulation, the ground plate was pushed upward to deform the flatfoot instead of being loaded downward by the tibia and fibula. Half of the subject's weight (31 kg) was applied to the ground plate as an evenly distributed upward pressure load. Regarding tendon forces, only the Achilles tendon force was examined [6]. The Achilles force was assumed to be 50 % of the ground reaction force [4], which is half of the body weight. Therefore, the Achilles force was calculated as 25 % of the body weight, or 151.9 N. The Achilles force was applied as a concentrated force load at the position of the backside of the calcaneus, as shown in Fig. 3a. Throughout the simulations, the top surfaces of the tibia and fibula were fixed in space (Fig. 3a).

All solid parts, except the ground plate, were meshed with a 4-node linear tetrahedron "C3D4" element, and the wire parts were meshed with a 2-node linear truss "T3D2" element. The ground plate was meshed with an 8-node linear brick "C3D8R" element. The complete model, as shown in Fig. 3b, consists of a total of 50,914 nodes and 139,763 elements.

3 Simulation Results and Discussion

Three simulations were performed using implicit dynamic analysis and the geometrical nonlinearity was turned on in Abaqus®. The first simulation was a normal balanced standing scenario before surgical correction of the flatfoot. The simulated plantar stress distribution was compared to an actual measurement. The second and third simulations were surgical corrections of MCO and LCL. The simulation results were compared before and after surgery.

3.1 Simulation Results of Balanced Standing

A balanced standing simulation with a duration of 3 seconds was performed using the flatfoot model. Simulated stress distributions on the skeleton and plantar tissue surface are shown in Fig. 4a–c. To validate the simulation results, actual measurements of plantar stress during balanced standing were taken using an Emed-M® pressure platform system with the same subject used for the CT scan. Three measurements were taken for both feet, and the average stress of the right foot was calculated and is shown in Fig. 4d. For the skeleton, the simulation results showed large stresses at the talo-navicular, naviculo-cuneiform, 1st tarso-metatarsal, and metatarsal-phalangeal joints. For the plantar tissue surface, the simulation results showed large stresses appeared at the hindfoot area under the heel, which agreed with the measurement, and the forefoot area under the sesamoid bone, which is not found in actual measurement. However, with the actual measurements, large stresses also appeared at the center area of the forefoot. In both the simulation and actual measurement, the great toe experienced some stress; however, in the simulation, stress was also observed at the areas under the fourth and fifth distal phalanxes. The differences between the simulation and the actual measurements were due to the initial geometry of the encapsulated soft tissue used for the simulation. The CT scan was taken while the subject was lying on the CT table with his lower limb fixed by a custom-made device. During CT scan, both feet were subjected to $5.7 \pm 2.6\,\%$ of body weight [10]. This initial loading makes the initial geometry of the plantar surface relatively flat, in contrast to the naturally curved state in which the forefoot and hindfoot usually have a lower profile than the other areas of the foot. There are two main factors affecting the stress distribution on the plantar tissue surface: the profile of the plantar surface and the profile of the skeleton. During balanced standing, low profile areas on the plantar surface contact the ground plate earlier than other areas and, therefore, result in larger

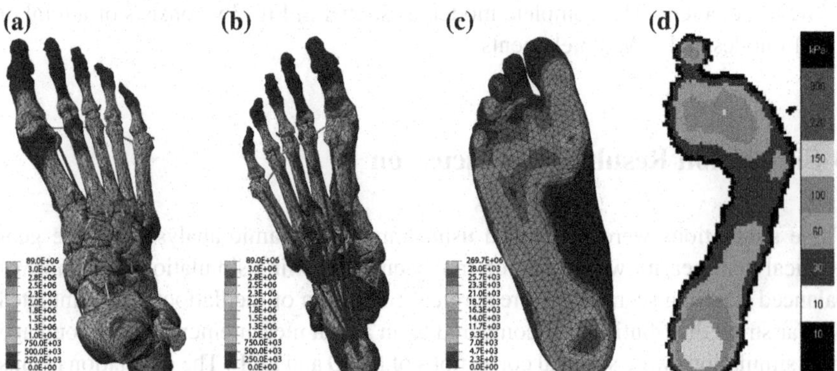

Fig. 4 Simulation results of balanced standing. Skeletal stress distribution from a (**a**) dorsal view and (**b**) plantar view. Stress distribution on the plantar tissue surface in simulation (**c**) and actual measurement (**d**). The unit of stress is Pascal or Pa

deformation and stress at the end of the standing period. On the other hand, a low profile of the skeleton indicates that less soft tissue is present between the profile and the ground plate, which results in larger stress once the deformation exceeds a certain threshold under this profile. Because the tissue geometry used in this work included a flat plantar surface, this model could not reproduce the effects of the profile of the plantar surface. The effect of the skeleton profile can clearly be seen by examining the stress distribution (Fig. 4c): low profile areas (under the heel and sesamoid bone) generated large stresses. The effects of the plantar surface profile can be introduced to the model by using a natural and undeformed tissue geometry. However, it is difficult to ensure the stability of the foot without initial loading during a CT scan.

3.2 Simulation Results of MCO Surgery

According to [12], MCO surgery is performed with an oscillating saw at a right angle to the lateral border of the calcaneus and is inclined posteriorly approximately 45° to the plantar surface of the hindfoot. The posterior fragment is shifted 10 mm medially, and the osteotomy is closed by inserting one cannulated screw. The same surgery was simulated using the proposed FE model. The simulation was performed in two steps. In the first step, the calcaneus was cut into two parts at the approximate position and angle shown in Fig. 5a. The medial shifting of the posterior fragment was simulated with all tissues attached. Two boundary conditions were applied on the two fragements of the calcaneus. One is to fix the anterior fragment (colored dark red in Fig. 5) and the other is to displace the posterior fragment. The shifted geometries of the calcaneus and the encapsulated tissue are shown in Fig. 5b, c. A back-view of the original geometry of the encapsulated tissue is presented in Fig. 5d for comparison. The geometry correction produced by the surgery can be clearly seen by comparing Fig. 5c, d. The corrected geometries were then imported into a new model for the second simulation step. The stress generated in the first step was discarded, as only the deformed geometries were of interest. In the new model, the two separated

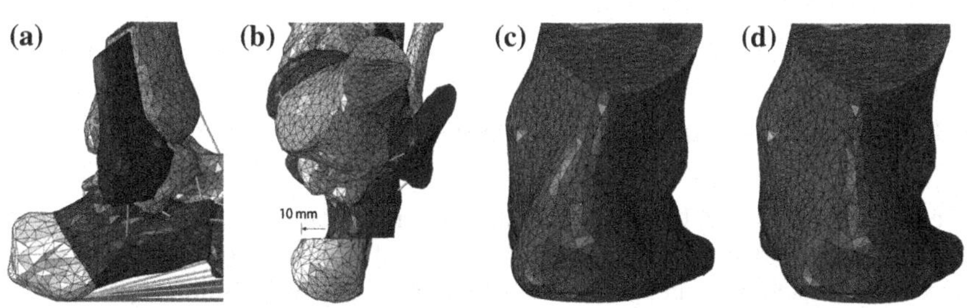

Fig. 5 The first step of the surgical simulation of MCO. The calcaneus was cut into two parts (**a**) and the posterior fragment was medially shift 10 mm (**b**). Foot geometry after (**c**) and before (**d**) shifting

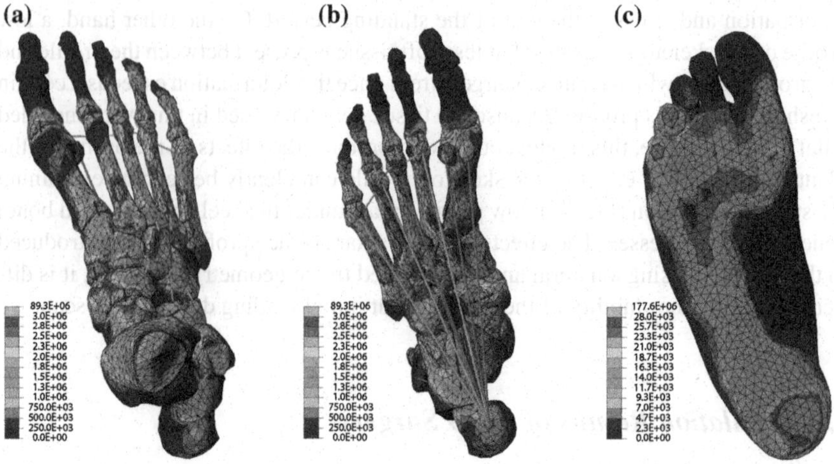

Fig. 6 Simulation results of balanced standing after MCO surgery. Stress distributions on skeleton from a (**a**) dorsal and (**b**) plantar view. Stress distribution on plantar tissue surface (**c**). The unit of stress is Pascal or Pa

calcaneus parts were merged into one part instead of inserting a cannulated screw. As presented in the previous section, the same interactions and constraints and loading and boundary conditions were applied in the new model. A 3 s balanced standing simulation was then performed, and the stress distributions on the skeleton and plantar tissue surface generated by the simulation are shown in Fig. 6. Compared with the results in Fig. 4, we found that the stress around the talo-navicular joint was alleviated, and large stresses were shifted from the medial area (the 1st metatarsal bone) to the center and lateral areas (the 3rd, 4th, and 5th metatarsal bones) after MCO surgery. On the plantar surface (Fig. 6c), a large amount of stress was still present under the heel area, but the amplitude of the stress had increased. In addition, the stresses under the 4th and 5th distal areas had also increased compared to the results before MCO surgery (Fig. 4c). Meanwhile, the stress at the mid-foot area was slightly reduced after MCO surgery.

3.3 Simulation Results of LCL Surgery

According to [12], in LCL surgery, the calcaneus is osteomized at 4 mm proximal to the calcaneocuboid joint. A wedge shaped bicortical iliac crest bone graft is laterally placed in the osteotomy site. After closure of the osteotomy and suitable positioning of the correction, fixation is accomplished with two Steinmann pins or one cannulated screw. In the first step of the simulation, we osteomized the calcaneus into two parts at the required position and then applied boundary conditions to move the two parts away from each other with an opening distance of 10 mm, as shown in Fig. 7a, b.

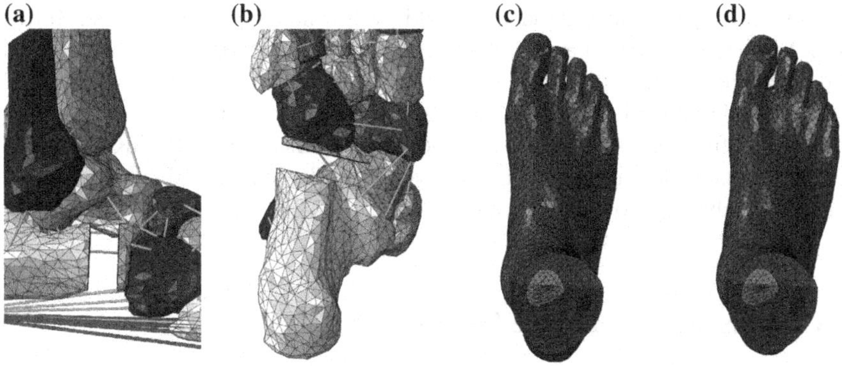

Fig. 7 The first step of the surgical simulation of LCL. The cut calcaneus after surgical opening in a (**a**) side-view and (**b**) plantar view. Foot geometry after (**c**) and before (**d**) surgical opening

The foot geometry was corrected according to the surgical opening of the calcaneus, as shown in Fig. 7c. Compared with the original geometry (Fig. 7d), the correction rotated the forefoot medially around the ankle, and the total length of the foot was increased, as implied by the name of the surgery. The corrected geometries were then imported into a new model for the second simulation step. In the new model, a bone graft was inserted into the osteotomy site and was tied with both fragments of the calcaneus, as shown in Fig. 8a. A 3 s balanced standing simulation was performed and the stress distributions obtained by the simulation are presented in Fig. 8b–d. Compared to the stress distribution before surgery (Fig. 4), we found that LCL surgery also alleviated stress around the talo-navicular joint and shifted high stress from the medial area to the center and lateral areas. This was very clear based on the stress

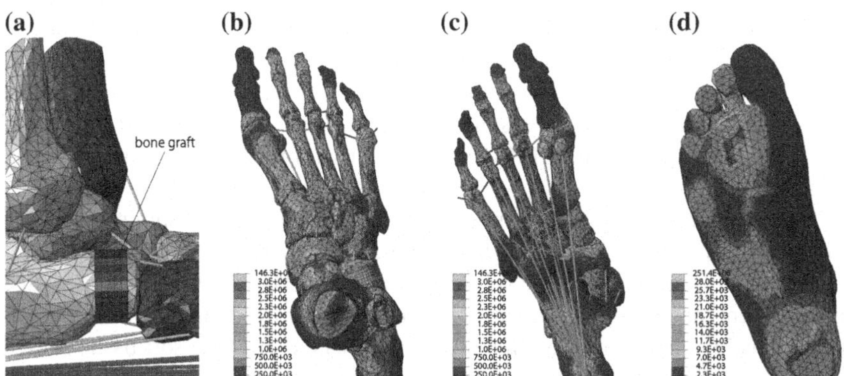

Fig. 8 The second step of the surgical simulation of LCL: a bone graft inserted in the osteotomy site (**a**), simulated stress distributions on the skeleton from a (**b**) dorsal and (**c**) plantar view, and (**d**) on the plantar surface. The unit of stress is Pascal or Pa

distribution on the plantar tissue surface (Fig. 8d), where high stresses were shifted from the medial sesamoid area to the center of the forefoot and under the 2nd and 3rd distal areas. Comparing the results of the two surgical simulations (Figs. 6 and 8), we found that the LCL surgery alleviated more stress around the talo-navicular joint and shifted more stress to the 2nd and 3rd metatarsal bones than MCO surgery. On the plantar tissue surface, LCL surgery also results in more stress being shifted from the medial area to the center area.

4 Conclusions and Future Works

An FE model of a flatfoot deformity was presented to study surgical simulation for the improvement of optimal individualized treatments. The modeling procedure began with a CT scan of the subject with flatfoot and was followed by generation of the geometries of the skeleton and encapsulated tissue. The major ligaments and plantar fascia were manually created to connect the bones. The constraints and interactions were defined to tie different tissue parts together and apply contact interactions. Finally, the loading and boundary conditions were defined to impose loads and motions to certain parts of the foot to activate the simulation.

Three simulations were performed using the FE model. First, the balanced standing or weight-bearing simulation was performed, and the stress distribution on the plantar surface was compared to actual measurements to validate the model. The discrepancies between the results of the simulation and the actual measurements suggest that the naturally curved plantar surface is preferred to obtain an accurate stress distribution on the plantar surface in the simulation. The second simulation was MCO surgery, in which the calcaneus was osteomized and shifted 10 mm medially. The balanced standing simulation was performed on the corrected flatfoot model, and the results showed stress alleviation around the talo-navicular joint and stress shifting from the medial area to the center and lateral areas. The third simulation was LCL surgery, in which the calcaneus was osteomized, and a bone graft was inserted into the osteotomy site. A balanced standing simulation was also performed on the LCL-corrected model, and the results showed the same alleviation and shifting of the stress distribution as with MCO surgery, but with more obvious improvement than with MCO surgery.

This paper presents a preliminary study for developing optimal surgical planning for individual patients with flatfoot deformities, and there is much room for improvement of this FE model and these surgical simulations. The material properties used in the current model were linear elasticity and nonlinear hyperelasticity. During balanced standing simulations, oscillations were observed after the soft tissue started to contact the ground plate, and it took 2 or 3 s to resolve the oscillations. To eliminate the oscillations, viscosity should be considered for the encapsulated soft tissue and appropriate viscosity parameters need to be determined. Surgical simulations of MCO and LCL with different shifting and opening procedures will be investigated to determine the optimal osteotomy site and shifting or opening dimension. An FE model and simulation of healthy foot will be established and performed, respectively, to generate criteria for evaluating the performance of surgical corrections of flatfoot deformity.

Acknowledgments This work was supported by MEXT-Supported Program for the Strategic Research Foundation at Private Universities (2013–2017), in part by JSPS Grant-in-Aid for Scientific Research 15H02230, and also in part by MEXT KAKENHI 26860404, JSPS, Japan.

References

1. Wang, Z., Imai, K., Kido, M., Ikoma, K., Hirai, S.: A finite element model of flatfoot (pes planus) for improving surgical plan. In: 36th Annual International Conference of the IEEE Engineering in Medicine and Biology Society, Chicago (2014)
2. Niu, W., Yang, Y., Fan, Y., Ding, Z., Yu, G.: Experimental modeling and biomechanical measurement of flatfoot deformity. In: Proceedings of 7th Asian-Pacific Conference on Medical and Biological Engineering, vol. 19, pp. 133–138. Springer, Heidelberg (2008)
3. Blackman, A.J., Blevins, J.J., Sangeorzan, B.J., Ledoux, W.R.: Cadaveric flatfoot model: ligament attenuation and Achilles tendon overpull. J. Orthop. Res. **27**(12), 1547–1554 (2009)
4. Lewis, G.S.: Computational modeling of the mechanics of flatfoot deformity and its surgical corrections. Ph.D. Dissertation, Pennsylvania State University (2008)
5. Iaquinto, J.M., Wayne, J.S.: Effects of surgical correction for the treatment of adult acquired flatfoot deformity: a computational investigation. J. Orthop. Res. **29**(7), 1047–1054 (2011)
6. Cheung, J.T.M., Zhang, M.: Finite element modeling of the human foot and footwear. ABAQUS Users' Conference, pp. 145–159. Cambridge (2006)
7. Qiu, T., Teo, E., Yan, Y., Lei, W.: Finite element modeling of a 3D coupled foot-boot model. Med. Eng. Phys. **33**(10), 1228–1233. Elsevier (2011)
8. Isvilanonda, V., Dengler, E., Iaquinto, M., Sangeorzan, B.J., Ledoux, W.R.: Finite element analysis of the foot: model validation and comparison between two common treatments of the clawed hallux deformity. Clin. Biomech. **27**(8), 837–844. Elsevier (2012)
9. Ozen, M., Sayman, O., Havitcioglu, H.: Modeling and stress analyses of a normal foot-ankle and a prosthetic foot-ankle complex, Acta Bioeng. Biomech. **15**(3), 19–27. Wroclaw University of Technology (2013)
10. Kido, M., Ikoma, K., Imai, K., Maki, M., Takatori, R., Tokunaga, D., Inoue, N., Kubo, T.: Load response of the tarsal bones in patients with flatfoot deformity. In vivo 3D study. Foot Ankle Int. **32**(11), 1017–1022 (2011)
11. Netter, F.H.: Atlas of Human Anatomy, 5th edn. pp. 51–525. Elsevier (2011)
12. Trnka, H.J., Easley, M.E., Myerson, M.S.: The role of calcaneal osteotomies for correction of adult flatfoot. Clin. Orthop. Relat. Res. **365**, 50–64. Lippincott Williams and Wilkins (1999)

A Study of Meditation Effectiveness for Virtual Reality Based Stress Therapy Using EEG Measurement and Questionnaire Approaches

Gamini Perhakaran, Azmi Mohd Yusof, Mohd Ezanee Rusli, Mohd Zaliman Mohd Yusoff, Imran Mahalil and Ahmad Redza Razieff Zainuddin

Abstract Various approaches are available to evaluate the effectiveness of stress therapy. In this research, we compared virtual reality based stress therapy and imaginary technique which includes cultural elements such as typical Malaysian environment in 3D, Mozart, soothing breathing exercise and audio. It examines meditation effectiveness between virtual reality based stress therapy and imaginary technique using Electroencephalograph. The effectiveness of the virtual reality therapy and imaginary technique are measured by NeuroSky eSense Meditation level. Findings for both approaches indicated that there are positive changes in participants' meditation state. Moreover, the virtual reality participants were observed to be in a better meditation state (significantly different) compared to the imaginary participants at the end of the study.

Keywords Stress • Virtual reality therapy (VRT) • Electroencephalograph (EEG) • Esense meditation

---

G. Perhakaran (✉) · A.M. Yusof · M.E. Rusli · M.Z.M. Yusoff · I. Mahalil · A.R.R. Zainuddin
College of Information Technology, Universiti Tenaga Nasional, Putrajaya Campus, Jalan IKRAM-UNITEN, 43009 Kajang, Selangor, Malaysia
e-mail: gamini.perhakaran@yahoo.com

A.M. Yusof
e-mail: azmiy@uniten.edu.my

M.E. Rusli
e-mail: ezanee@uniten.edu.my

M.Z.M. Yusoff
e-mail: zaliman@uniten.edu.my

I. Mahalil
e-mail: imranmahalil@gmail.com

A.R.R. Zainuddin
e-mail: ahmadredzarazieff_redza@yahoo.com

Y.-W. Chen et al. (eds.), *Innovation in Medicine and Healthcare 2015*, Smart Innovation, Systems and Technologies 45,
DOI 10.1007/978-3-319-23024-5_33

1 Introduction

Stress is a state of mental or emotional strain resulting from adverse circumstances. It is a force of nature that enables the individuals' to respond in various way towards stress that can affect the person and their surroundings [1, 2]. Based on previous researches, VRT (Virtual Reality Technology) has been used to treat Post Traumatic Stress Disorder (PTSD) and were found to be an effective treatment tool. VRT also has been identified to be effective to stress related disorder compared to standard cognitive behavioral program [3, 4]. In our previous research, comparative study was done between VRT and imaginary technique for stress therapy. The research was evaluated using questionnaires. Responses from the questionnaire resulted that the virtual reality based stress therapy system was more effective compared to imaginary technique [5]. In this paper, we have adopted a new approach of evaluation that is by using a dedicated brainwave device called Electroencephalograph (EEG) as an assessment tool.

Besides that, this system incorporates the elements of comforting audio, immersive visualization using upgraded Head Mounted Display (HMD) with higher resolution specification compared to previous research [5]. In addition to that, the EEG [6] is being integrated to obtain the brainwave signal level while using the system. In medical approach, brainwaves signals are obtained using conventional EEG which uses multiple electrode and electrolyte gels. Fortunately, in the latest EEG, dry electrodes EEG are used, and it has been developed by companies such as Neuro Vigil Inc. [7], Emotiv [8] and NeuroSky [9]. This dry electrodes EEG is more ease to use compared to conventional EEG as mentioned earlier. In this study, NeuroSky EEG device has been used to evaluate the meditation level of the participants while using VRT and imaginary technique. The headset in this EEG method consists of sensors which can indicate mental calmness level known as "Meditation". It also capture the brain wave electrical signals using a mobile application EEG analyzer [10].

Virtual reality (VR) is a computer simulated environment that consists of virtual objects in a virtual world. Users can visualize and immerse in a virtual environment using HMD, audio and haptic devices. Burdea and Coiffet categorized VR into three types of system: immersive, non-immersive and hybrid [11]. In this research, the study is conducted under an "immersive" category. In an "immersive" category, the computer generated images replaces a real world view and what to be viewed is determined by users' head position and orientation in a real-time mode. In order to increase the immersion level, audio and interaction devices are also used. While venturing in the virtual world, users are attached with a device called NeuroSky Mindset EEG Meditation level.

NeuroSky's e-Sense meters display the reading of high cognitive mental states. The Mindset is a sensor placed on the user's forehead. It is able to measure "Attention" and "Meditation" meter values respectively along with raw EEG data. The research focused on "Meditation" state only. It measures the user's level of relaxation and calmness. The brain's mental processes will result reduction of the meter, while, an increased meter is the resulted from brain's relaxation state. Sense of calm and peace are related with clear mind and thoughts. In many occasions, closing eyes will result in an increase of the meditation meter as well [12].

2 Background

Imagination technique was found to be effective [13] for a meta-analysis of imagery rehearsal for post-trauma nightmares. Similarly, VRT has been found to be effective in various system and it has a potential to be used for treating people with traumatic disorder, stress and phobias of medical field. In general, VRT has been used and positive result for stress related disorder has been obtained compared to a standard cognitive behavioral program [4]. The scope of VRT in a medical field is widened by now that it has been implemented for a brain injury rehabilitation where positive outcomes have been obtained [14]. In another related research, meta-analysis collected from the experiment shows that VRT has potential for treating anxiety and several phobias [15].

Lately, virtual reality has been integrated with brain-computer interface (BCI) using EEG [16]. The findings from this integration had proven that EEG signals using BCI could interface with virtual reality application accordingly [17]. Furthermore, emotional data has been acquired using EEG signal under an audio-visual induction environment [18]. Previous research shows that emotion state was evaluated using Derogatis Stress Profile (DSP) questionnaire [5, 19]. The mental state was indicated by NeuroSky Mindset a simplified EEG for detecting the correct behaviors' to increase players' Meditation level from eSense meters [20]. The headset calculates the raw EEG through a ThinkGear chip to produce the eSense Meters (Attention and Meditation) output per second to the computer [21]. Another study conducted using NeuroSky Mindset shows that Meditation level changes at different places such as the highest meditation was obtained at garden compared to other places as in [22].

In this paper, an approach using EEG brainwave signals from NeuroSky Mindset is used to evaluate the mental emotional state while undergoing the treatment using VRT system and imaginary technique.

3 System Specifications

Nowadays, there are many platforms are available to develop 3D models and virtual environments. Examples of these platforms are Cryengine, Unreal Engine, Unity 3D, Autodesk Maya, Blender and etc. In this research, an open source game engine platform known as Unity 3D was chosen. This engine is able to produce a natural 3D environment with a realistic world effect such as the vegetation and nature's physics as shown in Fig. 1. The natural sound was also embedded [5, 23].

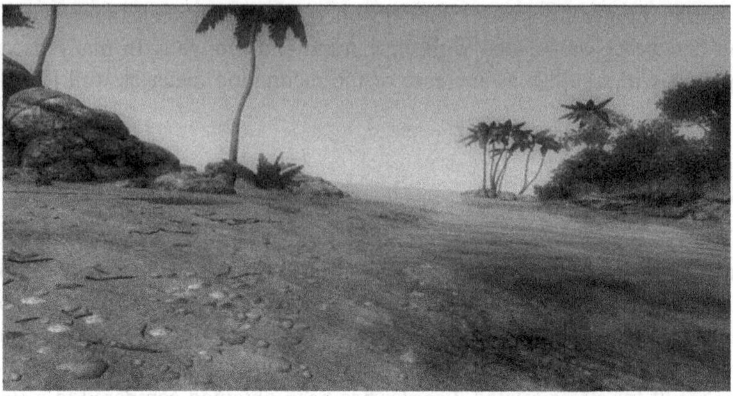

Fig. 1 VRT Environment

As mentioned earlier, the integration of brain-computer interface (BCI) using Mindwave mobile EEG with VRT environment are used in this experiment to capture the meditation level of eSense meter [12]. Mindwave mobile is a headset as shown in Fig. 2. The headset signal from the participants is captured using the SDK called ThinkGear developed by NeuroSky Inc. [21, 24]. The brainwave signals are acquired by this ThinkGear to calculate the attention and meditation level. NeuroSky has also provided an application called an EEG Analyzer to record the collected data in an excel format for future references and studies. This application can only run on Android devices [10].

These two types of meters (attention and mediation) are scaled from 1 to 100 and it is being trademark as eSense. Attention meter indicates the strength of users'

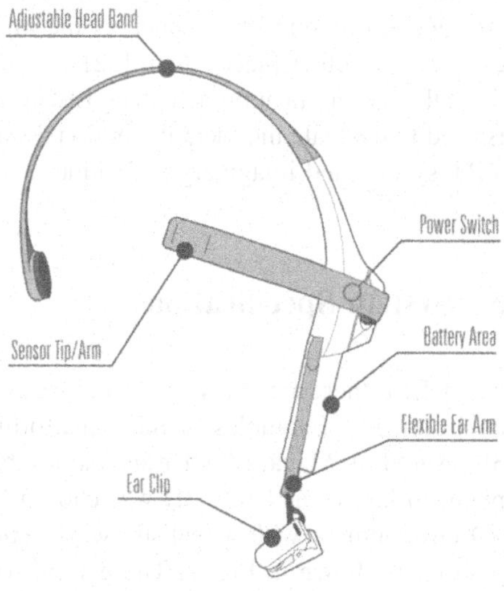

Fig. 2 NeuroSky Mindwave mobile

Table 1 Meditation level interpretation

Meditation level	Specification
01–20	Strongly lowered
21–40	Reduced
41–60	Neutral
61–80	Slightly elevated
81–100	Elevated

mental state such as during deep concentration. The level and the specification of mental states [12] is listed in Table 1.

4 Research Methodologies

In this experiments, 30 participants volunteered for the study. During the VRT session, 15 participants sat in a comfortable chair while wearing a HMD, wireless headphone and NeuroSky Mindset Mobile. The HMD was connected to a desktop computer running the VRT application that comes with 5 min relaxation script. Another group of 15 participants were experimented using an imaginary technique. Thus, the only difference between these two experiments setup is that a HMD is not available to imaginary technique. The flow chart of the experiment and analysis implemented is shown in Fig. 3.

As stated earlier, a Mindwave Mobile EEG and a mobile application (EEG Analyzer) are installed to Android device [10]: a Lenovo S860 Smartphone to obtain the EEG data coming from the EEG headset. This mobile application is connected to the Mindwave Mobile EEG via Bluetooth. The application runs as the participant wears the device and it gets connected in real time. The analyzer

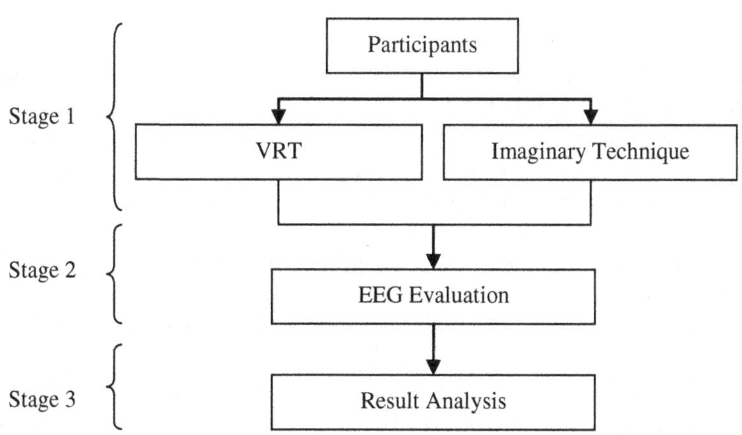

Fig. 3 The flow chart of the VRT and Imaginary Technique Evaluation

displays the mind data such as meditation level and attention level. The meditation level and attention level meter are displayed in real time chart and the captured data in the mobile application are saved and exported to Dropbox servers in *.cvs format after each of the session.

In order to measure the mean value of the meditation levels (χ) of VR-based and imaginary therapies, Eq. (1) is used where n represents the total number of participants and χ_1, χ_2, χ_3 and χ_n represents the meditation level for each seconds from all participants respectively.

The formula in computing meditation mean is as follows:

$$\bar{x} = \frac{x_1 + x_2 + x_3 = \cdots + x_n}{n} \tag{1}$$

where:

x meditation level per second

n total number of participant

First stage: The participants will be going through a VRT session or an Imaginary technique. The Mindwave Mobile EEG is placed at the participants head for capturing data while Bluetooth connection will be activated on the mobile.

Second stage: After the session has been completed the data captured from the participants are transferred to Dropbox. The participants' experiment session is completed here.

Final stage: In this stage, the results from the conducted VRT and imaginary session are analyzed.

5 Result and Analysis

Meditation Level. Figure 4 shows the eSense Meditation mean level for all the 30 participants throughout the 5 min VRT session and imaginary technique (i.e. 15 participants each). In this Fig. 4, a similarity of graph pattern between the two therapies from second 45 to 169 have been identified. This pattern similarity happens during the point of relaxation breathing exercise where a relaxation script is being played via a headphone [5, 25].

Box Plot in Fig. 5 shows 50 is the mean values of meditation level from all participants of each technique respectively. The box plot shows that meditation level of VRT session is more stable compared to the imaginary technique with high fluctuation. So, this suggest that VRT session has been more effective for a stress therapy.

From a column chart as shown in Fig. 6, the meditation level mean of the participants falls between the ranges of 40–60. According to the eSense meter stated

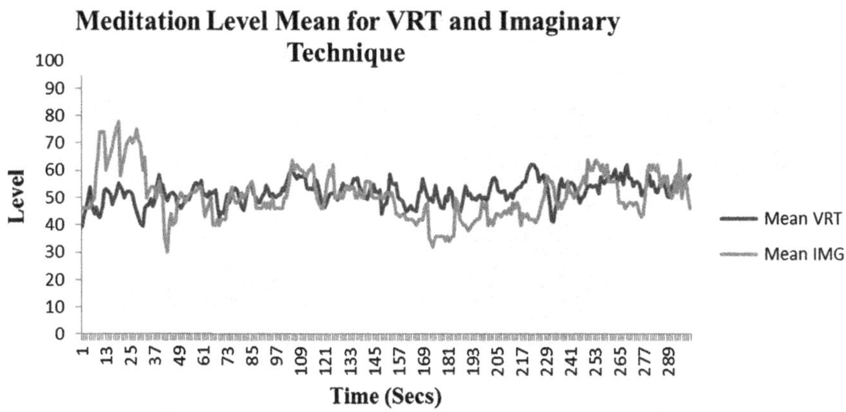

Fig. 4 Meditation Level Mean

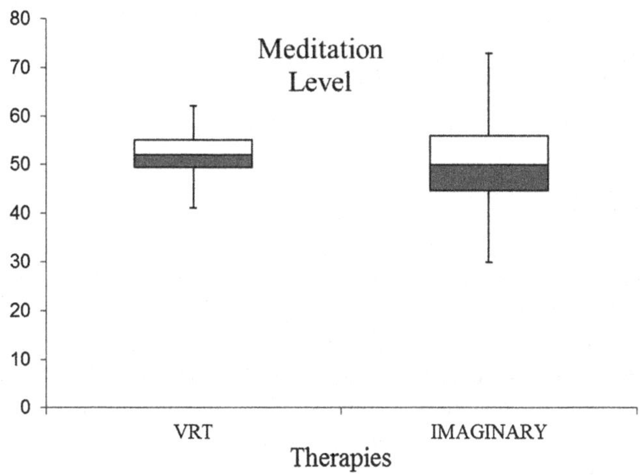

Fig. 5 Meditation Levels in Different Techniques

in Table 1, this range suggests that the participants are at the "neutral" state. The meditation level mean for both VRT and Imaginary session are shown in Fig. 6 which indicates the meditation level effectiveness.

A t-test analysis between the two therapies technique (i.e. VRT and Imaginary) was conducted for the 15 participants' mean meditation value at each second. Based on this analysis, the p-value for VRT and imaginary technique is shown in Table 2. The analysis shows that there is a significant different where it suggests that VRT technique has been more effective between the therapies.

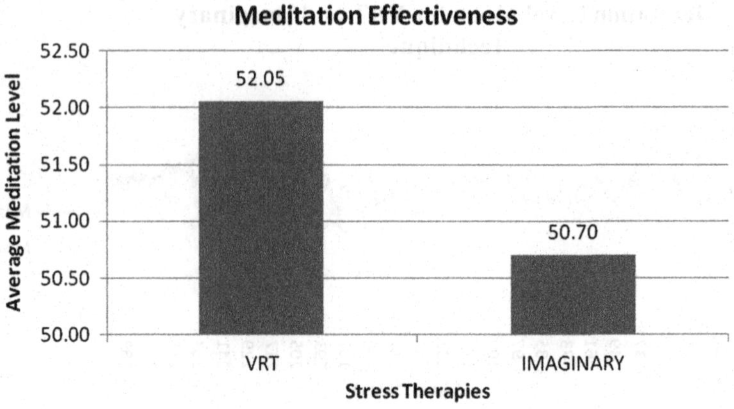

Fig. 6 The eSense Meditation level Mean

Table 2 p-Value of VRT and Imaginary Technique (95 % Confident Interval)

p-Value
6.772e-03

6 Conclusion

Several conclusions can be derived from the findings on study of meditation effectiveness for virtual reality based stress therapy and imaginary technique using EEG Measurement and Questionnaire Approaches: First, based on questionnaire approach referred to [5], the participants' result concluded that the VRT to be more effective compared to Imaginary technique. Next, the measurement of meditation level using EEG approach results a stable neutral state (40–70) for VRT which means a positive effectiveness of stress therapy compared to fluctuating result (20–80) in imaginary technique. In conclusion, both result from EEG and questionnaire reflected that VRT is more effectiveness for stress therapy. Note that the findings using questionnaire is not being discussed in detail here. Please refer research [5] which carried out using the same methodologies on a similar platforms (i.e. VRT and Imaginary). This also suggest that EEG produces a similar result to questionnaire and data collected from the EEG is valid and reliable for experimental purposes.

References

1. Gaware, V.M., Chavanke, A., Dolas, R.T.: Stress and its management. A Review **661**(2), 155–180 (2013)
2. Singh, D.P.: Control of workplace stress : a study. Int. J. Educ. Appl. Res. **2**(2), 165–172 (2012)
3. Difede, J., Cukor, J., Cukor, J., Jayasinghe, N., Jayasinghe, N., Patt, I., Jedel, S., Spielman, L., Giosan, C., Hoffman, H.G.: Virtual reality exposure therapy for the treatment of posttraumatic stress disorder following September 11, 2001. J. Clin. Psychiatry **68**(11), 1639–1647 (2007)
4. Baños, R.M., Guillen, V., Quero, S., García-Palacios, A., Alcaniz, M., Botella, C.: A virtual reality system for the treatment of stress-related disorders: a preliminary analysis of efficacy compared to a standard cognitive behavioral program. Int. J. Hum Comput Stud. **69**(9), 602–613 (2011)
5. Mahalil, I., Rusli, M. E., Yusof, A. M., Zaliman, M., Yusof, M., Razieff, A. R.: Virtual Reality-based Technique for Stress Therapy, pp. 295–300 (2014)
6. Nunez, P.L.: The brain wave equation: a model for the EEG. Math. Biosci. **21**(3–4), 279–297 (1974)
7. Neurovigil, Inc—iBrain Device. http://neurovigil.com/index.php/technology/ibrain-device. Accessed 20-May 2015
8. Emotiv I EEG System I Electroencephalography. https://emotiv.com/. Accessed 20 May 2015
9. Biosensors and Algorithms I ECG I EEG I NeuroSky. http://neurosky.com/. Accessed 20 May 2015
10. EEG Analyzer. http://store.neurosky.com/products/eeg-analyzer. Accessed 12 May 2015
11. Burdea, G.C., Coiffet, P.: Virtual Reality Technology, Volume 1. Wiley, New York (2003)
12. Neurosky, NeuroSky's eSense ™ Meters and Detection of Mental State, pp. 1–5 (2009)
13. Casement, M.D., Swanson, L.M.: A meta-analysis of imagery rehearsal for post-trauma nightmares: effects on nightmare frequency, sleep quality, and posttraumatic stress. Clin. Psychol. Rev. **32**(6), 566–574 (2012)
14. Rose, F. D.: Virtual reality in rehabilitation following traumatic brain injury. In: 1st European Conference on Disability, Virtual Reality Association and technology, pp. 5–12 (1996)
15. Parsons, T.D., Rizzo, A.A.: Affective outcomes of virtual reality exposure therapy for anxiety and specific phobias: a meta-analysis. J. Behav. Ther. Exp. Psychiatry **39**(3), 250–261 (2008)
16. Bayliss, J.D., Ballard, D.H.: A virtual reality testbed for brain-computer interface research. IEEE Trans. Rehabil. Eng. **8**(2), 188–190 (2000)
17. Bayliss, J.D.: Use of the evoked potential P3 component for control in a virtual apartment. IEEE Trans. Neural Syst. Rehabil. Eng. **11**(2), 113–116 (2003)
18. Murugappan, M., Rizon, M., Nagarajan, R., Yaacob, S., Zunaidi, I., Hazry, D.: EEG feature extraction for classifying emotions using FCM and FKM. Int. J. Comput. Commun. **1**(2), 21–25 (2007)
19. Derogatis Tests .Com. http://www.derogatis-tests.com/dsp_synopsis.asp. Accessed 21 May 2015
20. Report F., Iyengar, D.: Improving Players 'Control Over the Neurosky Brain-Computer Interface (2011)
21. ThinkGear Connector User Guide, (2010)
22. Al-Barrak, L., Kanjo, E.: NeuroPlace: making sense of a place. In: 4th Augmented Human International Conference Augmented, pp. 186–189 (2013)
23. Redza, A., Zainudin, R., Yusof, A. M., Rusli, M. E., Zaliman, M., Yusof, M., Mahalil, I.: Stress treatment: the effectiveness between guided and non-guided virtual reality setup, pp. 374–379 (2014)
24. Neurosky, MindWave User Guide (2011)
25. Mahalil, I., Rusli, M. E., Yusof, A. M., Zaliman, M., Yusoff, M., Razieff, A. R.: Study of Immersion Effectiveness in VR-based stress therapy, pp. 380–384 (2014)

Part VI
Statistical Signal Processing and Artificial Intelligence

Late Onset Bipolar Disorder Versus Alzheimer Disease

Darya Chyzhyk, Marina Graña-Lecuona and Manuel Graña

Abstract The aging of population is increasing the prevalence of some previously rare neuropathological condition, such as the Late Onset of Bipolar Disorder (LOBD). Bipolar Disorder appears at youth or even earlier in life, so that its appearance at sixty years or later is a rare event that can be confused with degenerative diseases such as Alzheimer's Disease (AD). A study designed inby the Hospital Universitario de Alava devoted to find diagnostic differences between these populations, in order to help improve diagnostic accuracy. In this paper we comment on some of the works that we have been carrying on this data.

1 Introduction

Bipolar disorder (BD) is a chronic mood disorder associated with cognitive, affective and functional impairment, often appearing at youth (around age 20 years), or even earlier [13], which has been considered as a risk factor for developing dementia [14, 15]. However, dementia syndrome arising as a result of a history of bipolarity does not correspond to the criteria of Alzheimer's disease (AD) [7]. On the other hand, late onset (i.e. age > 60 years) of BD [6] poses diagnostic quandaries in clinical practice, as it may be difficult to differentiate from behavioral impairment associated with Alzheimer's disease (AD), because both are progressive neuropsychiatric illnesses with overlapping symptoms and neuropathology, including cognitive impairment, emotional disturbances, neuroinflammation, excitotoxicity and upreg-

M. Graña-Lecuona · M. Graña · D. Chyzhyk (✉)
Computational Intelligence Group, University of the Basque Country,
UPV/EHU, San Sebastian, Spain
e-mail: daria.chizhik@gmail.com

M. Graña
ENGINE Centre, Wrocław University of Technology,
Wybrzeże Wyspiańskiego 27, 50-370 Wrocław, Poland

D. Chyzhyk
CISE Department, University of Florida, Gainesville, USA

Y.-W. Chen et al. (eds.), *Innovation in Medicine and Healthcare 2015*,
Smart Innovation, Systems and Technologies 45,
DOI 10.1007/978-3-319-23024-5_34

ulated brain metabolism [17]. While the established viewpoint considers that AD and BD are distinct and unrelated clinical entities, there is a trend in recent years to question whether there is a link between both disorders based on the overlapping symptoms and the increased successful use of BD well-established treatments to treat dementia [3, 9]. Inflammation and oxidative stress have been found as common pathopshysiological processes underlying AD [1, 19] and BD [8, 10, 11], as well as many other neuropsychological illness, such as depression and mania [5]. These disorders seem to be epigenetically linked to decrease transcriptional activity. It has been observed that in BD and AD patients the frontal cortex exhibits an altered epigenetic regulation related to neuroinflammation, synaptic integrity and neuroprotection. Contributing oxidative stress to the pathogenesis of both diseases through similar mechanisms. New findings identifying the relative role of inflammation and the localization of effects could help in identifying new therapeutic routes for treatment and diagnosis. The study was designed to investigate the feasibility of identifying these effects differentiating LOBD from AD by means of machine learning approaches, either on the clinical variables or imaging data or both. The approach is closely related to predictive CAD systems, which have been proposed to improve the diagnostic accuracy complementing the neuropsychological assessments carried out by expert clinicians [18, 20, 21].

The paper structure is as follows: Sect. 2 contains a description of the materials of the study, including patient population, imaging performed and other variables gathered for the study. Section 3 contains a description of the kind of computational processes tested on these data, with some overall results. Section 4 gives our conclusions.

2 Materials

Patients with memory complaints included in the present study with AD and LOBD were referred to the psychiatric unit at Alava University Hospital, Vitoria from the hospital catchment area. All patients were living independently in the community. Healthy volunteers with an MMSE score of >26 were either recruited from the community through advertisements, or nonrelated members of the patient's families or caregiver's relatives. Selected subjects underwent a standard protocol including: clinical evaluation, a cognitive and a neuropsychological evaluation, and brain imaging (MRI). Cognitive status was screened in all groups with the Mini-mental State Examination (MMSE) and Cambridge cognitive examination (CAMCOG). All patients gave their written consent to participate in the study, which was conducted according to the provisions of the Helsinki declaration. After written informed consent was obtained, venous blood samples (10 mL) were collected from the volunteers, after which all the MRI imaging, mood scales and cognitive tests were performed.

Fifty-seven elderly subjects were included in the present study. The subjects were divided in three groups. The AD group included 20 subjects fulfilling the

NINDS-ADRDA criteria for probable AD. The BD group included 12 subjects fulfilling DSM IV's criteria [14], all of them were bipolar I with a late onset of the disease. The healthy control group included 25 subjects without memory complaints. Subjects with psychiatric disorders (i.e. major depression) or other conditions (i.e. brain tumors) were not considered for this study. Demographic information for AD, BD, HC subjects, respectively: Age mean(SD) years is 78.65 (4.79), 69.55(7.58), 71.65 (8.55). Gender male/female 8/12, 7/5, 12/13. MMSE scores 19 (14–24), 25 (22–28), 29 (27–30). CAMCOG (mean, SD) 58.68 (19.50), 75.36 (11.40), 92.88 (8.14). Medications (n) Lithium (0, 0, 0), Risperidone (3, 3, 0), Quetiapine (1, 3, 0), Olanzapine (0,3,0). Patients were functionally assessed by the Functional Assessment Staging procedure (FAST). Patients with greater functional impairment show increments in cognitive loss. FAST ranks patients in 16 stages. Stage 1 marks subjects without difficulties, while Stage 7(f) marks patients unable to hold up his/her head. The last eleven stages are subdivisions of FAST between the late stages 6 and 7. FAST was administered by the study clinician.

Structural MRI and Diffusion-weighted imaging (DWI) data were obtained on a 1.5 T scanner (Magnetom Avanto, Siemens). Study protocol consists of 3D T1-weighted acquisition (isometric $1 \times 1 \times 1$ mm, 176 slices, TR = 1900 ms, TE = 337 ms and FOV = 256/76 %), a 3D Flair sequence (isometric $1 \times 1 \times 1$ mm, 176 slices, TR = 5000 ms, TE = 333 ms and FOV = 260/87.5%) and diffusion weighted sequence (slice thickness = 5 mm, 19 slices, TR = 2700 ms, TE = 88 ms, matrix 120/100, 3 averages, b = 1000 and 30 gradient directions) allowing fast acquisition minimizing the risk movement artifacts due to the agitated nature of the subjects [12].

Diffusion-weighted imaging (DWI) is an MRI method that produces in vivo MR images of biological tissues weighted with the local characteristics of water diffusion, allowing to study the integrity of the WM fibers [2, 16]. Diffusion is a real-valued second order tensor that can be estimated from the DWI signals obtained using six or more non-collinear gradient directions. The visualization of the diffusion tensor at each voxel site represented in its eigen-vector coordinate system with eigen-values is called Diffusion tensor imaging (DTI). Scalar measures of water diffusion computed from DTI are the fractional anisotropy (FA), mean diffusivity (MD), radial diffusivity (RD), and others giving information about the magnitude of the diffusion process at each voxel, but losing directional information. Data preprocessing, except non-linear registration, have been performed using FSL software (http://www.fmrib.ox.ac.uk/fsl/), includes skull stripping, affine and non-linear registration, eddy current correction of DWI, and corregistration between structural and diffusion data for localization.

For each subject in the study, we have measured the following 3 categories of non-imaging variables. In order to reduce circularity effects, variable normalization (standardization) was carried out independently at each cross-validation folder. Neuropsychological variables (NEURO): Cognitive performance has been assessed with a battery of neuropsychological tests covering the following cognitive domains: executive function, learning and memory, and attention. The index for each cognitive domain is the mean of the standardized scores of the tests covering that domain. Biological markers (BIO): We selected biological markers for analysis based on the relevant BD and AD literature, such as studies on inflammation. After extracting plasma from blood samples inflammatory cytokines Interleukins 1 and 6 (IL-1, IL-6) and Tumor Necrosis Factor (TNFα) were determined by enzyme immunoassay (EIA). Clinical observations (CLIN): The Neuropsychiatric Inventory (NPI) [34] was developed to provide a means of assessing neuropsychiatric symptoms and psychopathology of patients with Alzheimer's disease and other neurodegenerative disorders. The NPI assesses 10 (10-item NPI) or 12 (2-item NPI) behavioral domains common in dementia.

3 Summary Description of Methods

The analysis performed has been in general a process of feature extraction and classification, where we try to identify the most discriminant features as the most significative from the point of view of the biological understanding of the differences between LOBD and AD and providing insights into the mechanisms. The study of the ancillary variables, that is, the ones describing the clinical, neurological and blood biomarkers, has not been very conclusive. In fact, the best classification result is achieved when the clinical variables are used for classification with several state-of-the-art classifiers. Clinical achieves 85 % accuracy in a 10-fold cross-validation procedure, while adding other variables to the feature classification set does not improve results. The biological biomarkers are very poor discriminants (below 70 % accuracy in 10-fold cross-validation), which is consistent with the hypothesis that LOBD and AD share the inflammation as the biological process underlying the symptoms. However, the clinical classification results involve some degree of circularity, because they are directly correlated with the diagnostic decision. For instance, the importance of variables shown in Fig. 1 computed on a CART tree for the discrimination of controls versus LOBD patients, shows that FAST is the most important measure, which is not uncorrelated with the diagnostic decision. On the other hand, the inflammation biomarkers have surprisingly low discriminant power.

Regarding image data, our general procedure has consisted in selecting significant voxels from the volumes which are then used as features for classification. The classification results are some kind of post-hoc analysis providing the value of the selected pixels. We have found that DTI data is most discriminant than anatomical information. In the first works, [3] the selection process was performed on the FA and MD voxel representation, achieving surprisingly high classification, i.e. 100 % accuracy with SVM classifiers in a leave-one-out process. The feature selection process consisted in computing the Pearson's correlation between the categorical variable and the voxel value across subjects. The distribution of the absolute values is used to select the voxels having values above some percentile of the distribution. Changing the percentile provides feature vectors of different sizes. In this regard some circularity of the analysis leads to the high classification results shown in Fig. 2, because we are selecting pixels which are either correlated or anticorrelated with the classification of the volume.

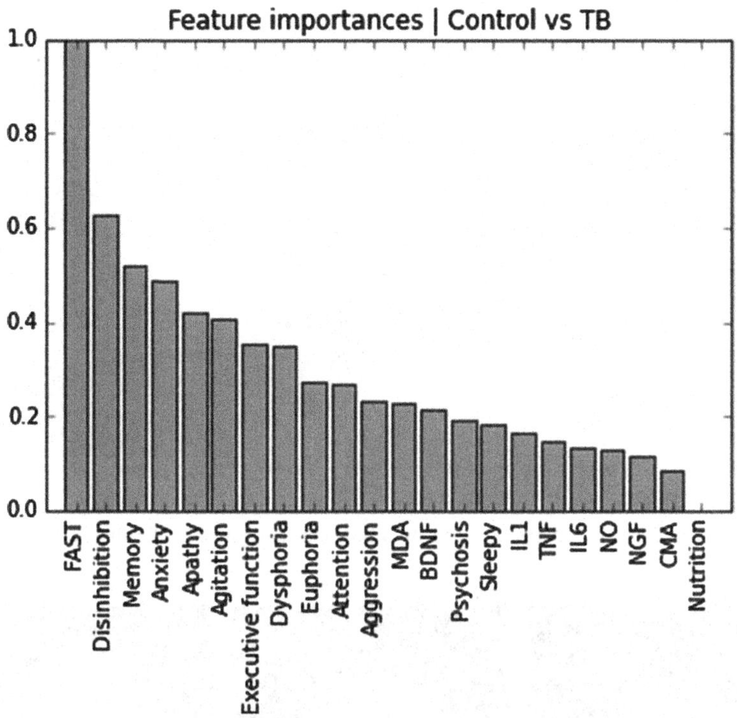

Fig. 1 Importance of ancillary variables in the discrimination of HC versus LOBD

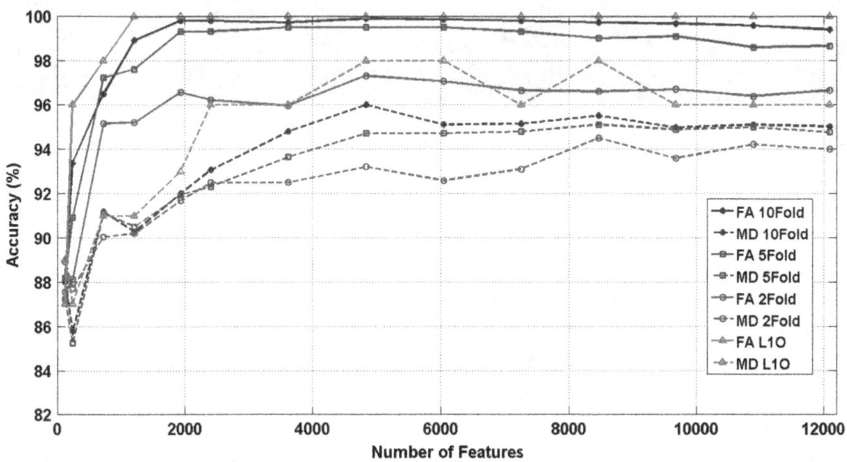

Fig. 2 Average accuracy on FA and MD data in the discrimination of LOBD versus AD reported in [3] for increasing feature vector size and cross-validation number of folders. L1O means Leave-one-out cross-validation

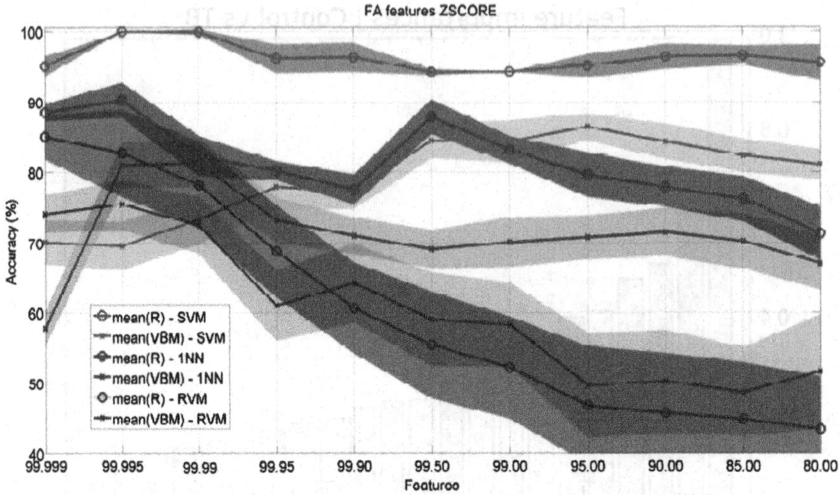

Fig. 3 Comparison of features obtained by VBM and the residuals of lattice autoassociative memories

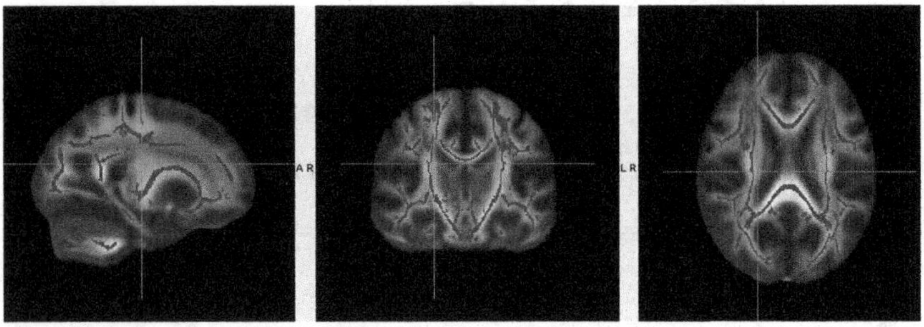

Fig. 4 TBSS preliminary results on the discrimination of LOBD and AD on FA data

Another process consisted in the computation of a lattice associative memory recall residuals as the features for classification [22], the lattice associative memory is built to store complete volumes, so that they can be recalled from the memory, serving also as content addressable storage. The selection of the residuals for classification is performed by Pearson's correlation and compared with other feature extraction. The comparison with feature selection based on a Voxel Based Morphometry (VBM) shows enhanced results, as can be appreciated in Fig. 3. Therefore, diffusion information which is relevant to the integrity of the white matter seems to provide strong clues to the discrimination of LOBD and AD.

Further analysis [4] has been then carried by performing the selection of voxels highly correlated with biomarker variables, by means of the eigenanatomy approach which performs canonical correlation analysis to find sparse eigendecomposition of the data, where the selected voxels can be used as features for classification. That way we test the feasibility of finding which brain white matter locations are more discriminant. Moreover, blood biomarker can be giving some clue as to what it is happening in the brain at the molecular level. Results find that regions of the brain highly correlated with the oxidative biomarker MDA are the most discriminant, however results are far from the 100 % accuracy.

4 Conclusions and Further Work

The discrimination of LOBD and AD is an interesting problem, because they share many cognitive traits, and biological causes, such as inflammation. In fact, our results on the ancillary variables, i.e. clinical, neurological tests and biological markers are rather disappointing, suggesting the difficulty of the problem at hand. The imaging data seems to be more fruitful, giving good results in some cases and pointing to localization that may give clues for medical research. We are still processing and working on the data. For instance, new results applying track based statistics (TBSS) illustrated in Fig. 4 are on the way, and may give further clues to the understanding of the subtle differences between LOBD and AD.

Acknowledgments The data was provided by A Besga from Hospital Universitario de Alava according to ethical committee permissions. This research has been partially funded by grant TIN2011-23823 of the Ministerio de Ciencia e Innovación of the Spanish Government (MINECO), with FEDER funds. The Basque Government grant IT874-13 for the research group. Manuel Graña was supported by EC under FP7, Coordination and Support Action, Grant Agreement Number 316097, ENGINE European Research Centre of Network Intelligence for Innovation Enhancement. Darya Chyzhyk has been supported by Basque Government post-doctoral grant No. Ref.: POS-2014-1-2, MOD:POSDOC.

References

1. Akiyama, H., Barger, S., Barnum, S., Bradt, B., Bauer, J., Cole, G., et al.: Inflammation and Alzheimer's disease. Neurobiol. Aging **21**(3), 383–421 (2000)
2. Basser, P.J., Mattiello, J., LeBihan, D.: MR diffusion tensor spectroscopy and imaging. Biophys. J. **66**(1), 259–267 (1994)
3. Besga, A., Termenon, M., Graña, M., Echeveste, J., Perez, J., Gonzalez-Pinto, A.: Discovering Alzheimer's disease and bipolar disorder white matter effects building computer aided diagnostic systems on brain diffusion tensor imaging features. Neurosci. Lett. **520**(1), 71–76 (2012)
4. Besga-Basterra, A., Chyzhyk, D., González-Ortega, I., Savio, A., Ayerdi, B., Echeveste, J., Graña, M., González-Pinto, A.: White matter anatomical correlates with biomarkers discriminating between Alzheimer's disease and late onset bipolar disorder by eigenanatomy on fractional anisotropy imaging. Curr. Alzherimer Res. (2015) (in press)
5. Castanon, N., Lasselin, J., Capuron, L.: Neuropsychiatric comorbidity in obesity: role of inflammatory processes. Neuroendocr. Sci. **5**, 74 (2014)
6. Depp, C., Jeste, D.: Bipolar disorder in older adults: a critical review. Bipolar Disord. **6**, 343–367 (2004)

7. Forcada, I., Mur, M., Mora, E., Vieta, E., Bartras-Faz, D., Portella, M.: The influence of cognitive reserve on psychosocial and neuropsychological functioning in bipolar disorder. Eur. Neuropsychopharmacol. **25**(2), 214–222 (2015)
8. Goldstein, B., Kemp, D., Soczynska, J., McIntyre, R.: Inflammation and the phenomenology, pathophysiology, comorbidity, and treatment of bipolar disorder: a systematic review of the literature. J. Clin. Psychiatry **70**(8), 1078–1090 (2009)
9. Graña, M., Termenon, M., Savio, A., Gonzalez-Pinto, A., Echeveste, J., Pérez, J.M., Besga, A.: Computer aided diagnosis system for Alzheimer disease using brain diffusion tensor imaging features selected by pearson's correlation. Neurosci. Lett. **502**(3), 225–229 (2011)
10. Leboyer, M., Soreca, I., Scott, J., Frye, M., Henry, C., Tamouza, R., Kupfer, D.: Can bipolar disorder be viewed as a multi-system inflammatory disease? J. Affect. Disord. **141**(1), 1–10 (2012)
11. Lee, S.Y., Chen, S.L., Chang, Y.H., Chen, P., Huang, S.Y.: Inflammation's association with metabolic profiles before and after a twelve-week clinical trial in drug-naive patients with bipolar II disorder. PLoS One **8**(6), e66847 (2013)
12. Liu, Y., Spulber, G., et al.: Diffusion tensor imaging and tract-based spatial statistics in Alzheimer's disease and mild cognitive impairment. Neurobiol. Aging **32**, 1558–1571 (2011)
13. Martinez-Cengotitabengoa, M., Mico, J., Arango, C., Castro-Fornieles, J., Graell, M., Paya, B., et al.: Basal low antioxidant capacity correlates with cognitive deficits in early onset psychosis. a 2-year follow-up study. Schizophr. Res. **156**(1), 23–29 (2014)
14. Ng, B., Camacho, A., et al.: A case series on the hypothesized connection between dementia and bipolar spectrum disorders: bipolar type VI? J. Affect. Disord. **107**(1–3), 307–315 (2008)
15. Ng, B., Camacho, A., Lara, D., Brunstein, M., Pinto, O., Akiskal, H.: A case series on the hypothesized connection between dementia and bipolar spectrum disorders: bipolar type VI? J. Affect. Disord. **107**(307–315) (2008)
16. Pierpaoli, C., Jezzard, P., Basser, P.J., Barnett, A., Di Chiro, G.: Diffusion tensor MR imaging of the human brain. Radiology **201**(3), 637–648 (1996)
17. Rao, J., Harry, G., Rapoport, S., Kim, H.: Increased excitotoxicity and neuroinflammatory markers in postmortem frontal cortex from bipolar disorder patients. Mol. Psychiatry **15**, 384–392 (2010)
18. Salas-Gonzalez, D., Górriz, J.M., Ramírez, J., López, M., Illan, I.A., Segovia, F., Puntonet, C.G., Gómez-Río, M.: Analysis of SPECT brain images for the diagnosis of Alzheimer's disease using moments and support vector machines. Neurosci. Lett. **461**(1), 60–64 (2009)
19. Sardi, F., Fassina, L., Venturini, L., Inguscio, M., Guerriero, F., Rolfo, E., Ricevuti, G.: Alzheimer's disease, autoimmunity and inflammation. the good, the bad and the ugly. Autoimmun. Rev. **11**(2), 149–153 (2011)
20. Savio, A., Chyzhyk, M.G.S.D., Hernandez, C., Graña, M., Sistiaga, A., Lopez de Munain, A., Villanua, J.: Neurocognitive disorder detection based on feature vectors extracted from VBM analysis of structural MRI. Comput. Biol. Med. **41**, 600–610 (2011)
21. Segovia, F., Górriz, J.M., Ramírez, J., Salas-González, D., Álvarez, I., López, M., Chaves, R., Padilla, P.: Classification of functional brain images using a GMM-based multi-variate approach. Neurosci. Lett. **474**(1), 58–62 (2010)
22. Termenon, M., Graña, M., Besga, A., Echeveste, J., Gonzalez-Pinto, A.: Lattice independent component analysis feature selection on diffusion weighted imaging for Alzheimer's disease classification. Neurocomputing **114**, 132–141 (2013)

Short-term Prediction of MCI to AD Conversion Based on Longitudinal MRI Analysis and Neuropsychological Tests

Juan Eloy Arco, Javier Ramírez, Juan Manuel Górriz, Carlos G. Puntonet and María Ruz

Abstract Nowadays, 35 million people worldwide suffer from some form of dementia. Given the increase in life expectancy it is estimated that in 2035 this number will grow to 115 million. Alzheimer's disease is the most common cause of dementia and it is of great importance diagnose it at an early stage. This is the main goal of this work, the development of a new automatic method to predict the mild cognitive impairment (MCI) patients who will develop Alzheimer's disease within one year or, conversely, its impairment will remain stable. This technique will analyze data from both magnetic resonance imaging and neuropsychological tests by utilizing a t-test for feature selection, maximum-uncertainty linear discriminant analysis (MLDA) for classification and leave-one-out cross validation (LOOCV) for evaluating the performance of the methods, which achieved a classification accuracy of 73.95 %, with a sensitivity of 72.14 % and a specificity of 73.77 %.

1 Introduction

The ability to diagnose and predict Alzheimer's disease (AD) at an early stage has great impact on the possibility for improving treatment choices of this disease. For this reason, in recent years there has been a large increase in the number of studies attempting to develop systems that help in the diagnosis of AD [1–4]. In [5], a technique was proposed for predicting future clinical changes of MCI patients by using both baseline and longitudinal multimodality data. The main drawback of this

J.E. Arco (✉) · M. Ruz
Department of Experimental Psychology, University of Granada, Granada, Spain
e-mail: jearco@correo.ugr.es

J. Ramírez · J.M. Górriz
Department of Signal Theory Networking and Communications,
University of Granada, Granada, Spain

C.G. Puntonet
Department of Architecture and Computer Technology, University of Granada,
18071 Granada, Spain

Y.-W. Chen et al. (eds.), *Innovation in Medicine and Healthcare 2015*,
Smart Innovation, Systems and Technologies 45,
DOI 10.1007/978-3-319-23024-5_35

study is the request of having multimodality data across different time points for each subject, which limits the size of subjects that can be used for the study. Most existing research focuses on only a single modality of biomarkers for diagnosis of AD and MCI, although recent studies have shown that different biomarkers may provide complementary information for the diagnosis of AD and MCI [6, 7].

Despite the brilliant solutions presented by these approaches, all of them are focused on classifying AD or MCI patients from healthy controls. Since the earlier the diagnosis of this disease, the more effective the treatment, in this study we propose a method to compare between MCI patients who had converted to AD within 12 months and MCI patients who had not converted to AD within 12 months, in order to predict whether the patient will develop the disease or not. Once the images have been preprocessed, the whole brain is then partitioned into 116 regions of interest (ROIs) in terms of the Automated Anatomical Labeling (AAL) atlas, and the mean intensity and standard deviation value of each region was acquired by averaging the intensities and standard deviations values within that region. These extracted values along with the two neuropsychological tests (MMSE and ADAS-Cog) make the dataset. To reduce its size, a Student's t-test selects the most important features, i.e. those with greater discrimination power. Once this is achieved, MLDA algorithm is used for classification, evaluating the performance with a Leave-One-Out cross validation technique (LOOCV).

The organization of the rest of the paper is as follows. Details or our method based on both MR images and neuropsychological tests and MLDA algorithm for classification are mentioned below. A description of the data used in the preparation of this article is done in Sect. 2. The method consists of four stages. In Sect. 3.1 we focus on the source of information, which is based on an anatomical atlas for MRI and direct scores in the case of neuropsychological tests. It is necessary to select the right features not to overtrain the system, since this can cause a decrease in its performance and an increase in the computation time. That is the purpose of Student's t-test, which is described in Sect. 3.1. The classification algorithm and the techniques to evaluate its performance are available in Sect. 3.3. The experimental results are provided in Sect. 5, and a discussion of research contributions and practical advantages in addition to the conclusions are available in Sects. 6 and 7.

2 Database

The data used in the preparation of this article were obtained from the Alzheimer's Disease Neuroimaging Initiative (ADNI) database. The primary goal of ADNI has been to test whether serial MRI, PET, other biological markers, and clinical and neuropsychological assessments can be combined to measure the progression of MCI and early AD. Determination of sensitive and specific markers of very early AD progression is intended to aid researchers and clinicians to develop new treatments and monitor their effectiveness, as well as lessen the time and cost of clinical trials. In this paper, only ADNI subjects with all corresponding MRI, MMSE and ADAS-Cog baseline data are included. This yields a total of 134 MCI subjects who had at least three longitudinal scans (baseline image, and two subsequent images six months and twelve months after) including 73 MCI converters who had converted to AD within 12 months and 61 non-converters who had not converted to AD within 12 months.

3 Methods

3.1 Feature Extraction

In Alzheimer's disease, the hippocampus is one of the first regions of the brain to become damaged and that is why it is used as a marker of early AD in a vast number of studies, therefore it is logical that some approaches focus on the study of changes in it. In [8], the classification accuracy of a system was tested using the hippocampal volume as an only feature. Volumes were normalized by the total intracranial volume computed by summing SPM5 segmentation, averaging left and right volumes for more robustness with respect to segmentation errors as proposed in [9]. Hippocampal shape is another feature used in other approaches. More specifically, [10] described a new method to automatically discriminate between patients with Alzheimer's disease or mild cognitive impairment using spherical harmonics (SPHARM) coefficients to model the shape of the hippocampi. These coefficients are a mathematical approach to represent surfaces with spherical topology, which can be seen as a 3D analog of Fourier series expansion.

Another approach is based on a labeled atlas for grouping the voxels into anatomical regions and was employed in [11]. The number of available atlases is large but this work uses AAL (Automated Anatomical Labeling), [12], a predefined anatomical atlas formed by 116 regions of interest (ROI), meaning which has not been specifically designed for studying patients with AD so its areas do not necessarily represent pathologically homogeneous regions. Once the structural images were segmented into gray matter density (GMD) and white matter density (WMD), individual GMD and WMD maps were partitioned into the 116 regions of AAL. Then both the mean and standard deviation of the GMD/WMD values of each region was then extracted by averaging the GMD/WMD values of all voxels within that region. Thus, each subject has a total of 464 features from grey matter and white matter images and 2 more features from neuropsychological tests, resulting on 466 features for each session.

3.2 Feature Selection

Not all the features are equally effective. Some of them may become irrelevant or redundant for the classification process. From this arises the necessity to select a small set of features with the greatest discriminative power to improve the performance of the final classifier [13, 14] and to speed up computation [15, 16]. PCA (Principal component analysis, [17]) and ICA (Independent component analysis, [18]) are two methods widely used in literature [19, 20]. The former is a statistical procedure that uses an orthogonal transformation to convert a set of observations of possibly correlated variables into a set of values of linearly uncorrelated variables, which are known as principal component. The latter focus on separating a multivariate signal into additive non-Gaussian and statistically independent subcomponents. However, a different approach was adopted in this work, using a filter ranking based on two-sample two-tailed t-tests. For each feature of the complete data set, a decision test was performed for the null hypothesis that the data in features vector of both classes (MCI-C and MCI-NC) come from independent random samples from normal distributions with equal means but unknown variances, at the 5 % significance level. The alternative hypothesis is that the data in both vectors come from populations with unequal means. Mathematically, the test statistic is:

$$t = \frac{\overline{x} - \overline{y}}{\sqrt{\frac{S_1^2}{n} + \frac{S_2^2}{m}}} \tag{1}$$

where $\overline{x}$ and $\overline{y}$ are the means of each group, S_1 and S_2 are the sample standard deviations and n and m are the number of features for each group. This process was developed on the training set of each LOOCV fold. Thus, features whose p-values were less than the significance level were selected meaning that from the whole 116 brain regions, only 26 of them had an adequate discriminative power for use in the classification process (Fig. 1).

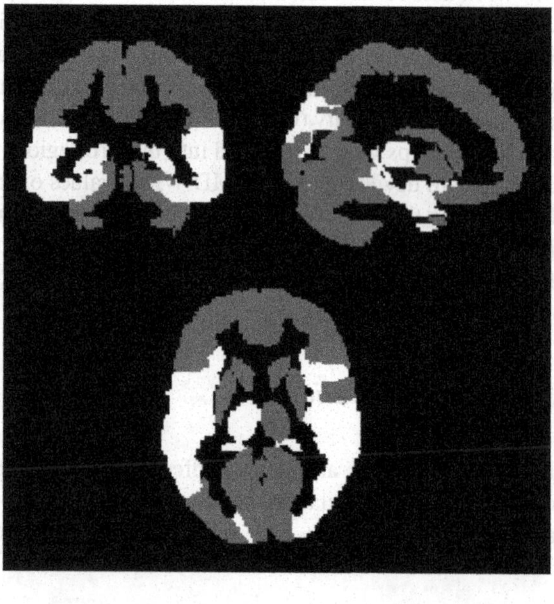

Fig. 1 Map of the brain regions chosen by the feature selection process (*white colour*). Some of the 28 areas with greater power of discrimination are the hippocampus, amygdala, thalamus, insula, temporal medial, temporal superior and occipital inferior

3.3 Classification

Although in the literature there are more commonly used algorithms (i.e., SVM), in this work a variation of Linear Discriminant Analysis (LDA) was employed. LDA is a classification method that projects high-dimensional data onto a line and performs classification in this one-dimensional space. The projection maximizes the distance between the means of the two classes while minimizing the variance within each class. This defines the Fisher criterion, which is maximized over all linear projections, w:

$$J(w) = \frac{|m_1 - m_2|^2}{s_1^2 + s_2^2} \tag{2}$$

where m represents a mean, s^2 represents a variance, and the subscripts denote the two classes. Therefore, the main objective of LDA is to find a projection matrix that maximizes the ratio of the determinant of the between-class scatter matrix to the determinant of the within-class scatter matrix. As in PCA, the eigenvalues are of great importance in the correct separation of the classes. Following the complete mathematical procedure described in [21], Eq. 2 can be rewritten as follows:

$$J(w) = \frac{w_k^T S_B w}{w_k^T S_W w} = \frac{\lambda_k w_k^T S_B w_k}{w_k^T S_W w_k} = \lambda_k \; con \; k = 1 \ldots d \tag{3}$$

where S_B is the "between classes scatter matrix", S_W is the "within classes scatter matrix" and w_k is the eigenvector associated to the eigenvalue λ_k. Consequently, to maximize the solution the eigenvector associated with the largest eigenvalue must be considered.

However, the traditional LDA cannot be directly used when the within-class scatter matrix is singular, as in the case of limited samples and high dimensional feature space. In this work, the dimension of feature space was still higher than the number of samples. In order to avoid these critical issues, [22] proposed a maximum uncertainty LDA-based approach (MLDA) to overcome the instability of the S_W matrix. It is based on the maximum entropy covariance selection method developed to improve quadratic classification performance on limited sample size problems.

The proposed method considers the issue of stabilizing the S_W estimate with a multiple of the identity matrix by selecting the largest dispersions regarding the S_W average eigenvalue. This selection algorithm expands only the smaller and consequently less reliable eigenvalues of within-class scatter matrix S_W. Thus, it is necessary to replace S_W matrix, as follows:

$$S_W^* = S_P^*(N - g) = (\Phi \Lambda^* \Phi^T)(N - g) \tag{4}$$

where S_P is the covariance matrix, Φ and Λ are the eigenvalues and eigenvectors of the covariance matrix, respectively, N is the number of training patterns from both classes and g is the total number of classes. It is a straightforward method that overcomes both the singularity and instability of the within-class scatter matrix S_W when LDA is used in limited sample and high dimensional problems, so that's the reason why we chose it for this work.

4 Performance Evaluation

In a general classification problem, the goal is to learn a classifier that performs well on unseen data drawn from the same distribution as the available data. One common way to estimate generalization capabilities is to measure the performance of the learned classifier on test data that has not been used to train the classifier. When a large test data set cannot be held out or easily acquired, resampling methods, such as cross validation, are commonly used to estimate the generalization error [23]. Leave-one-out cross validation (LOOCV) was used to estimate the performance of the classifier. LOOCV involves separating the data so in each iteration there is only a test data while the remaining data are used to train the classifier. This means that on every fold of LOOCV, the most discriminative features are calculated and projected onto a one-dimensional space to properly determine the label of the testing sample.

Other measures to evaluate the performance of a classifier can be extracted from the confusion matrix. Accuracy is the proportion of the total number of predictions that are correct. Secondly, sensitivity (or true positive rate) measures the proportion of actual positives which are correctly identified. And finally, specificity (also called the true negative rate) measures the proportion of negatives which are correctly identified. It is desirable to have a classifier that gives high values of these three measures. In [24], ROC curve illustrates the performance of a binary classification as its discrimination threshold is varied. The curve is created by plotting the true positive rate (i.e. sensitivity) against the false positive rate (that is, 1-specificity) at various thresholds settings. This area can be interpreted as the probability that given a couple of patients (in our case, a mci converter and a non-converter patient), our algorithm classify them properly.

$$Accuracy = \frac{TP + TN}{TP + FN + TN + FP} \tag{5}$$

$$Sensitivity = \frac{TP}{TP + FN} \tag{6}$$

$$Specificity = \frac{TN}{TN + FP} \tag{7}$$

5 Results

The aim of this work was the development of a completely automatic method for prediction of Alzheimer's disease and it has been broadly achieved. The experiments carried out on the database composed by both structural MRI (segmented into gray matter density and white matter density) and neuropsychological tests (MMSE and ADAS-Cog). Thus, in each session there are two measures (mean and standard deviation) for each region of both segmented images besides the two neuropsychological tests. Several trials were made combining the different features yielding a value of accuracy equal to 73.95 %, with a sensitivity of 74.14 %, a specificity of 73.77 % and an area under the ROC curve of 0.7923.

Table 1 shows the results obtained by the LDA classification algorithm when data from MRI images (means and deviations) and neuropsychological tests (MMSE and ADAS-Cog) are used as input features. For MCI converters patients, the data from one and two sessions before their conversions (i.e. six and twelve months before the conversion session respectively) can be used separately and in combination of both sessions. Besides, the average conversion session was calculated for all these patients, resulting that this was the fourth session (month 18 of the longitudinal analysis). Therefore, the data used for MCI non converters patients were those relating to the second and the third sessions.

The results show that we can predict more reliably the development of Alzheimer's disease 6 months before it appears instead of 12 months before the diagnosis of this disease, something which otherwise is logical. Regarding the use of means and deviations of each atlas region, there are no major differences between choosing one or

Table 1 Results obtained using gray matter, white matter and neuropsychological tests from sessions 6/12 months before conversion (MCI-converters) and combining data from both sessions

GRAY MATTER + WHITE MATTER				
Features used	Sensitivity (%)	Specificity (%)	Accuracy (%)	AUC
6 months before conversion				
Means + Tests	65.67	72.13	68.75	0.7913
Deviations + Tests	65.67	70.49	67.97	0.7962
Means + Deviations + Tests	65.67	72.13	68.75	0.7839
12 months before conversion				
Means + Tests	67.24	63.93	65.55	0.7671
Deviations + Tests	68.97	62.3	65.55	0.7646
Means+ Deviations + Tests	67.24	65.57	66.39	0.7674
6 + 12 months before conversion				
Means + Tests	74.14	73.77	73.95	0.7923
Deviations + Tests	72.41	73.77	73.11	0.7911
Means + Deviations + Tests	74.14	73.77	73.95	0.7925

the other. However, combining the data from two previous sessions to the diagnosis, both accuracy and specificity and sensitivity increases considerably (almost 10 percentage points), while the area under the ROC curve remained almost unchanged. A t-test was used to compare the different experiments, resulting in that they are statistically significant, with a *t-value* exceeding 600 and a *p-value* less than 0.0001.

6 Discussion

In this study, we introduce a new method for discriminating MCI patients who will be diagnosed with Alzheimer's disease (up to a year before that it happens) from MCI patients whose impairment will remain constant in this period of time. Using an atlas (AAL) for partitioning the brain into 116 anatomical regions, a t-test for feature selection and LDA as classification algorithm our method achieved a high accuracy (73.95 %), and the AUC was 0.79. Other methods [10, 20] achieved accuracies above 90 %, which are superior to those achieved in our work. It is necessary to clarify the complexity of the problem we faced and the great potential our method has shown. The development of an automated system for prediction of Alzheimer's disease in an early stage is not a new challenge. However, this work represents a step further in predicting this disease because only patients with mild cognitive impairment are considered, because subjects who developed Alzheimer's disease at some point in our study are only considered from sessions before conversion. Therefore, our method is able to find significant differences in patients whose clinical diagnosis is identical, using a very simple approach in which the features are based on statistical measures from anatomical regions of the brain.

Thus, this system can be used as an aid in the diagnosis of Alzheimer's disease because is fully automatic, so it is not required to choose a prior anatomical region where focuses the analysis since the entire brain is considered. The fact that it is only needed a nuclear magnetic resonance which is available in most of the diagnostic centers and that only a few minutes are necessary to collect the data from both neuropsychological tests are important advantages for using this technique for clinical diagnosis. A suggestion for future research might be to consider the contribution of each voxel separately, as Multi-Voxel Pattern Analysis (MVPA) proposes, a technique which allows to detect differences with higher sensitivity than conventional univariate analysis.

7 Conclusion

In the current study, we have developed a system to predict if MCI patients will develop Alzheimer's disease within a period of one year by combining data from magnetic resonance images (the mean and the standard deviation of each brain region proposed by the atlas AAL) and the results from two neuropsychological tests

(MMSE and ADAS-Cog), yielding an excellent performance (73.95 % accuracy and AUC = 0.79). This promising discrimination power suggests that this technique could be used as an aid in the diagnosis of AD, becoming a promising starting point for other more complex methods as multivariate pattern analysis. We conclude that it would be so interesting to repeat all the procedure of this work extracting the features from an anatomical atlas based on the most damaged regions by this disease instead of an anatomical atlas, since it could improve significantly the results.

Acknowledgments This work was partly supported by the MICINN under the TEC2012-34306 project and the Consejería de Innovación, Ciencia y Empresa (Junta de Andalucía, Spain) under the Excellence Project P11-TIC-7103.

References

1. Deskian, R.S., Cabral, H.J., Settecase, F., Hess, C.P., Dillon, W.P., Glastonbury, C.M., Weiner, M.W., Schmansky, N.J., Salat, D.H., Fischl, B., ADNI: Automated MRI measures predict progression to Alzheimer's disease. Neurobiol. Aging **31**(8), 1364–1374 (2010)
2. Liy, Y., Paajanen, T., Zhang, Y., Westman, E., Wahlund, L.O., Simmons, A., Tunnard, C., Sobow, T., Mecocci, P., Tsolaki, M., Vellas, B., Muehlboeck, S., Evans, A., Spenger, C., Lovestone, S., Soininen, H.: Automated MRI measures predict progression to Alzheimer's disease. Neurobiol. Aging **31(8)** (2010) 1375–1385
3. Chincarini, A., Bosco, P., Calvini, P., Gemme, G., Esposito, M., Olivieri, C., Rei, L., Squarcia, S., Rodriguez, G., Bellotti, R., Cerello, P., de Mitri, I., Retico, A., Nobili, F.: Local MRI analysis approach in the diagnosis of early and prodromal Alzheimer's disease. Neuroimage **102**(2), 657–665 (2011)
4. Nazeri, A., Ganjgahi, H., Roostaei, T., Nichols, T., Zarei, M.: Imaging proteomics for diagnosis, monitoring and prediction of Alzheimer's disease. Neuroimage **58**(12), 469–480 (2011)
5. Zhang, D., Shen, D., ADNI: Predicting future clinical changes of MCI patients using longitudinal and multimodal biomarkers. PLoS One **7(3)** (2012)
6. Apostolova, L.G., Hwang, K.S., Andrawis, J.P., Green, A.E., Babakchanian, S., Morra, J.H., Cummings, J.L., Toga, A.W., Trojanowski, J.Q., Shaw, L.M., Jr., Jack C.R., Jr., Petersen, R.C., Aisen, P.S., Jagust, W.J., Koeppe, R.A., Mathis, C.A., Weiner, M.W., Thompson, P.M.: 3D PIB and CSF biomarker associations with the hippocampal atrophy in ADNI subjects. Neurobiol. Aging **31** (2010) 1284–1303
7. Fjell, A.M., Walhovd, K.B., Fennema-Notestine, C., McEvoy, L.K., Hagler, D.J., Holland, D., Brewer, J.B., Dale, A.M.: CSF biomarkers in prediction of cerebral and clinical change in mild cognitive impairment and Alzheimer's disease. J. Neurosci. **30**, 2088–2101 (2010)
8. Cuingnet, R., Gerardin, E., Tessieras, J., Auzias, G., Lehricy, S., Habert, M., Chupin, M., Benali, H., Colliot, O., ADNI: Automatic classification of patients with Alzheimer's disease from structural MRI: a comparison of ten methods using the ADNI database. Neuroimage **56** (2011) 766–781
9. Chupin, M., Hammers, A., Liu, R., Colliot, O., Burdett, J., Bardinet, E., Duncan, J., Garnero, L., Lemieux, L.: Automatic segmentation of the hyppocampus and the amygdala driven by hybrid constraints: method and validation. Neuroimage **46**(3), 749–761 (2009a)
10. Geradin, R., Chtelat, G., Chupin, M., Cuingnet, R., Desgranges, B., Kim, H.S., Niethammer, M., Dubois, B., Lehricy, S., Garnero, L., Francis, E., Colliot, O.: Multidimensional classification of hippocampal shape features discriminates alzheimer's disease ang mild cognitive impairment from normal aging. Neuroimage **47(4)** (2009) 1476–1486

11. Magnin, B., Mesrob, L., Kinkingnéhun, S., Pélégrini-Isaac, M., Colliot, O., Sarazin, M., Dubois, B., Lehéricy, B., Benali, H.: Support vector machine-based classification of Alzheimer's disease from whole-brain anatomical mri. Neuroradiology **51**(2), 73–83 (2009)
12. Tzourio-Mayer, N., Landeau, B., Papathanassiou, D., Crivello, F., Etard, O., Delcroix, N., Mazoyer, B., Joliot, M.: Automated anatomical labeling of activations in SPM using a macroscopic anatomical parcellation of the MNI MRI single-subject brain. Neuroimage **15**, 273–289 (2002)
13. Yan, J., Li, T., Wang, H., Huand, H., Wan, J., Nho, K., Kim, S., Risacher, S., Saykin, A.J., Shen, L.: Cortical surface biomarkers for predicting cognitive outcomes using group l2,1 norm. Neurobiol. Aging **36**(1), S185–S193 (2015)
14. Raymer, M.L., Punch, W.F., Goodman, E.D., Kuhn, L.A., Jain, A.K.: Dimensionality reduction using genetic algorithms. IEEE Trans. Evolut. Comput. **4**(2), 164–171 (2002)
15. Cui, X., Beaver, J.M., Charles, J.S., Potok, T.E.: Dimensionality reduction particle swarn algorithm for high dimensional clustering. In: IEEE Swarm Intelligence Symposium, vol. 1, pp. 1–6 (2008)
16. Salcedo-Sanz, S., Pastor-Snchez, A., Prieto, L., Blanco-Aguilera, A., Garca-Herrera, R.: Feature selection in wind speed prediction systems based on a hybrid coral reefs optimization—extreme learning machine approach. Energy Convers. Manag. **87**, 10–18 (2014)
17. Jolliffe, I.T.: Principal Component Analysis, 2nd edn. Springer (1973)
18. Hyvärinen, A.: Fast and robust fixex-point algorithms for independent component analysis. IEEE Trans. Neural Netw. **10**, 626–634 (1999)
19. Álvarez, I., Górriz, J.M., Ramírez, J., Salas, D., López, M., Puntonet, C., Segovia, F.: Independent component analysis of spect images to assist the Alzhimer's disease diagnosis. In: The Sixth International Symposium on Neural Networks (ISSN 2009). Advances in Intelligent Soft Computing, vol. 56, pp. 411–419 (2009)
20. Dai, Z., Yan, C., Wang, Z., Wang, J., Xia, M., Li, K., He, Y.: Discriminative analysis of early Alzheimer's disease using multi-modal imaging and multi-level characterization with multi-classifier (m3). Neuroimage **59**(3), 2187–2195 (2012)
21. Welling, M.: Fisher Linear Discriminant Analysis. http://www.ics.uci.edu/~welling/classnotes/papers_class/Fisher-LDA.pdf (2010)
22. Thomaz, C., Boardman, J., Hil, D., Hajnal, J.V., Edwards, A., Rutherford, M., Gillies, D., Ruckert, D.: Whole brain voxel-based analysis using registration and multivariate statistics. In: Proceedings of the 8th Medical Image Understanding Analysis (MIUA'04), vol. 1, pp. 73–76 (2004)
23. Rao, R.B., Fung, G.: On the dangers of cross-validation. An experimental evaluation. Siemens Medical Solutions, 588–596 (2008)
24. Hanley, J.A., McNeill, B.J.: The meaning and use of the area under a receiver operating characteristic (ROC) curve. Radiology **143**(1), 29–36 (1982)

Ensemble Tree Learning Techniques for Magnetic Resonance Image Analysis

Javier Ramírez, Juan M. Górriz, Andrés Ortiz, Pablo Padilla and Francisco J. Martínez-Murcia for the Alzheimer Disease Neuroimaging Initiative

Abstract This paper shows a comparative study of boosting and bagging algorithms for magnetic resonance image (MRI) analysis and classification and the early detection of Alzheimer's disease (AD). The methods evaluated are based on a feature extraction process estimating first-order statistics from gray matter (GM) segmented MRI for a number of subcortical structures, and a learning process of an ensemble of decision trees. Several experiments were conducted in order to compare the performance of the generalization ability of the ensemble learning algorithms for different complexity classification tasks. The generalization error converges to a limit as the number of trees in the ensemble becomes large for boosting and bagging. It depends on the strength of the individual trees in the forest and the correlation between them. Bagging outperforms boosting algorithms in terms of classification error and convergence rate. The improvement of bagging over boosting techniques increases with the complexity of the classification task. Thus, bagging is better suited for discrimination of mild cognitive impairment (MCI) from healthy controls or AD subjects than boosting techniques.

1 Introduction

Alzheimer's disease (AD) is the most common type of dementia in the elderly. It accounts for an estimated 60–80 % of cases [1]. The hallmark pathologies of AD are the progressive accumulation of beta-amyloid plaques outside neurons in the brain and protein tau tangles inside neurons. Diagnosis of the AD is most commonly made by physicians who obtain a medical and family history, including psychiatric history and history of cognitive and behavioral changes. In addition, the physician conducts cognitive tests as well as physical and neurologic examinations including brain imaging techniques such as a magnetic resonance image (MRI) assessment.

J. Ramírez (✉) · J.M. Górriz · A. Ortiz · P. Padilla · F.J. Martínez-Murcia
Department of Signal Theory, Telematics and Communications University of Granada, 18071 Granada, Spain
e-mail: javierrp@ugr.es

Y.-W. Chen et al. (eds.), *Innovation in Medicine and Healthcare 2015*,
Smart Innovation, Systems and Technologies 45,
DOI 10.1007/978-3-319-23024-5_36

Boosting and bagging are popular methods for improving the accuracy of classification algorithms. They are based on a learning process of an ensemble consisting of weak learners. One of the most popular boosting algorithms is AdaBoost [2, 3], which has been applied in neuroimaging for MRI subcortical surface-based analysis [4], automated hippocampal segmentation [5] or automated mapping of hippocampal atrophy [6] in AD patients. However, no other boosting algorithms have been studied in depth for AD detection and/or compared with the AdaBoost algorithm. In this paper, a number of boosting algorithms are considered for MRI image analysis in an ensemble tree learning framework, and a study is carried out to compare then to bagging for different AD complexity classification tasks.

2 Materials and Methods

2.1 Dataset

Data used in the preparation of this article was obtained from the Alzheimer's disease neuroimaging initiative (ADNI) database (http://adni.loni.usc.edu/). The ADNI was launched in 2003 by the National Institute on Aging (NIA), the National Institute of Biomedical Imaging and Bioengineering (NIBIB), the Food and Drug Administration (FDA), private pharmaceutical companies and non-profit organizations, as a $60 million, 5-year public-private partnership. The primary goal of ADNI has been to test whether serial MRI, positron emission tomography (PET), other biological markers, and the progression of mild cognitive impairment (MCI), and early AD. Determining sensitive and specific markers of very early AD progression is intended to aid researchers and clinicians to develop new treatments, as well as reduce the time and cost of clinical trials. The Principal Investigator of this initiative is Michael W. Weiner, MD, VA Medical Center and University of California, San Francisco. ADNI is the result of efforts of many co-investigators from a broad range of academic institutions and private corporations, and subjects have been recruited from over 50 sites across the U.S. and Canada. The initial goal of ADNI was to recruit 800 adults, ages 55–90, to participate in the research: approximately 200 cognitively normal older individuals to be followed for three years, 400 people with MCI to be followed for three years and 200 people with early AD to be followed for two years. For up-to-date information, see www.adni-info.org.

In this work, only 1.5 T weighted MRI data from normal subjects, MCI and AD patients was used. Table 1 shows the demographic details of the subjects who compose the dataset used in this work. General inclusion/exclusion criteria are as follows:

1. Normal control (NC) subjects: Mini-mental state examination (MMSE) scores between 24–30 (inclusive), a clinical dementia rating (CDR) of 0, non-depressed, non MCI, and nondemented. The age range of normal subjects will be roughly matched to that of MCI and AD subjects. Therefore, there should be minimal enrollment of normals under the age of 70.

Table 1 Sociodemographic data and neuropsychological test summary

	#Patients	Sex M/F	Mean age/std.	Mean MMSE/std.
NC	229	119/110	75.97/5.0	29.00/1.0
MCI	401	258/143	74.85/7.4	27.01/1.8
AD	188	99/89	75.36/7.5	23.28/2.0

2. MCI subjects: MMSE scores between 24–30 (inclusive), a memory complaint, have objective memory loss measured by education adjusted scores on Wechsler Memory Scale Logical Memory II, a CDR of 0.5, absence of significant levels of impairment in other cognitive domains, essentially preserved activities of daily living, and an absence of dementia.
3. Mild AD: MMSE scores between 20–26 (inclusive), CDR of 0.5 or 1.0, and meets NINCDS/ADRDA criteria for probable AD.

2.2 MRI Data Preprocessing

Image data preprocessing, segmentation and co-registration of T1-weighted MRI images from the ADNI database have been performed according to the block diagram shown in Fig. 1. Initially, images from the ADNI database were nor skull-stripped neither spatially normalized. Thus, all the images had to be pre-processed and co-registered before segmentation. The whole process has been performed using the voxel-based morphometry (VBM) [7] toolbox for statistical parametric mapping (SPM) [8, 9].

Once the image has been segmented, the system uses a brain atlas [10] consisting of 106 regions of interest (ROIs) $R_i, i = 1, 2, \ldots, 116$, to extract the mean μ_i and the standard deviation σ_i for each region of interest (ROI) from GM-segmented MRI $I_{GM}(\mathbf{x})$:

$$\mu_i = \frac{1}{N_i}\sum_{j=1}^{N_i} I_{GM}(\mathbf{x}_{i,j}) \qquad \sigma_i = \sqrt{\frac{1}{N_i - 1}\sum_{i=1}^{N_i}(I_{GM}(\mathbf{x}_{i,j}) - \mu_i)^2} \tag{1}$$

where $\mathbf{x}_{i,j}$ denote the jth voxel belonging to R_i and N_i the number of voxels of the ith ROI.

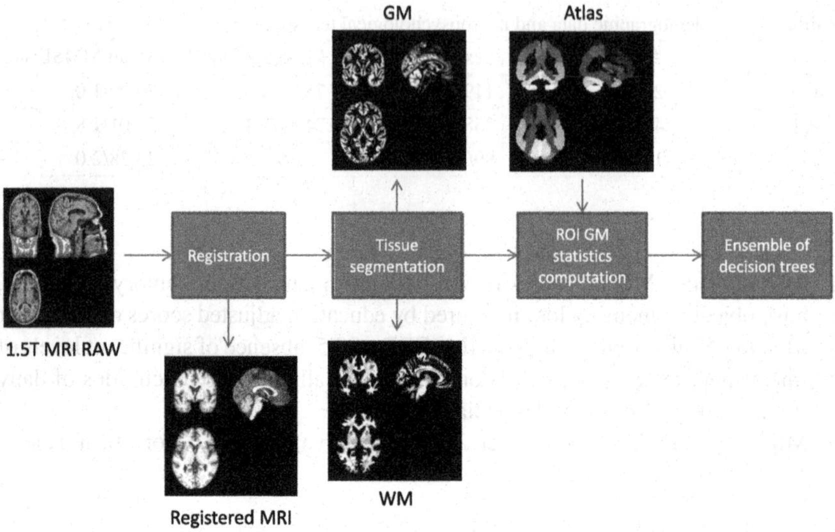

Fig. 1 MRI preprocessing and feature extraction

2.3 Ensemble Learning Methods

Various ensemble classification methods have been proposed in recent years for improved classification accuracy [11]. In ensemble classification, several classifiers are trained and their results are combined through a voting process. Perhaps, the most widely used such methods are boosting and bagging. Boosting is based on sample re-weighting but bagging uses bootstrapping.

Boosting is a powerful learning technique, originally designed for classification problems, that can be extended to regression as well. It combines the outputs of many weak classifiers to produce a more robust ensemble. The most popular boosting algorithm called AdaBoost.M1 was originally proposed by Freund and Schapire [2, 3]. Given a vector of predictor variables $\mathbf{x}_n$ for observation n and associated binary class labels y_n, the algorithm trains learners $h_t(\mathbf{x})$ sequentially and computes the weighted classification error:

$$\epsilon_t = \sum_{n=1}^{N} d_n^{(t)} I(y_n \neq h_t(\mathbf{x}_n)) \tag{2}$$

where $d_n^{(t)}$ is the weight of observation n at step t. Then, Adaboost increases the weight for misclassified observations in an iterative fashion in which the next learner $t+1$ is trained on the data with updated weights $d_n^{(t+1)}$. After training, a new observation vector $\mathbf{x}$ is classified my means:

$$f(\mathbf{x}) = \sum_{t=1}^{T} \alpha_t h_t(\mathbf{x}) \tag{3}$$

where

$$\alpha_t = \frac{1}{2} \log \frac{1 - \epsilon_t}{\epsilon_t} \tag{4}$$

There are many different boosting alternatives to AdaBoost algorithm. Logitboost works similarly to AdaBoostM1, except that it minimizes the binomial deviance [12] instead of the exponential loss. It reduces the weight for misclassified observations with large values of $y_n f(\mathbf{x}_n)$. The benefits of Logitboost when compared to AdaBoost is that it can provide better average accuracy for poorly separable classes. GentleBoost or Gentle AdaBoost [12] is a hybrid method combining several features of AdaBoost and LogitBoost. It minimizes the exponential loss like AdaBoost but every weak learner fits a regression model to class labels y_n.

Bagging [13] is another type of ensemble learning method. It can be combined with a weak learner such a decision tree. In fact, the random forest classifier [11] uses bagging, or bootstrap aggregating, to form an ensemble of classification and regression tree (CART)-like classifiers $h_t(\mathbf{x})$, where each one is trained by a bootstrap replica obtained by randomly selecting N observations out of N with replacement, where N is the dataset size, and $\mathbf{x}$ is a vector of predictor variables [11]. For classification, each tree in the random forest casts a unit vote for the most popular class for input $\mathbf{x}$. The output of the classifier is determined by a majority vote of the trees. This method is not sensitive to noise or overtraining, as the resampling is not based on weighting. Furthermore, it is computationally more efficient than methods based on boosting and somewhat better than simple bagging [14].

3 Results

The motivation of this work is to evaluate and compare popular ensemble learning methods for classification tasks of increasing complexity in the context of a research project focusing the development of computer-aided diagnosis (CAD) systems for Alzheimer's disease. The study starts with a database of 229 NC, 401 MCI and 188 AD subjects. The classification tasks are: (i) NC versus AD, (ii) NC versus MCI, and (iii) MCI versus AD. For the three classification tasks, balanced datasets were defined in order to avoid inflated performance estimates occurring on imbalanced datasets [15].

The first experiment compares the classification error of ensembles consisting of an increasing number of decision trees that were trained using AdaBoost.M1, LogitBoost, GentleBoost and Bagging, for each of the three classification tasks. Figure 2 shows the loss of the ensemble as a function of the number of trees in the ensemble for NC versus AD, NC versus MCI, and MCI versus AD classification. The classification

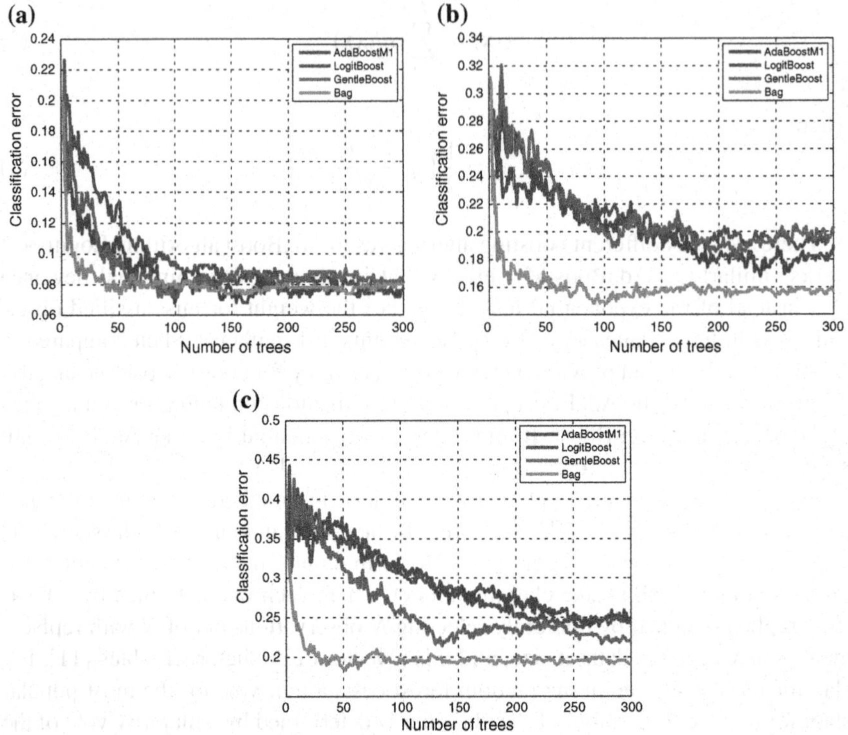

Fig. 2 Classification error as a function of the number of trees in the ensemble for: (**a**) NC versus AD, (**b**) NC versus MCI, and (**c**) MCI versus AD

error was obtained by leave-one-out cross-validation. Note that, the generalization error converges to a limit as the number of trees in the ensemble becomes large. Moreover, the generalization error depends on the strength of the individual trees in the forest and the correlation between them. Bagging performs better than boosting method in terms of classification error and convergence rate. For the reduced complexity NC versus AD classification task, all the ensemble learning methods yield similar error rates around 0.08 %. However, bagging attains convergence with less trees in the ensemble, thus reducing the training and evaluation complexity of the classifier. The same behavior is observed for higher complexity tasks. Bagging outperforms boosting methods specially when the label confidence decreases and the complexity of the classification task increases.

In a second experiment, the accuracy, sensitivity and specificity of the classification tasks were obtained for an ensemble of 300 decision trees using leave-one-out cross-validation. Figure 3 shows the results of this analysis. It can be concluded that for NC versus AD classification there are minor differences in performance between the ensemble learning techniques tested. However, when the complexity of the clas-

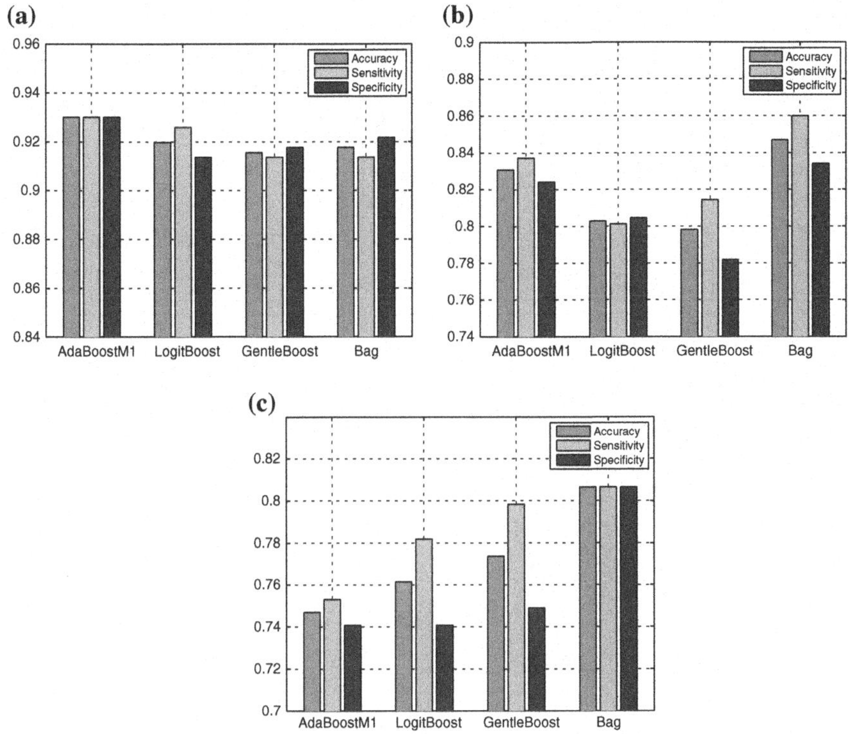

Fig. 3 Accuracy, sensitivity and specificity of ensemble learning methods: (**a**) NC versus AD, (**b**) NC versus MCI, and (**c**) MCI versus AD

sification tasks increases in NC versus MCI and MCI versus AD classification, bagging yields again the best results.

Finally, the receiver operating characteristics (ROC) and the area under the curve (AUC) were obtained for the different ensemble learning algorithms and each of the three classification tasks. Figure 4 shows the tradeoff between the sensitivity and specificity of the classifier as the decision threshold is tuned. It can be concluded that:

- For NC versus AD classification, AdaBoost.M1, LogitBoost and GentleBoost boosting methods as well as bagging yield similar results with AUC values ranging from 0.96 to 0.97.
- For higher complexity NC versus MCI and MCI versus AD classification problems, bagging outperforms boosting algorithms with ROC curves shifted up and to the left in the ROC space. Bagging yields an AUC of 0.92 for NC versus MCI outperforming boosting with a maximum AUC of 0.87 for GentleBoost. Similar improvements are obtained in discriminating MCI from AD patients with bagging reporting an AUC of 0.88 while the best boosting algorithm, GentleBoost, yields 0.82.

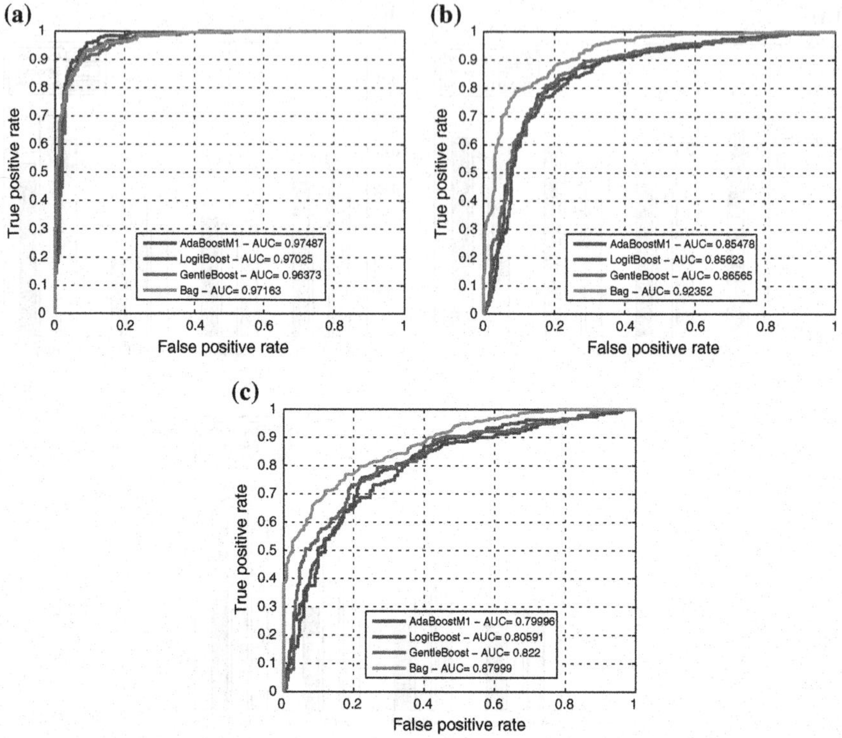

Fig. 4 ROC and AUC of ensemble learning methods: (**a**) NC versus AD, (**b**) NC versus MCI, and (**c**) MCI versus AD

As a conclusion, it was found that bagging and boosting provides similar classification results for reduced complexity classification task. When the complexity of the classification task increases, bagging outperforms boosting methods followed by GentleBoost learning. Independently of the complexity of the classification task, bagging performs better than boosting with a reduced number of trees in the ensemble.

Finally, an analysis related to the out-of-bag estimate of the feature relevance was carried out in order to check if the ensemble methods are focusing on the most relevant ROIs for the detection of the Alzheimer's disease. Figure 5 shows a map of the out-of-bag feature relevance index for mean features and standard deviation features. These maps show the brain areas where degeneration is observed in the population under study.

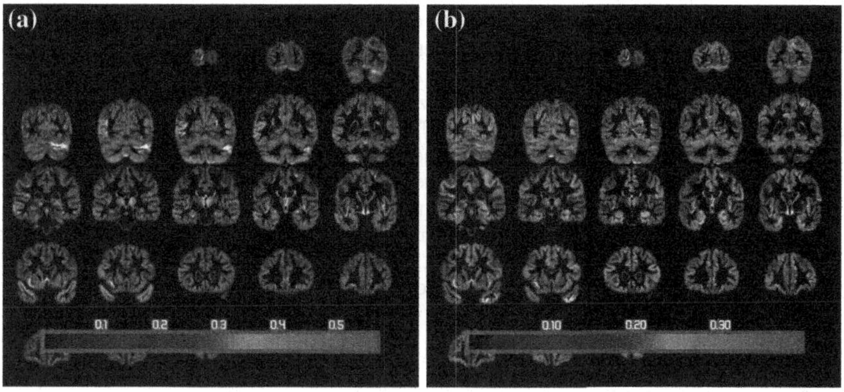

Fig. 5 Out-of-bag estimate of the feature relevance for NC versus AD. (**a**) Mean and (**b**) Standard deviation features

4 Conclusions

A comparative study of boosting and bagging algorithms for magnetic resonance image (MRI) analysis and classification was presented in this paper. A database collected from ADNI consisting of 1.5 T weighted MRI data from 229 NC subjects, 401 MCI and 188 AD patients was used. Three different complexity classification tasks were studied: NC versus AD, NC versus MCI and MCI versus AD. For the three classification tasks, balanced datasets were defined in order to avoid inflated performance estimates occurring on imbalanced datasets. Three boosting algorithms: AdaBoost.M1, LogitBoost and GentleBoost, as well as bagging were compared within an ensemble tree learning process. It was found that the generalization error converges to a limit as the number of trees in the ensemble becomes large. It depends on the strength of the individual trees in the forest and the correlation between them. Bagging performs better than boosting method in terms of classification error and convergence rate. In terms of complexity of the classification task, bagging and boosting provides similar classification results for reduced complexity classification task (i.e., NC versus AD). However, when the complexity of the classification task increases (in NC versus MCI or MCI versus AD), bagging outperforms boosting methods followed by GentleBoost learning. Independently of the complexity of the classification task, bagging performs better than boosting with a reduced number of trees in the ensemble.

Acknowledgments This work was partly supported by the MICINN under the TEC2012-34306 project and the Consejería de Innovación, Ciencia y Empresa (Junta de Andalucía, Spain) under the Excellence Project P11-TIC-7103.

Data collection and sharing for this project was funded by the Alzheimer's Disease Neuroimaging Initiative (ADNI; National Institutes of Health Grant U01 AG024904). ADNI is funded by the National Institute on Aging, the National Institute of Biomedical Imaging and Bioengineering, and through generous contributions from the following: Abbott, AstraZeneca AB, Bayer Schering

Pharma AG, Bristol-Myers Squibb, Eisai Global Clinical Development, Elan Corporation, Genentech, GE Healthcare, GlaxoSmithKline, Innogenetics, Johnson and Johnson, Eli Lilly and Co., Medpace, Inc., Merck and Co., Inc., Novartis AG, Pfizer Inc., F. Hoffman-La Roche, Schering-Plough, Synarc, Inc., as well as non-profit partners the Alzheimer's Association and Alzheimer's Drug Discovery Foundation, with participation from the U.S. Food and Drug Administration. Private sector contributions to ADNI are facilitated by the Foundation for the National Institutes of Health (www.fnih.org). The grantee organization is the Northern California Institute for Research and Education, and the study is coordinated by the Alzheimer's Disease Cooperative Study at the University of California, San Diego. ADNI data are disseminated by the Laboratory for Neuro-Imaging at the University of California, Los Angeles. This research was also supported by NIH grants P30 AG010129, K01 AG030514, and the Dana Foundation.

References

1. Association, A.: alzheimer's disease facts and figures. Alzheimer's & Dementia **10**(2014), e47–e92 (2014)
2. Freund, Y., Schapire, R.E.: A decision-theoretic generalization of on-line learning and an application to boosting. J. Comput. Syst. Sci. **55**, 119–139 (1997)
3. Schapire, R., Freund, Y., Bartlett, P., Lee, W.S.: Boosting the margin: a new explanation for the effectiveness of voting methods. Ann. Stat. **26**, 1651–1686 (1998)
4. Zhiwei, H., Zhifang, P., Hongtao, L., Wenbin, L.: Classification of Alzheimer's disease based on cortical thickness using adaboost and combination feature selection method. In: Computing and Intelligent Systems. Communications in Computer and Information Science. Springer, Berlin (2011)
5. Morra, J., Zhuowen, T., Apostolova, L.G., Green, A.E., Toga, A., Thompson, P.: Comparison of adaboost and support vector machines for detecting alzheimer's disease through automated hippocampal segmentation. IEEE Trans. Med. Imag. **29**, 30–43 (2010)
6. Morra, J., Tu, Z., Apostolova, L., Green, A., Avedissian, C., Madsen, S., Parikshak, N., Toga, A., Jack, C., Schuff, N., Weiner, M., Thompson, P.: Automated mapping of hippocampal atrophy in 1-year repeat MRI data from 490 subjects with alzheimer's disease, mild cognitive impairment, and elderly controls. NeuroImage **45**, S3–S15 (2009)
7. Structural Brain Mapping Group, D.o.P.: VBM manual. University of Jena, Germany (2010)
8. Ashburner, J., Friston, K.J.: Voxel-based morphometry—the methods. Neuroimage **11**, 805–821 (2000)
9. Good, C.D., Johnsrude, I.S., Ashburner, J., Henson, R.N.A., Friston, K.J., Frackowiak, R.S.J.: A voxel-based morphometric study of ageing in 465 normal adult human brains. Neuroimage **11**, 805–821 (2000)
10. Alemán-Gómez, Y., Melie-García, L., Valdés-Hernandez, P.: Ibaspm: toolbox for automatic parcellation of brain structures. In: 12th Annual Meeting of the Organization for Human Brain Mapping (2006)
11. Breiman, L.: Random forests. Machine Learning **45**, 32–35 (2001)
12. Friedman, J., Hastie, T., Tibshirani, R.: Additive logistic regression: a statistical view of boosting. Ann. Stat. **28**, 337–407 (2000)
13. Breiman, L.: Bagging predictors. Mach. Learn. **24**, 123–140 (1996)
14. Ramírez, J., Górriz, J., Segovia, F., Chaves, R., Salas-Gonzalez, D., López, M., Álvarez, I., Padilla, P.: Computer aided diagnosis system for the alzheimer's disease based on partial least squares and random forest SPECT image classification. Neurosci. Lett. **472**, 99–103 (2010)
15. Wei, Q., Dunbrack, R.L.: The role of balanced training and testing data sets for binary classifiers in bioinformatics. PLoS One **8**, e67863 (2013)

Part VII
Smart Medical and Healthcare System 2015 Workshop

Integrating Electronic Health Records in Clinical Decision Support Systems

Eider Sanchez, Carlos Toro and Manuel Graña

Abstract Electronic Health Records (EHR) are systematic collections of digital health information about individual patients or populations. They provide readily access to the complete medical history of the patient, which is useful for decision-making activities. In this paper we focus on a secondary benefit of EHR: the reuse of the implicit knowledge embedded in it to improve the knowledge on the mechanisms of a disease and/or the effectiveness of the treatments. In fact, all such patient data registries stored in EHR reflect implicitly different clinical decisions made by the clinical professionals that participated in the assistance of patients (e.g. criteria followed during decision making, patient parameters taken into account, effect of the treatments prescribed). This work proposes a methodology that allows the management of EHR not only as data containers and information repositories, but also as clinical knowledge repositories. Moreover, we propose an architecture for the extraction of the knowledge from EHR. Such knowledge can be fed into a Clinical Decision Support System (CDSS), in a way that could render benefits for the development of innovations from clinicians, health managers and medical researchers.

Keywords Electronic health record • Clinical decision support system • Knowledge extraction • Semantic model

---

E. Sanchez (✉) · C. Toro
Vicomtech-IK4 Research Centre, Mikeletegi Pasealekua 57, 20009 San Sebastian, Spain
e-mail: esanchez@vicomtech.org

E. Sanchez
Biodonostia Health Research Institute, P. Doctor Begiristain S/N, 20014 San Sebastian, Spain

E. Sanchez · M. Graña
University of the Basque Country UPV/EHU, Computational Intelligence Group, Computer Science Faculty, P. Manuel Lardizabal 1, 20018 San Sebastian, Spain

M. Graña
ENGINE Centre, Wrocław University of Technology, Wybrzeże Wyspiańskiego 27, 50-370 Wrocław, Poland

Y.-W. Chen et al. (eds.), *Innovation in Medicine and Healthcare 2015*,
Smart Innovation, Systems and Technologies 45,
DOI 10.1007/978-3-319-23024-5_37

1 Introduction

Electronic Health Records (EHR) are systematic collections of digital health in-formation about individual patients or populations. They include demographical data, medical history, medication and allergies records, immunization status, laboratory test results, radiological images, vital signs, personal statistics, such as age and weight, and even billing information. The main objective of EHR is to make patient clinical information as well as all their medical history available for future clinicians that will be treating this patient. In such way, the diagnosis could be improved and the prescribed treatments could be better suited to each patient.

During the last years the medical community has identified EHR as valuable as-sets and hard work has been done in order to improve and integrate them in clinical and hospital environments [1, 2–4]. In particular, interoperability has been broadly addressed, so that EHR of a patient visiting different Health Systems can travel safely with the patient integrating the information along the way. Different EHR standards have been defined, such as CEN/ISO 13606, HL7 (RIM, CDA) and OpenEHR [1, 2, 4, 5]. Such standards determine the structural characteristics of EHR, as well as the ones needed for communication purposes with other EHR. Results obtained at research and technological levels have been successful, so that interoperability of EHR management systems is a reality nowadays, even though they are still not implemented in most clinical or hospital environments.

Nevertheless, such vision does not take advantage of the complete potential offered by EHR [6]. In particular, all patient data registries stored in EHR implicitly reflect different clinical decisions made by the clinical professionals that participated in the assistance of patients. More in detail:

- Which patient parameters have been used in each decision (e.g. which medical tests have been performed, which treatments were prescribed, which interventions carried out, etc.).
- Which criteria have been followed during such decisions (whether such criteria follows clinical guidelines and protocols).
- Which has been the result of the decisions made on the patient (e.g. the effect of the prescribed treatments, the success versus failure of such a treatment).

Thus, the exploitation and reuse of the implicit knowledge in EHR could also be used to improve the knowledge on the mechanisms of a disease or the effectiveness of the treatments. At a clinical level such necessity is clear: nowadays the mechanisms of quite a lot of relevant diseases as well as the treatments applied to fight them are still unknown. For instance, oncology and neurology could be two domains in which such knowledge is still needed.

This paper proposes a methodology that allows the management of EHR not only as data containers and information repositories, but also as clinical knowledge repositories. The main objectives are: (i) to improve and enlarge the knowledge of the mechanisms of a disease, (ii) to evaluate the effectiveness of the applied therapies and interventional procedures, (iii) to evaluate whether the clinical practice developed follows clinical guidelines and protocols, (iv) to identify similar patients for facilitating enrolment of patients in clinical studies in general, (v) to identify groups of similar patients for the stratification of the patient population, (vi) to measure the quality of the clinical practice developed by a clinical team, and (vii) to generate preliminary evidence of a certain hypothesis (e.g. a certain treatment is not effective or valid for patients of a certain type) that could lead to start clinical studies.

In this paper we propose an architecture for the extraction of the knowledge from EHR. Additionally, we also propose feeding such knowledge into a Clinical Decision Support System (CDSS), in order to handle the knowledge in such a way that could be useful for clinicians, health managers and medical researchers alike.

This paper is structured as follows: Sect. 2 introduces EHR and CDSS. Section 3 proposes the methodology for the semantic modelling of EHR and the knowledge extraction. Section 4 proposed a methodology for reusing such knowledge to provide clinical decision support. Finally, Sect. 5 discusses some relevant aspects of our approach.

2 Related Concepts

EHR systems, as well as CDSS are introduced in this Section, in order to provide the relevant concepts regarding the aspects covered in this paper.

2.1 Electronic Health Record

According to the definition provided by the Institute of Medicine (IOM) Electronic Health Records (EHR) are defined as "a longitudinal collection of electronic information about the health status of patients, introduced or generated by members of the medical team in a health organization or hospital". The main characteristics of EHR are the following: (i) persistence of the information during every step of the clinical assistance, (ii) unambiguous patient identification, by means of a universal identifier for each patient, (iii) interoperability with other systems, (iv) standardization of information storage, (v) representation of the contents in an understandable manner by other healthcare professionals, (vi) usability, easy to use by all healthcare professionals, (vii) legal value of every document contained, signed by the corresponding responsible, and (viii) security and privacy of the data.

EHR are intended to provide a benefit in different domains, such as (i) healthcare: EHR stores all patient data; (ii) teaching: the information contained is useful for the learning of clinical cases; (iii) research: patient data can be reused for performing clinical studies; (iv) management: the costs of clinical procedures, patient billing, and clinical and economic indicators can be calculated based on patient data, and (v) legal: the assistance provided to a patient can be certified and the legal responsible in cases of failure or are identified.

Different EHR standards have been developed. Health Level 7 (HL7), for in-stance, is a Standards Developing Organization (SDO) oriented to heath information and interoperability. HL7 develops different standards, covering areas such as messaging and data interchange, rules, syntax, visual integration, context, clinical document architecture, functional model, and labelling. For EHR, the HL7 Version 3 is currently the most applied. It is based on a Reference Information Model (RIM) [7] and covers specially messaging aspects. Clinical Document Architecture (CDA) complements the RIM, focusing on the data structure of the EHR.

OpenEHR is an open standard detailed for the development of a complete and interoperable computational platform for clinical information [7]. The technical specifications of information, service and clinical models are detailed. A dual model is implemented, formed by a Reference Model (information) and an Archetype Model (formal definition of clinical concepts). An archetype is formed by three different parts: (i) descriptive information (identifier, code of the clinical concept described and metadata); (ii) restriction rules (regarding cardinality, structure and content), and (iii) ontological definitions (vocabulary).

ISO EN 13606 is formed by 5 parts: (i) Reference Model: a general model of information to communicate with the clinical history of a patient; (ii) Specification of the archetype model: a generic model of information and a representation language for the individual instances of archetypes (archetype description language, ADL [8]; (iii) Reference archetypes and term lists: a normative section with the list of codified terms to be used in the attributes of the reference model and an informative section in which examples archetypes are presented to show how to map using ISO 13606 structures the clinical information codified in HL7 v3 or OpenEHR, (iv) Security characteristics that individual instances must comply, and (v) Inter-change model: contains a set of models for communication purposes based messages and services. ISO 13606 has adopted the Dual Model of OpenEHR for the representation of every health data introduced in the EHR, which has 2 parts. (i) The first one is the reference model: a generic class model that represents the generic properties of the information in the EHR [9], following the different perspectives of the company, the information, computational, engineering and technology. The second is the archetype model: the definition of the clinical content of the data. Archetypes are metadata used to represent the specific characteristics of clinical data. They are a formal definition of a clinical concept based on the reference model.

The relationship between HL7, OpenEHR and ISO EN 13606, reported by Schloeffel [7], is depicted in Fig. 1.

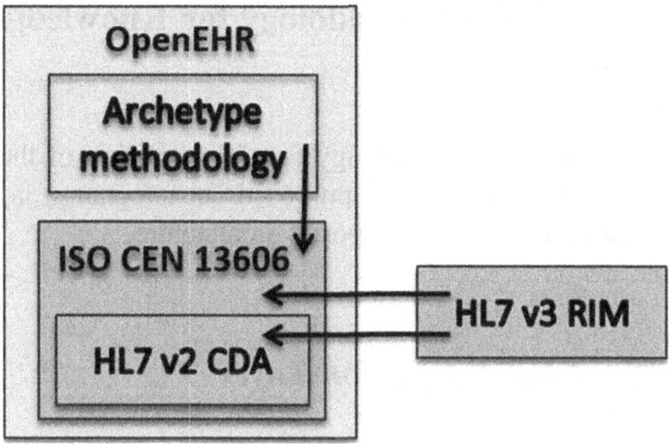

Fig. 1 Relationship of standards HL7, OpenEHR and ISO EN 13606 by Schloeffel (Schloeffel, 2006)

2.2 Clinical Decision Support Systems

We adhere to the definition of CDSS given in [10] stating that CDSS are active intelligent systems that use patient clinical data to generate case specific advice. According to [11], the main task of CDSS consists of the retrieval of relevant knowledge and patient data (coming from medical devices, evidence provided by the medical community, and clinical guidelines and protocols) and their analysis to perform some action, often the generation of recommendations. The target user can be a physician or any other medical professional, a medical organization, a patient or patient's caregivers or relatives. The goals of CDSS are: (i) to facilitate assessment of patient data, (ii) to foster optimal decision making, problem solving and acting, in different contexts and tasks (such as diagnosis and treatment), ensuring that decision makers have all the necessary knowledge to make a correct decision, and (iii) to reduce medical errors [12, 13]. A wide variety of tools can be included in CDSS, some examples are: (i) computerized alerts and reminders, (ii) clinical guidelines, (iii) order sets, (iv) patient data reports and dashboards, (v) documentation templates, (vi) diagnostic support, and (vii) clinical workflow tools [14]. The technologies in which such tools and interventions are based are sparse (e.g. data mining techniques, communication protocols, knowledge acquisition techniques, semantic representation and reasoning, etc.).

We will focus on Knowledge-based CDSS, which benefit from a symbolic representation of knowledge about a particular domain, and the ability for reasoning about solutions of problems within that domain, [15]. The general model of Knowledge-based CDSS proposed by Berner et al. [12] consist of 4 elements: (i) an input, (ii) an output, (iii) a Knowledge Base and (iv) a reasoning engine.

Knowledge-based CDSS in our approach are focused in two main functionalities: generation of recommendations [16, 17] and the management of the underlying knowledge that will drive such recommendations [18].

3 Proposed Methodology for Knowledge Extraction from EHR

We propose a methodology for the extraction of the implicit knowledge in EHR. Two different layers are proposed: an integration layer and a semantization layer. Figure 2 depicts the proposed architecture.

3.1 EHR Integration Layer

This layer is intended to provide the corresponding modules capable of integrating the information contained in different EHR (i.e. EHR of different types, structures, standards, origins). Each EHR will develop a different integration module.

The main idea underlying this approach is the requirement of no information loss from the current existing EHR (i.e. interoperable EHR) to the proposed semantic EHR. In our approach we intend to build novel EHR that could be easily integrated to existing systems currently running in hospitals and clinical organizations.

Taking into account legal issues of data protection and privacy, the system will be provided of an anonimization layer that will ensure that all data processed is stripped of personal data. This process is followed by data extraction and clustering of data fields. Clustering processes will be qualitative due to the heterogeneous nature of the data in the HER, conventional quantitative clustering do not deal well with categorical or descriptive data. To this end, a tool to be considered is the

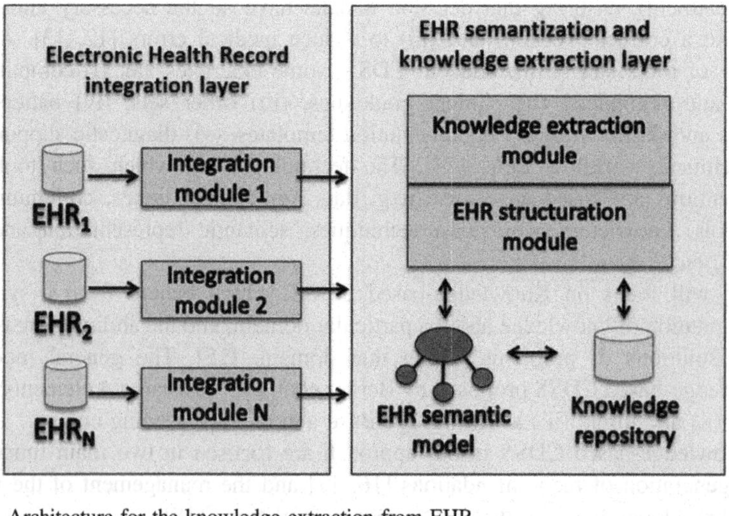

Fig. 2 Architecture for the knowledge extraction from EHR

Formal Concept Analysis [19], based on a lattice approach to the discovery of semantic classes and ontology creation. This approach only requires the existence of some kind of ordering, and is able to work on very heterogenous data. Also the recent advances include some kinds of adaptive processes which allow the semantic ontology to evolve in time with the new data.

3.2 EHR Semantization and Knowledge Extraction Layer

The main objective of this layer is to extract the knowledge from the EHR and store it in a knowledge repository in which it is represented in a way that will allow future reuse and reasoning over it.

3.2.1 EHR Structuration Module

We propose a new semantic model for the representation of the contents of the EHR. Our model extends the Dual Model (of ISO EN 13606 and OpenEHR) with a triple approach in which not only the patient, the disease and the performed medical tests are represented (dual approach), but also a decision model is represented. The decision model contains both, the decision made and the context of such decision: (i) patient data (socio-demographic data, data from anamnesis and data from the medical tests performed to the patient), (ii) decision criteria considered during decision-making, (iii) the objective of the decision (e.g. fast recovery, survival without surgery, avoid blood transfusion), and (iv) the result of the decision (level of success achieved with regard to the objective searched).

The works reported in [18, 17] are aimed to mine the experience present in the history of interactions between doctors and patients. This approach is greatly benefitted by the formalization of the EHR, so that actual experiential events (decisions) can be readily extracted and traced by the entries in the EHR. Therefore, we propose the usage of Decisional DNA and SOEKS [20] to model decisions contained in the EHR.

3.2.2 Knowledge Extraction Module

The mining of the decision model will generate new knowledge in the system, such as the assessment of the effectiveness of the treatments prescribed. We propose the development of different algorithms for the knowledge extraction from EHR. The development of natural language processing algorithms will be a key success factor for such mining. Some approaches have been previously developed, specially regarding codification of clinical terms into different terminologies (i.e. SNOMED CT, CIE-9, CIE-10, UMLS, etc.). However, error rates are still high.

4 Integration of EHR into CDSS

We intend to benefit from the architecture proposed in [18, 17] for Semantically enhanced CDSS (S-CDSS), based on:

- The user layer
- Data, knowledge and experience repositories.
- A multiagent architecture consisting of 9 distinct agents: majordomo, data handling, data translation, knowledge and decision, experience handling, reasoning, application, user characterization, and standards and interoperability.

A new agent in the architecture, the EHR integration agent, will implement the architecture proposed in the previous section (Fig. 3).

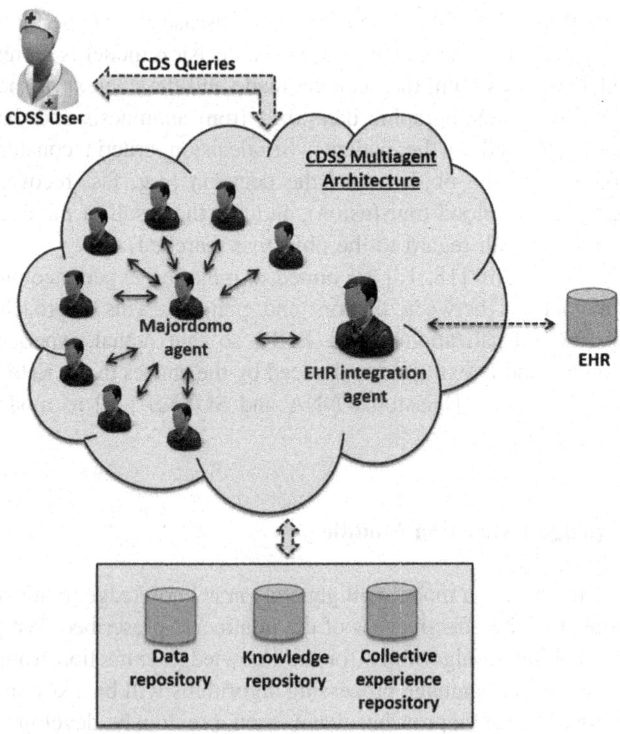

Fig. 3 Integration of EHR into CDSS

5 Conclusions

In this paper we have proposed an architecture for the semantization of EHR, that allows knowledge extraction and reuse from EHR. Additionally, we have also presented a methodology for integrating such Semantic EHR into CDSS. We are actually planning the validation of this approach on real data provided by private companies, or made available for research at the Internet, such as the ones provided by OpenMRS (http://openmrs.org/).

Acknowledgements M Graña was supported by EC under FP7, Coordination and Support Action, Grant Agreement Number 316097, ENGINE European Research Centre of Network Intelligence for Innovation Enhancement

References

1. Sumita, Y., Takata, M., Ishitsuka, K., Tominaga, Y., Ohe, K.: Building a reference functional model for EHR systems. Int. J. Med. Inform. **76**(9), 688–700 (2007)
2. Blobel, B.: Advanced and secure architectural EHR approaches. Int. J. Med. Inform. **75**(3–4), 185–190 (2006)
3. Martínez Costa, C., Menárguez-Tortosa, M., Fernández-Breis, J.T.: Clinical data interoperability based on archetype transformation. J. Biomed. Inform. **44**(5), 869–880 (2011)
4. Martínez-Costa, C., Menárguez-Tortosa, M., Fernández-Breis, J.T.: An approach for the se-mantic interoperability of ISO EN 13606 and OpenEHR archetypes. J. Biomed. Inform. **43**(5), 736–746 (2010)
5. Garde, S., Hovenga, E., Buck, J., Knaup, P.: Expressing clinical data sets with openEHR archetypes: a solid basis for ubiquitous computing. Int. J. Med. Inform. **76**(3), S334–S341 (2007)
6. Bakker, A.: Access to EHR and access control at a moment in the past: a discussion of the need and an exploration of the consequences. Int. J. Med. Inform. **73**(3), 267–270 (2004)
7. Schloeffel, P., Beale, T., Hayworth, G., Heard, S., Leslie, H.: The relationship between CEN 13606, HL7, and openEHR. In: Proceedings of HIC 2006 and HINZ 2006, p. 24 (2006)
8. Eichelberg, M., Aden, T., Riesmeier, J., Dogac, A., Laleci, G.B.: A survey and analysis of electronic healthcare record standards. ACM Comput. Surv. **37**(4), 277–315 (2005)
9. Kalra, D., Ingram, D.: Electronic health records. In: Zieliaski, K., Duplaga, M., Ingram, D., (eds.) Information Technology Solutions for Healthcare, Health Informatics, pp 135–181. Springer, London (2006)
10. Liu, J., Wyatt, J.C., Altman, D.G.: Decision tools in health care: focus on the problem, not the solution. BMC Med. Inform. Decis. Mak. **6**(4) (2006)
11. Greenes, R.A: Clinical Decision Support: The Road Ahead. Elsevier Science, Boston (2011)
12. Berner, E.S., La Lande, T.J.: Overview of Clinical Decision Support Systems. In: Berner, E.S. (ed.) Clinical Decision Support Systems, Theory and Practice, 1, 2nd edn. Springer, New York (2007)
13. Peleg, M., Tu, S.W.: Decision support, knowledge representation and management in medicine. In: 2006 IMIA Yearbook of Medical Informatics: Assessing Information—Technologies for Health, pp 72–80. Schattauer Verlagsgesellschaft GmbH, Stuttgart (2006)
14. Osheroff, J.A., Teich, J.M., Middleton, B.F., Steen, E.B., Wright, A., Detmer, D.E.: A roadmap for national action on clinical decision support. JAMIA **14**(2), 141–145 (2007)

15. Carson, E.R., Collison, P.O., Kalogeropoulos, D.A.: Towards knowledge-based systems in clinical practice: development of an integrated clinical information and knowledge management support system. Comput. Methods Programs Biomed. **72**, 65–80 (2003)
16. Sanchez, E., Toro, C., Artetxe, A., Graña, M., Sanin, C., Szczerbicki, E., Carrasco, E., Guijarro, F.: Bridging challenges of clinical decision support systems with a semantic approach. A case study on breast cancer. Pattern Recogn. Lett. **34**(14), 1758–1768 (2013)
17. Sanchez, E., Toro, C., Graña, M., Sanin, C., Szczerbicki, E.: Extended Reflexive Ontologies for the generation of clinical recommendations. Cyberntetics Syst. **46**(1–2), 4–18 (2015)
18. Sanchez, E., Peng, W., Toro, C., Sanin, C., Graña, M., Szczerbicki, E., Carrasco, E., Guijarro, F., Brualla, L.: Decisional DNA for modeling and reuse of experiential clinical assessments in breast cancer diagnosis and treatment. Neurocomputing **146**(25), 308–318 (2014)
19. Poelmans, J., Ignatov, D.I., Kuznetsov, S.O., Dedene, G.: Formal concept analysis in knowledge processing: a survey on applications. Expert Syst. Appl. **40**(16), 6538–6560 (2013)
20. Sanin, C., Szczerbicki, E.: Decisional DNA and the Smart Knowledge Management System: A process of transforming information into knowledge. In: Gunasekaran, A. (ed.) Techniques and Tools for the Design and Implementation of Enterprise Information Systems, pp. 149–175. IGI, New York (2008)

An Ad-Hoc Image Segmentation of Subcutaneous and Visceral Adipose Tissue from Abdomino-Pelvic Magnetic Resonance Images

Oier Echaniz, Borja Ayerdi, Alexandre Savio and Manuel Graña

Abstract Overweighted people and children with obesity has reached the epidemic ranges in developed and near-development countries. They are a serious public health issue, with big economic impact. Looking for remedies, studies are being carried out to test the impact of several treatments on overweight children health. Such studies require the longitudinal measurement of fat deposits in the abdomino-pelvic regions along the study treatment. Because such studies involve large populations, these measurements requires automated procedures for reliable unbiased estimations of fat volume. This paper describes an ad-hoc image segmentation process developed in the framework of a study on the impact of physical exercise on the visceral and subcutaneous adipose tissue. Several Magnetic Resonance Imaging (MRI) modalities focused in fat visualization have been used in this study, which produce hiperintense values for fat tissues, and are combined by the proposed algorithm. Validation in this paper is qualitative, because we do not have ground truth manual segmentations for quantitative validations.

1 Introduction

The number of overweighted people and obese children in many developed and in process of development countries has reached epidemic ranges. They constitute a serious public health issue [4]. Obese children have 5 times more risk of developing resistance to insulin and type-2 diabetes than not obese children. In addition, the great majority of overweight children have at least one cardiovascular (CV) risk factor [3]. Although most CV problems commonly associated with obesity appear at adult life,

O. Echaniz (✉) · B. Ayerdi · A. Savio · M. Graña
Grupo de Inteligencia Computacional (GIC), Universidad Del País Vasco (UPV/EHU), San Sebastian, Spain
e-mail: oier.etxaniz@gmail.com

A. Savio · M. Graña
ENGINE Centre, Wrocław University of Technology,
Wybrzeże Wyspiańskiego 27, 50-370 Wroclaw, Poland

Y.-W. Chen et al. (eds.), *Innovation in Medicine and Healthcare 2015*,
Smart Innovation, Systems and Technologies 45,
DOI 10.1007/978-3-319-23024-5_38

their origins seem to come from earlier life stages [2]. Hence, measures of CV risk factors during infancy are able to predict the development of coronary lesions in the adult life [1]. The accumulation of liver fat is intimately linked to the visceral fat and the resistance to insulin. Given that physical exercise improves the sensibility to insulin and is capable of reducing the visceral fat in obese children, our hypothesis is that moderate to high intensity physical exercise will reduce liver fat, improve body composition and health in obese children.

To test this hypothesis a comparison between the quantity of adipose tissue before and after the exercise periods is needed. Since manual segmentation is a hard, time consuming task that may introduce bias due to operator fatigue. Automatic segmentation methods are the most accurate tools [5] required to perform large scale studies. This method should provide a quantification of the total Visceral (VAT) and Subcutaneous Adipose Tissue (SAT) volume in order to compare both sequences.

The main objective of this work was to develop an automated method to segment VAT and SAT from abdomio-pelvic magnetic resonance images (MRI) in a large number of subjects, before and after treatment, so that we can improve our understanding of the relation between the treatments and the evolution of adipose tissue distribution. Also this procedure allows the quantitative test of the study hypothesis. For the segmentation method to be successful the result has to be accurate, reproducible and, above all, comparable to manual segmentation, which we will demonstrate with visual data presented in the following sections.

2 Materials

Acquisition protocol MRI is performed with a 1.5-T magnet (Magnetom Avanto, Siemens Medical Systems) equipped with a phased-array surface coil and a spine array coil. For hepatic fat quantification, two different 3D in and opposed-phase gradient-echo data acquisition with Dixon reconstruction sequences are used in breath-hold: a two-point Dixon and a recently commercialized multi-echo Dixon with six-echoes in and opposed-phase values that provides a more accurate liver fat estimation. Liver fat is quantified as the percentage of relative signal intensity loss of the liver on opposed images with the screening Dixon, whereas with the multi-echo Dixon a fat percentage map is automatically calculated. Visceral and subcutaneous fat volume is calculated on the six-echo Dixon fat only resultant volumetric images, from the hepatic dome to the lumbosacral union.

Data The cohort of subjects analyzed for this work contains 24 children, boys and girls, 9 and 11 years old. These children are diagnosed with obesity or overweight (IOFT). They come from several schools from Vitoria-Gasteiz. Around 160 children grouped by the body mass index (BMI), age and gender will be randomly chosen for this ongoing project.

3 Methods

Data preparation The image data were transferred to personal computers in Digital Imaging and Communication in Medicine (DICOM) format. For a better analysis we transform the images to a one-file format called nifti, which is used in neuroimaging and can be used, as in this case, in other medical imaging areas. The image data were unorganized, different sequences together and children with no marked separation. To create a proper structured database and transform the images to a proper usable format we used our open source library available on github under Neurita's copyright.

Algorithm A fully automated method to determine VAT and SAT was implemented in R (R-project http://www.r-project.org). The main steps of the process are as follows:

1. Cleaning the body by histogram filtering
2. For each slice
   (a) Remove arms by connected components analysis
   (b) adipose tissue segmentation, we compute the Total Adipose Tissue (TST) regions and we separate the SAT and VAT for analysis.
3. Compute fat volume

3.1 Cleaning the Body

First of all, the image can have artifacts or noisy areas. To avoid them we remove low intensity areas, retaining areas with higher intensity which are our areas of interest for the detection of fat in adipose tissues. To clean this images we are using the mean of the intensity distribution, as we can see in Fig. 1 the distribution is a long tail distribution and the mean value is perfectly adequate to clean it, removing the noisy part that falls below it. As a result we do not need to use a computational expensive algorithm (Fig. 2).

3.2 Remove Arms

The strategy followed to remove arms is to obtain the biggest connected component in the image as shape of the body and left everything else. To this end we fill all holes in the image. We compute the connected components in this image, keeping the one with the biggest area. Following the normal procedure to remove arms it will follow as seen in Fig. 3. To remove hands and obtain the main application area morphologic methods are used. Figure 3a threshold to remove unwanted artifacts and to separate the background from the body tissue. Figure 3b shows all connected areas are filled

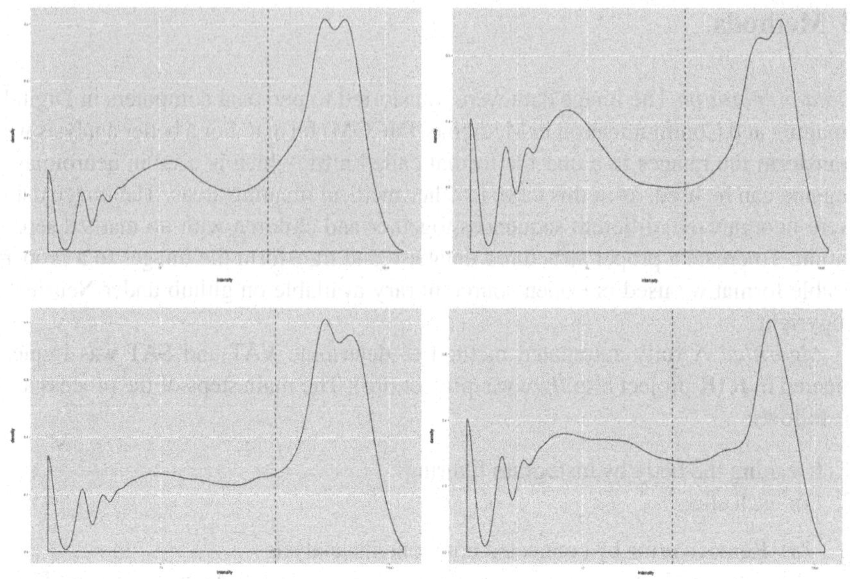

Fig. 1 MRI volume intensity histograms of several subjects with the mean intensity highlighted (*red line*). Noise removal is performed retaining values above the mean

being the biggest one shown in Fig. 3c, which is our working area to find VAT. The other are the hands, as we do not need them we will remove them and apply our application area to the first cleaned image to obtain our Fig. 3d slice with the Total Adipose Tissue (TAT).

Sometimes it can happen that the body is touching the arms. You can detect if by the body is attached to the arms in many ways. The easiest way is to check if the connected component corresponding to the body is touching the boundaries of the image. If so, we know for sure that the arms weren't removed from the body with the matrix label. To remove the arm we apply some morphological operators. First, we perform erosion to detach the arm from the body and second we perform dilation on the body component to recover the body size discarding the arms. This process is illustrated in Fig. 4

3.3 Known Issues

There is one specific situation where we need to create a custom method, it is when the SAT connected component does not closed around the visceral region, this happens around the navel and can span 3–5 slices depending on its size. The issue can

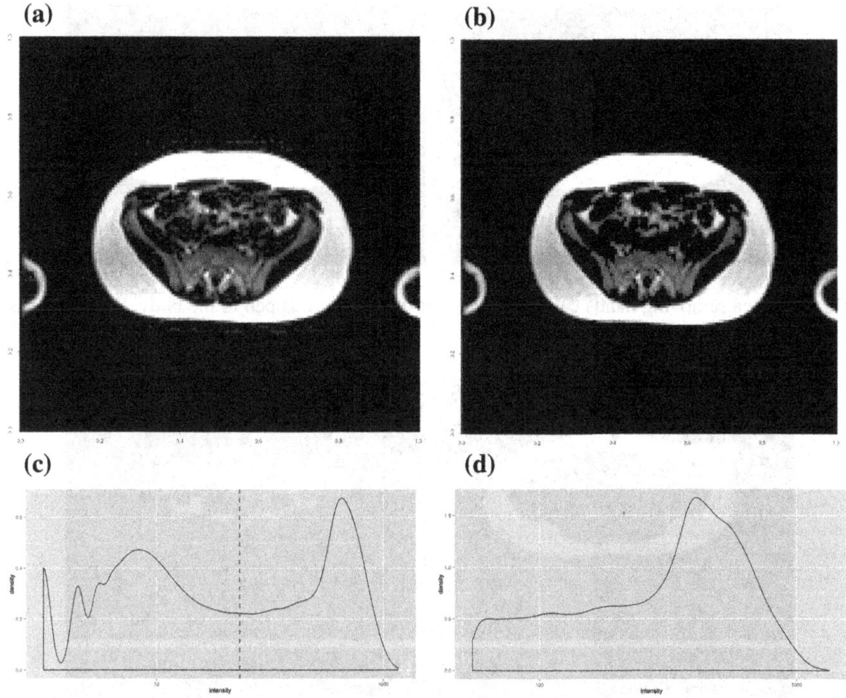

Fig. 2 MRI volume intensity histograms of a subject (**c**) before and (**d**) after applying the mean threshold with the mean intensity highlighted (*red line*). The image in (**a**) has been processed to highlight the noise which appears around the body. Noise pixels are removed in (**b**) after filtering

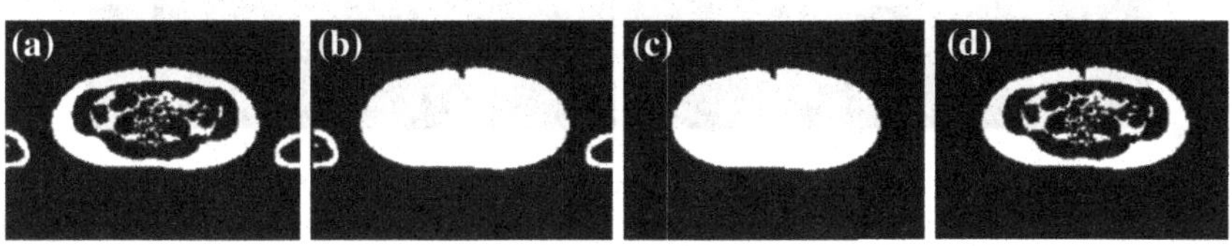

Fig. 3 To remove hands and obtain the main application area morphologic methods are used (**a**) threshold to remove unwanted artifacts and to separate the background from the body tissue. (**b**) After that all connected areas are filled being the biggest one (**c**) our application area. The other are the hands, as we do not need them we will remove them and apply our application area to the first cleaned image to obtain our (**d**) slice with the Total Adipose Tissue (TAT)

be easily solved; when detecting the body is not a complete enclosing figure, we perform a dilation to close the gap, and the circle will become complete, after that we can perform an erosion to recover the initial circle size. In Fig. 3a, b, it can be seen how a not completed circle can be filled.

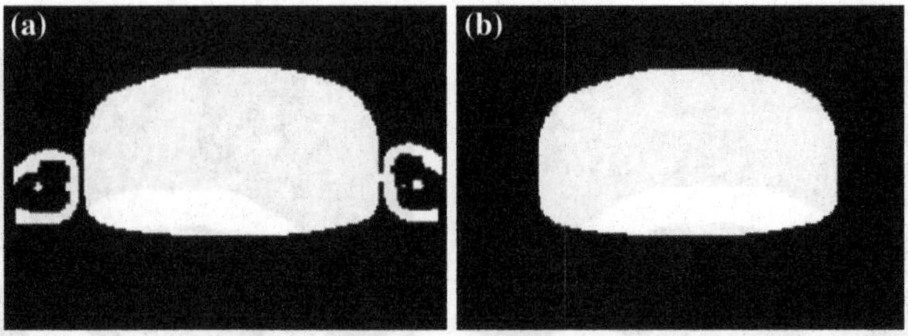

Fig. 4 When removing hands can happened that the arms are appen to the body. With morphological operators can be solved

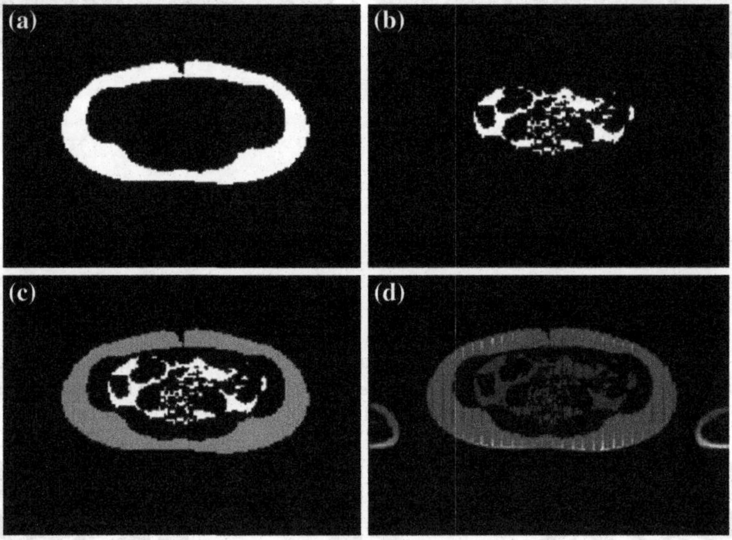

Fig. 5 After obtaining the TAT we need to separate (**a**) SAT and (**b**) VAT. After obtaining the proper segmentation we localize them in the same mask (**c**) and also paint it overlaid on the original image (**d**)

3.4 Adipose Tissue Segmentation

The final mask provides us with the localization of the total adipose tissue (TAT), from this mask and the thresholded slice in Fig. 3a we localize two type of adipose tissues, SAT and VAT. To segment both adipose tissues first the SAT is separated and then VAT is calculated using $VAT = TAT - SAT$. To calculate SAT matrix labels are localized in the TAT mask, and the biggest object is identified as the SAT region. Illustration is provided in Fig. 5.

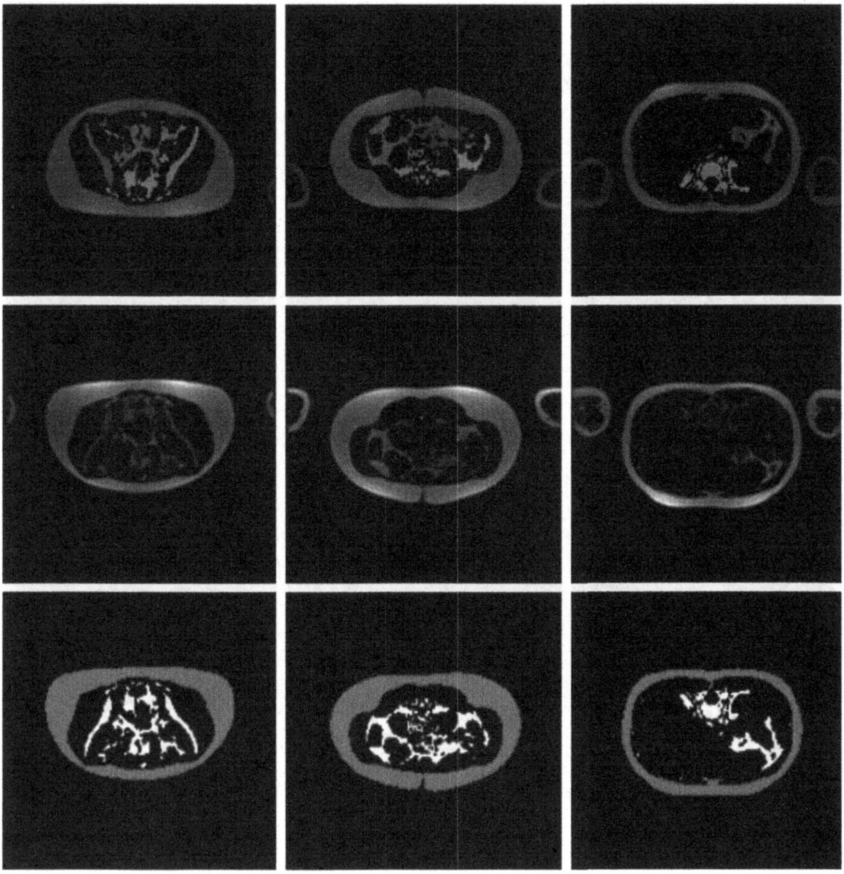

Fig. 6 subject A. We select 3 axial slices with some critical feature. *First row* shows handlabeled fat pixels. *Second row* shows the original slice intensity. *Third row* shows the result of the segmentation, *orange color* for the SAT and white for the VAT

4 Results

SAT and VAT volume is calculated on the six-echo Dixon adipose tissue only resultant volumetric images, from the hepatic dome to the lumbosacral union. An automatic segmentation algorithm segments the subcutaneous and the visceral fat from the rest of the tissues, specially bones. The result of the automatic segmentation is visually checked and manually corrected when needed. We do not have ground truth so the validation is made visually and corrections manually when needed. Figures 6 and 7 show specific results in selected slices which have some critical feature, such as the navel.

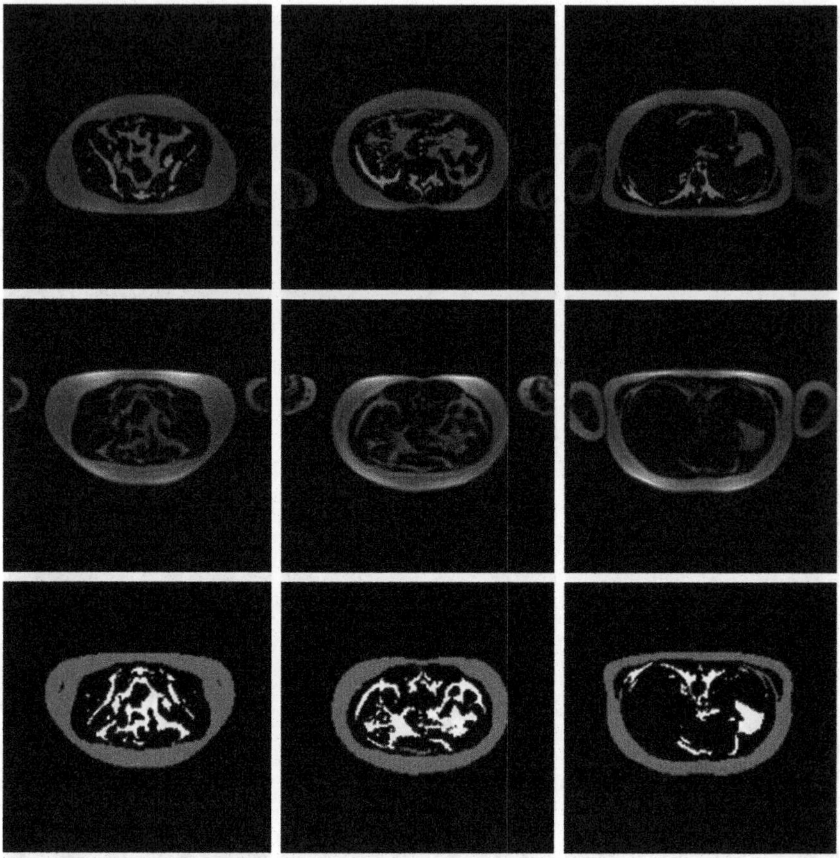

Fig. 7 subject B. We select 3 axial slices with some critical feature. *First row* shows handlabeled fat pixels. *Second row* shows the original slice intensity. *Third row* shows the result of the segmentation, *orange color* for the SAT and white for the VAT

5 Conclusions

The realization of large scale studies about children obesity requires the processing of huge quantities of MRI data, in order to segment and quantify the evolution of the fat deposited in the subcutaneous and visceral adipose tissues. This paper reports an ad hoc segmentation algorithm working on specific fat visualization MRI sequences, which provide good contrast of fat voxels. Results have been visually validated by the medical personnel involved in the project, and we are planning the quantitative validation requiring the manual segmentation, which is a big effort from the human operators.

Acknowledgments This research has been partially funded by grant TIN2011-23823 of the Ministerio de Ciencia e Innovación of the Spanish Government (MINECO), and the Basque Government grant IT874-13 for the research group. Alexandre Savio and Manuel Graña were supported by EC under FP7, Coordination and Support Action, Grant Agreement Number 316097, ENGINE European Research Centre of Network Intelligence for Innovation Enhancement.

References

1. Labayen, I., Ruiz, J.R., Ortega, F.B., Harro, J., Merenakk, L., Oja, L., Veidebaum, T., Sjostrom, M.: Insulin sensitivity at childhood predicts changes in total and central adiposity over a 6-year period. Int. J. Obes. **35**(10), 1284–1288 (2011)
2. Labayen, I., Ortega, F.B., Sjostrom, M., Ruiz, J.R.: Early life origins of low-grade inflammation and atherosclerosis risk in children and adolescents. J. Pediatr. **155**(5), 673–677 (2009)
3. May, A.L., Kuklina, E.V., Yoon, P.W.: Prevalence of cardiovascular disease risk factors among US adolescents, 1999–2008. Pediatrics **129**(6), 1035–1041 (2012)
4. Ogden, C.L., Carroll, M.D., Flegal, K.M.: High body mass index for age among US children and adolescents, 2003–2006. JAMA **299**(20), 2401–2405 (2008)
5. Ross, R.: Advances in the application of imaging methods in applied and clinical physiology. Acta Diabetolog. **40**(Suppl 1), S45–50 (2003)

Automated Segmentation of Subcutaneous and Visceral Adipose Tissues from MRI

Borja Ayerdi, Oier Echaniz, Alexandre Savio and Manuel Graña

Abstract Our objective is to create an automatic image segmentation system of the abdomino-pelvic area allowing quick adipose tissue segmentation demanding minimal intervention of the human operator. The algorithm tackling with this problem is a process encompassing several image processing techniques including morphological operators (erosion, dilatation), binarization, connected-component labeling, holes filling techniques, watershed transform, achieving accurate segmentation results. We have performed computational experiments over 24 anonymized human magnetic resonance image datasets, consisting of 60 slices each, of the abdomino-pelvic area. Right now the evaluation is visual, because we still haven't got the manual delineation serving as ground truth, so that we can't calculate the accuracy, sensitivity or specificity values. Medical expert examination of the obtained results are encouraging, comparable to manual segmentation. This automatic method could save a lot of time allowing the realization of large scale studies.

1 Introduction

Overweight and childhood obesity in developed countries has become epidemic and constitute a huge problem in the public health system [4]. Children with obesity are 5 times more likely to develop insulin resistance and type 2 diabetes mellitus than non-obese ones. Moreover, the majority of children with overweight has at least one cardiovascular (CV) risk factor [3]. Although most CV problems commonly associated with obesity are manifested in adulthood, its origins appear in early stages of life [2]. Thus, CV risk factors measured in childhood predict the development of

B. Ayerdi (✉) · O. Echaniz · A. Savio · M. Graña
Computational Intelligence Group, University of the Basque Country (UPV/EHU), San Sebastián, Spain
e-mail: ayerdi.borja@gmail.com

A. Savio · M. Graña
ENGINE Centre, Wrocław University of Technology, Wybrzeże Wyspiańskiego 27, 50-370 Wrocław, Poland

Y.-W. Chen et al. (eds.), *Innovation in Medicine and Healthcare 2015*, Smart Innovation, Systems and Technologies 45,
DOI 10.1007/978-3-319-23024-5_39

coronary lesions in adulthood, suggesting that some of these lesions causing CV risk factors may already be occurring in childhood [1].

The accumulation of liver fat is closely linked to visceral adipose tissue (VAT) and insulin resistance. Since exercise improves insulin sensitivity and is able to reduce VAT in overweight children. The work in this paper is developed in the framework of a study whose hypothesis is that exercise of moderate to high intensity (between ventilatory thresholds) will reduce liver fat and improve body composition and cardiovascular health in overweight children. To test this hypothesis is needed a comparison between the quantity of adipose tissue before and after the exercise periods. Since manual segmentation is hard and time consuming task, and given the high volume of data that will be generated by the project, an automatic segmentation method is required. This method should provide a quantification of the total VAT and Subcutaneous Adipose Tissue (SAT) volume in order to compare both sequences.

The MRI for this study has been conducted in a Magnetom Avanto equipment, Siemens Healthcare, 1.5 Tesla, of 33mt m maximum gradient amplitude, minimum rise time of 264 microseconds, high sink rate of 125 T/m/s, version syngo MR B17, Numaris/4 software. The equipment is located at the magnetic resonance unit of Osatek in Hospital Santiago in Vitoria (Álava University Hospital). The sequences were performed in supine position, in apnea without intravenous contrast injection, using phased array matrix body antennas and spine matrix.

The main objective of this work was to develop an automated method to distinguish different type of adipose tissue in a large number of subjects, before and after they are in treatment, so that we can improve our understanding of the relation between the treatments and the presence of adipose tissue. Image based volume quantification will allow to test the study hypothesis. For the method to be successful the result of the newly developed segmentation system have to be accurate, reproducible and, above all, comparable to manual segmentation, which we will demonstrate with visual data presented in the following sections. Section 2 describes the methods we have developed of automatic segmentation. Section 3 provides some visual results on different datasets, highlighting the issues that are solved robustly by the proposed algorithm. Section 4 gives some conclusions and future work to be done.

2 Methods

As we have described in the previous section several methods have been proposed in order to make VAT and SAT segmentation. In our case we are mainly working with fat signal and pve images. Our proposed method works as follows: We load the entire volume of MRI data from fat and fat partial volume (fat_pve) sequences, however the data are processed one axial slice at at time. For each axial slice the segmentation process is an heuristic sequence of image processing operation, including different morphological operators (erode, dilate, open, close), thresholding to obtain binary masks, finding blobs by connectivity analysis, filling holes in a binary image,

Algorithm 1 Automated fat segmentation method

- Load volume (fat_signal and fat_pve)
- For each slice:

1. Binarize fat signal applying a threshold (see Fig. 1a)
2. Apply small erosion (disk, R=1) (see Fig. 1b)
3. Find largest connected component (see Fig. 1c)
4. Fill Image holes by rows. (see Fig. 1d)
5. Apply big erosion (disk, R=20) (see Fig. 1d)
6. Watershed segmentation of the results of step 4.
7. Select the unique watershed region labels so that watershed region is included in the eroded image mask obtained in step 5.
8. Compose a binary image mask with this regions selected in step 7. (see Fig. 1e)
9. Find largest connected component.
10. Make a small erosion and get the perimeter pixels (width 5) by subtracting the eroded image from the original. (see Fig. 1f)
11. Apply the fat mask to extract the visceral region from the fat partial volume signal, denoted L.
12. Binarize L applying a threshold. (Fig. 1g)
13. Sum to the binarized L the perimeter mask obtained in step 10.
14. Apply small erosion (disk, R=1)
15. Find largest connected component. (Fig. 1h)
16. Fill the center of the biggest blob
17. Apply small erosion (disk, R=1)
18. Find largest connected component. (see Fig. 1i)
19. Compute image closing (disk, R=10)
20. Calculate VAT and SAT areas. (see Fig. 1j)

performing watershed segmentation, calculating some objects perimeter, etc. The detailed process description is given in Algorithm 1, with illustration of some key steps given in Fig. 1. All this experiments are carried out in Matlab R2013a.

First, we have images that correspond to fat content by design of the imaging sequences. Therefore, creating masks that cover fat regions is relatively easy, almost any threshold would do. The fat image allows easy separation of visceral and peripheral fat, however fat quantification is better done on the pve signal. The steps in the process are intended to solve some of the issues found in the available images. We discuss some:

- Removal of arms: they appear in many slices as separate regions, but in some of them they are touching the body. Strong erosion and selection of the biggest blob in the image are intended to separate arms from the body and ensure that the body is selected.
- Removal of connections of the peripheral body fat with innermost visceral fat. Strong erosion breaks this link. Also, computing the inside region of the body by filling the peripheral fat blob and computing the difference, allows to separate peripheral fat from the visceral fat.

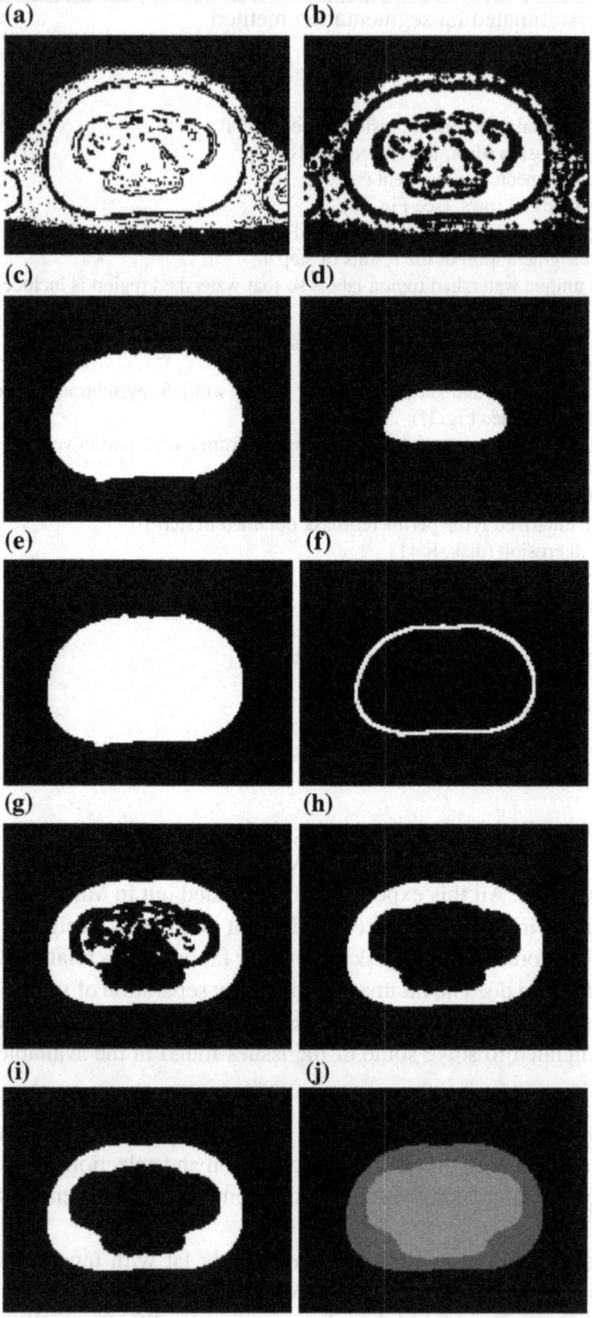

Fig. 1 Visualization of the steps in Algorithm

- Filling the gaps corresponding to the navel, which breaks the peripheral fat region in some slices. This is achieved by applying a closing morphological operator which fills the gaps.

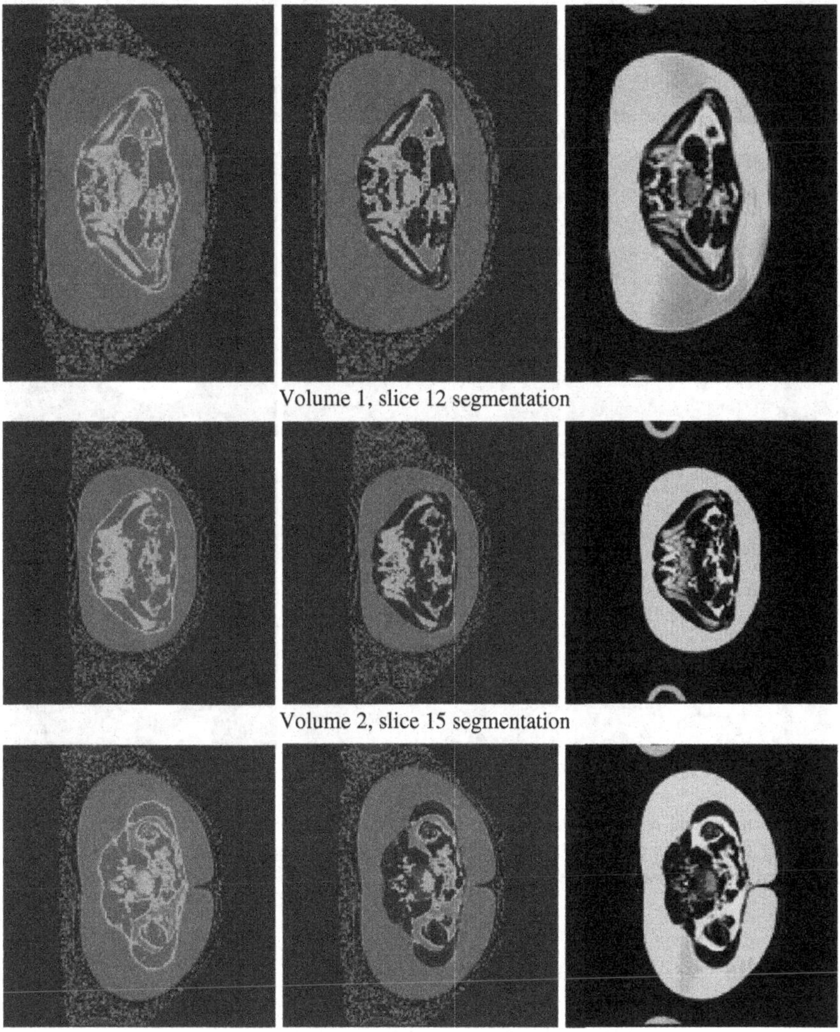

Volume 1, slice 12 segmentation
Volume 2, slice 15 segmentation
Volume 3, slice 16 segmentation

Fig. 2 Some visual results of the algorithm, *left* to *right*, computing the mask on the fat signal, extracting the regions of partial volume fat signal, resulting segmentation, *pink* corresponds to abdominal fat, and *green* to visceral fat

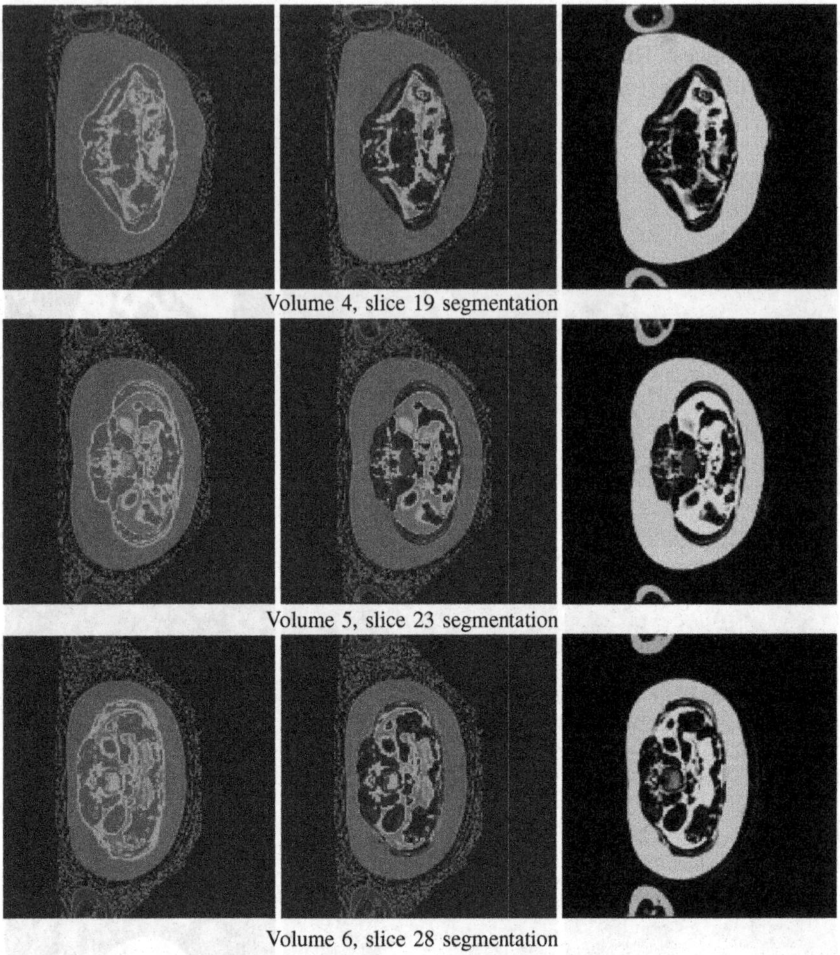

Volume 4, slice 19 segmentation
Volume 5, slice 23 segmentation
Volume 6, slice 28 segmentation

Fig. 3 Some visual results of the algorithm, *left* to *right*, computing the mask on the fat signal, extracting the regions of partial volume fat signal, resulting segmentation, *pink* corresponds to abdominal fat, and *green* to visceral fat

3 Results

In this section we are showing some visual results. As we said in the previous sections we haven't got the ground truth so our way to validate our results right now is visually. We are displaying one sample slice from one volume at each row in Figs. 2 and 3. From left to right, first image corresponds to VAT and SAT areas. Second picture shows coloured original image overlapped by a red and green mask. Red mask shows segmented SAT area while green mask corresponds to VAT area. The rightmost image we are plotting the original fat signal image in a grayscale level and overlapped again SAT and VAT areas in red and green respectively. We are showing different slices on different volumes to demonstrate that our method is working for different volumes and conditions.

4 Conclusions

A large study (n > 1000) on the effect of execs on the fat contained in adipose tissues of children at risk of obesity requires some automated fat segmentation and quantification in order to test the study hypothesis. We have developed a robust VAT and SAT automatic segmentation algorithm. The results look promising even if we still haven't got the ground truth and we can't extract numerical results (accuracy, specificity, ROC, etc.). As future work we are planning to start working with more subjects (>100) and have their ground truth mask segmented by clinical experts.

Acknowledgments This research has been partially funded by grant TIN2011-23823 of the Ministerio de Ciencia e Innovación of the Spanish Government (MINECO), and the Basque Government grant IT874-13 for the research group. Alexandre Savio and Manuel Graña were supported by EC under FP7, Coordination and Support Action, Grant Agreement Number 316097, ENGINE European Research Centre of Network Intelligence for Innovation Enhancement

References

1. Labayen, I., Ruiz, J.R., Ortega, F.B., Harro, J., Merenakk, L., Oja, L., Veidebaum, T., Sjostrom, M.: Insulin sensitivity at childhood predicts changes in total and central adiposity over a 6-year period. Int. J. Obes. **35**(10), 1284–1288 (2011)
2. Labayen, I., Ortega, F.B., Sjostrom, M., Ruiz, J.R.: Early life origins of low-grade inflammation and atherosclerosis risk in children and adolescents. J. Pediatr. **155**(5), 673–677 (2009)
3. May, A.L., Kuklina, E.V., Yoon, P.W.: Prevalence of cardiovascular disease risk factors among US adolescents, 1999–2008. Pediatrics **129**(6), 1035–1041 (2012)
4. Ogden, C.L., Carroll, M.D., Flegal, K.M.: High body mass index for age among US children and adolescents, 2003–2006. JAMA **299**(20), 2401–2405 (2008)

Enabling a Smart and Distributed Communication Infrastructure in Healthcare

Chrystinne Oliveira Fernandes, Carlos José Pereira de Lucena, Carlos Alberto Pereira de Lucena and Bruno Alvares de Azevedo

Abstract The search for innovative solutions within the health care context has largely motivated the conduct of scientific research in this area. Despite the technological resources available nowadays, there are still many problems in the hospital environment. We propose a solution to assist medical teams in performing their activities. It is a platform of information distribution that focus on the status of patients' health and is meant to be easily accessed by health care professionals. It also supports the automatic collection of vital patient data by using Arduino microcontrollers, medical sensors and wearables. In addition, it performs an automatic detection process of anomalies in a patient's condition in real time and sends alerts to the health care providers in charge, through the use of software agents. We conducted a case study in a Brazilian hospital in the city of Rio de Janeiro. In this experiment, a medical team used our platform. We observed that any solution should have good usability in order to be adopted as a tool by health care professionals in their work routine.

Keywords Healthcare · Medical systems · E-health · Sensors · Wearables · Micro-controllers · Monitoring · Internet of things · Software agents

C.O. Fernandes (✉) · C.J.P. de Lucena · C.A.P. de Lucena · B.A. de Azevedo
Pontifical Catholic University of Rio de Janeiro (PUC-Rio), Rio de Janeiro, Brazil
e-mail: cfernandes@inf.puc-rio.br

C.J.P. de Lucena
e-mail: lucena@inf.puc-rio.br

C.A.P. de Lucena
e-mail: azevedo@puc-rio.br

B.A. de Azevedo
e-mail: lucenapucdesign@gmail.com

Y.-W. Chen et al. (eds.), *Innovation in Medicine and Healthcare 2015*,
Smart Innovation, Systems and Technologies 45,
DOI 10.1007/978-3-319-23024-5_40

1 Introduction

There are many researches aimed at achieving technological innovations that can help improve the development of the health care area. The application of such innovations in this field is essential to reduce costs and help replace costly and expensive procedures with more effective techniques that can bring numerous benefits to society.

The hospital environment is faced with some challenges, such as the large number of patients per healthcare provider; the need to collect vital patient data continuously and react as quickly as possible in case the patients' condition worsens. Commonly, professionals involved in a patient's treatment face an inflexible work routine and need to meet other health care providers to discuss the patients' outcome, diagnosis and treatment modalities, among other things.

Our goal is to provide a solution that will help to reduce cost and time spent by these professionals in performing such tasks. We also aim at assisting them in providing services with greater agility and quality. In order to solve, or minimize, some of these problems, we built a platform for effective communication and distribution of information within the health care context. We named this solution Remote Patient Monitoring System (RPMS).

Our solution supports automatic collection of vital data by using Arduino microcontrollers, medical sensors and wearables. Furthermore, it supports remote and autonomous monitoring of the patients' health condition by using software agents; it provides automatic detection of abnormalities in a patient's vital data, and it sends alerts to the health care professionals.

The RPMS incorporates the use of smart devices and different software techniques in order to save hospital resources. The RPMS comprises a prototype based on Internet of Things (IoT) technologies. IoT is field within Computer Science that has grown substantially over recent years. It broadens the established concept of the internet, from a network that connects people to a wider network that allows for the connection between people and things, and between things, with little or no human intervention. Within the IoT context, "things" are real-world entities that are part of the IoT network. These things can vary from simple objects, such as a chair, appliances or cars, including living entities, for instance, plants, animals and persons. Our solution adopts a modeling strategy based on reactive software agents to build the IoT application.

We conducted a case study that resulted in the development of the platform, enabling remote patient monitoring and detection of anomalies in the patients' health status in real time. The platform was deployed in a real environment, in a Brazilian hospital in the city of Rio de Janeiro. During this experiment, a medical team could make use of the platform's features and contribute to the refinement of our solution by giving their feedback. We observed that any solution in such environment needs to offer a usability property in order to be effectively used by the medical team.

The remainder of this paper is organized as follows: Sect. 2 describes the theoretical fundamentals and related work, and discusses aspects of IoT and Multi-Agent Systems (MAS). Section 3 describes the research method used in this study. Section 4 presents the details of the conducted case study. Section 5 concludes this paper with final remarks and future work.

2 Theoretical Fundamentals and Related Work

This project takes a multidisciplinary approach, involving a variety of research areas, such as the IoT, Artificial Intelligence (AI), Multi-Agent Systems (MAS) and Design. Building on these areas, we designed and constructed an e-health system to assist remote patient monitoring activity. Before discussing the solution in detail, we present a brief overview of fundamental concepts that support the features in this work. One can define IoT as a global network of smart devices that can sense and interact with their environment using the Internet for their communication and interaction with users and other systems [1]. IoT application developers may rely on a variety of communication technologies. In this work, we use RFID (Radio-Frequency IDentification), Arduino micro-controllers and sensors.

RFID is an automatic identification technology based on radio signals, used for sensing and communication [2]. A RFID system consists of two components: the transponder, which is located on the object to be identified and the interrogator or reader, which, depending on the technology used, may be a read-only or read-write device. The reader and transponder are the main components of every RFID system [3]. Arduino is a modular open-source prototyping platform. It consists of a microcontroller that can be programmed to process input and output of external electronic components connected to it. It is an embedded computing device that allows to build systems to interact with the environment through hardware and software [1]. Developers can use different types of sensors to collect useful data in IoT applications in the e-health context. These sensors can provide a variety of vital data, including heartbeat rate, blood glucose (to monitor diabetic patients), temperature, humidity, liquid level, oxygen level, carbon dioxide level, patient activities (with an accelerometer) and many others.

Another area involved in this work is MAS. According to Ferber, MAS are systems those contains agents, objects and an environment. An agent is an autonomous entity that has skills to achieve its goals. They are software entities that can act, perceive its environment and communicate with each other. In this context, agents can be reactive or cognitive. Cognitive agents are those that can form plans for their behaviors, whereas reactive agents are those that just have reflexes [4].

Exploring scientific productions in e-health domain, we find some papers with similar approaches to our, such as Su and Wu's proposal [5]. It presents the implementation of a distributed information infrastructure that offers: An automatic notification process to the professionals in charge of patients' care about abnormalities in their health status; remote medical advice; and the possibility of holding health continuous monitoring using intelligent agents. Su and Wu proposed a mobile and ubiquitous monitoring system that allows immediate analysis of physiological patient data besides personalized and real time feedback on their condition by sending alarms and reminders. In this solution, patients can be assessed, diagnosed and treated remotely and ubiquitously.

In [6], the Su and Chu's approach focuses on the design and development of a mobile multi-agent based distributed information system to allow automatic fetal monitoring in real time from any location using a PDA, smart phone, laptop, or desktop computer. According Su and Chu, the benefits of Mobile Agents (MA) consist of overcoming the limitations of client devices, customizability, higher survivability, asynchronous and autonomous computing, local data access and interoperability, processing decentralization, communication and computational resource optimization, and the support for designing applications that interact with human users.

According Mohammadzadeh et al. [7], innovations in the field of information technology in healthcare applications such as mobile health systems are very important to gain full benefits of E-Health. Apply remote medical diagnosis and monitoring system provides health care professionals access to central database and patient information. Mobile health could be a solution to overcome barriers of health service personnel, timely access to health information related to patient especially in emergencies and prevent tests duplication, delay and error in suitable treatment to patient.

3 Methodology

In order to perform an in-depth analysis and clarify research challenges regarding patient monitoring through an IoT view, we have defined research questions followed by a case study to explore design and implementation issues.

3.1 Research Questions

1. What are the benefits of automatic data collection through sensors?
2. What types of anomalies could be detected automatically by using our solution?
3. Which benefits remote storage of patient data can bring?

4 Case Study: Remote Patient Monitoring

4.1 Problem Definition and Proposed Solution

Scientific research within the context of healthcare is a complex task. Dealing with such sensitive issues as patients' health and the risks involved in their medical treatment encompass challenges of diverse natures. Barriers to conducting research in this area are not limited to strictly technical matters. The direct involvement of patients in any scientific research demands the definition of ethical protocols. Moreover, healthcare staff and patients may be involved in design stages of a software development process, since their perspectives might contribute with practical design issues. However, these parties may have little spare time for collaborating with the research.

We observe that in many cases the patient monitoring is done reactively. In this case, the medical team only takes action after detecting a decline in the patient's health. We define the term Anomaly Detection Interval (ADI) as the time interval between the moment that the patient had complications in their health status and the time of its detection by health professionals. We define as anomalies noticeable deviations in patients' health status, which requires professional intervention at the instant they occur. The physical monitoring is one of the factors that contribute to raising the ADI, since the healthcare provider needs to displace himself to the location of patients and then collect vital data for the assessment of their condition.

As a proposed solution for patient monitoring, the RPMS is an IoT application that supports automatic collection and patient data distribution. It comprises a mobile app that provides access to patient data remotely stored and helps to visualize it in real-time. This system makes use of software agents for anomaly detection and dynamic reconfiguration in response to changes in the environment.

4.2 Goals

We defined the following goals to guide the development of the prototype solution, aiming: 1—To minimize the ADI; 2—To automate the process of collecting vital patient data; 3—To allow remote monitoring of patient's vital data; 4—To share health-related information about a patients' treatment with medical staff and external collaborators; 5—To provide the medical team with data analysis and a collaborative diagnoses; 6—To allow automatic detection of abnormalities in a patient's health status;

4.3 Results

RPMS Architecture. The RPMS is structured in three layers (Fig. 1).

L1—Data Distribution Layer. Our solution uses a cloud-based platform to distribute patient data called Parse [8]. Parse is a free remote data storage service that offers functionalities for saving data objects, file storage, push notifications and user management. It allows data portability, offering a way to import data and export an application's entire data set, in the same format as the REST API.
L2—Data Communication Layer. Performs the communication of the IoT application (L3) with the cloud-based platform (L1) through a REST API. We use a technology called Temboo to provide this communication. The Temboo is a platform used to facilitate building applications and interacting with various APIs [9]. It has the Parse library that supports code creation for consume the services offered by this cloud platform. We also use another Temboo library called Twilio to send alerts to health professionals via SMS.
L3—Data Management Layer. Comprises the IoT application with its six modules (M1-M6). It is responsible for the entire information processing in RPMS. These modules are described as follows:

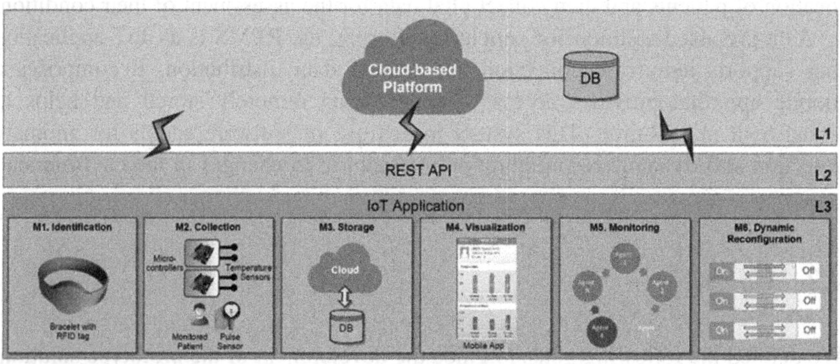

Fig. 1 The RPMS architecture with its three layers (L1-L3). The IoT application (L3) interacts with a cloud-based platform (L1) through a REST API (L2)

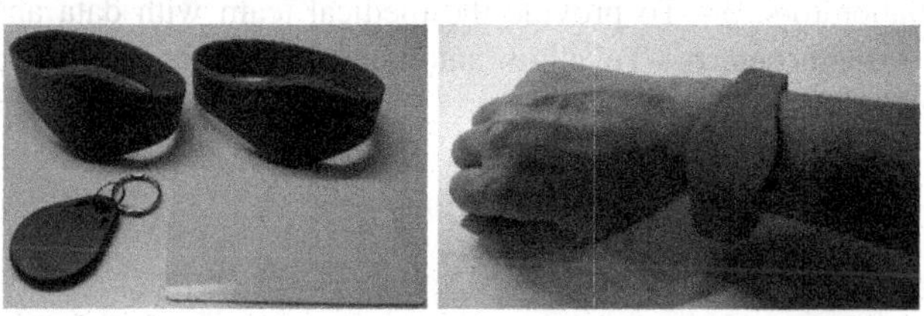

Fig. 2 Accessories that can be used for patient's identification, containing RFID tags

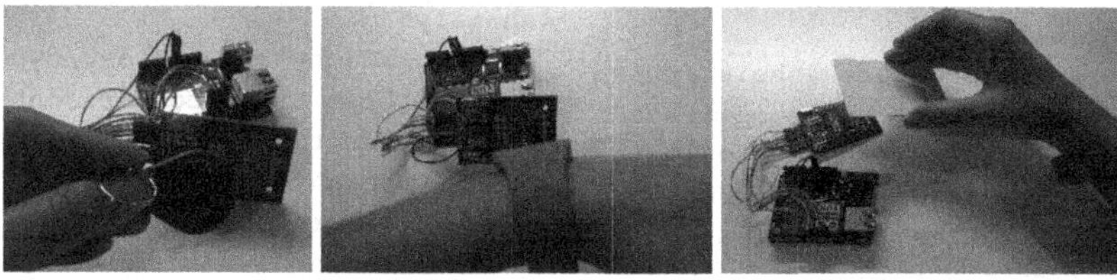

Fig. 3 Readings of accessories with RFID tags through our hardware prototype

M1. Patient's Identification: We utilize an RFID system that includes a wearable bracelet-type device with an RFID tag (Fig. 2) and an RFID reader (Fig. 4). In such case, a patient uses a bracelet in order to be identified it in the system by a health professional (Fig. 3).
M2. Collection: Our application collects automatically patient data such as pulse and body temperature by using a hardware prototype. The prototype comprises an Arduino with wireless and Ethernet network interface, a temperature sensor and a heartbeat sensor (Fig. 4). We implement the M1 and M2 modules in the C++ programming language, by using the Arduino Integrated Development Environment (IDE) [10].
M3. Storage: Once collected, the system transmits the patients' data to a cloud database service if connectivity is available. Otherwise, the application persists data locally and transmits them later on.
M4. Visualization: When health professionals read a patient's bracelet using a device such as a smartphone or a tablet, the data of this patent can be quickly visualized in their device. The RFID reading triggers the initialization of this module displaying patient records. Any authorized person can access it from a smartphone. The application requests data from the cloud platform and exhibits at the smartphone in line charts. The plotted data is updated in real-time, in interval time settings previously. The Fig. 6f shows an example of charts corresponding to patient temperature and heartrate data.

We named our mobile application MedData. In addition to exhibit patient records in chart lines and real time, MedData also has many other features to facilitate patient monitoring. MedData's features are presented in detail in the next subsections.

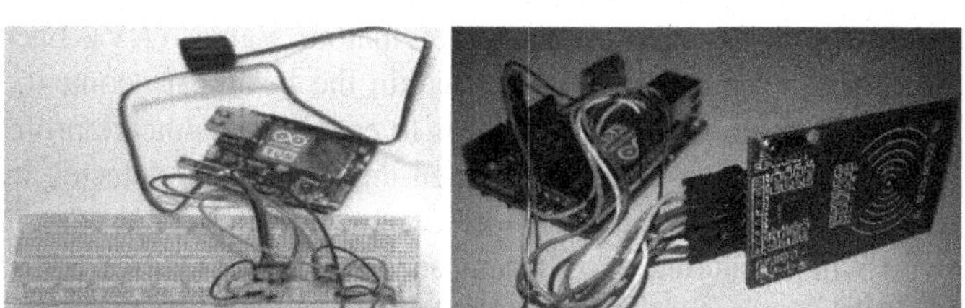

Fig. 4 (On the *left*) Prototype for monitoring patients containing temperature and pulse sensors. (On the *right*) Prototype for patients' identification with RFID technology

```
<anomaly>
    <type>Bradyarrhythmia</type>
    <criteria type="comparison">
        <function symbol="<"/>
        <data>Heartrate</data>
        <value>50</value>
    </criteria>
</anomaly>

<anomaly>
    <type>Tachyarrhythmias</type>
    <criteria type="comparison">
        <function symbol=">"/>
        <data>Heartrate</data>
        <value>110</value>
    </criteria>
</anomaly>

<anomaly>
    <type>Hypothermia</type>
    <criteria type="comparison">
        <function symbol="<"/>
        <data>Temperature</data>
        <value>35</value>
    </criteria>
</anomaly>

<anomaly>
    <type>Hyperthermia</type>
    <criteria type="comparison">
        <function symbol=">"/>
        <data>Temperature</data>
        <value>38</value>
    </criteria>
</anomaly>
```

Fig. 5 The XML document encoding the types of anomalies

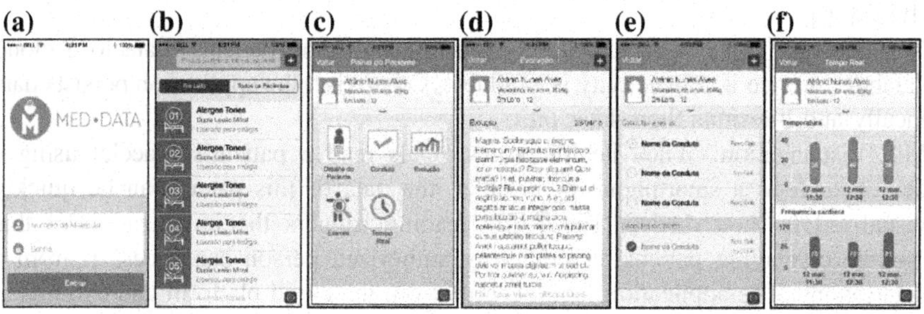

Fig. 6 **a** Login. **b** General board. **c** Patient dashboard with real-time. **d** Patient evolution. **e** Patient evolution. **f** Patient records shown in real-time

M5. Monitoring: This module constantly monitors the collected patient data through reactive agents that should react in case of anomalies detection. The system has a mandatory configuration step for each patient that supports the anomalies detection mechanism as follows: an administrator user defines the Desired Value Range (DVR) for each sensor (e.g., expected temperature and pulse values). We call the values that are outside this range Anomalous Values (AV). Each of these anomalies receives a representative label within the healthcare context, so that it makes sense to a domain expert. The goal is to enable a healthcare professional to identify quickly any problem occurring when the anomaly is detected by the system. In addition, the administrator must assign a professional to handle each anomaly, who will be alerted of its occurrence through e-mail or SMS by using agents. In RPMS, the criteria used by the reactive agents for the diagnosis of a specific patient are prescribed and maintained by the responsible physician and encoded in XML format [6] (Fig. 5).

Considering technologies used in the development of system, we use the Java language. To implement software agents in the Monitoring module (M5), we used the JADE (Java Agent Development Framework) framework [11]. The adoption of the JADE addresses issues related to interoperability, scalability, and openness in heterogeneous e-health environments because this framework is a Foundation for Intelligent Physical Agents (FIPA)-compliant agent development platform [6].
M6. Dynamic reconfiguration: The collection module is context sensitive, i.e., the system can react dynamically in response to changes in the environment. The displacement from a patient to a new environment can invalidate the defined data range for the anomalies. In this case, the application will need to be reconfigured. The user can reconfigure them through the application interface or the system cans reconfigure itself autonomously by intelligent agents. In the latter case, the agents will exchange information, so that new agents can learn the environment configuration, by querying other agents that already know the environment conditions.

MedData Application. The mobile application MedData was developed during the year of 2014, in Pontifícia Universidade Católica do Rio de Janeiro (PUC-Rio), involving the departments of Informatics and Design of this university. Currently, the MedData is in its third development version.

In the first version, MedData was developed to run on iOS system and its data entry interface was text-based. This version was applied to a real hospital environment. The pilot project of MedData was conducted for a period of 6 months during the year 2014. It was applied in the ward of a Brazilian tertiary hospital, in Rio de Janeiro. The hospital was the National Institute of Cardiology. The test was implemented and supervised by Dr. Bruno Azevedo, belonging to the clinical staff of the medical team. This ward is made up of thirty beds spread over five staff doctors and ten interns.

The first step of deployment of the system was perform a brief training of medical team and interns. As the training's result, the users were able to perform the tasks assigned to them. However, already at this stage, it became clear that the usability of the MedData should be redesigned. In order to quickly adopt the MedData and promote its immediate use by the medical staff, the entire team was informed about the need for daily updates of patient data, such as laboratory tests results, discharge, transfer beds etc. Throughout the experiment, the rate of MedData use was constantly observed. After the first 2 months, there was a decrease around 20 % in the patient data updates. This drop occurred despite incentives for the use of MedData, warning that the integration of clinical data across the medical team would result in patient safety.

Some hypotheses have been suggested to the progressive decline of MedData employment: 1—Approximately 50 % of staff had Android operating system, which precluded the adoption of MedData since its inception; 2—The use of tablets was rare in the ward, about 5 % of the team, which made the data entry required only by smartphones. In this regard, when there was the need of complete fields with multiple characters, e.g., first and last name, there was a report of impracticality to perform this task on a smartphone; 3—The ward, where the pilot project was carried out, already had an electronic medical record system, which is filled through desktop and is not integrated with MedData. Therefore, the completion and use of MedData represented another task to be performed during the daily medical routine.

The medical routine, either in an outpatient or hospital—emergency department, wards and intensive care units, has the characteristic of being dynamic, fast and with many crucial tasks to be performed. Any optional process or step that do not clarify its immediate utility will have difficulty in their insertion in this daily routine [12, 13].

After testing MedData's first version and based on the difficulties encountered on this pilot and the reporting of users, we decided to redesign the application towards a second version. In the second version, MedData could run on multiple operating systems such as iOS and Android. The second change of greatest impact was the method of data input used by the medical team. To facilitate the data entry process, we supported it via voice commands. Based on the analysis of the interface testing with users during the pilot project, the new technology applied was aimed at recognizing and translating all the data inserted by voice and image into text, so it can be understand by the rest of the medical team. Regarding interface Design, the whole success of the use of the application depends on the easiness of use of the application. In a medical environment, anything that requires extra work is not used.

Although the second version is being tested, we have developed the third version of the MedData. In this release, we evolve the data entry step to allow automatic collection of patient records. Now we have three ways to collect patient data: via text, via voice and by using hardware prototypes mentioned and illustrated above (Fig. 4). We aim to evolve these prototypes to support the use of other medical sensors.

5 Conclusions and Future Work

Considering the current stage of our project, we can answer the defined research questions as follows. First, concerning our proposed approach for automatic data collection through sensors, we can list the following benefits: collection using sensors is a more efficient process of gathering vital patient data than manual data collection processes; also, automatic data collection is less prone to errors than manual collecting process; It saves medical resources; It can bring greater clinical safety to a patient that needs continuous monitoring; It exhibits trend curves as patients' response to a medical intervention, e.g., a therapeutic response to a newly introduced medicine; positive psychological factor for patients regarding security of being monitored.

Second, our platform is a support tool for medical diagnosis, acting proactively in anomalies detection and prevention of diseases. Once the system alerts the physician about the occurrence of anomalous values in patient data monitored in real-time, thus specialists can work in a more proactive way. Analyzing values in patient data characterized as anomalies by software agents, specialists may find out the types of anomalies that the monitored patient could have. For example, considering heartrate, patients could have the following types of anomalies: 1—bradyarrhythmias as sinus bradycardia or atrioventricular block; 2—tachyarrhythmias, such as atrial fibrillation, supraventricular tachycardia and ventricular tachycardia. Analogously, with regard to patient's temperature, anomalous values could represent hypothermia, hyperthermia, fever, inflammatory conditions, infections, etc.

Third, we can list diverse benefits that remote storage of patient data can bring, such as: saving of medical resources; patient data availability; information sharing between experts to get a second opinion to possible treatments for it; backup of data made ease; access to patient data history, which can also assist in prevention of diseases; valuable information about the physiological behavior of each patient that being monitored. This information is displayed as trend curves and its analysis can anticipate physicians in the identification of an eminent clinical decompensation.

As future work, we consider using cognitive agents to work collaboratively on resource sharing, promoting effective resource management by using argumentation techniques. They could perform recommendations, such as which patient should be next in line for medical care or which patient needs to receive, more urgently, medical assistance such as a nursing professional. Agents can also perform activities such as predicting potential patient's health conditions that can lead to anomalies. Lastly, we expect to evolve our platform to handle security aspects aiming at protect data against attacks, as well to assure privacy and confidentiality of this data.

Acknowledgements This work was supported by grants from CAPES.

References

1. Doukas, C.: Building Internet of Things with the ARDUINO. CreateSpace Independent Publishing Platform (2012)
2. Atzori, L., Iera, A., Morabito, G.: The internet of things: a survey. Comput. Netw. **54**, 2787–2805 (2010)
3. Finkenzeller, K.: RFID Handbook: Fundamentals and Applications in Contactless Smart Cards and Identification. Wiley, New York (2003)
4. Ferber, J.: Multi-agent systems: an introduction to distributed artificial intelligence. Addison-Wesley, Reading (1999)
5. Su, C.-J., Wu, C.-Y.: JADE implemented mobile multi-agent based, distributed information platform for pervasive health care monitoring. Appl. Soft Comput. **11**, 315–325 (2011)
6. Su, C.-J., Chu, T.-W.: A mobile multi-agent information system for ubiquitous fetal monitoring. Int. J. Environ. Res. Public. Health. **11**, 600–625 (2014)
7. Mohammadzadeh, N., Safdari, R.: Patient monitoring in mobile health: opportunities and challenges. Med. Arch. **68**, 57–60 (2014)
8. Parse.: https://parse.com/ (2015)
9. Temboo.: https://www.temboo.com/(2015)
10. Arduino.: http://www.arduino.cc/ (2015)
11. JAVA Agent DEvelopment Framework (JADE). http://jade.tilab.com/ (2015)

12. Edwards, P.J., Moloney, K.P., Jacko, J.A., Sainfort, F.: Evaluating usability of a commercial electronic health record: A case study. Int. J. Hum. Comput. Stud. **66**, 718–728 (2008)
13. Viitanen, J., Hyppönen, H., Lääveri, T., Vänskä, J., Reponen, J., Winblad, I.: National questionnaire study on clinical ICT systems proofs: physicians suffer from poor usability. Int. J. Med. Inf. **80**, 708–725 (2011)

Ultrasound Image Dataset for Image Analysis Algorithms Evaluation

Camilo Cortes, Luis Kabongo, Ivan Macia, Oscar E. Ruiz and Julian Florez

Abstract The use of ultrasound (US) imaging as an alternative for real-time computer assisted interventions is increasing. Growing usage of US occurs despite of US lower imaging quality compared to other techniques and its difficulty to be used with image analysis algorithms. On the other hand, it is still difficult to find sufficient data to develop and assess solutions for navigation, registration and reconstruction at medical research level. At present, manually acquired available datasets present significant usability obstacles due to their lack of control of acquisition conditions, which hinders the study and correction of algorithm design parameters. To address these limitations, we present a database of robotically acquired sequences of US images from medical phantoms, ensuring the trajectory, pose and force control of the probe. The acquired dataset is publicly available, and it is specially useful for designing and testing registration and volume reconstruction algorithms.

Keywords Ultrasound • Dataset • Registration • Reconstruction • Datafusion • Tracking • Verification • Validation • Evaluation • Medical images

---

C. Cortes (✉) · L. Kabongo · I. Macia · J. Florez
eHealth and Biomedical Applications, Vicomtech-IK4, San Sebastián, Donostia, Spain
e-mail: ccortes@vicomtech.org

L. Kabongo
e-mail: lkabongo@vicomtech.org

I. Macia
e-mail: imacia@vicomtech.org

J. Florez
e-mail: jflorez@vicomtech.org

C. Cortes · O.E. Ruiz
Laboratorio de CAD CAM CAE, Universidad EAFIT, Medellín, Colombia
e-mail: oruiz@eafit.edu.co

C. Cortes · L. Kabongo · I. Macia
Biodonostia Health Research Center, San Sebastián, Donostia, Spain

Y.-W. Chen et al. (eds.), *Innovation in Medicine and Healthcare 2015*,
Smart Innovation, Systems and Technologies 45,
DOI 10.1007/978-3-319-23024-5_41

1 Introduction

The real-time nature, low-cost and non-invasiveness of US imaging makes it attractive not only for early and simple diagnosis but also more and more as a real-time source of imaging to guide minimally invasive interventions. Nevertheless, due to the poor signal-to-noise ratio that US images present, it is cumbersome to design and test the required image analysis algorithms that are required in patient intra-operative registration, volume reconstruction, data fusion and navigation, among others.

Designing and testing algorithms for image guided interventions require datasets that enable evaluation of their accuracy, performance and sensitivity to design parameters. Reference [1] indicates that public US image datasets are required to evaluate the performance of such algorithms.

Most current public US image datasets (e.g. [2, 3] do not include information of the US *probe* (ultrasound transducer) poses along their acquisition. This means that the images are not spatially tracked, which prevents their use image guided procedures that require spatial information. The scientific community has published some tracked US image datasets [1, 4] to address such limitation.

Reference [4] presents US manually-acquired images from brain tumours of patients with the objective of testing US registration algorithms *with respect to* (w.r.t.) Magnetic Resonance Imaging (MRI) scans of the patients. In [1], the CIRS Abdominal Phantom Model 057® is manually scanned with a probe that is tracked with an optical tracking system. Reference [1] presents US images acquired by varying image acquisition parameters such as frequency, focal depth, gain, power, dynamic range, etc. Although the mentioned data is valuable, manual acquisition of US image datasets implies arbitrary and imprecise control of the pose and force of the sensing device. The consequent variable quality of the image limits the use of these datasets in image guided intervention evaluation environments.

Our Literature Survey in the domain of Ultrasound shows no existing dataset acquired with a machine-controlled, repeatable and systematic manner. Such datasets would be useful for evaluating algorithms for: interventional US registration with pre-operative imaging or planning, US registration for automatic annotation and segmentation of reconstructed volumes, US-based navigation based on image fusion or re-slicing, US-based planning using volume reconstruction, automatic feature extraction and classification, among others.

The desirable characteristics of a dataset for ultrasound for image analysis algorithms include: (1) Tracked and non-tracked frame captures for random image registration, (2) Reconstructed data for volumetric exploration, (3) Multiple source acquisition for image fusion, (4) Tissue identification and segmentation for modelling and simulation, (5) Intra-scan constant—and variable—quality of acquisition and (6) Ground Truth measurements of targeted areas.

Based on these observations, our contribution aims to produce a public and documented image dataset of medical phantoms containing: (a) The complete tracked sequence of robot—acquired US images while the US probe force and pose are precisely controlled, (b) Volume reconstruction from the controlled US images, and (c) A set of individually tracked US images targeting phantom features (e.g., lesions, anatomical landmarks, etc.) from ad hoc poses of the probe (i.e. not considered in item (a)). Geometric specifications of the scanned medical phantoms are available from the providers for comparison and verification purposes.

2 Materials and Methods

2.1 Problem Description

In this section, we state the problem of acquiring sequences of US images along with the poses of the US probe w.r.t. the phantom *coordinate system* (CS). The acquisition methodology of such image dataset allows using it for the evaluation of image analysis algorithms. The hardware required to generate such datasets includes: (1) a robotic arm, (2) a US machine, (3) an optical tracking system and (4) a set of medical phantoms to be scanned. The goal is to obtain the robotically acquired US image sequences of the medical phantoms by controlling the pose and force of the US probe (). Downstream effects include the repeatability, controllability of such dataset acquisitions. This problem can be formally stated as follows (Fig. 1).

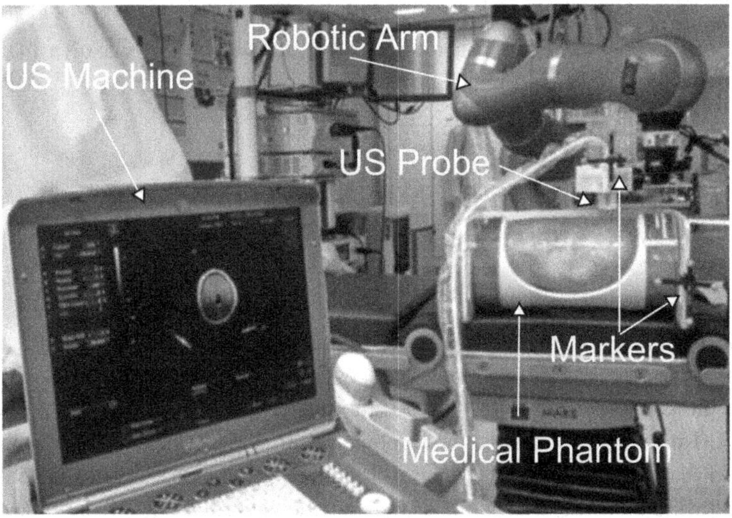

Fig. 1 System to acquire a controlled ultrasound image dataset

Given:

1. A KUKA LWR IV + lightweight robot R [5] able to recreate the dynamics of a spring-damper system with stiffness and damping matrices K and $D \in \mathfrak{R}^{+6x6}$ by using its Cartesian Impedance control [6]. The desired stiffness and damping along the axes of translation and rotation of the robot task space (*x, y, z, a, b, c*) are indicated by the components of matrices $K = diag\{k_x, k_y, k_z, k_a, k_b, k_c\}$ and $D = diag\{d_x, d_y, d_z, d_a, d_b, d_c\}$. The robot provides estimates of the force and torque that is being exerted at the tip of the *Robot End-Effector or tool* (REE).
2. A NDI Polaris Spectra *Optical Tracking System* (OTS) O that estimates the pose of a set of arrays of passive markers $A = \{a_0, \ \cdots, \ a_g\}$ installed on the desired object to track. The OTS O computes the set $T^O(t) = \{T^O_0(t), \ \cdots, \ T^O_g(t)\}$ where each $T^O_i(t)$ is a matrix $\in \mathfrak{R}^{4x4}$ that describes the pose of markers $a_i (\in [0, g])$ w.r.t. the O reference CS.
3. An ultrasound scanning machine GE Voluson i® with probe P (model 9L-RS), which produces a sequence of 2D greyscale images I_i of the region scanned by P.
4. A set of medical phantoms $M = \{m_0, \ \cdots, \ m_h,\}$ that are US-compatible and mimic the physical properties of various tissues and organs of human bodies. A cylindrical hull bounds the *baby phantom* (BP) and a rectangular prism bounds the *abdominal phantom* (AP). Both phantoms are manufactured by CIRS®.

Goal:

A set $H = \{h_0, \ \cdots, \ h_n\}$ of tracked US images $h_i = \left[I_i, \ T_P^{ref}{}_i\right]$ for each of the m_j phantoms acquired under pose and force control of P. The tracked image $h_i = \left[I_i, \ T_P^{ref}{}_i\right]$ consists of an US image I_i plus a transformation matrix $T_P^{ref}{}_i$, which describes the pose of P w.r.t. a reference CS defined by the CS of a marker a_j attached to the m_j scanned medical phantom (Fig. 2).

2.2 *Ultrasound Image Calibration, Acquisition and Processing*

In order to calibrate, capture and process the US images, we have used the software PLUS (Public software Library for Ultrasound imaging research) [7]. Before acquiring the tracked US images, it is necessary to find the transformation T_I^P that relates the CS of the US image I w.r.t. the marker attached to the US probe P to track it. Knowing T_I^P enables the computation of the 3D position of each of the pixels of the US images of the dataset. Finding T_I^P requires the steps described in the following calibration section. depicts a schematic diagram of the objects and coordinate systems involved in the calibration and acquisition procedures.

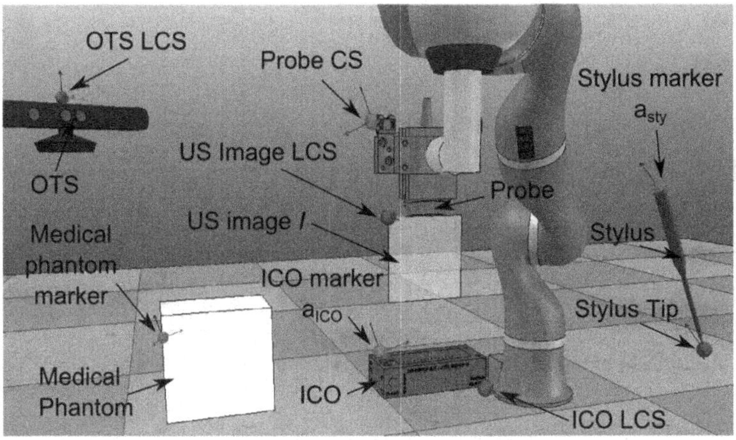

Fig. 2 Schematic diagram of the objects and CS involved in the US image calibration and acquisition procedures. *Red* CS represent marker a_i CS and *blue* CS represent local coordinate systems

Calibration. The calibration procedures are described in detail in [7], and therefore, we briefly discuss them here:

1. Time Axis Calibration: Estimates the time offsets between the data streams provided by the OTS and the US machine. This calibration allows relating US image I_i with the corresponding $T_{P_i}^{ref}$ pose.
2. Stylus Tip Computation: Estimates the transformation $T_{tip}^{a_{sty}}$ of the stylus (narrow elongated rod with a sharp tip) tip w.r.t. the marker a_{sty} CS installed on the stylus to track it. This calibration is necessary to measure the stylus tip coordinates (translation component of T_{tip}^{ref}) w.r.t. a reference CS defined by a marker a_i.
3. Image Calibration Object and OTS Registration: Estimates the transformation $T_{ico}^{a_{ico}}$ of the image calibration object (ICO) *Local CS* (LCS) w.r.t. the CS of marker a_{ico} installed on the ICO to track it. $T_{ico}^{a_{ico}}$ is computed by using a landmark-based registration method using the stylus. Knowing $T_{ico}^{a_{ico}}$ allows expressing the coordinates of the ICO calibration fiducials (N-shaped patterns formed by nylon wires) w.r.t. the OTS, which is a precondition to compute T_I^P.
4. US Image and OTS Registration: Estimates the rigid transformation T_I^P that relates: (a) the coordinates of the ICO fiducials observed in images I_i with (b) the known coordinates of the ICO fiducials w.r.t. the *P* CS (). The details of this algorithm are described in [8].

Image Acquisition Parameters. The ultrasound machine has been configured with the following image acquisition parameters: Receiver frequency = 12.00–2.5 MHz (penetration mode), Depth = 14 cm, Focal Points = 1, Gain = 0 (Fig. 3).

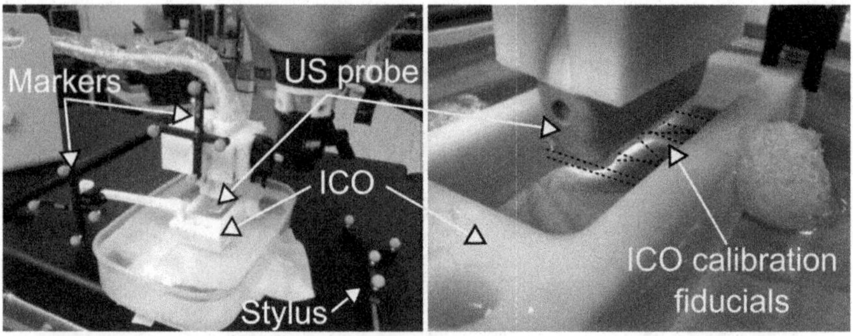

Fig. 3 Registration of the US image CS with respect to the probe CS

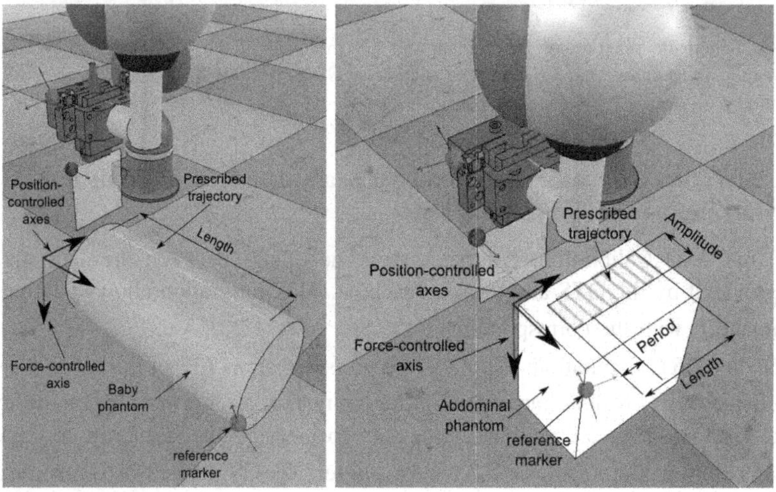

Fig. 4 *Left* Prescribed trajectory to scan the BP. *Right* Prescribed trajectory to scan the AP

2.3 Motion Control of the Robot

To achieve the desired position-force control of P during the robotic-assisted scans, a hybrid position-force controller is implemented on top of the robot Cartesian-Impedance controller. In the force-controlled task subspace of the robot, conditions that allow P to keep contact with the surface of the medical phantom are imposed. To apply the desired force along axis i of R task space, k_i should be zero and a force set point f_i is commanded along axis i. In the position-controlled task subspace, conditions that allow P to traverse the region to be scanned are imposed. To control the position along axis i of R task space, k_i should be assigned with a high magnitude. To guarantee smooth movements, the components of D are assigned with high values.

Table 1 Features of the desired trajectory to scan the BP (Fig. 4 left)

Scan	Length (m)	*V* (m/s)	$norm(\vec{F})$ (N)
1	0.19	0.00100	15
2	0.19	0.00125	15

Table 2 Features of the desired trajectory to scan the AP (Fig. 4 right)

Scan	Length (m)	Amplitude (m)	Period (m)	*V* (m/s)	$norm(\vec{F})$ (N)
1	0.15	0.05	0.0375	0.00125	10
2	0.15	0.045	0.03	0.00125	10

According to the mentioned requirements, we have extended the control module for robot trajectory that we presented in [9] to include force constraints in the desired REE trajectories as follows:

The REE trajectory $E = \{ c(\alpha)_0, \cdots, c(\alpha)_b \}$ is composed by a set of parametric curve segments $c(\alpha)(\alpha \in [0, 1])$, which keep at least C^0 continuity among themselves. Each $c(\alpha)$ is defined by: (a) The minimum set of poses $Q = \{ Q_0, \cdots, Q_s \}$ to define uniquely the desired curve geometry and rotations of the REE, (b) the desired linear velocity $V \in \Re^+$ to go from the initial to the final pose of the segment, and (c) the desired force and torque $\vec{F} \in \Re^6$ to be exerted by the REE while traversing the curve segment.

Prescribed Scanning Trajectories. The BP can be scanned by moving *P* along a straight line parallel to the longitudinal axis of the phantom. The orientation is commanded to keep the probe normal to the phantom surface along the traversed line. The force is commanded to be exerted along the longitudinal axis of *P*. Table 1 summarizes the features of the trajectories to scan the BP.

The AP can be scanned by following a trajectory that resembles a square wave on a plane parallel to the surface of the phantom. The orientation of the REE was programmed to keep the probe normal to be trajectory plane. The force set-point is imposed along the probe longitudinal axis and avoids the deformation of the internal structures of the phantom. Table 2 summarizes the features of the trajectories to scan the AP.

3 Results and Discussion

The results corresponding to the US probe and image calibration processes are presented in Table 3, and the dataset is publicly available at: http://www.vicomtech.org/demos/us_tracked_dataset/.

Comparing our results with those discussed in reference [7], we conclude that the performed calibrations are suitable to acquire tracked US scans.With respect to

Table 3 Us probe calibration

Calibration:	Result:
Time axis	Video stream lags 170.7 ms respect to the OTS stream
Stylus tip computation	$T_{tip}^{a_{sty}}$ is computed with an average error of 0.378038 mm
ICO and OTS registration	$T_{ico}^{a_{ico}}$ is computed with an average error of 0.647239 mm
US Image and OTS registration	T_I^P is computed with an average error of 0.379253 mm

the performance of the implemented hybrid position-force controller, the following metrics are computed to quantify the achievement of the constraints imposed on the trajectories E to scan the medical phantoms:

1. The position error metric (PE): is the Hausdorff distance between the prescribed and traversed trajectory of the REE.
2. The average orientation error (AOE): $u \in \Re^3$ is the representation in exponential map notation [10] of the necessary rotation matrix to go from the orientation in the current REE pose Q_{REE} to the prescribed orientation in pose $Q_i = c(\alpha_i)$ (where α_i represents the parameter value to evaluate $c(\alpha)$). $\|u\|$ is used as a measurement of the REE orientation error. The AOE corresponds to the average of the all the obtained $\|u\|$ while traversing E.
3. The average force error (AFE): is the average magnitude of the difference between desired and exerted force vectors.
4. The average linear velocity error (ALVE): is the average of the differences between the desired and presented linear velocities of the REE. The ALVE metric, does not consider the velocity in the direction of force-controlled axes.

The results of these performance metrics for each scan are presented in Table 4. From results in Table 4, we conclude that the implemented controller allowed scanning the medical phantoms fulfilling the constraints that we imposed on E for each scan.This means that the obtained datasets H do present different levels of quality in function of the linear speed (in the case of BP scans) or number of sweeps (in the case of the AP scans) imposed on the trajectory to acquire them.

In addition to the mentioned datasets H, we include in our database: (a) volume reconstructions V_H from the H datasets generated with the PLUS software (Fig. 5) and (b) a set of tracked ultrasound single frames S_M of the various landmarks, organs and lesions that the phantoms present acquired in different poses of the probe with respect to the images in dataset H.

Table 4 Error metrics related to the accomplishment of constraints in E

Scan	PE (m)	AOE (deg)	AFE (N)	A LVE (m/s)
BP Scan 1	0.00314	0.51620	0.55560	0.00001
BP Scan 2	0.00298	0.50808	0.56241	0.00001
AP Scan 1	0.00368	0.43935	0.65519	0.00004
AP Scan 2	0.00314	0.38477	0.62012	0.00002

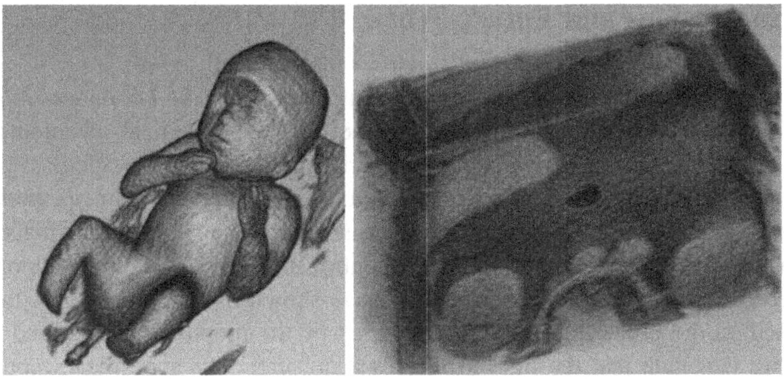

Fig. 5 Volume rendering in 3D Slicer of the BP (*left*) and AP (*right*) of the reconstructed volumes

These datasets provide ground truth information for testing:

1. Volume reconstruction: Image sequences H can be re-sampled to obtain lower-quality datasets to test (tracked and non-tracked) volume reconstruction algorithms (e.g. volume reconstruction with hole-filling algorithms). In this case, V_H volumes serve as reference reconstructions for quantitative comparison purposes.
2. Registration:

   (a) 3D-2D registrations: Volumes V_H and single tracked images S_M can be used to test 3D-2D registrations. By using T_I^P and T_P^{ref}, the pose T_I^{ref} of an US image I (in S_M) with respect to the reference coordinate system can be computed. Note that T_I^{ref} provides the true transformation between S_M and V_H. Then, the estimated transformation provided by the registration algorithm can be compared to T_I^{ref} in order to measure the registration accuracy.

   (b) 3D-3D registrations: Volumes V_H can be used to test 3D-3D registrations. Regions $V_H{'}$ can be extracted from V_H, and then, an arbitrary rigid transformation T can be applied to $V_H{'}$. The registration algorithm should estimate the transformation T.

3. Feature detection: Phantom specifications and volumes V_H can be used as guides to annotate frames in sequences H that contain the desired features to detect. Annotated frames serve as training datasets for feature detection algorithms. Validation can be performed with images S_M or by images obtained by re-slicing V_H.
4. Segmentation: Phantom-based validation of trained automatic and atlas-based 3D segmentation algorithms using H and V_H.

4 Conclusions and Future Work

This article presents a public database of sequences of tracked US images in http://www.vicomtech.org/demos/us_tracked_dataset/ of two medical phantoms that allow the evaluation of image analysis algorithms for procedures such as: patient intra-operatory registration and reconstruction, among others. The methodology proposed to obtain such tracked images consists in using an optical tracking system and a robot under hybrid position/force control to scan the phantoms along prescribed trajectories of the US probe. We have shown that the constraints that we imposed on the probe trajectories are fulfilled by the proposed system, and therefore, we conclude that the tracked images acquisition was systematic, repeatable and controlled. In this way, the acquired tracked US images overcome the limitations of manually acquired datasets. This work is an initial approach to provide relevant data for applying image analysis algorithms to ultrasound in interventional context. As an extension to this work a short term contribution will be the acquisition of existing phantoms under CT and MRI for multi-modal reconstruction, fusion and registration. Future work also consists of the automatic generation of trajectories for the robotic scanning of static and dynamic targets.

References

1. Shivaprabhu, V.R., Enquobahrie, A., Mullen, Z., Aylward, S.: Accelerating ultrasound image analysis research through publically available database. In: SPIE Medical Imaging, pp. 867517–867517 (2013)
2. Balocco, S., Gatta, C., Ciompi, F., Wahle, A., Radeva, P., Carlier, S., Unal, G., Sanidas, E., Mauri, J., Carillo, X., et al.: Standardized evaluation methodology and reference database for evaluating IVUS image segmentation. Comput. Med. Imaging Graph. **38**(2), 70–90 (2014)
3. Tian, J., Wang, Y., Huang, J., Ning, C., Wang, H., Liu, Y., Tang, X.: The digital database for breast ultrasound image. In: 11th Joint International Conference on Information Sciences (2008)
4. Mercier, L., Del Maestro, R.F., Petrecca, K., Araujo, D., Haegelen, C., Collins, D.L.: Online database of clinical MR and ultrasound images of brain tumors. Med. Phys. **39**(6), 3253–3261 (2012)
5. Bischoff, R., Kurth, J., Schreiber, G., Koeppe, R., Albu-Schäffer, A., Beyer, A., Eiberger, O., Haddadin, S., Stemmer, A., Grunwald, G., et al.: The KUKA-DLR Lightweight Robot arm-a new reference platform for robotics research and manufacturing. In: Robotics (ISR), 2010 41st International Symposium on and 2010 6th German Conference on Robotics (ROBOTIK), pp. 1–8 (2010)
6. Albu-Schäffer, A., Ott, C., Hirzinger, G.: A unified passivity-based control framework for position, torque and impedance control of flexible joint robots. Int. J. Robot. Res. **26**(1), 23–39 (2007)
7. Lasso, A., Heffter, T., Rankin, A., Pinter, C., Ungi, T., Fichtinger, G.: PLUS: Open-source toolkit for ultrasound-guided intervention systems. IEEE Trans. Biomed. Eng. **10**, 2527–2537 (2014)
8. Carbajal, G., Lasso, A., Gómez, Á., Fichtinger, G.: Improving N-wire phantom-based freehand ultrasound calibration. Int. J. Comput. Assist. Radiol. Surg. **8**(6), 1063–1072 (2013)

9. Cortes, C.A., Barandiaran, I., Ruiz, O.E., Mauro, A.D.: Robotic research platform for image-guided surgery assistance. In: Proceedings of the IASTED International Conference Biomedical Engineering (BioMed 2013), Innsbruck, Austria, pp. 427–434 (2013)
10. Grassia, F.S.: Practical parameterization of rotations using the exponential map. J. Graph. Tools **3**(3), 29–48 (1998)

Approaches of Phase Lag Index to EEG Signals in Alzheimer's Disease from Complex Network Analysis

Shinya Kasakawa, Teruya Yamanishi, Tetsuya Takahashi, Kanji Ueno, Mitsuru Kikuchi and Haruhiko Nishimura

Abstract The brain is organized as neuronal assemblies with hierarchies of complex network connectivity, and its function is consider to be arisen by synchronized rhythmical firing of neurons. Recently, it is suggested that some of the mental disorders are related to the alterations in the network connectivity in the brain and/or of the strength on synchronized rhythm for brain waves. Here we attempt to analyze electroencephalograms of Alzheimer's disease by Phase Lag Index (PLI) as an index of the synchronization on signals. By regarding values of PLI as the network connectivity among electrodes, we construct a network for PLI in the brain. So, a clustering coefficient describing structural characteristics of the network are also discussed.

Keywords EEG Analysis · Phase Lag Index · Alzheimer's Disease · Synchronization Phenomena · α Wave

1 Introduction

Even if the generation mechanism of brain waves is different in a frequency, a common mechanism is underlying basically [1]. The rhythms of brain waves are arisen from the source of the generation in the thalamus, and the reticular nucleus of the

S. Kasakawa (✉) · T. Yamanishi
Department of Management Information Science, Fukui University of Technology,
Gakuen, Fukui 910–8505, Japan
e-mail: sin0831b@gmail.com

T. Takahashi · M. Kikuchi
Research Center for Child Mental Development, Kanazawa University,
Takaramachi, Kanazawa 920–8640, Japan

K. Ueno
Department of Neuropsychiatry, Faculty of Medical Sciences,
University of Fukui, Eiheiji-cho, Fukui 910–1193, Japan

H. Nishimura
Graduate School of Applied Informatics, University of Hyogo,
Chuo-ku, Kobe650–0044, Japan

Y.-W. Chen et al. (eds.), *Innovation in Medicine and Healthcare 2015*,
Smart Innovation, Systems and Technologies 45,
DOI 10.1007/978-3-319-23024-5_42

thalamus plays the leading role in rhythm formation. The membrane potential fluctuation arisen from rhythmic depolarization and hyperpolarization compositions in the thalamus/cortical projection neuron group makes the shift to synchronization by the signal from reticular nucleus of the thalamus. The greater petrosal nerve soma in a cerebral cortex evolves rhythms of brain wave by input from that fluctuation. The frequency of brain wave rhythms depends on individual arousal levels or states of the brain function. For example, we find mainly alpha wave (8–13 Hz) when a person closes his eyes or remains quiet. The synchronized rhythm event is closely connected with actions or states of brain for animals, and plays a very important role in the successful execution of various functions of the brain [2, 3].

At present, there are several powerful methods on analyzing the synchronization. For a frequency analysis, a Hilbert Huang Coherence (HHC) method from a Hilbert Huang transform has been proposed on analyzing the degree of synchronization with high temporal frequency resolution [4, 5]. Temporal frequency resolution of HHC was found to be higher than that of traditional coherence methods for analysis of non-stationary signals. On the other hand, phase synchronization indexes like Phase Locking Value (PLV) [6, 7], Phase Lag Index (PLI) [8–13], and weighted Phase Lag Index (wPLI) [14, 15] have been suggested as phase analyses on the synchronization.

PLV or PLI's series estimate on the direct quantification of frequency-specific synchronization between pair time trail signals. For instance, the analysis of PLV revealed the synchronizations of the large-scale distance in the gamma band for epileptic patients [7]. On PLI's series Netherlands groups are strenuously investigating and bring continuously exceptional results. Stam and collaborators implied the difference of PLI with electroencephalography (EEG) signals of Alzheimer's disease (AD) and of healthy control for the average of all paris of 21 channels electrodes at β rhythm band [8].

For AD, it is suggested that not only the synchronized rhythms of the brain but also the connections of neural network are abnormal. Delbeuck has reviewed the growing amount of research articles on AD including a disconnection syndrome, and implied that AD pathology would be the consequence of a disturbance of the brain's effective connectivity suggesting abnormal interactions between neuronal system [10]. So, it is important for the research in AD to quantitatively estimate the connectivity using EEG or magnetoencephalography (MEG) signals, and to find relationships of its evaluation value with the degree of AD.

In this paper, we estimate a degree of the synchronization on EEG signals by using PLI. Here the computational effort of PLI is light compared with HHC, and does not have a sensitive response to volume conduction or common source effects [8, 14]. So, the quantitative evaluation of AD is attempted from the estimation of PLI using EEG data of AD with Mini-Mental State Examination (MMSE) scores[1] [11]. Also, it is possible to generate adjacency matrix from any threshold value and to analyze on the brain network from the graph theory by regarding PLI value as the strength of

[1]MMSE is used to screen for cognitive impairment and gives quantitative measure of cognitive status for adults.

Table 1 Information on groups of AD for MMSE score and HC subjects

	All subjects	AD MMSE > 15	MMSE ≤ 15	HC
Total number	16	7	9	18
Male/Female	5/11	2/5	3/6	7/11
Average age years (range)	59.3 (43–66)	57.7 (43–64)	60.4 (55–66)	57.5 (51–67)
Average MMSE score (range)	15.5 (10–26)	19.7 (16–26)	12.3 (10–15)	NA

functional connections between the brain area. We try to investigate the difference in brain networks with healthy control persons and the Alzheimer's disease ones.

The paper is organized as follows: Sect. 2 describes the materials and methods for analyses of EEG data. Section 3 shows results the difference in PLI with HC and AD, and also discusses the correlations of PLI or the clustering coefficient with MMSE score. Section 4 provides a summary and considers topics for future research.

2 Materials and Methods

2.1 Subjects and EEG Data Recording

The personnel organization for the study have been designed by 34 subjects, 16 with AD; and 18 healthy control (HC) subjects [16]. The detailed information on each group of AD and HC is shown in Table 1 All subjects have been provided an informed consent with documents before the research, and the assessment of AD and the cognitive function in AD has used Diagnostic and Statistical Manual of Mental Disorders, Fourth Edition (DSM-IV)[2] [17] and MMSE for Japanese, respectively. Here we partitioned AD group into 2 subgroups by MMSE score, namely low MMSE score group (≤15) and high MMSE score group (>15).

EEG data have been recorded with 18-channel system (EEG–4518, Nihon-Koden, Tokyo, Japan) at 16 electrodes sites together with both ear lobes as the reference of physically link, which were assigned by the International 10–20 System [16]. The subjects were comfortably seated on a chair in an electrically shielded, soundproof, light-controlled room, and they were eyes-closed wakefulness during EEG recoding of 10–15 min. The sampling frequency was 200 Hz. The bandpass filter and the time constant were 1.5–60 Hz and 0.3 s, respectively.

For our analyses, the continuous 60 s, artifact-free epochs have been extracted from within EEG data by an expert electroencephalographer who was blined to the group identity of the subjects, and by double-check of another expert under same as above mentioned condition.

[2]DSM-IV is the fourth edition of the manual published by the American Psychiatric Association to provide the standard classification of mental disorders used by mental health professionals.

2.2 Phase Lag Index

For the measurement of phase synchronizations, characteristics of synchronous on brain waves in a different brain area can be quantitatively estimated from calculating indexes like PLV or PLI. PLV is not suitable on the estimation of the synchronization between signals observed at different two points. The reason is that PLV cannot classify whether the signal propagated from the common source or from different source. At some time t_i, it is observed signals of the phase $\phi_x(t_i)$ and $\phi_y(t_i)$ in the points x and y, respectively. Then, the difference of the phase $\Delta\phi_{xy}(t_i)$ at some time t_i is written as

$$|\Delta\phi_{xy}(t_i)| = \left|\phi_x(t_i) - \phi_y(t_i)\right| \leq \text{const}\,, \tag{1}$$

and also

$$\Delta\phi_{\text{mod}}(t_i) = \Delta\phi_{xy}(t_i) \mod 2\pi\,. \tag{2}$$

The PLI on the signals between the observed two points $x - y$ is defined as

$$\text{PLI}_{xy} = \left|\frac{1}{T}\sum_{i=1}^{T} sign\left(\Delta\phi_{\text{mod}}(t_i)\right)\right|\,. \tag{3}$$

Here PLI in Eq. (3) is moderately synchronous near 1, but is random near 0. From Eqs. (1) and (2), the value of PLI on case which it observes the signals with a common source at different points becomes 0 because $\Delta\phi_{xy}(t_i)$ is 0, and $\Delta\phi_{\text{mod}}(t_i) = 0$. Also, $\Delta\phi_{xy}(t_i) = \pi$ in Eq. (1) on the observation at the point located in an opposite side of the electric dipole, where a signal source is assumed dipole model. As PLI_{xy} becomes 0, the index PLI omits signals from the common source.

2.3 Complex Network Analysis

Depending on the network structure, we can classify graphs as follows.

- Complete graph
  A network in which each node is linked to all other nodes.
- Random graph [18]
  A network in which two randomly selected nodes are linked with a certain binding rate.
- Watts-Strogatz (WS) model (small-world model) [19]
  A network in which the average distance (the average number of nodes) between nodes is small, and the clustering (proportion of nodes adjacent to a random node that are also adjacent to each other) is high.

- Scale free model [20]
  A network in which, in addition to small average distance and high clustering, the number of links from a node follows a power law.

Examples of these graphs with 20 nodes are shown in Fig. 1.

Here the value of a clustering identifies the structure of these networks quantitatively and is described as

$$C = \frac{1}{N} \sum_{i \in N} \frac{2c_i}{k_i(k_i - 1)}, \tag{4}$$

with a total number of a node N in a graph [21, 22]. c_i and k_i are a local clustering coefficient and a degree of the node i, respectively, and are given as

$$c_i = \frac{1}{2} \sum_{j,h \in N} a_{ij} a_{ih} a_{jh}, \tag{5}$$

$$k_i = \sum_{j \in N} a_{ij}. \tag{6}$$

In Eqs. (5) and (6), a represents an adjacency matrix.

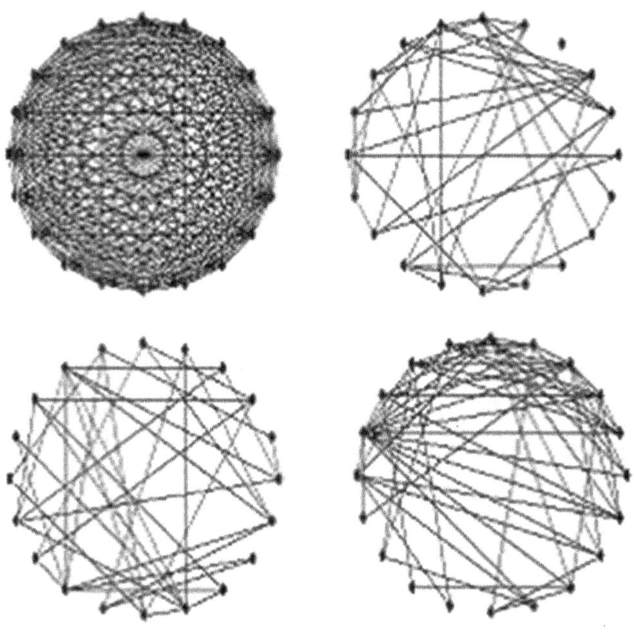

Fig. 1 Graphs of typical networks. In the *top* row are complete (*left*) and random (*right*) graphs; in the *bottom* row are Watts-Strogatz (*left*) and scale free (*right*) models

2.4 Statistical Analysis

The test for certification on group differences in PLI and the clustering coefficient were processed at two-tailed t-tests for independent samples without assuming equal variance, where a test of equal variance was carried by F-test. In this paper, a significance level of $\alpha < 0.05$ is chosen.

3 Results

3.1 Phase Lag Index AD Versus HC

We first estimated PLI on each typical rhythm bands for EEG, namely δ wave (2–4 Hz), θ wave (4–8 Hz), α wave (8–13 Hz), β wave (13–30 Hz), and γ wave (30–60 Hz) using HERMES as a toolbox for EEG/MEG analyzer on MATLAB of Mathworks [23]. Figure 2 shows the average of PLI for AD group and HC group on all pairs of electrodes, where the average of PLI over 0.1 (PLI $\geq \Lambda$ at $\Lambda = 0.1$) was drew at the solid line with the purple color for AD group and with green color for HC group.

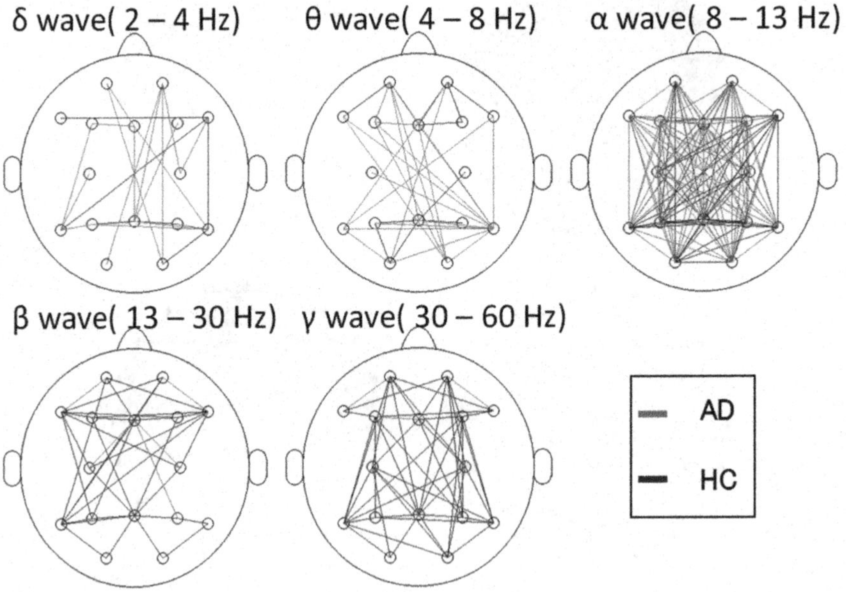

Fig. 2 Network graph on the average of PLI value of AD group and HC group for each frequency band. The *purple* colored *solid line* for AD group and the *green* colored one for HC group were drew at the averaged PLI $\geq \Lambda$ at $\Lambda = 0.1$

In Fig. 2, the synchronization was slightly high for the AD group compared with HC group at δ wave and θ wave. On the other hand, HC group had high PLI value and was synchronous complicatedly in the brain rather than AD group at β wave and γ wave. In particular, synchronousness for HC group at these waves was high on the frontal lobe part. We also found that both AD and HC groups had high synchronization at α wave.

3.2 Phase Lag Index and Mini-Mental State Examination

The relation between the synchronization and the cognitive function estimated on MMSE score was examined using PLI value of AD group. We have obtained the results of 120 ways for each wave from the combination of pairs for 16 electrodes. Figure 3 shows scatter charts on MMSE in term of PLI at the coefficient of determination R^2 over 0.6, $R^2 > 0.6$, on the correlation of PLI with MMSE score. It was found that there was high correlations at α wave on electrode pairs Fp2–T6 and P3–F7.

3.3 Complex Network Analysis on AD and HC

We estimated the clustering coefficient in Eq. (4) of the network given from the strength of PLI on each group. Let us the adjacency matrix a_{ij} in Eqs. (5) and (6) to be taken as

$$a_{ij} = \begin{cases} 1 & \text{for } PLI_{ij} \geq \Lambda\,, \\ 0 & \text{otherwise}\,. \end{cases} \tag{7}$$

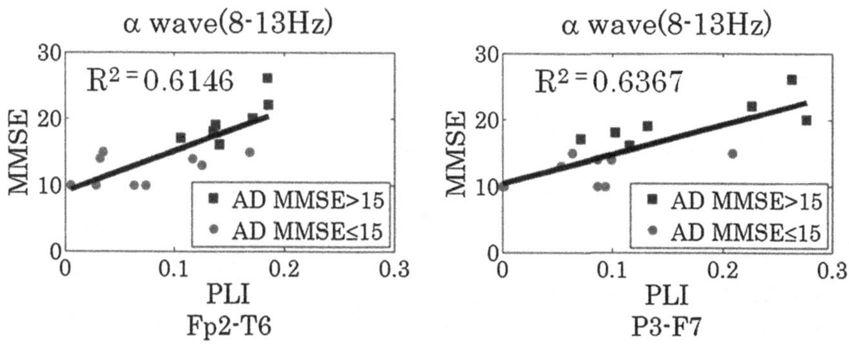

Fig. 3 Scatter charts of PLI and MMSE score. The results were chosen at the coefficient of determination $R^2 > 0.6$ on the correlation of PLI with MMSE score. The *blue* and *red* points indicated AD subject with *low* MMSE score and *high* one, respectively. The result on the method of least squares was represented at a *black line*

with any threshold Λ. Then, we obtained the clustering coefficient C in terms of the threshold Λ.

It was implied the results on the average of the clustering coefficient C for AD group with low, high MMSE score and HC group by the threshold value every 0.1 for the range from 0.1 to 0.9 in Fig. 4. Figure 4 implied no difference in the clustering coefficient of the AD group and HC group at δ and θ waves. On the other hand, there was a large difference in the clustering coefficient in AD group with low MMSE score and AD group with high MMSE score in the threshold value more than 0.2 at α wave. Also, the value of the clustering coefficient in order of highest to lowest became the average clustering coefficient of HC group, AD group with high MMSE score, and the AD group with low MMSE score for a threshold value greater than 0.2 at γ waves.

The statistical analysis of results on clustering coefficient are summarized in Table 2 by the two-tailed independent t-test with F-test as test of the homogeneity of variance at α and γ waves. From Table 2, we were able to see that a significantly difference of the clustering coefficient between AD group with low MMSE score and with high MMSE score on the threshold value 0.1 and 0.2 at α wave. Also, there is a significant difference of the cluster coefficient in AD groups with HC group on the threshold value 0.1 at γ waves.

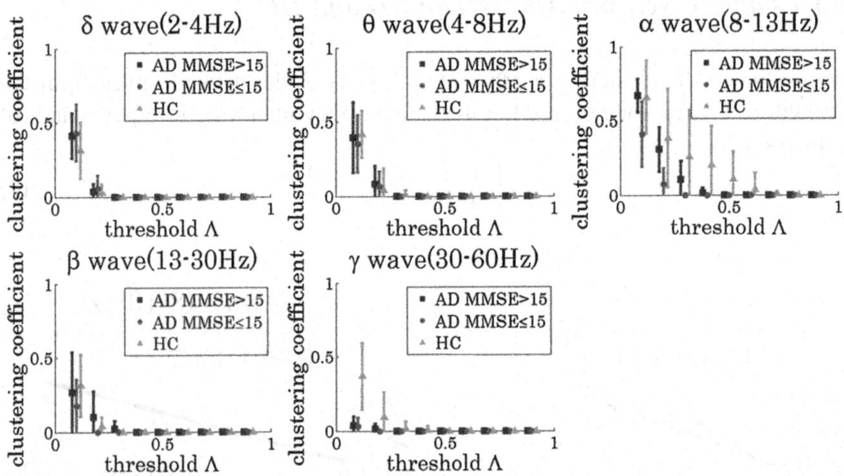

Fig. 4 The results on the average of the clustering coefficient C as function of the threshold Λ every 0.1 for the range from 0.1 to 0.9 on AD group with *low*, *high* MMSE score and HC group at each wave. The *red* colored *circle*, the *blue* colored squire, and the *green* colored *triangle* points with bars of the standard deviation indicated AD group with *low*, *high* MMSE score and HC group, respectively

Table 2 The two-tailed independent t-tests without assuming equal variance after giving F-test for the certification on group differences in the clustering coefficient at any threshold value among AD group with low, high MMSE score, and HC group. Here a significance level was taken as $\alpha < 0.05$

Threshold	AD MMSE>15		AD MMSE ≤ 15		T value	P value
(Wave Frequency)	AVE	SD	AVE	SD		
0.1(8-13Hz)	0.6707	0.1068	0.4084	0.2191	-2.6966	0.0174
0.2(8-13Hz)	0.3067	0.1499	0.0733	0.1068	-3.3982	0.0043
Threshold	AD MMSE>15		HC		T value	P value
(Wave Frequency)	AVE	SD	AVE	SD		
0.1(30-60Hz)	0.0361	0.0593	0.3703	0.2255	-5.5874	1.30E-05
Threshold	AD MMSE ≤ 15		HC		T value	P value
(Wave Frequency)	AVE	SD	AVE	SD		
0.1(30-60Hz)	0.0313	0.0585	0.3703	0.2255	-5.7990	8.86E-06

4 Summary and Discussion

We investigated on differences of network characteristics on AD with HC by calculating PLI from EEG data. For PLI at high frequency rhythms like β or γ waves, we found that HC group had strong synchronousness within the whole brain rather than AD group. Our result consists with the result of Stam and collaborators which showed the average PLI in β wave becoming significantly lower in AD group compared with HC group [8]. On the other hand, we obtained that AD group strongly synchronized more than HC group at low frequencies like δ or θ waves. The strength of synchronization at different wave frequencies seems to be relevant to an anomaly of the network in the brain for AD compared with HC.

Also, PLI-dependence on MMSE score has been shown at two electrode pairs, Fp2–T6 and P3–F7, in α wave and has been obtained at positive correlations. It is expected that the score of MMES as the assessment of cognitive function can be guessed from the estimation of PLI between these electrodes. We have calculated the average of the clustering coefficient for each group, AD with low MMSE score, AD with high MMSE score, and HC group at each brain wave. Comparing averaged values of each group with other groups, it was implied significant difference on AD group between low and high MMSE score at α wave. From these results, the synchronous strength at α wave can be consider to influence the score of MMSE.

In summary on this study, we implied an availability for the assessment and the severity of AD regarded as the pathophysiology with the anomaly of the network obtained from our analysis on EEG signals.

As future work, we will attempt to increase the number of AD subjects and to raise the statistical precision on the relation of the synchronous strength with the cognitive function. Furthermore, establishments of the index that can determine the cognitive function early will be aimed by using some analyses from other indexes with high potential like weighted PLI or directed PLI [24].

Acknowledgments The works of ones of authors, T.Y. and H.N., were supported by a Grant-in-Aid for Scientific Research (C-25330293) from the Japan Society for the Promotion of Science.

References

1. Schaul, N.: The fundamental neural mechanisms of electroencephalography. Electroencephalogr. Clin. Neurophysiol. **106**, 101–107 (1998)
2. Sakamoto, K., et al.: Discharge synchrony during the transition of behavioral goal representations encoded by discharge rates of prefrontal neurons. Cereb. Cortex **18**, 2036–2045 (2008)
3. Riehle, A., et al.: Spike synchronization and rate modulation differentially involved in motor cortical function. Science **278**, 1950–1953 (1997)
4. Huang, N.E. et al.:The empirical mode decomposition and the hilbert spectrum for nonlinear and nonstationary time series analysis. In: Proceedings of the Royal Society of London, vol. A454, pp. 903–995 (1998)
5. Kondo, E. et al.: Synchronization Analysis using the Hilbert Huang Coherence, IEICE Technical Report, MBE2014-29, 7–12 (2014)
6. Tass, P., et al.: Detection of *n:m* phase locking from noisy data: application to magnetoencephalography. Phys. Rev. Lett. **81**, 3291–3294 (1998)
7. Lachaux, J.-P., et al.: Measuring phase synchrony in brain signals. Hum. Brain Mapp. **8**, 194–208 (1999)
8. Stam, C.J., Nolte, G., Daffertshofer, A.: Phase lag index: assessment of functional connectivity from multi channel eeg and meg with diminished bias from common sources. Hum. Brain Mapp. **28**, 1178–1193 (2007)
9. Prince, M., Albanese, E., Guerchet, M., and Prina, M.: World Alzheimer Report 2014, Alzheimer's Disease International (2014)
10. Delbeuck, X., Van der Linden, M., Collette, F.: Alzheimer's disease as a disconnection syndrome? Neuropsychol. Rev. **13**, 79–92 (2003)
11. Folstein, M.F., Flostein, S.E., McHugh, P.R.: Mini-mental state a practical method for grading the cognitive state of patients for the clinician. J. Psychiatr. Res. **12**, 189–198 (1975)
12. Stam, C.J., et al.: Graph theoretical analysis of magnetoencephalographic functional connectivity in alzheimer's disease. Brain **132**, 213–224 (2009)
13. Tewarie, P., et al.: Structural degree predicts functional network connectivity: a multimodal resting-state fMRI and MEG study. NeuroImage **97**, 296–307 (2014)
14. Vinck, M., et al.: An improved index of phase-synchronization for electrophysiological data in the presence of volume-conduction, noise and sample-size bias. NeuroImage **55**, 1548–1565 (2011)
15. Hardmeier, M., et al.: Reproducibility of functional connectivity and graph measures based on the phase lag index (pli) and weighted phase lag index (wPLI) derived from high resolution EEG. PLOS ONE **9**(e108648), 1–10 (2014)
16. Mizuno, T., Takahashi, T., Cho, R.Y., Kikuchi, M., Murata, T., Takahashi, K., Wada, Y.: Assessment of EEG dynamical complexity in alzheimer's disease using multiscale entropy. Clin. Neurophysiol. **121**, 1438–1446 (2010)
17. American Psychiatric Association: Diagnostic and statistical manual of mental disorders, 4th edn. American Psychiatric Association, Washington (1994)
18. Erdös, P., Renyi, A.: On random graphs. Publ. Math. (Debrecen) **6**, 290–297 (1959)
19. Watts, D.J., Strogatz, S.H.: Collective dynamics of small-world networks. Nature **393**, 440–442 (1998)
20. Barabási, A.-L., Albert, R.: Emergence of scaling in random networks. Science **286**, 349–352 (1999)
21. Boccaletti, S., Latora, V., Chavez, M., Hwang, D.-U.: Complex networks: structure and dynamics. Phys. Rep. **424**, 175–308 (2006)
22. Arenas, A., Díaz-Guilera, A., Kurths, J., Moreno, Y., Zhou, C.: Synchronization in complex networks. Phys. Rep. **469**, 93–153 (2008)
23. Niso, G., et al.: HERMES: towards an integrated toolbox to characterize functional and effective brain connectivity. Neuroinformatics **11**, 405–434 (2013)
24. Stam, C.J., van Straaten, E.C.W.: Go with the flow: Use of a directed phase lag index (dPLI) to characterize patterns of phase relations in a large-scale model of brain dynamics. NeuroImage **62**, 1415–1428 (2012)

Part VIII
Healthcare Support System

A Benchmark on Artificial Intelligence Techniques for Automatic Chronic Respiratory Diseases Risk Classification

Sebastián A. Ríos, Fabián García Tenorio and Angel Jimenez-Molina

Abstract A major public health problem is the chronically respiratory ill patients. To create a more preventive and anticipatory system for these patients we can use artificial intelligence techniques. This work tackle the problem of developing a model for automatic classification of patients with risk of having a respiratory crisis on the biggest paediatric Public Hospital in Santiago, Chile. We present a benchmark of different approaches to create a model. The models were developed with history of biomedical signals for 45 patients from 0 months to 15 years old. We are able to identify to approaches which have a remarkable performance.

1 Introduction

Health systems from different countries have agreed on the need of tackling the challenge of chronic diseases by the mean of a more preventive, personalized and anticipatory health service. This requires to encourage chronic patients and caregivers to make them protagonists of their healthcare, assuming responsibility to keep themselves on controlled states without collapsing health centers. This implies to realize the metaphor of a continuous healthcare provisioning, that is, providing healthcare everywhere, anytime and to anyone [1].

To realize an anticipatory and personalized health care service, it is needed, for instance, to remotely monitor if the vital signs of chronic patients are in a normal range. Another example is to identify the level of humidity (or other environmental conditions) of the patient's bedroom during winter. Based on specific data and other information from the patients it is possible to develop artificial intelligence models to predict whether a patient have a high risk of having a health crisis or not.

This paper provides a benchmarking on different artificial intelligence techniques to predict patients' risk level of developing a crisis state. This is done by making

S.A. Ríos (✉) · F.G. Tenorio · A. Jimenez-Molina
Industrial Engineering Department, Business Intelligence Research Center,
University of Chile, Santiago, Chile
e-mail: sebastian@rios.tv

Y.-W. Chen et al. (eds.), *Innovation in Medicine and Healthcare 2015*,
Smart Innovation, Systems and Technologies 45,
DOI 10.1007/978-3-319-23024-5_43

use of real patients' data provided by a public pediatric hospital from the city of Santiago, Chile, which provides around 300,000 attentions per year, the majority of them from a segment of the population that corresponds to the smaller income.

The models used were: Fuzzy Reasoning, Naive Bayes, Decision Trees, Artificial Neural Networks (ANN), Support Vector Machines (SVM), and Logit (this is logistic regression).

2 Related Work

Remote patient monitoring (MRPM) is defined as the continuous or frequent periodic measurement of physiological processes of a patient, such as blood pressure, heart rate or respiratory rate, among others. The most obvious application of this approach lies within the monitoring of patients with chronic diseases. Recently, autonomous computational health services that incorporate artificial intelligence, like machine learning, to assist health professionals in the interpretation of medical data and decision making [7] have appeared. Such services implement models using data mining techniques over biosensors, such as clustering applied to real and historical data, predicting real-time health status of a patient, or performing pre-diagnoses [4, 10].

Recent literature on MRPM systems shows a great diversity in techniques used to implement either the detection of physiological bio-signals, communication of data captured from biosensors to mobile devices, servers or cloud, or the interpretation and analysis of bio-signals. An important set of these solutions focus on patients with heart problems and hypertension, and some include data mining techniques analyzing information captured by a portable electrocardiogram (ECG). For instance, the MobiHealthcare system is based on a server architecture, and stores data in a repository for big data, where data mining is applied [9]. Also, the Multi-Touch Diagnostic ECG system uses a multimodal analysis engine and displays the ECG information, pre-processed by data mining techniques, in three dimensions over a mobile device [8]. At a more advanced level is the Mobile Cardiac Wellness Application, which is a back-end repository; uses data mining techniques on ECG information to uncover knowledge patterns; it can process and evolve its knowledge; provides planning intervention; provides advisory services and delivers health status feedback to users about their health [6].

3 Developed Models

In this section we explain the data set used for the benchmark, the referential ranges established with medical expert criteria, the evaluation methodology used; and finally, the models developed are briefly explained.

3.1 Dataset Description

Our dataset has information about 45 paediatric patients with chronic respiratory diseases from Exequiel Gonzlez Corts Hospital (EGCH). These patients are hospitalized in two units at the hospital: paediatrics and critical patients.

To develop our models we selected those patients that have been under mechanical ventilation with nasal cannula or normal environmental breathing, i.e., without mechanical assistance of any kind, as this disrupts vital signs of patients. As a result we used 31 patients to conduct our study.

A record of this dataset contains information on three elements: (a) characterization of the patient, (b) vital signs and (c) ventilation type. In patient characteristics are features like: age, sex, diagnosis and other ratings. The vital signs recorded are: temperature (TEMP), heart rate (HR), respiratory rate (RR), oxygen Saturation (SAO2) and pressure (PRES).

Vital signs are registered every two to four hours, depending on whether the patient is in the critical care unit or paediatric unit, respectively.

The table below has an abstract, both in terms of rows and columns, the data we have of a particular patient. Of course it is not necessary to identify those patients for our models is why working with anonymized data.

3.2 Evaluation Methodology

We used two strategies to train and evaluate the results of the models. Both are based on cross validation: (a) without individualization of records and (b) with individualization of records. The first approach takes all records from all patients to a single bag of data. Then we use the first 80 % of the data to train and the next 20 % to evaluate the performance. In the second approach we take 80 % of records of a specific patient to train the models; afterwards, we compute the performance on the rest of their records (for all patients, of course). The first approach is similar to what medical expert are doing most of the time when they use rules like a *triage* to set up a priority, they relay that all people behaves similarly. Of course, this method is the opposite of a personalized health system. Thus, we also developed the second approach, where models are specifically trained to a patient. Our aim is to create a virtual agent to do a periodic monitoring of the health of a specific children in the future.

Nevertheless, we evaluated all models developed (except the fuzzy reasoning model) using both evaluation strategies. In the case of the fuzzy reasoning model explained in the following section, we can only apply the first evaluation strategy. Since we try to mimic medical expert criteria, this model does not individualize patients.

We used well known performance measures to evaluate the results: Precision, Accuracy, Sensitivity, Specificity and F-measure.

3.3 Fuzzy Reasoning Model

To support family members and medical team, we needed to embed part of the medical team knowledge into the software. To do so, we chose to develop a fuzzy reasoning model which captures the medical expert experience. This way, the software will be able to provide recommendations regarding the risk level of patients.

Our model begins with the development of a score schema to characterize different states on the vital sings (see Table 1). For example, if the patient only exhibit a high or low temperature, we assign it a score of 1. However, if the patient shows a low heart rate, then the system assigns a score of 3. Of course, for each vital sign we defined the normal range (with medical expert knowledge as shown in previous section), thus, it is possible to know when the vital sign is high, low or normal.

Once the score schema was established, we defined the correspondence between the combination of vital signs scores and the risk of a respiratory crisis (see Table 2). Therefore, the system can provide a risk assertion based on this information. In Table 2 an altered vital sign means that is not in the normal range (RN).

Finally, we can formalize this knowledge in the form of functions shown in the Eqs. (4)–(6). These equations define three membership functions to denote high range (RA), normal range (RN) and low range (RB) of a variable. Afterwards, we used these equations as a fuzzy reasoning model.

$$RA_i = \text{High Range for Indicator i, with } i \in \{T, RR, HR\} \tag{1}$$

$$RN_i = \text{Normal Range for Indicator i, with } i \in \{T, RR, HR\} \tag{2}$$

$$RB_i = \text{Low Range for Indicator i, with } i \in \{T, RR, HR\} \tag{3}$$

$$RA_i(x) = \begin{cases} 0 & \text{if } x < c_i \\ \frac{(d_i - x)}{(c_i - d_i)} & \text{if } c_i \leq x \leq d_i \\ 1 & \text{if } x > d_i \end{cases} \tag{4}$$

Table 1 Score scheme when bio-signals are deviated from normal ranges

Score scheme	Biosignal state
1	Temp. high or Temp. low
2	High heart rate
2	High respiratory rate
2	SAO2 90–93 (CR)
2	SAO2 94–95 (NCR)
3	Low heart rate
3	Low respiratory rate
4	SAO2 90–93 (NCR)
5	SAO2 < 90

Table 2 Mapping risk level with health indicators

Risk level	Chronic respiratory diseases (CR)	Non-chronic diseases (NCR)
Low (2–3 points)	Altered heart rate	Altered heart rate
Low (2–3 points)	Altered respiratory rate	Altered respiratory rate
Low (2–3 points)	SAO2 90–93	SAO2 94–95
Medium (4–5 points)	SAO2 90–93 and ((HR) or (RR) altered)	SAO2 94–95 and ((HR) or (RR) altered)
Medium (4–5 points)	High HR and altered RR	High HR and altered RR
Medium (4–5 points)	High RR and altered HR	High RR and altered HR
Medium (4–5 points)	Altered temperature and low HR	Altered temperature and low HR
Medium (4–5 points)	Altered temperature and low RR	Altered temperature and low RR
Medium (4–5 points)	–	SAO2 90–93
High (≥6 points)	Low (HR) and Low (RR)	SAO2 90–93 and ((HR) or (RR) altered)
High (≥6 points)	SAO2 <90	Low HR and Low RR
High (≥6 points)	High HR and low RR and altered temp	High HR and low RR and altered temp
High (≥6 points)	High RR and low HR and altered temp	High RR and low HR and altered temp
High (≥6 points)	–	SAO2 <90

$$RN_i(x) = \begin{cases} 0 & \text{if } x < a_i \text{ or } x > d_i \\ \frac{(x-a_i)}{(b_i-a_i)} & \text{if } a_i \le x \le b_i \\ 1 & \text{if } b_i \le x \le c_i \\ \frac{(d_i-x)}{(d_i-c_i)} & \text{if } c_i \le x \le d_i \end{cases} \tag{5}$$

$$RB_i(x) = \begin{cases} 0 & \text{if } x > b_i \\ \frac{(b_i-x)}{(b_i-a_i)} & \text{if } a_i \le x \le b_i \\ 1 & \text{if } x < a_i \end{cases} \tag{6}$$

For each vital sign i we denote its inferior limit as Min_i and its upper limit as Max_i. Afterwards, we introduce flexibility on these measures by defining two variables to each limit: $FlexMin_i$ and $FlexMax_i$ respectively. Finally, we can write the parameters for the membership functions in Eqs. (4) and (6) as following:

$$a_i = Min_i * (1 - FlexMin_i) \text{ for each } i \in \{T, RR, HR\} \tag{7}$$

$$b_i = Min_i * (1 + FlexMin_i) \text{ for each } i \in \{T, RR, HR\} \tag{8}$$

$$c_i = Max_i * (1 - FlexMax_i) \text{ for each } i \in \{T, RR, HR\} \tag{9}$$

$$d_i = Max_i * (1 + FlexMax_i) \text{ for each } i \in \{T, RR, HR\} \tag{10}$$

Now, we need to define when a vital sign is qualified as high, low or in a middle range. Each membership function takes values between 0 and 1. Therefore, we need to establish a value p_{ik} which is the probability that a vital sign i belongs to the membership function k.

Medic's reasoning changes depending on the combination of values from the vital signs. Therefore, let SV be the set of vital signs $\{T, RR, HR, SAO2\}$, we called SV^{-i} the set of vital signs without the vital sign i. Therefore, we can define p_{ik}^{norm} if SV^{-i} is in the normal range with probability 1. In the case, at least one vital sign SV^{-i} is not in the normal range, it will be used p_{ik}^{risk} as shown in Eq. (11).

$$p_{ik} = \begin{cases} p_{ik}^{norm} & \text{if } \sum_{m \in SV^{-i}} RN_m = 3 \\ p_{ik}^{risk} & \text{if this is not fulfilled} \end{cases} \tag{11}$$

$$P_t^1 = \begin{cases} 1 & \text{if } RN_t < p_{rn,t} \text{ with } rn \text{ normal range} \\ & \text{and } t \text{ temperature values} \\ 0 & \text{otherwise} \end{cases} \tag{12}$$

$$P_{fc}^2 = \begin{cases} 2 & \text{if } RA_t > p_{ra,hr} \text{ with } ra \text{ high range} \\ & \text{and } hr \text{ heart rate values} \\ 0 & \text{otherwise} \end{cases} \tag{13}$$

$$P_{fr}^2 = \begin{cases} 2 & \text{if } RA_{rr} > p_{ra,rr} \text{ with } ra \text{ high range} \\ & \text{and } rr \text{ respiratory rate values} \\ 0 & \text{otherwise} \end{cases} \tag{14}$$

$$P_{SAO2}^2(x, y) = \begin{cases} 2 & \text{if } x \leq SAO2 \leq y \\ 0 & \text{otherwise} \end{cases} \tag{15}$$

$$P_{fc}^3 = \begin{cases} 3 & \text{if } RB_{hr} > p_{rb,hr} \text{ with } rb \text{ low range} \\ & \text{and } hr \text{ heart rate values} \\ 0 & \text{otherwise} \end{cases} \tag{16}$$

$$P_{fr}^3 = \begin{cases} 3 & \text{if } RB_{rr} > p_{rb,rr} \text{ with } rb \text{ low range} \\ & \text{and } rr \text{ respiratory rate values} \\ 0 & \text{otherwise} \end{cases} \tag{17}$$

$$P_{SAO2}^4 = \begin{cases} 4 & \text{if } 90 \leq SAO2 \leq 93 \\ 0 & \text{otherwise} \end{cases} \tag{18}$$

$$P^6_{SAO2} = \begin{cases} 6 & \text{if } SAO2 < 90 \\ 0 & \text{otherwise} \end{cases} \tag{19}$$

Finally, to develop a fuzzy reasoning model we just need to establish a criterion to assign the scores shown in Table 1. These are defined from Eqs. (12) to (18). Afterwards, we are able to define our fuzzy reasoning model as shown in Eq. (20). This is the final fuzzy reasoning model used for the benchmarks.

$$\begin{aligned} PG = P^1_t + P^2_{fc} + P^2_{fr} + P^3_{fc} + P^3_{fr} + \\ + (1 - CR) * (P^2_{SAO2}(94, 95) + P^4_{SAO2}) + \\ + CR * P^2_{SAO2}(90, 93) + P^6_{SAO2} \end{aligned} \tag{20}$$

$$\text{with } CR = \begin{cases} 1 & \text{if chronic respiratory patient.} \\ 0 & \text{otherwise} \end{cases}$$

3.4 Classification Techniques

Five mathematical models were used in our benchmarks. We left a side their formal definition or any equation intentionally since they are well known techniques.

Naive Bayes We also developed a Naive Bayes classifier which is based on the Bayes theorem and several assumptions like attributes independence. It was commonly used in text retrieval but there are several medical applications that also use it, for example in automatic medical diagnosis [11].

Descision Trees Decision trees is a well known classification and regression technique. It is a supervised learning technique, which can be used since we have a supervised dataset. The main purpose of a decision tree is to create a set of rules over a set of variables which can be used to predict or classify a target variable [2].

Artificial Neural Networks The Artificial Neural Network (ANN) belong to the family of statistical learning algorithms. Its origins are inspired by biological neural networks which is model with neurons (or perceptrons) and interconnections between those. ANN is widely used for a variety of problems like handwritten recognition, speech recognition, computer vision, etc. [5].

In our work we used an ANN with a hidden layer, and we used back propagation training method.

port Vector Machines This model belongs to the supervised learning family, it is commonly used for classification and regression. The technique uses records marked as part of a class or part of another class; this way, it creates a model that assign new records the label of one of those classes [3].

A SVM can also be used for non-linear classification using Kernel functions which map the inputs of the SVM into high-dimensional feature spaces.

Logistic Regression This model it is commonly known as logit regression or logit model. This model is used to classify binary variables.

4 Benchmark Results and Discussion

As mentioned before, the models were evaluated following two strategies: (a) without individualization of patient's records and (b) individualizing the history of patient records. We present firstly benchmark results considering strategy (a) and secondly (b).

Benchmark results without individualizing records are presented in Table 3. Best results are obtained with a logit model with specificity of 91.34 % and similar sensitivity with 91.36 %. Although, these are a very good results, we need to continue working to enhance these numbers. In this case when the model marks a patient with high risk of a respiratory crisis it is very probable this is true. Similarly when the models label a patient as without risk it is highly probable this is true. Of course, a perfect technique should have *sensitivity* = *specificity* = 100 %; In addition, logit model is close to it. Besides shows very high values in precision and accuracy. Therefore, based on these evidence the models should behave very stable; which is a desire result for a classification technique.

On the contrary, the worst technique was the Naive Bayes classifier with a specificity of 62.79 % and a sensitivity of 38.90 %. Which in all experiments marked the worst performance. Therefore, we can observe that F measure in Bayes case is 49.14 % which is a very low result while F measure of Logit is 91.11 %, which is a very high value; this way, our recommendation it is that Naive Bayes it is not useful to solve this classification problem.

The second best technique was the ANN with a high sensitivity (77.89 %) and a medium specificity (59.70 %). A high sensitivity means that false negative cases are a small fraction, in other words, if the model marks a patient with high risk of a chronic respiratory crisis the probability to be true is high. Moreover, the other performance measures are very high (precision, accuracy and F-Measure).

Table 3 Benchmark results without individualization of records (%)

	Fuzzy Res.	Naive Bayes	ANN	SVM	Logit	Dec. Tre
Accuracy	79.3	49.41	81.35	65.24	88.17	67.07
Precision	51.8	66.70	92.86	72.97	90.86	74.63
Sensitivity	56.6	38.90	77.89	70.96	91.36	76.32
Specificity	78.0	62.79	59.70	43.37	91.34	48.83
F–measure	53.2	49.14	84.72	71.95	91.11	75.47

Table 4 Benchmark results with individualization of records (%)

	Naive Bayes	ANN	SVM	Logit	Dec. Tree
Accuracy	51.66	79.25	51.06	84.19	64.85
Precision	NaN	79.65	49.62	77.80	63.45
Sensitivity	0.00	76.67	82.08	94.17	64.38
Specificity	100	81.68	22.02	74.85	65.3
F–Measure	NaN	78.13	61.85	85.20	63.91

An unexpected result is that the fuzzy reasoning model has the second best specificity (78.0 %) after the logit model. However, all other measures are lower than the specificity measures of ANN, SVM, Logit and Decision Trees; which place this technique just over the worst. A fuzzy reasoning is expected to have much better performance on a supervised data set of discrete cases, but it only shows a F-Measure of 53.2 %, which is not sufficient to use this technique in a practice.

In the second case, when individualized records were used to train the models, evaluation results are drastically affected, see Table 4. In this case, although we can use the fuzzy reasoning model, we decided to leave it aside since the set up parameters of the model were established using all records without individualizing them. Therefore, it is not correct to compare it with the other models which were trained following the second strategy.

In this case, the best technique continues to be the logit model followed by the ANN. This model present a high specificity 94.17 % (even higher than the value of the first evaluation strategy), but its specificity is only 74.85 %, much lower than the one obtained in previous experiments. Finally, the F-measure is also lower with 85.20 % (approximately 6 % lower than earlier).

The second best technique is again the ANN which also exhibit lower performance measures. However, this time accuracy, precision and specificity measures are closer to logit measures. The only strong difference between these two models is on the sensitivity.

The SVM and Decision Trees performance measures are far from ANN and logit measures. But, the worst model is again Naive Bayes. This occurs because the technique once trained, it labels every record as "no risk"; thus, recall is 0 % but specificity is 100 % and precision is "not a number" or undefined value, since there is a division by 0. In this case, this technique is not suitable to be used in this kind of applications.

5 Conclusions

As mentioned before, the evaluation with individualization of patients' history is the one that better fit the main problem of a health system which should be personalized and anticipative. Models, should be developed having these principles to implement a really innovative solution.

We have been experiencing an explosion of new bio-signals sensing technologies from non invasive sensors like fabric-sensors to devises like iPhone 6 which has several sensors already built in the phone. Other sensing technology developed using Arduino, Raspberry PI, Edison (Intel) and so on are also available. All these technologies will enable people to have a personal history dataset of bio-signals in the near future.

To have a personalized and more anticipative health care system one solution is to create software services which can automatically classify the risk of crisis on different patients. However, which is the best model is always a question unanswered. We decided to perform a benchmark on several artificial intelligence techniques to answer this question. To do so, we focused our study on the major public paediatric hospital in Santiago, Chile. We focused on children with chronic respiratory diseases, which is a major health problem in the city. We created a dataset with history of 45 patients (anonimized) to developed our experiments. Afterwards, we implemented six different classification models: Fuzzy Reasoning, Naive Bayes, Artificial Neural Networks (ANN), Support Vector Machines (SVM), Logit, and Decision Trees. Besides, we developed two evaluation strategies: one that is similar to what medical expert do today (as-is), and a personalized method (to-be).

The results of our experiments in both evaluation scenarios show that the best models for this problem is the Logit model and the second best model is the ANN. Results in the personalized evaluation approach are worst. We think this is due to lesser amount of records per patients to train the models. Thus, we are creating a new dataset with more patients and more history (several episodes of crisis) to again perform our benchmarks.

Acknowledgments This work was supported by CONICYT programmes: IDeA FONDEF project code: CA13i-10300, and FONDECYT project code: 11130252. Also, authors would like to thank the continuous support of "Instituto Sistemas Complejos de Ingeniería" (ICM: P-05-004- F, CONICYT: FBO16).

References

1. Arnrich, B., Mayora, O., Bardram, J., Trster, G.: Pervasive healthcare: paving the way for a pervasive, user-centered and preventive healthcare model. Methods Inf. Med. **49**(1), 67–73 (2009)
2. Cha, S.-H., Tappert, C.C.: A genetic algorithm for constructing compact binary decision trees. J. Pattern Recogn. **4**(1), 1–13 (2009)
3. Cortes, C., Vapnik, V.: Support-vector networks. Mach. Learn. **20**(3), 273–297 (1995)
4. Erazo, L., Ríos, S.A.: A benchmark on automatic obstructive sleep apnea screening algorithms in children. Procedia Comput. Sci. **35**, 739–746 (2014)
5. Ferreira, C.: Designing neural networks using Gene expression programming. Adv. Soft Comput. **34**, 517–535 (2006)

6. Fortier, P., Viall, B.: Development of a mobile cardiac wellness application and integrated wearable sensor suite. In: The Fifth International Conference on Sensor Technologies and Applications, pp. 301–306 (2011)
7. Fotiadis, D.I., Likas, A., Protopappas, V.: Intelligent Patient Monitoring, 1st edn. Wiley, New York (2006)
8. Lin, K.-J., Zhang, J., Zhai, Y., Xu, B.: The design and implementation of service process reconfiguration with end-to-end qos constraints in soa. Serv. Oriented Comput. Appl. **4**(3), 157–168, (2010)
9. Miao, F., Miao, X., Shangguan, W., Li, Y.: Mobihealthcare system: body sensor network based m-health system for healthcare application. E-Health Telecommun. Syst. Netw. **1**(1), 12–18 (2012)
10. Patil, D., Wadhai, V. M., Gund, M., Biyani, R., Andhalkar, S., Agrawal, B.: An adaptive parameter free data mining approach for healthcare application. Int. J. Adv. Comput. Sci. Appl. **3**(1), 55–59 (2012)
11. Rish, I.: An empirical study of the naive bayes classifier. IJCAI Workshop Empirical Methods AI **3**(22), 41–46 (2001)

Toward Non-invasive Polysomnograms Through the Study of Electroencephalographic Signal Correlation for Remotely Monitored Cloud-Based Systems

Claudio Estevez, Diego Vallejos, Sebastián A. Ríos and Pablo Brockmann

Abstract Sleep disorders affect a great percentage of the world population, particularly in large cities. The polysomnography is a commonly administered test that helps diagnose sleep disorders. Polysomnograms have many sensors that gather data for approximately 8 h, which generate vast amounts of data and consumes valuable local resources. An alternative that can save local resources, while generating patient data backups, and can even pre-diagnose patients, is having a centralized health center with a cloud architecture. One hurdle that this technology might experience is social acceptance. Polysomnograms have 20–30 sensors, where approximately half are composed of electroencephalographic sensors. This can be very bothersome, and more importantly adds unnecessary redundancy. In sleep tests/studies electroencephalograms are used to determine the sleep stages of the patient, and are studies reveal that a single electrode placed in the back of the head has a an average correlation of 94 % with the remaining sensors. Therefore, the sensors can be significantly reduced for remote cloud-based health monitoring.

Keywords Cloud-computing · e-Health · Electrode · Electroencephalogram · Health · Monitoring · Network · Polysomnography · Remote · Sensor · Sleep disorder

C. Estevez (✉) · D. Vallejos
Electrical Engineering Department, Universidad de Chile, Santiago, Chile
e-mail: cestevez@ing.uchile.cl

S.A. Ríos
Industrial Engineering Department, Universidad de Chile, Santiago, Chile

P. Brockmann
Department of Pediatric Cardiology and Pulmonology, School of Medicine, Pontificia Universidad Católica de Chile, Santiago, Chile

P. Brockmann
Sleep Center, Pontificia Universidad Católica de Chile, Santiago, Chile

Y.-W. Chen et al. (eds.), *Innovation in Medicine and Healthcare 2015*,
Smart Innovation, Systems and Technologies 45,
DOI 10.1007/978-3-319-23024-5_44

1 Introduction

Sleep disorders affect a large percentage of the world population. Very often sleep disorders arise when the patient's circadian rhythm in unsynchronized with their daily activities, particularly in children. Many chronic cases in children are under-reported or untreated [3]. Many countries lack the resources to provide massive polysomnography tests, which is a method of detecting sleep disorders. Only the more vulnerable are subjected to these tests. The vulnerability is determined by a simple open-loop model based the age (children and elderly). This model is sub-optimal, but there are alternatives to determine vulnerability based on a closed-loop model with massive low-cost polysomnographic tests that can feedback indicators that help determine which patients are more vulnerable. The key is a low-cost autonomous centralized healthcare system.

Technology and health are rapidly fusing together. This interaction has served as a catalyst to the fast growing field of e-Health. A novel architecture for next-generation telecommunication systems is to have a centralized health data center [1, 8] with a cloud-computing backbone that stores and analyzes patient data, as portrayed in Fig. 1. To analyze vast amount of data a specialized platform called data warehousing must be implemented. In this case, the raw data enters the data staging area where using extraction, transformation and loading techniques (ETL) the warehouse is generated. Afterwards, data mining techniques attempt to discover disease patterns and other relevant information to assist medics, generate automatic alarms, etc. This information can exit in the form of a pre-diagnostic (premature diagnostic). A pre-diagnostic is defined, in this context, as a predictive assessment that attempts

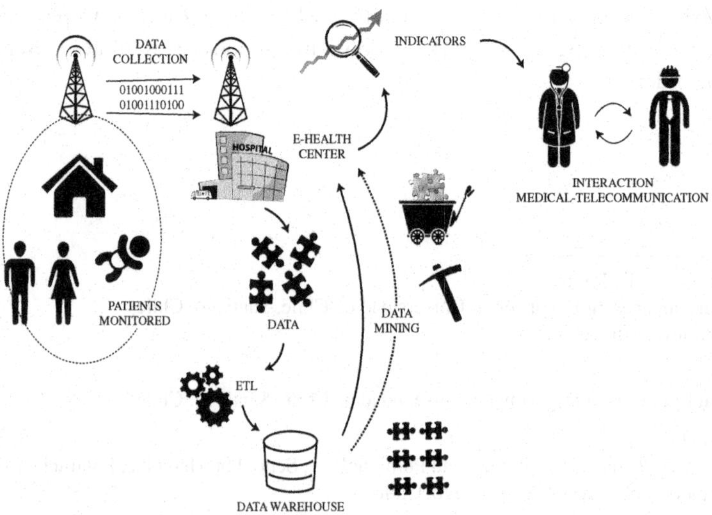

Fig. 1 Respiratory diseases remote monitoring cloud-computing model

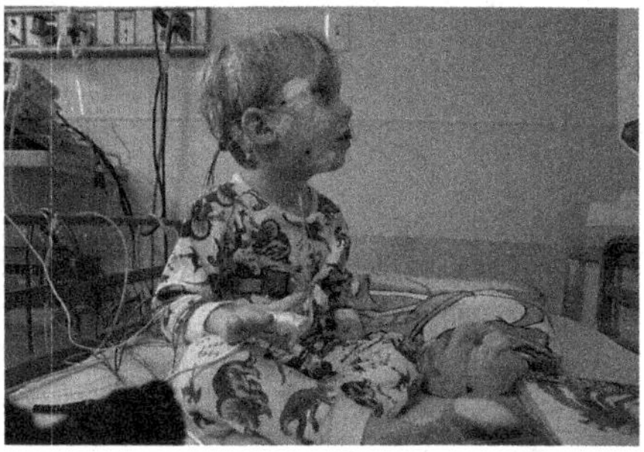

Fig. 2 A pediatric patient prepared for a polysomnogram by a trained respiratory therapist. *Note* Picture used under the Creative Commons (CC) license. *Author* Robert Lawton

to conjecture a diagnosis based on a set of measurable physical states, symptoms, or events. The pre-diagnosis is obtained using data mining techniques, which essentially correlates the data patterns of cases where the patient is known to suffer a disorder or disease with the data patterns where the diagnosis is still unknown, which are performed with a supervised learning methodology guided by medical doctors and/or experts in the field. One expected attribute of pre-diagnostic is the degree of confidence (of presence of illness), such that the cases with higher probability of illness are considered vulnerable and are treated with higher priority.

The success of the remotely monitored cloud-based e-Health system is heavily dependent on how invasive the polysomnograms are. Even for polysomnograms performed in hospitals, the results can be more representative of undisturbed sleep behavior if the sensor network was non-invasive. Having an uncomfortable and highly perceptive measuring setup will alter the results. An inconspicuous monitoring system will not only yield experimental data that is closer to the actual encephalographic sleep activity but it is more likely to be socially accepted. This is an important issue, particularly in remote applications, as there is no medical supervision. In Fig. 2 it can be observed that a pediatric patient is connected to a polysomnogram and the amount of wiring can be overwhelming. Nearly half of the polysomnogram's wiring corresponds to electroencephalographic sensors. Therefore, if the amount of these sensors is reduced it can significantly improve social acceptance.

2 Electroencephalographic Signal Correlation Study

An electroencephalogram (EEG) records electrical activity, using electrodes, along the scalp by measuring voltage fluctuations resulting from ionic current flows within the neurons of the cortex [2, 4, 7]. Polysomnographic data is recorded in (or can be exported to) the European data format (EDF), which is an open and non-proprietary format, this allows files to be easily imported and analyzed. EDF files have a header (coded in ASCII) followed by binary data. Each data sample is coded as a 16-bit integer using two's complement and little-endian notation. The sampling rates vary depending on the sensor, but are in the order of 100 samples per second. Since each

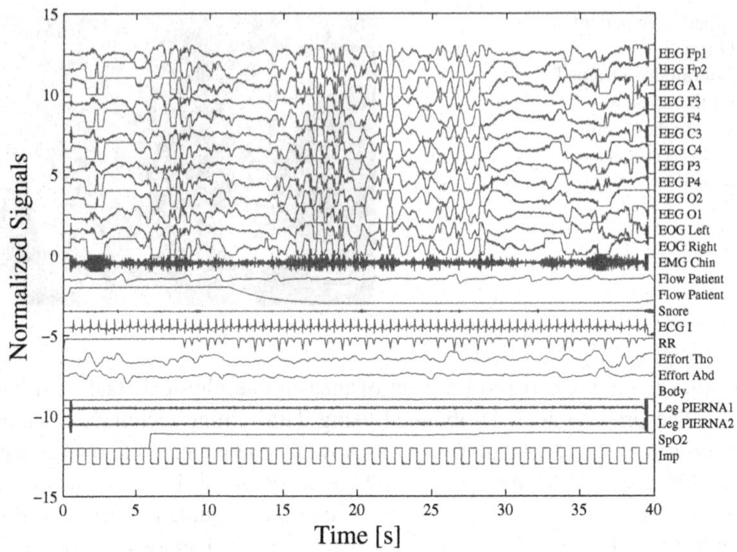

Fig. 3 40-s extract of a polysomnogram stored in an EDF file

sample contains 16 bits, this translates to up to 3.2 kbps per sensor. An extract of a polysomnogram is shown in Fig. 3.

A typical polysomnogram has 8–9 h (i.e., while patient sleeps) of data and occupies approximately 200 MB per test. The information is stored in blocks (typically with one second of data) where each sensor has a recurrent fixed size, i.e., it occupies N samples in every block. Not all sensors have the same amount of samples per block, as different sensors sample at different rates. The header contains the samples per block per sensor information. It is recommended that the data per block (for all signals) does not exceed 61440 bytes. If a block is expected to surpass this limit, it is recommended to reduce the duration of the block. EEG data is sampled at a rate of 100 samples per second.

The EEG signals, which are shown in the top portion of Fig. 3, are highly correlated. As mentioned earlier, the main purpose of EEG sensors in the polysomnogram is to determine in which sleep stage the patient is in. There are 4 stages where the last is a rapid-eye movement (REM) stage (usually when patients dream), and the first 3 are non-REM stages. During all these stages, EEG signals have different patterns, but within a stage the individual sensors produced nearly similar measurements (the correlation between sensors is fairly high) and therefore redundant. The removal of the redundancy is not trivial if the objective is to retain the sensors that provide the most information, i.e., the more unique information. This work describes a methodological algorithm that determines where are the best locations for sensors, for a specific amount of sensors. In this work, the setup consists of eleven sensors, but the method is explained such that it can be reproducible with any amount of sensors. To organize the methodology Sect. 2.1 first explains the overall process and then the details of steps 2 and 3, which are considered the more complex steps.

2.1 Sensor Reduction Algorithm

To reduce the amounts of sensors needed for the polysomnogram an algorithm was designed. This algorithm is organized into steps, which are: building a correlation matrix, categorizing the sensors into groups, and finding the centroid sensor. The set of centroid sensors composed the reduced set of sensors.

1. Correlation Matrix: The correlation between one sensor and every other sensor is computed, and repeated for all the available sensors building a correlation matrix where the diagonal is composed of ones.
2. Group Categorization: The sensors are grouped into every possible combination of group sizes and for every combination the group correlation is computed. The combination of groups that produces the highest overall correlation is the chosen arrangement for that particular group-sensor setup. This is explained in more detail ahead.
3. Centroid Sensor: Once the sensors have been allocated into groups, the sensor with the highest group correlation (correlation between a sensor and every other sensor of the group) will determine the sensor that is closest to the centroid, i.e., the sensor that best represents the group.
4. Steps 2 and 3 are repeated for every group-sensor setup.

Group Categorization (step 2) Categorization is the process of selecting groups of sensors that exhibit similar traits. The groups are not necessarily composed of equal amount of sensors. Removing this restriction broadens the possibilities and therefore yields better results. To select the reduced set of sensors that best represent the entire original set of sensors, a methodical sequential algorithm was designed. The algorithm methodology behaves as follows. First all combinations for a specific group-sensor setup are determined. For example, all possible combinations of 11 sensors categorized into 4 groups are (each number represents the number of sensors in that group):

8-1-1-1	6-2-2-1	5-2-2-2
7-2-1-1	5-3-2-1	4-3-2-2
6-3-1-1	4-4-2-1	3-3-3-2
5-4-1-1	4-3-3-1	

This gives 11 possible combinations for the 4–11 setup. Any other combination, if sorted in descending order, will already be contained in this list. After all combinations are found, these are used as masks for the search of the highest group-combination correlation. The sensors are placed in the mask and the correlation is computed, then the order of the sensors is changed and the correlation is recomputed. This sequential process continues until the correlation of all the possible arrangements of sensors have been computed. The algorithm can be optimized to eliminate repetitions. For example, in a 2–3 setup with a 2-1 mask, the arrangement {S1 S2} S3, will produce the same correlation as the arrangement {S2 S1} S3, as

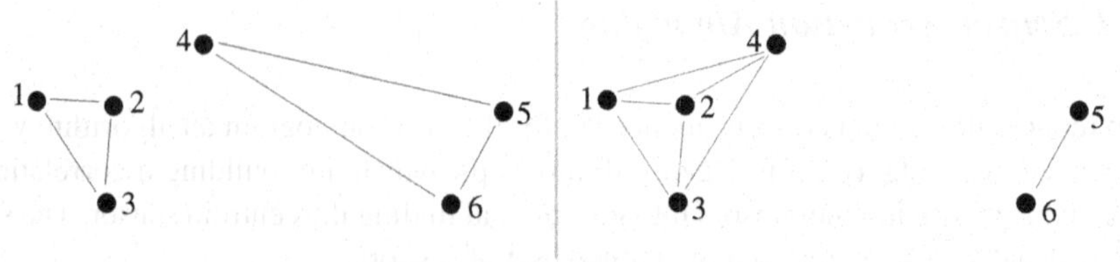

Fig. 4 Groups selecting process based on the overall correlation

the correlation {S1 S2} is the same as the correlation {S2 S1}. Though in this work all possible arrangements, even redundant, were considered.

To better illustrate graphically the effect of selecting the overall highest correlated arrangement, observe Fig. 4. It is illustrating two sequences of a 2–6 setup. The algorithm is comparing the correlation of the arrangement {S1 S2 S3} {S4 S5 S6}, with the arrangement {S1 S2 S3 S4} {S5 S6}. In this example, the latter case produced a greater correlation and therefore kept for the comparison with the next arrangement. If no arrangement produces a greater overall correlation, these groups are used for the next (centroid sensor) step. For the case where there are groups of one sensor, rather than using the correlation with itself (always gives 1), the average correlation with the other sensor is subtracted to 1. This gives more weight to the sensors that are isolated from the remaining sensors.

It should be mentioned that fuzzy clustering techniques were also considered in a correlation maximization scheme rather than distance minimization (distance minimization is explained in [5, 6]). This was discarded because to implement fuzzy clustering a continuous space is required to compute the distances (or correlations), rather than discrete samples. In our case selecting a random point in our space of correlations is analogous to inserting virtual sensors and slowly shifting these toward the centroids. To do this the correlation from the virtual sensors to every other sensor has to be known, which is not the case.

Centroid Sensor Once the groups have been identified, the next step is to find the sensor that is closest to the geometrical center, i.e., the sensor that has a greatest correlation to the remaining sensors of its group, such that it best represents the group. This is simply done by computing the correlation to every other sensor in the group and the sensor that has the greatest overall correlation is the closest to the centroid. This step is illustrated in Fig. 5. In this example, sensor 2 is chosen as the centroid sensor.

In the case where two (or more) nodes are equidistant to the group centroid, then the sensors with the lowest correlation to every other sensor (outside the group) is chosen as the centroid sensor. The reason for taking the lowest correlated sensor with respect to the outside nodes is because the original objective is to search for unique sensors that represent an area.

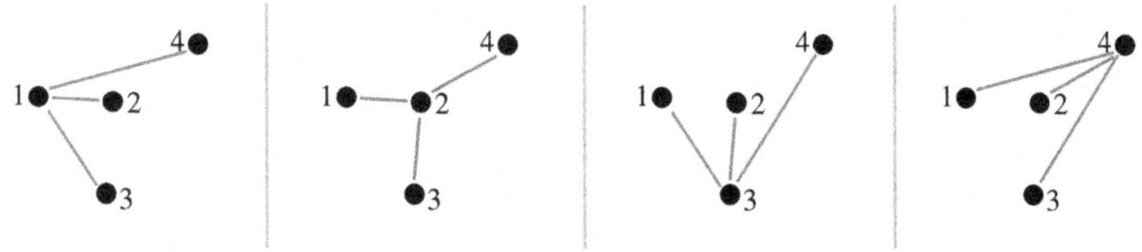

Fig. 5 Identifying sensor that is closest to the geometrical center

This section described the process of sensor selection. To summarize, using a group-sensor setup, the amount of sensors needed for EEG are reduced from the total available amount of sensors to the group amount, where the centroid sensor represents the group. The results obtained are discussed ahead.

3 Results and Discussion

In this section the results are presented and explained. Our medical facility is equipped with an Alice 5 polysomnogram, which has 11 EEG sensors in total that can be placed in different parts of a human head. Following the EEG 10–20 system, data was gathered from 78 different patients. The data was exported to EDF format and analyzed using the MATLAB software. The correlation matrix obtained (step 1, from Sect. 2.1) is summarized in Table 1.

The group categorization and centroid sensor selection (steps 2 and 3) yielded the results shown in Table 1 for the 11 sensors that were studied. Figure 6 shows the original set of sensors employed in the measurements, which are located 10 % from the midline in each side of the head (Table 2).

Table 1 EEG Sensor Correlation Matrix

	A1	C3	C4	F3	F4	FP1	FP2	O1	O2	P3	P4
A1	1	0.8962	0.9488	0.8926	0.9479	0.8907	0.9442	0.9070	0.9565	0.9018	0.9512
C3	0.8962	1	0.7333	0.8127	0.6927	0.9401	0.9192	0.9514	0.8787	0.8222	0.7040
C4	0.9488	0.7333	1	0.6803	0.8316	0.9230	0.9447	0.9364	0.9320	0.6569	0.8083
F3	0.8926	0.8127	0.6803	1	0.7450	0.9545	0.9265	0.9435	0.8562	0.7033	0.6271
F4	0.9479	0.6927	0.8316	0.7450	1	0.9311	0.9575	0.9276	0.8913	0.5946	0.7378
FP1	0.8907	0.9401	0.9230	0.9545	0.9311	1	0.9557	0.9361	0.9169	0.9387	0.9171
FP2	0.9442	0.9192	0.9447	0.9265	0.9575	0.9557	1	0.9161	0.9359	0.9160	0.9361
O1	0.9070	0.9514	0.9364	0.9435	0.9276	0.9361	0.9161	1	0.9531	0.9721	0.9469
O2	0.9565	0.8787	0.9320	0.8562	0.8913	0.9169	0.9359	0.9531	1	0.8954	0.9735
P3	0.9018	0.8222	0.6569	0.7033	0.5946	0.9387	0.9160	0.9721	0.8954	1	0.7231
P4	0.9512	0.7040	0.8083	0.6271	0.7378	0.9171	0.9361	0.9469	0.9735	0.7231	1

Fig. 6 All available sensors, no reduction performed

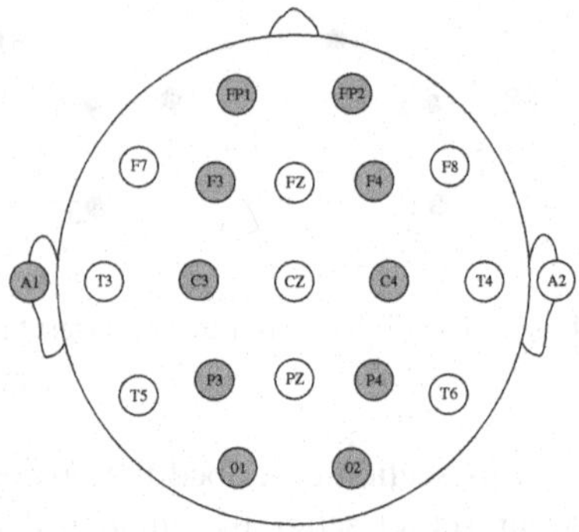

Table 2 Sensor placement to obtain maximum amount of information

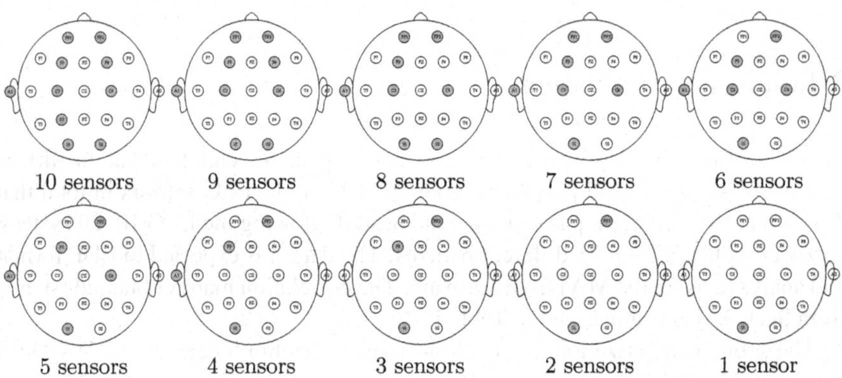

An interesting observation is that the sensor that exhibited the highest correlation with the remaining sensors is not located on the midline-center (or, from the available sensors, at either side of the midline at the center), but rather on the back of the head. This is an interesting result because there is a possibility that a single sensor in the lower back of the head, where a sensor might be less bothersome, will be sufficient to determine the sleep stages of the patient. Reducing significantly the amount of sensors needed. One essential analysis that must be made is the amount of information encompassed by each additional sensor, i.e., how representative of the other sensors are (or is) the selected nodes. Observing the case where the system was reduced to a single sensor (O1), the average correlation between this sensor and the remaining sensors is 0.939 (~6 %), where the minimum is 0.907. So, arguably, it can be concluded that one sensor is sufficient to determine the sleep stages of a patient. If a second sensors is used (FP2), and the averages and combined in parallel, that is: $Corr_{O1}||Corr_{FP2} = 1 - (1 - Corr_{O1})(1 - Corr_{FP2})$ then a value of 0.996 (<1 %) is obtained. The results for all x-11 group sensor correlations are shown in Fig. 7. Figure 8 shows the (1—correlation) difference, which gives better understanding of the overall correlation increment pattern. The set of 10 and 11 sensors are not shown

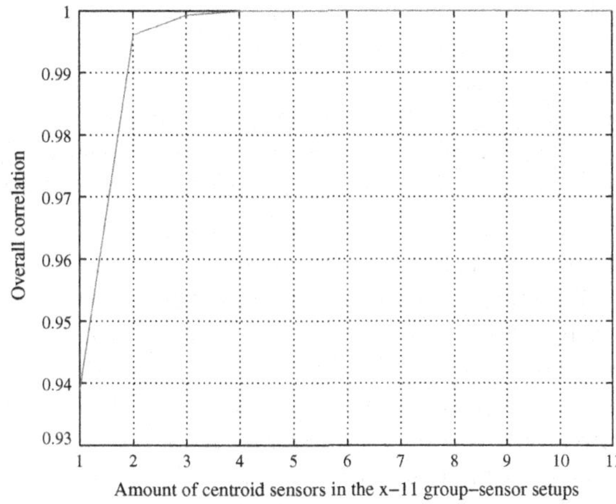

Fig. 7 Correlation of the centroid sensors that composed the x-11 group sensor setups

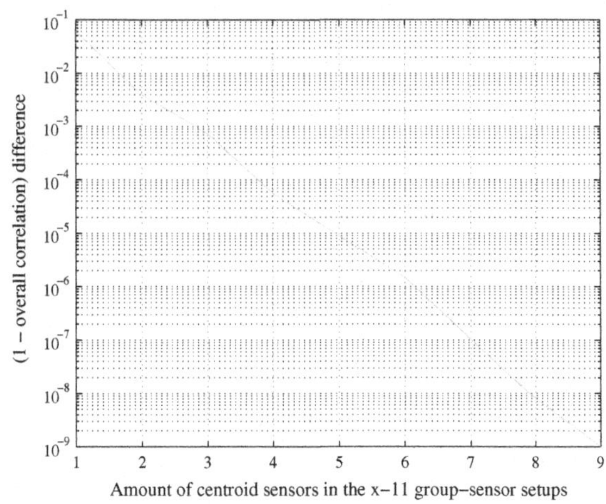

Fig. 8 (1—correlation) difference of the centroid sensors that composed the x-11 group sensor setups

because, to the accuracy of our calculations, 10 nodes yields 100 % correlation and 11 sensors by definition have 100 % correlation, so the difference in these two cases is zero (in log scale $-\infty$).

4 Conclusions

A strategy for the reduction of the amount of EEG sensors is presented. This algorithm is reproducible with any amount of sensors, so it can accommodate data from polysomnograms that have higher or lower amount of sensors. The algorithm is organized into 4 steps: Construction of the correlation matrix, group categorization, centroid sensor search, and repeat for all (or desired) group-sensor setups. This process can be used to reduce the amount of sensors currently employed in polysomnograms. For our particular setup, it was shown that the system only requires a few sensors for over 99 % correlation. A single sensor will have 94 % correlation average with all the sensors used for these tests and a minimum on over 90 %. This is an excellent indicator that the amount of sensors used in polysomnography can be drastically reduced with very little loss in effectiveness. With the data from one (or few) sensors it is sufficient to determine the sleep stages of the tested patient, which is the main purpose of the EEGs in the polysomnographic test.

From a broader point of view, it can be concluded that polysomnographic tests can have higher social acceptance if the amount of sensors is reduced. This itself can help this technology expand from the hospitals to remote locations via cloud-based health networks that are connected to an e-Health monitoring center. Fewer sensors also reduce the amount of storage required to save and process the collected data. This eases the load (or even enables the implementation) of data warehouses that compute pre-diagnostics based on a trained system. The system training would be a collaborative work between engineering and medical doctors. Pre-diagnostics can be used to identify the more vulnerable patients and set priorities to medical treatment access. This can replace the obsolete open loop model of prioritizing by age that is mentioned in the introduction. Additionally, since the system is designed to return a pre-diagnostic, opposed to a full diagnostic (by human), the remote unit does not need all the sensors, i.e., reduce EEG sensors and eliminate other sensors that do not contribute much information. This will reduce the cost of the remote testing unit. Finally, by having numerous low-cost remote testing units distributed throughout the general population, the amount of patients that can be tested will significantly increase reaching a greater number of vulnerable patients.

Acknowledgments This work is partially funded by project FONDEF No. CA13i-10300, and project FONDECYT No. 11130573.

References

1. Falchuk, B., Famolari, D., Fischer, R., Loeb, S., Panagos, E.: The mHealth stack: technology enablers for patient-centric mobile healthcare. Int. J. E-Health Med. Commun. (IJEHMC) **1**(1), 1–17 (2010)
2. Gilmore, R.L.: American-electroencephalographic-society guidelines in electroencephalography, evoked-potentials, and polysomnography. J. Clin. Neurophysiol. **11**(1), 1–142 (1994)
3. Ivanenko, A., Massey, C.: Assessment and management of sleep disorders in children. Psychiatr. Times **23**(11) (2006)
4. Niedermeyer, E., da Silva, F.H.L.: Electroencephalography: Basic Principles, Clinical Applications, and Related Fields. Wolters Kluwer Health (2005)
5. Ruspini, E.H.: A new approach to clustering. Inf. Control **15**(1), 22–32 (1969)
6. Ruspini, E.H.: Numerical methods for fuzzy clustering. Inf. Sci. **2**(3), 319–350 (1970)
7. Sanei, S., Chambers, J.A.: EEG Signal Processing. Wiley, Chichester (2008)
8. Yu, W.D., Bhagwat, R.: Modeling emergency and telemedicine heath support system: a service oriented architecture approach using cloud computing. Int. J. E-Health Med. Commun. (IJEHMC) **2**(3), 63–88 (2011)

Work with Iodine-125: 8 Years Experience in Brachy-Therapy Sources Production Lab

C.D. Souza, F.S. Peleias Jr, M.E.C.M. Rostelato, C.A. Zeituni, R. Tiezzi, B.T. Rodrigues, A. Feher, J.A. Moura and O.L. Costa

Abstract Prostate cancer represents about 10 % of all cases of cancer in the world. Brachytherapy has been extensively used in the early and intermediate stages of the illness. This radiotherapy method reduces the damage to surrounding healthy tissues by concentrating radiation in the target area. The present study presents some of our challenges of working with radioactive iodine, such as, reaction pH and chemical characteristics. It also introduces a new method for manufacturing iodine-125 sources that is being implemented in a production laboratory. This new facility will provide these sources to Brazil hospitals for a lower cost.

Keywords Brachytherapy · Prostate cancer · Iodine-125 · Cancer treatment

1 Introduction

1.1 Cancer in Brazil and in the World

Malignant tumors are responsible for a high mortality rate worldwide. The World Health Organization (WHO) estimated that 2030 will have 21.4 million new cases, 13.2 million cancer deaths and 73 million people living with the disease. Prostate cancer is the second most common among men, after lung cancer. Currently, cancer is the second cause of death in most countries [1, 2].

Although not commonly discussed, the economic and social impacts of cancer are enormous. The implications for patients, family and society in general are pain, suffering, disability and death. It consumes a vast amount of resources devoted to the diagnosis and treatment and reduce the human labor potential.

C.D. Souza (✉) · F.S. Peleias Jr · M.E.C.M.Rostelato · C.A. Zeituni
R. Tiezzi · B.T. Rodrigues · A. Feher · J.A. Moura · O.L. Costa
Instituto de Pesquisas Energéticas E Nucleares (IPEN/CNEN—SP), São Paul, Brazil
e-mail: carladdsouza@yahoo.com.br

Y.-W. Chen et al. (eds.), *Innovation in Medicine and Healthcare 2015*,
Smart Innovation, Systems and Technologies 45,
DOI 10.1007/978-3-319-23024-5_45

1.2 Brachytherapy and Iodine-125 Seeds

Brachytherapy is a form of radiation therapy in which the radiation source is placed close to or in contact with the region to be treated. The dose is continuously released for a short period of time (temporary implants) or during the decay of the source (permanent implants). The lesion receives the major part of the radiation dose, protecting healthy surrounding tissues [3].

The brachytherapy with iodine-125 seeds can be used as a permanent implant (prostate) or temporary (eyes and brain). It consists of:

- a core which contains the iodine-125 and a radiological marker;
- a biocompatible material capsule that surrounds the core.

Treatment of prostate cancer by brachytherapy has curative purposes. According to the literature results, 95 % of patients treated with these seeds are free of disease after 12 years of treatment. Moreover, as this protects healthy surrounding tissues, side effects occurrence are low when compared to other procedures. For prostate cancer, only 15 % of patients shown altered sexual activity and less than 1 % have had urinary incontinence. At surgery these numbers increase to 45 % for sexual impotence and 8 % for urinary incontinence [4].

Seed implantation procedure is non-surgical and has low impact on heathy tissues. Most patients can go back to normal activity within 1–3 days, with little or no pain [4]. Iodine-125 is fixed on a silver substrate (3 mm length and 0.5 mm diameter) placed inside a titanium tube of 0.8 mm outside diametrer, 0.05 mm wall thickness and 4.5 mm length. Silver is also used as an x-ray marker.

1.3 Brachytherapy Group of IPEN

Treatment of prostate cancer with permanent iodine-125 seed implantation increased significantly in recent years. The technique is indicated for cancer patients in early and intermediate stages [5]. In a prostate cancer treatment, about 100 units of seed are used. They are imported for $60.00 a unit, preventing the use in public funded hospitals [6].

A multidisciplinary team was established at the Nuclear and Energy Research Institute—Radiation Technology Center (CTR-IPEN /SP) to develop a national iodine-125 seed and installation for local production. The manufacture of seeds in Brazil will make the treatment costs cheaper and feasible for more patients.

Iodine-125 is deposited on a silver wire and them, placed inside a titanium capsule. For the implementation of routine production, it is necessary to develop a methodology for the deposition of radioactive iodine on the silver wire (core) in order to develop an efficient, inexpensive and reliable method.

The objectives of this paper is to present some of the issues that we have working with iodine-125 and our new chemical reaction to be implemented in the routine production of iodine-125 seeds used in brachytherapy.

2 Bibliographic Review

2.1 Iodine-125 Seeds

The literature on the techniques used in the production of iodine-125 seeds is found in articles (with few details about the fixation method), patents or in commercial catalogs with summary descriptions, in order to protect industrial secrets. Section 2.2 summarizes the patents and articles.

2.2 Important Articles and Patents

The first iodine-125 seed were developed in 1965 by Lawrence in a patent entitled "Therapeutic metal seed containing the radioactive isotope within disposed on the carrier and method of manufacture" [7]. The dimensions and shape of the seed are described as in Fig. 1. For core, the author recommends nylon, silicone rubber, Teflon or polyester resin. palladium-103, cesium-131 and iodine-125 can be used as radioactive isotopes. Gold and tungsten are suggested as radiological markers. Stainless steel and titanium are suitable for coating material.

The second patent obtained was in 1982, by Kubiatowicz with title "Radioactive iodine seed" [8]. The author suggests using silver chloride or silver bromide to perform the ion exchange, resulting in silver iodide (AgI^{125}). It is recommended to reduce blue and ultraviolet light exposure.

Four iodine-125 depositions in silver examples are described. In the first example, five silver wires of 70 mm length and 0.25 mm diameter are in contact a1 mol/L sodium chloride solution. The silver wire is connected to a positive electrode. The platinum foil negative electrode is connected and a electric current is applied. This process, known as electroplating, creates a silver chloride layer on the substrate. They were then cut into 3 mm long pieces and placed in a 0.2 mL sodium iodide (NaI^{125}) and a 0.01 mol/L sodium hydroxide solution. Non-radioactive iodine in the form of NaI combined with NaOH solution (known as a carrier) was added to the solution. After stirring for 17 h, the cores are sealed within a titanium capsule. The author claims 97 % fixation efficiency.

In the second example, 3 mm long and 0.5 mm diameter silver wires are placed in contact with 1 mol/L sodium chloride solution. The container is connected to the positive electrode. A platinum foil is used as negative electrode. The electric current was applied during 6.5 h. A silver chloride layer is produced on the silver wires surface. The deposition is done shown in the first example.

In the third example, 3 mm long and 0.5 mm diameter silver wires are placed in a glass container with a 6 mol/L hydrochloric acid and a 1 mol/L sodium chlorite or hypochlorite. After stirring for 1 h at room temperature, a silver chloride layer is formed on the wires. The cores are placed in a iodine-125 (NaI^{125}) and 10^{-4} mol/L sodium hydroxide solution. Non-radioactive iodine, in the form of NaI, is added as carrier. The solution is stirred for 19 h in absence of light. The author reports 97 % fixation efficiency. The cores are inserted inside a titanium capsule and sealed by plasma welding.

In the fourth example, 18 silver wires 3 mm long and 0.5 mm diameter are placed in a vessel containing a platinum foil connected to the negative pole, and a platinum wire connected to the positive pole. The NaI^{125} solution is diluted with 1.5 mL NaOH with pH 10. A 25 μA current is applied for 2 hours under constant stirring. The fixation efficiency is 97 %.

Manolkar et al. in the article "Comparison of methods for preparation of ^{125}I brachytherapy source cores for the treatment of eye cancer" [9], describes two types of seeds. In the first method, a silver wire positioned in a vial containing 30 μL of a sodium iodide solution (3.5 mCi/1.3 × 10^{14} Bq) and of 650 μL of a sodium sulfite with 0.001 mol/L. The solution was then placed in a magnetic stirrer. A platinum wire was connected to the negative electrode and the silver wire to the positive electrode. Electric current flow through the system causing iodine-125 to deposit onto silver. In the second model, alumina beads were treated with 10^{-3} mol/L sodium nitrate. Then they were immersed in a 30 μL of iodine-125 and 0.1 mL Chloramine-T dissolved in 10^{-3} mol/L of sodium nitrate. The solution was stirred for 4 h at room temperature. The beads were washed in sodium nitrate, and dried at room temperature.

In several publications [10–12] the group headed by Cieszykowska published two new methods for iodine-125 seeds preparation. The first is an ophthalmic applicator with iodine-125 fixated in a silver shell by electrolysis. The source is hermetically sealed within an acrylic capsule. The dose rate measurements indicate that the total activity was incorporated. In the second method, the authors use the internal electrolysis on two types of silver substrates: cores with dimensions of 3 mm in length and 0.5 mm in diameter and 30 mm entire wire length. The cell used for fixation consists of a silver anode inserted in a platinum cup (cathode) with 20 mL activated sodium iodide in 0.01 mol/L sodium hydroxide solution. The results indicate that the silver wire should first be coated with iodine-125 (99 % efficiency) and then cut into pieces 3 mm length.

In 2009, Saxena et al. published the article "Development of a new I-125 design brachytherapy seed for its application in the treatment of eye and prostate cancer" [13] that describes a seed made with silver spheres (diameter 0.5 mm) coated with palladium. Radioactive sodium iodide in sodium hydroxide solution is in contact for a time and temperature not stipulated by the author. After, the spheres are washed with distilled water at 50 °C and coated with polystyrene. The author claims 85 % efficiency.

Saxena published in 2012 the article "Development of the 125I source for its application in bone densitometry" which describes a source with silver core coated with palladium. Little information about the process are given. The authors use a 250 μL iodine solution with activities between 100–200 mCi (3.7–7.4 × 10^{15} Bq) per mL. The reaction was performed under 65 °C temperature for 6 h with 35 μg carrier solution. The author affirms 76 % efficiency [14].

Since the surface treatment influences the fixation efficiency, Lee et al. published the article "Surface treatments of silver iodide rods with enhanced adsorption for I-125 brachytherapy seeds". Various binders, abrasives treatments and oxidizing compounds were tested. The best ones were: binder phosphate (0.417 mol/L), nitric acid as abrasive and hydrogen peroxide (0.063 mol/L) as the oxidant [15].

2.3 Iodine-125 Characteristics

Iodine-125 is produced in nuclear reactor from Xenon-124. It decays by electron capture and internal conversion to Tellurium-125. Photons of 25.2, 22.1 and 35.5 keV (average 29 keV) are emitted. Due to the low energy emission, the photons have little penetrating power. Its half-life is 59.43 days [16].

3 Methodology

This work methodology will be presented with analysis of important items discovered through literature and during the execution of the experiments. They are:

- "Iodine-131 has the same chemical behavior of iodine-125"
  Many researchers do their tests with iodine-131 by stating that both are iodine and so results are comparable. Iodine-131 needs a smaller neutron flux to be produce than iodine-125. During the development of the project "*Comparison of fixation methods of radioactive iodine on silver substrate for making sources used in brachytherapy*" [17] this assumption was used. The new method developed in that work presented a 99.83 % yield with iodine-131. Repeating the exact method with iodine-125 yielded only 18 % efficiency.
- Chemical Parameters to be considered
  For the reaction to occur as expected, it is necessary to study the important chemical parameters. No reaction occurs without the addition of any solution, that is, the silver substrate itself doesn't react with the radioactive solution.
  The silver substrate is purchased already cut into small 3 mm pieces. The composition is 100 % pure silver. However, the silver, having a high oxidation potential, forms silver oxide Ag_2O when in contact with air. Thus, for the reaction to occur, it is required to strip the surface or depositing another compound that exchange efficiently with the radioactive iodide.

After that study, a new fixation method was created. Iron (III) is a relatively strong oxidant ($E^0 = 0.77$ V) showing similar reduction potential to the pair Ag^+/Ag ($E^0 = 0.80$ V) [18]. Then, a $FeCl_3$ solution may be used for preparing AgCl coated substrates because as the Fe^{3+} oxidizes the metallic silver to Ag^+, an adhesive silver chloride layer is formed on its surface. After this process, the cores will react with NaI^{125} solution resulting in AgI^{125} [18]. The new iodine-125 method uses treated silver nuclei with ferric chloride solutions with 10^{-4} to 10^{-1} mol/L in ethanol/water 1:1 (v/v) acidified in hydrochloric acid. The reaction occurs under stirring during 10 h.

4 Results and Discussion

4.1 "Iodine-131 Has the Same Chemical Behavior of Iodine-125"

The explanation for this fact is that the solutions of the two iodines are made in completely different ways. The iodine-131 solution made by IPEN is sparked on sodium hydroxide with pH 12 and has about 19 % iodates which are converted by the sodium borohydride solution. The Iodine-125 solution is imported by IPEN and the company does not inform which method is used on production (after several attempts to contact).

By comparing the total amount of iodine in one reaction (about 10^{-9} g) with impurities one can realize the importance of knowing how the material was made. For example, 1 % impurity in 1 g of solution results in 0.01 g which is much greater than the total radioactive iodine. This is one of the reasons why the behavior of radioactive iodine is anomalous and the experiments should not be performed with other isotopes assuming similar behavior. Further studies are under development.

4.2 Chemical Parameters to Be Considered

In this work, etching will be done by ¾ peroxide hydrogen and ¼ sulfuric acid solution (volume ratio). After this process, a solution capable of oxidizing silver to Ag^+ will be inserted. Etching the surface results in a slight decrease in volume, but is easy to control.

The primary radioactive iodine solution, in the form of sodium iodide (NaI), is acquired with 50 mCi (1.85×10^{15} Bq), diluted in NaOH solution, pH 12, in small volumes (about 0.05 mL). This volume is completed to 500 μL with NaOH solution with the same pH. As a result, for each batch of radioactive iodine five experiments with 100 mL and 10 mCi (3.7×10^{14} Bq) may be performed. Each experiment will be performed with 10 silver cores, following the activity indication of 1 mCi

(3.7×10^{13} Bq) per core. The NaI is completely soluble under the experiment conditions—solubility of sodium iodide in water, 184 g/100 mL at 25 °C (0,644 g/350 μL—volume used in the experiments) and 294 g /100 mL at 70 °C with pH between 8 and 9.5.

The basic medium is known to be appropriate, following the premise that disfavors the iodide binding in iodine gas [19, 20]. But new studies [21] are showing an increase in yield with the decrease of pH. To this end, various solutions with different pH were made using hydrochloric acid and sodium hydroxide. They were added to a glass vial with 500 μL of known pH solution and 20 μL of radioactive solution. The result is shown in Table 1.

The results suggest that the medium may not influence the results. It must also be considered the iodine species that hinder reaction dynamics, such as, IO^{3-}, IO^{-1} and IO^{4-}. Its formation is favored by acid pH. To prevent the formation of these compounds, pH control should be extremely strict. Other iodine ions, such as, I^{3-} and I^{5-} can be converted into I- with a reducing agent [22].

The most reactive metals are those that have great tendency to lose electrons forming positive ions. Chemical reactivity of non-metals varies with the electronegativity (the ability of an atom to attract electrons). The more electronegative the element is, the more reactive it will be. The more reactive non-metals are, the greater is the tendency for receiving electrons, thus negative ions are formed easier In this case, iodine is more electronegative than hydroxyl (OH^-). But the OH^- concentration is much greater than the iodide, which impairs the formation of NaI^{125}. The consumption of OH^- ions cause a sudden drop in pH, which might be an explanation for iodine loss during the course of the reaction (40 % mean activity loss) since the acidic pH may promote formation of highly volatile iodine gas [19, 22].

In conclusion, it is clear that the knowing if the pH influence the experiment is imperative. In our case, pH makes no difference in volatilization and changes the fixation results completely. Preformed in pH 12 our experiment yield 40 % activity. In pH 3, the numbers rise to 80 %.

Table 1 Test analysis of radioactive material loss performed with different pH

	pH	Activity μCi	Activity μCi after 24 h	Loss percentage (%)	Mean value
NaOH	14	321	304	5.29	3.90 % basic
	12	325	319	1.84	Medium
	10	779	754	3.21	Average loss
	8.1	970	919	5.26	
HCl	7	753	728	3.32	2.65 % acid
	4.7	449	445	0.89	Medium
	3.1	71	70	1.41	Average loss
	1.1	904	859	4.98	

Table 2 Iodine-125 yield for 5 experiments and method average yield

Experiment number	Total Iodine-125 activity	Total Iodine-125 incorporated in 10 seeds	Yield %
1	10 mCi/3.7·1014 Bq	7.8 mCi/2.9·1014 Bq	78
2	10 mCi/3.7·1014 Bq	8.6 mCi /3.2·1014 Bq	86
3	10 mCi/3.7·1014 Bq	6.8 mCi/2.5·1014 Bq	68
4	10 mCi/3.7·1014 Bq	9.3 mCi//3.4·1014 Bq	93
5	10 mCi/3.7·1014 Bq	7.7 mCi/2.8·1014 Bq	77
Total			80.4

4.3 *Results of the Experiments*

The new method presented 80 % iodine-125 yield. Table 2 presents medium values between 5 experiments.

5 Conclusion

Prostate cancer is one of the most common among men. New, innovative, easy and low cost treatment studies are at the utmost importance. In Brazil the high cost of brachytherapy seeds prevents the use in large scale. Our group is developing a new laboratory for local production.

We start our research based on premises that has being use for year in the field. After 8 years of challenge, we discover some new data such as: Iodine-131 should not be use instead of Iodine-125; study the dynamics of your reaction before deciding with pH to use considering all the chemical bindings that the iodine can made; pH may not change the volatilization at all.

Our new method presented 80 % yield. It is under implementation in our new laboratory.

References

1. Descoberta célula-tronco associada ao câncer de próstata. http://www.oncoguia.com.br/site/interna.php?cat=58&id=1813&menu=2 Accessed 3 Nov (2009)
2. Ministério Da Saúde. Instituto Nacional De Câncer: Incidência de Câncer no Brasil 2014. http://www.inca.gov.br/estimativa/2014/estimativa-24042014.pdf. Accessed 16 April (2014)
3. Podgorsak, E.B.: Radiation Oncology Physics: A Handbook for Teachers and Students. International Atomic Energy Agency, Vienna (2005)
4. Souza, C. D.: Braquiterapia com sementes de Iodo-125: manufatura e tratamento. Trabalho de conclusão (bacharelado—Física médica) Bachaleour required research (Medical physics)—Universidade Estadual Paulista, Instituto de Biociências, Botucatu, São Paulo (2009)
5. Srougi, M.A.: Próstata como ela é. Folha de São Paulo, São Paulo (2002)

6. Rostelato, M.E.C.M.: Estudo e Desenvolvimento de uma nova Metodologia para Confecção de Sementes de Iodo-125 para Aplicação em Braquiterapia. Tese (Doutoramento) Thesis (PhD)—Instituto de Pesquisas Energéticas e Nucleares—IPEN-CNEN/SP, São Paulo (2006)
7. Hazleton-Nuclear Science Corporation. Lawrence, D.C.: Therapeutic metal seed containing within a radioactive isotope disposed on a carrier and method of manufacture. US Patent 3.351.0497, Nov (1967)
8. Minnesota Mining And Manufacturing Company. Kubiatowicz, D.O.: Radioactive iodine seed. US Patent 4.323.055, 6 April (1982)
9. Manolkar, R.B., Sane, S.U., Pillai, K.T., Majali, M.A.: Comparison of methods for preparation of ^{125}I brachytherapy source cores for the treatment of eye cancer. Appl. Radiat. Isot. **59**, 145–150 (2003)
10. Cieszykowska, I., Mielcarski, M.: Seed-less iodine-125 ophthalmic applicator. Appl. Radiat. Isot. **58**, 15–20 (2002)
11. Cieszykowska, I., Piasecki, A., Mielcarski, M.: An approach to the preparation of iodine-125 seed-type sources. Nukleonika **50**(1), 17–22 (2004)
12. TECDOC-1512, International Atomic Energy Agency: Production Techniques and Quality Control of Sealed Radioactive Sources of Palladium-103, Iodine-125, Iridium-192 and Ytterbium-169. Vienna, 2006. ISBN 92–0–108606–7 (2006)
13. Saxena, S.K., Sharma, S.D., Dash, A., Venkatesh, M.: Development of a new design 125I-brachytherapy seed for its application in the treatment of eye and prostate cancer. Appl. Radiat. Isot. **67**, 1421–1425 (2009)
14. Saxena, S.K., Kumar, Y., Pillai, K.T.Dash: A.: development of a 125I source for its application in bone densitometry. Appl. Radiat. Isot. **70**, 470–477 (2012)
15. Lee, J.H., Choi, K.H., Yu, K.H.: Surface teratments of silver rods with enhanced iodide adsorption for I-125 brachytherapy seeds. Appl. Radiat. Isot. **85**, 96–100 (2014)
16. Kaplan, I.: Física nuclear, vol. 2. Guanabara Dois, Rio de Janeiro (1978)
17. Souza, C.D.: Comparação entre métodos de fixação do iodo radioativo em substrato de prata para confecção de fontes utilizadas em Braquiterapia. Dissertação (Mestrado) Dissertation (mSc)—Instituto de Pesquisas Energéticas e Nucleares—IPEN-CNEN/SP, São Paulo (2012)
18. Lide, D.R.: CRC Handbook of Chemistry and Physics: a Ready-Reference Book of Chemistry and Physical Data, 90 edn. CRC Press, Boca Raton (2009)
19. Mellor, J.W.: A comprehensive treatise on inorganic and theoretical chemistry. Longmans, Green and CO, Londres (1965)
20. Pomeroy, R., Kirschman, H.D.: The solubility of sodium iodide in sodium hydroxide solutions at 20°C. J. Am. Chem. Soc. **66**(2), 178–179 (1944)
21. Jiaheng, H.E., Jiang, L., Xingliang, L., Wenbin, Z., Jing, W., Zongping, M., Yuan, J.: Preparation of the radioactive source core of iodine-125 seed. Nucl. Sci. Tech. **20**, 231–234 (2009)
22. Kahn, M., Kleinberg, J.: Subcommittee on radiochemistry of national academy of sciences-national research council: radiochemistry of lodine. Technical Information Center, Energy Research and Development Administration, Tennessee (1977)

Comprehensible Video Acquisition for Caregiving Scenes—How Multimedia Can Support Caregiver Training

Yuichi Nakamura, Kazuaki Kondo, Taiki Mashimo, Yoshiaki Matsuoka and Tomotake Ohtsuka

Abstract Caregiving requires a variety of techniques that directly affect care-receivers' quality of life. However, caregivers have difficulties in objectively observing and confirming their skills and whether they are providing care-receivers with appropriate and acceptable care. Videotaping is often used in caregiver training for this purpose. This paper introduces a novel method for enhancing such videotaping using information media technology, capturing video using multiple cameras and editing the videos automatically into a single-stream video to achieve a recording purpose. The purpose is to provide an effective means of observing and learning caregiving from typical important points of view. Our experiments showed that videos obtained through our proposed method are effective for the intended purposes.

1 Introduction

Many kinds of interaction between caregivers and care-receivers occur in caregiving everyday. One of the most important problems for caregiver is to make their interactions smooth and comprehensible to care-receivers, because they directly affects care-receivers' the quality of life (QOL). Caregivers need specific skills and training in communication to enable care-receivers to understand their intentions fully. Videotaping has been used often for training. Caregivers can testing and improve skills that they have difficulty evaluating on their own. They can also learn how experts behave and pay attention in caregiving.

Y. Nakamura (✉) · K. Kondo · T. Mashimo
ACCMS, Kyoto University, Sakyo Kyoto, Japan
e-mail: yuichi@media.kyoto-u.ac.jp

K. Kondo
e-mail: kondo@media.kyoto-u.ac.jp

Y. Matsuoka
Faculty of Health Science, Aino University, Ibaraki Osaka, Japan

T. Ohtsuka
Nishikagawa Hospital, Mitoyo Kagawa, Japan

Y.-W. Chen et al. (eds.), *Innovation in Medicine and Healthcare 2015*,
Smart Innovation, Systems and Technologies 45,
DOI 10.1007/978-3-319-23024-5_46

While videotaping is a promising method for learning and training, it is tiresome, and skills must be recorded and paid attention to are often difficult to capture precisely. For this purpose, we propose video acquisition support in caregiving scenes by introducing recent media technologies, such as smart video capturing using multiple cameras and automatic editing of captured videos. Those techniques provide not only comprehensible videos but also different means of reviewing videos corresponding to different viewpoints.

One important point that we need to focus on is care-receiver's perception, e.g., how a care-receiver perceives a caregiver's approaches, how a care-receiver pays attention, how a care-receiver understands care. This viewpoint enables us to understand what kinds of reaction caregiving methods might cause, and why they occur. Another possible point is an experts' skill, e.g., to which portion experts pay attention most and how they make their intentions understood by care-receivers. We can also consider other viewpoints, for example, the perspectives on usability of equipment in caregiving settings.

With the help of video captured considering the above viewpoints, we can expect that caregivers and care-receivers' families have favorable opportunities for improving their skills with better understanding of care-receivers' characteristics. This leads to better care-receivers' QOL. In this paper, we demonstrate the potential of our scheme through preliminary experiments involving simple tasks that appear commonly in daily care.

In the following sections, we first present background and related works in Sect. 2, the purpose and general framework for taking caregiving videos in Sect. 3, and possible video capturing and editing techniques in Sect. 4. We describe our preliminary experiments showing the potential of our scheme in Sect. 5.

2 Background and Related Work

This research aims to provide training supports for human-centered care and care-related knowledge to various communities. Humanitude [1, 2] is a powerful methodology for caregiving. Its key idea is to consider the perceptual and cognitive characteristics of care-receivers, and to make full use of human communication channels for ensuring sufficient information can be shared among care-receivers and caregivers. Methods and skills for eye contact, touch, speech, and standing have been intensively discussed and put into practice. Practice of this methodology drastically reduces care-receivers' undesirable and often aggressive behaviors, improves caregivers' satisfaction, and accordingly improves care-receivers' QOL.

Based on this background, the idea arose that one effective way for supporting caregiving is to help caregivers understand care-receivers' nature by showing how the caregiving method changes care-receivers' perceptions and reactions. Recent devices and media technologies on capturing and editing videos have potential for supporting the above purpose. Topics on video acquisition and handling, e.g., automated video capturing, automated video editing, and video indexing and retrieval have been intensively explored, and their possibilities have been demonstrated. The application most related to the above purpose is automated lecture archiving and video content production [3–5]: automated cameras shoot at people or objects, and the system recognizes humans, objects, and events, which are then used for automated editing and summarizing [6].

In addition, wearable camera devices have been developed for a variety of purposes, such as Lifelog, daily healthcare, and remote medicine [7, 8]. First person vision (FPV), that is, taking videos or pictures with a small camera attached to the head or body, is closely related to our topic. We can record what we see and what we experience, and we can review the record on our demand, e.g., recalling daily events or looking for a lost object [9, 10]. We can expect that such technologies will provide substantial assistance in recording and utilizing caregiving scenes and enable us to understand how to meet care-receivers' demands.

3 Purpose of Capturing Caregiving Scenes

3.1 What Needs to be Captured

An essential problem is how we can notice and understand important points, when we are learning or practicing caregiving. For example, we need to know how a care-receiver perceives a caregiver's approach and touch and understand how their undesirable reactions such as Behavioral and Psychological Symptoms of Dementia (BPSD) are sometimes caused by caregiving. Those are tightly related to interactions between caregivers and care-receivers, spatial relationships and physical touches, and the facilities or environments in a care setting. Let us consider those aspects in the following.

Actions in interactions: Interactions between caregivers and care-receivers occur through several channels, including eye contact, facial expression, speech, and touch. It is important to see details in what signals and movements are taken in which ways, and to which portion attention has been paid. Figure 1 shows typical scene captures that are focused on the above points. Figure 1a–d show how the caregiver entered the sight of the care-receiver, initiated the interaction by talking to the care-receiver, touched the care-receiver on the leg, and conducted descriptive conversations, i.e., explained what the person was about to do, respectively.

Attention and perception: Perception and attention, i.e., how people pay attention to each other, what is perceived, and how it is recognized provides essential information in caregiving. Knowing care-receivers' perception and attention is particularly important, since caregivers must exercise considerable skill and effort to enable care-receivers with reduced sensory efficiency to understand their intentions. Figure 2 shows scene captures that explain perception and attention well. Figure 2a, b show where or to which object a care-receiver paid attention. Figure 2c shows an unde-

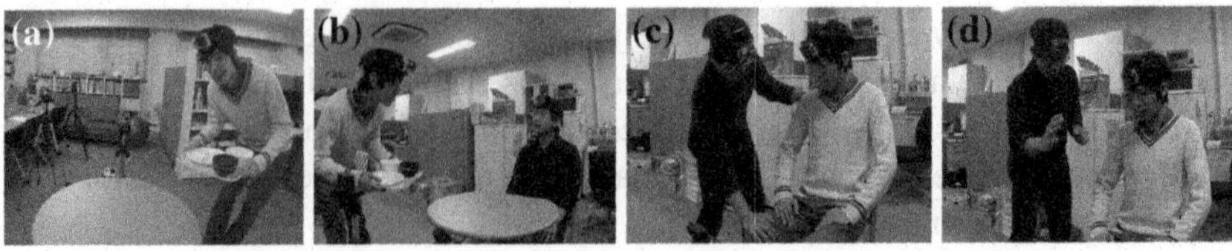

Fig. 1 Typical shots focusing on actions in interactions. **a** Catch sight, **b** talk to, **c** touch, **d** explanation

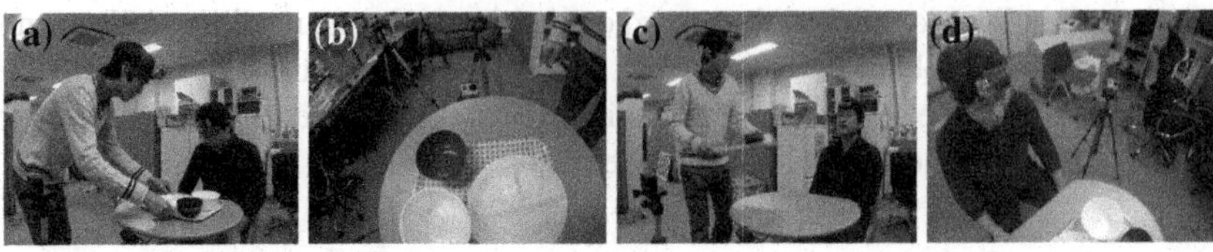

Fig. 2 Typical shots focusing on attention and perception. **a** Attention of a care-receiver, **b** target of attention, **c** not noticed by care-receiver, **d** attention of a caregiver

sirable example in which the care-receiver did not notice the caregiver's action, for which Fig. 1a, b already showed an improved example in which the caregiver successfully caught the eye of the care-receiver. Figure 2d shows where and what the caregiver paid attention to. Joint attention such as one person directing the other's attention is also an important factor.

Position and environment: The spatial and positional relationship of a caregiver and a care-receiver is also an important factor, and how facilities are used or affect the manner of caregiving is also useful information. Figure 3 shows typical scene captures relating to the above information. Figure 3a–c show an overview of the scene, a posture of a caregiver and a care-receiver, the spatial relationship to the objects, and how tools and furniture were arranged, respectively.

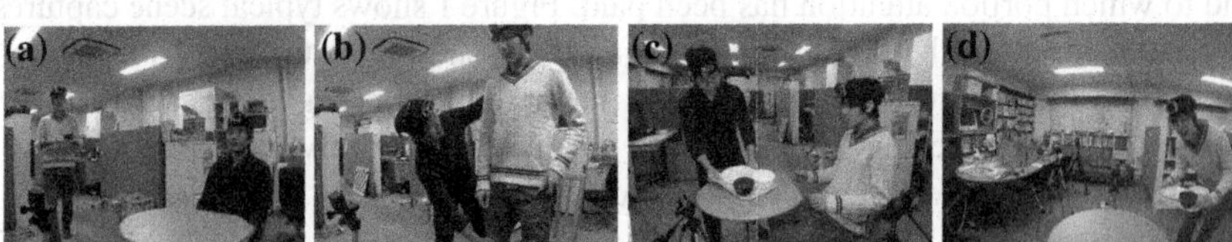

Fig. 3 Typical shots focusing on spatial relationships and environments. **a** Overview, **b** posture, **c** relationship to an object, **d** tool and furniture

3.2 How Scenes Need to be Presented

An audience naturally attempts to find continuity and causality among neighboring shots in a video. An appropriate combination of shots provides rich clues of cause-and-effect relationships, as well as specific information in each shot.

For example, a caregiver's skill at catching the sight of a care-receiver would be explained well by a combination of the shots of the caregiver's action of coming closer and getting into the view of a care-receiver, the action of touching the care-receiver, and the care-receiver's and the caregiver's faces, together with a subjective view of the caregiver from the care-receiver's viewpoint.

Typically, all shots cannot be packed into one video stream, because multiple cameras provide views of different targets simultaneously. Replaying all video streams in parallel also fails to provides a comprehensible explanation of a scene. Watching multiple videos in parallel is usually tiring, and it is difficult to pay attention to the correct portion.[1] For example, we have difficulty in watching both the caregiver's attention and the care-receiver's attention simultaneously. Consequently, we need video editing to present such scenes comprehensibly by choosing an appropriate shot at each moment. This kind of problem has been discussed well as "editing" in film studies [11], where we can find useful knowledge and techniques in actual movies and research.

The problem is how to invoke such knowledge and techniques to satisfy our purposes, some of which involve the following.

Overview of caregiving scene: This focuses primarily on how care actions and events occur in a scene, and what results are obtained.

How a care-receiver receives care: This focuses primarily on how a care-receiver perceives and understands a caregiver's actions, and on how a care-receiver accepts, misses, or rejects it.

How a caregiver applies skills for care: This focuses primarily on how a trainee or an expert approaches a care-receiver, what he or she pays attention to, and how he or she performs care actions.

Although those purposes are not always mutually exclusive, they sometimes conflict because it is very difficult to pay attention to different targets simultaneously.

4 Utilizing Knowledge of Film Studies and Media Technology

Film studies have proved that audience perception and understanding heavily depend on shots and editing schemas.

[1]We are assuming that people without professional skills are analyzing videos. For a person with video analytics skills, multiple views with complete information could be the most powerful tools.

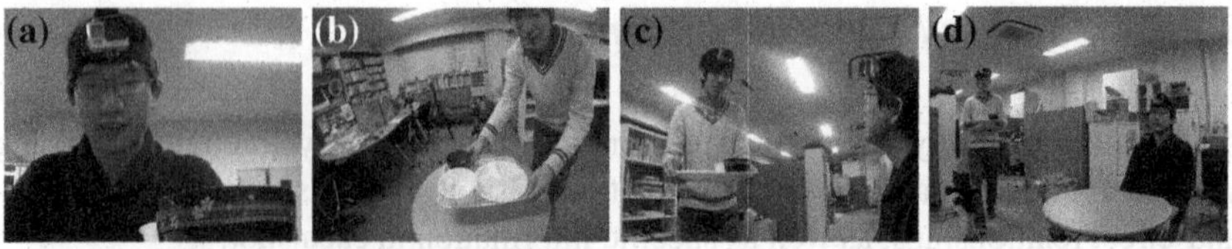

Fig. 4 Example of typical shot categories in Film Studies. **a** Close-up, **b** POV shot, **c** medium shot, **d** long shot

4.1 Category of Shots

Let us first consider shots. In film studies, shots are categorized based on target size in a screen e.g., close-up, bust, or medium shot. Another categorization of shots is based on viewing position and angle, e.g., point-of-view (POV) shot,[2] bird's-eye view, mobile-view shot.[3]

We need to choose appropriate shots for typical purposes. Figure 4 shows typical shots.

- A close-up shot, as shown in Fig. 4a, or a bust shot is preferable for showing facial expression and emotion of a care-receiver or a caregiver.
- A close-up shot, as shown in Fig. 4b, is most suitable for showing the target to which attention is paid. A POV shot can be an alternative. Other shots, such as a medium shot (c) or a bird's-eye view shot, would partially explain attention.
- Presenting touch or physical interaction between a care-receiver and a caregiver requires the same types of shot as the above.
- Explanation of spatial relationships between a care-receiver and a caregiver requires longer and wider shots such as (c) or (d). A bird's-eye view shot is also acceptable. Those shots play a role of an "establishing shot" that provides overview of a scene and its environment.
- Presenting postures and movements of a care-receiver or a caregiver requires the same types of shot as the above, though a combination of medium or closer shots could be alternatives.

We assume that those shots and their combinations have potential to explain care-giving scenes. What we need is to set up a camera for taking each of the above types of shots. Sufficiently many cameras must be located at appropriate locations with appropriate focal lengths.

[2]A camera is shooting at the scene simulating the persons sight from the position of his/her eyes.

[3]A camera is moving, typically dollying.

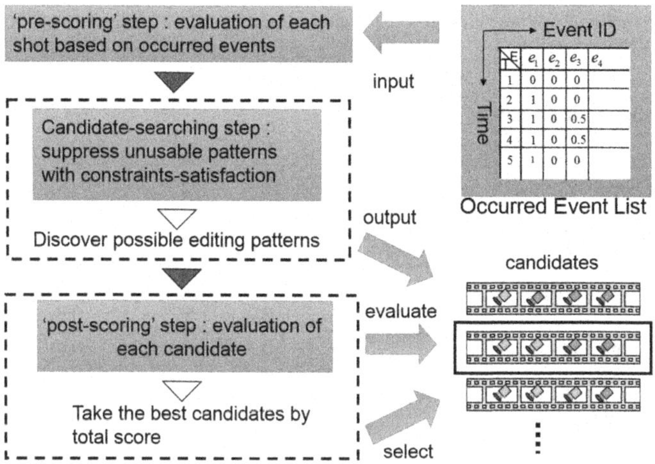

Fig. 5 Flow of computation

4.2 Editing Technique

As discussed above, we consider view switching among multiple cameras as an editing scheme. To simplify this process, we use the automated editing scheme proposed by Ogata et al. [6]. In that scheme, video editing is considered as the problem of assigning an appropriate shot to each video unit segment. Every possible pattern of assignment is listed and scored using evaluation functions, and the best pattern is chosen. Appendix A presents the formal description of this editing.

Figure 5 shows the flow of computation, which consists roughly of three steps, *pre-scoring*, *candidate searching*, and *post-scoring and selection*. The correspondence between the editing scheme and our purpose in videotaping can be explained briefly as follows.

In the pre-scoring step, the relevance of each shot at each time is evaluated based on the matching between characteristics of the shot and the purpose of videotaping. It is related to events occurring in the scene. Table 1 shows the rough idea. Basically, we assign better scores to the shots that match an editing purpose, i.e., the shots that should be paid attention for the editing purpose. For example, when a caregiver is talking to a care-receiver, the care-receiver's POV shot is assigned a high score if the purpose of video is to focus on the care-receiver's perception.

In the candidate-searching step, possible editing patterns that satisfy constraints are searched using a constraint programming. Some constraints are derived from common and conventional editing schemas in film studies, and others from the nature of human perception. For example, "prohibiting too frequent shot changes" is a typical rule for avoiding dizzying patterns that are difficult to understand. A substantial number of unnecessary editing patterns are drastically eliminated at this step.

Table 1 Example of editing rules (how each shot fits each purpose. Values range between 0 (no match) and 1 (best match))

Shot	(a)	(b)	(c)
Caregiver talks to care-receiver			
Long shot	0.8	0.3	0.5
Close-up of caregiver	0.3	0.3	0.7
...	...	...	...
POV of care-receiver	0.3	1.0	0.7
Caregiver serves something			
Long shot	0.7	0.2	0.3
Medium shot of caregiver	0.3	0.3	0.9
...	...	...	...
Close-up of care-receiver	0.5	0.5	0.7
POV of care-receiver	0.7	1.0	0.5

Editing purposes (what is focused)
(a) how the caregiver and the care-receiver behave (overview).
(b) how the care-receiver receives care (care-receiver's attention and reaction).
(c) how the caregiver gives care (caregiver's attention and caregiving skill).

In the post-scoring step, each editing pattern receives a final score. This score evaluates primarily the appropriateness of combinations of consecutive shots that are not fully fixed in the pre-scoring step. For example, a POV shot is preferable if it has a preceding close-up shot of the viewing person, because audience sometimes have difficulty in understanding whose POV it is.

After scoring is completed, the editing pattern, i.e., the shot sequence, that received the highest score, is selected as the result.

5 Preliminary Experiments

Objective: The objective of the experiments is to confirm that videos obtained using our scheme are comprehensible and help audiences notice the focused points. We chose two typical caregiving scenes, serving meal to a care-receiver and helping a care-receiver stand up. These two scenes frequently appear in daily caregiving, in which problems sometimes occur as a result of a care-receiver's reduced sight, attention, or memory capacity. We simulated the above two types of care scenes by some of the authors.

Shots and events: Two head-mounted cameras and four fixed cameras were used, as shown in Fig. 6. Head-mounted cameras are usually allowable in training, and are allowable if care-receivers are willing to cooperate to improve caregiving. However, the location of a fixed camera is often limited because of the spatial arrangements of a caregiving venue. We assumed the behaviors of the care-receiver and the caregiver

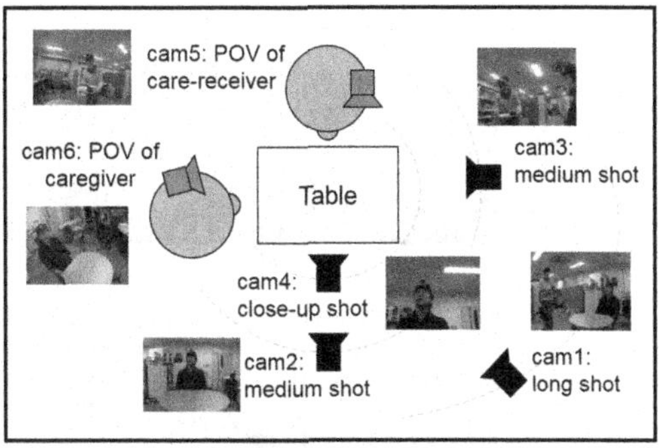

Fig. 6 Camera arrangement

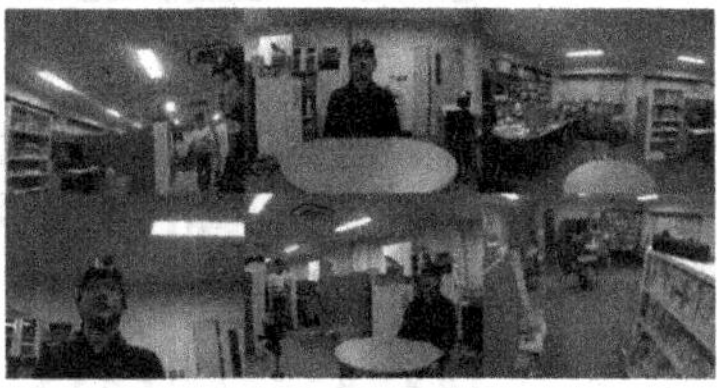

Fig. 7 Captured videos: all videos are presented in a tiled format

are observed sufficiently as events, e.g., speaking, walking, or touching (Fig. 7). For each recorded video, we manually detected those events and annotated them with time of occurrence. Automatic detection of events is left for future work.

Editing and purposes: We compared three purposes of videotaping: (a) focusing on how a caregiver and a care-receiver behaved and felt, (b) whether care was perceived sufficiently by the care-receiver, and (c) a caregiver's attention and skills. Table 1 contains an example of rules for each videotaping purpose.

Results: Figure 8 presents the obtained movies in a film strip view. Comparing (a), (b), and (c), we can see differences among the movies. Movie (a) presents an overview of how both persons behaved and felt. Movie (b) emphasizes the care-receiver perception: (b) at t_2 and t_3 show what the care-receiver looked when the caregiver talked to him, and (b) at t_4 indicates that the care-receiver probably understood that the lunch tray was served to the care-receiver. Movie (c), in contrast, emphasizes where the caregiver looked and how the caregiver behaved. Movie (c) at t_2 shows that the caregiver looked at the care-receiver's eye and confirmed eye contact, and movie (c) at t_4 shows how the caregiver checked the care-receiver's recognition.

To verify the above observations quantitatively, we asked eight participants to provide subjective evaluations, scoring each video according to the criteria shown in Fig. 9. For comparison, we added two types of video, a long shot without editing and a combination of all views replayed simultaneously, as shown in Fig. 7. The participants watched those movies and assigned scores based on whether the specified information is difficult or easy to discern from the movies.

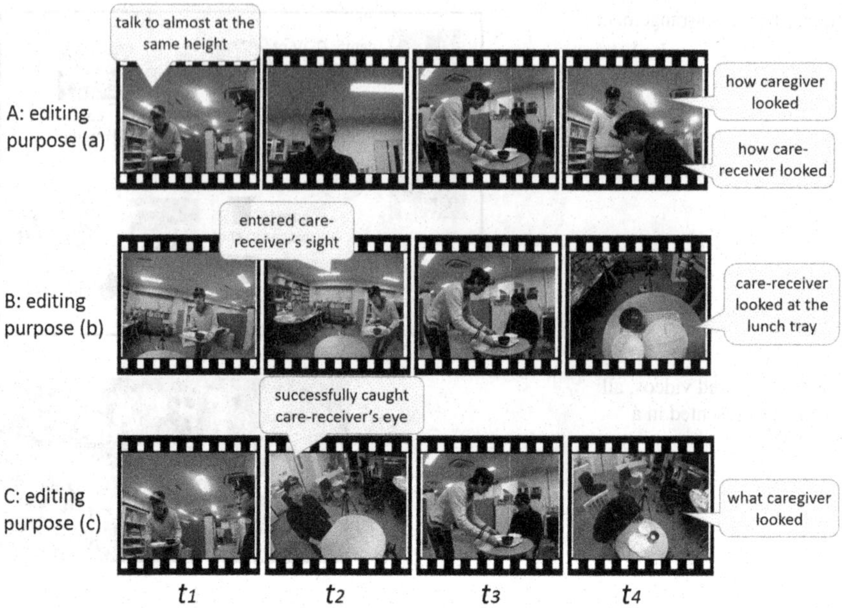

Fig. 8 Edited movies

The graph in Fig. 9 shows the results. Score 5 is the most positive (easy) and 1 is the most negative (difficult). The graph shows clear differences among videos. For each criterion, the difference between group "■ (suitable)" and group "● (not suitable)" is statistically significant at the 1 % level.

Notice that the simultaneous replay of all views in a tiled arrangement (P) obtained almost the worst score for any criterion, strongly supporting the necessity of editing. Long shot without editing (N) obtained good scores for C_1 and C_6, which request primarily overview and spatial information. Next, let us check how the obtained videos meet the editing purposes. The rectangles with thick lines enclosing P, N, or A-C below the graph show videos that are primarily related to the criteria, and the rectangles with thin lines show marginally related videos. Editing (a) obtained good scores for C_4, which is the primary purpose of editing (a); however, an overview of the scene (C_1) is not well indicated. Editing (b) obtained almost the best scores for C_2, C_5, and C_6, which are related to how the care-receiver perceived and received care. Editing (c) obtained almost the best scores for C_2, C_3, and C_7, which are related primarily to the caregiver's skills.

Discussion: The result supports our idea that appropriate video capturing and editing facilitates better understanding of care scenes. However, the participants for verification were not skilled, which can be considered to be the case of novice trainees or patients' family members. Systematic evaluation including skilled professionals is also necessary for future work.

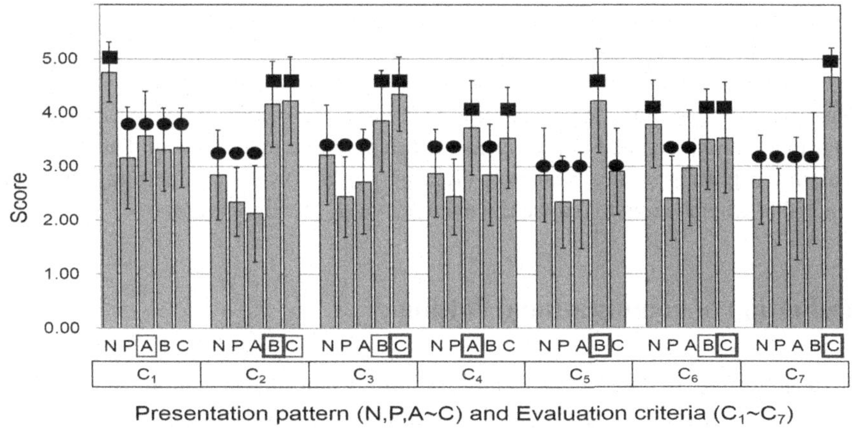

Videos
N:Long shot with no editing
P: Multiple video sare presented in tiled format and replayed simultaneously
A: Editing purpose (a)
B: Editing purpose (b)
C: Editing purpose (c)

Criteria
C_1: How care is given in the scene.
C_2: Degree to which eye contact is established andmaintained.
C_3:The the caregiver's position is appropriate when the caregiver talked to the care-receiver.
C_4:How the care-receiver feels
C_5:How the care-receiver perceives or recognizes the care
C_6:How the caregiver touches the care-receiver
C_7:Which object or place the caregiver looks at

Fig. 9 Subjective evaluation result

Moreover, we still need further work to ensure that our scheme will be applicable to actual caregiving scenes. More systematic evaluations for various situations are necessary. Image processing and speech recognition must be investigated to detect events, such as speech, touch, and important motions. Such automated event detection and design would substantially reduce the time and cost of actual practice. We also need a complete system design, including camera arrangement, for capturing sufficient information.

6 Conclusion

This paper introduced a novel scheme of video content acquisition and editing for caregiving scenes. The scheme utilizes knowledge of film studies and media technology for obtaining appropriate videos for typical purposes. The preliminary results are convincing in that the obtained video emphasizes the purpose of videos, such as understanding care-receiver's perception and caregiver's attention, and assists an audience in noticing important features.

We have substantial room for future work. Further experiments with a variety of caregiving scenes and video purposes are necessary, as is verification in actual training. In addition, we need to put further efforts into automating event detection and possibly capturing scenes more actively, e.g., pan/tilt or other camera movements, since this scheme aims to reduce the tiresome work of videotaping.

Definition of computational editing

In the following, we briefly introduce the editing scheme used in our method. Please see [6] for details. The definition is modified for clarity, but the computational scheme is the same.

The computational model of editing is composed formally of five elements:

$$\text{Editing} = \{S, V, E, O, C\} \tag{1}$$

The explanation of the above terms is as follows:

Shots (*S*): S is a set of shots i.e., $S = \{s_0, \dots, s_n\}$, where s_i is a shot, *e.g.*, "a bust shot of person A," "a long shot of person B,".

Shot assignment (*V*): V is a sequence of shot assignments to video segments, each of which has a length, e.g., 0.5 or 1 second. One shot in S is assigned to each video segment, i.e., $V = \{s_i, \dots, s_k\}$,

Events (*E*): E is a collection of events $\{e_i\}$ occurring in the scene, for example, "person A spoke," "person B laughed," or "person A touched person B." If e_i occurs at time t with a certainty of 0.9, we denote it as $e_i(t) = 0.9$.

Evaluation (*O*): O is a collection of objective functions $\{o_i(V, t)\}$, each of which assigns a score for a shot assignment at time t. The criterion can be comprehensibility, entertainment quality, or one of many other factors.

Constraints (*C*): C is a set of constraints. Some of the editing rules are constraints, *e.g.* "do not use shots longer than t_n seconds." The number of candidates can be reduced by applying the constraints.

The objective of this model is the optimization of G in the following formula.

$$G = \sum_{t=0}^{t_{max}} \sum_{i=0}^{i_{max}} o_i(V, t) \tag{2}$$

In other words, the objective is to find the best assignment of shots to video segments that maximizes evaluation value G based on O and satisfies constraints C. For this purpose, we first use a constraint programming to obtain candidates and select the best-scored editing.

References

1. Honda, M., Gineste, Y., Marescotti, R.: Introduction to Humanitude (in Japanese), Igaku Shoin (2014)
2. Phaneuf, M.: The concept of humanitude as applied to general nursing care, http://www.infiressources.ca/fer/depotdocument_anglais/the_concept_of_humanitude_as_applied_to_general_nursing_care.pdf (accessed April 15, 2015)
3. Atarashi, Y., et al.: Controlling a camera with minimized camera motion changes under the constraint of a planned camera-work. Proceedings of International Workshop on Pattern Recognition and Understanding for Visual Information Media **2002**, 9–14 (2002)
4. Ozeki, M., Nakamura, Y.: Evaluation of Self-Editing Based on Behaviors-for-Attention for Desktop Manipulation Videos, Proceedings IEEE International Conference on Multimedia and Expo, MA2-L5.2 (2006)
5. Yamaguchi, S., Ohnishi, Y., Nishino, K.: The design of an automatic lecture archiving system offering video based on teacher's demands. Intell. Interact. Multimed. Syst. Serv. Smart Innov. Syst. Technol. **14**, 599–608 (2012)
6. Ogata, R., Nakamura, Y., Ohta, Y.: Computational Video Editing Model based on Optimization with Constraint-Satisfaction. Proceedings Fourth Pacific-Rim Conference on Multimedia, CD-ROM, 2A1-2 (2003)
7. Garner, P., Collins, M., Webster, S., Rose, D.: The application of telepresence in medicine. BT Technol. J. **15**(4), 181–187 (1997)
8. Gemmell, J., Bell, G., Luede, R.: MyLifeBits: a personal database for everything. Commun. ACM **49**(1), 88–95 (2006)
9. Hodges, S., et al.: SenseCam: a Retrospective Memory Aid, Ubicomp 2006. LNCS **4206**, 177–193 (2006)
10. Berry, E., et al.: The use of a wearable camera, SenseCam, as a pictorial diary to improve autobiographical memory in a patient with limbic encephalitis: a preliminary report. Neuropsychol. Rehabil. **17**(4/5), 582–601 (2007)
11. Bordwell, D., Thompson, K.: Film Art: An Introduction, 5th edn. McGraw-Hill, New York (1997)

Care at the End of Life: Design Priorities for People with Dementia

Alastair S. Macdonald and Louise Robinson

Abstract This paper discusses pre-design stage research concerned with supporting excellence in end-of-life care (EoLC) for people with dementia (PwD). The discontinuation and replacement of previous with new EoLC guidance provides the opportunity for improving care package materials (CPMs) to support EoLC. Current CPMs tend largely to address governance, recording of treatment and consent for audit purposes. This research identified the need for CPMs to better reflect the complexities, coordination and communication needs between the patient (and those important to them) carers and physicians, and to anticipate discussions, scenarios and consequences of decision-making between all parties involved along a patient's uncertain trajectory at EoL: dementia adds another level of challenge. Findings from evaluating existing CPMs and surveying of new technological developments are discussed in this context.

Keywords End of life · Dementia · Technological design · Care package materials

1 Introduction

One of the consequences of an ageing population is that more people will require long-term care for illnesses such as dementia. This will lead to an increased need for end-of-life care (EoLC) for those with complex needs living in the community. Providing EoLC relies on the coordination of, and communication between, many kinds of professional and lay expertise to provide both treatment and palliative care in a variety of different settings and situations along uncertain trajectories of frailty

A.S. Macdonald (✉)
School of Design, The Glasgow School of Art, Glasgow, UK
e-mail: a.macdonald@gsa.ac.uk

L. Robinson
Newcastle University Institute for Ageing and Institute for Health and Society, Newcastle University, Newcastle upon Tyne, UK

Y.-W. Chen et al. (eds.), *Innovation in Medicine and Healthcare 2015*,
Smart Innovation, Systems and Technologies 45,
DOI 10.1007/978-3-319-23024-5_47

and illness [1]. EoLC for people living with dementia (PwD) adds another level of challenge: PwD already receive poorer EoLC compared to those with cancer, with more hospital admissions and worse pain control [2]. EoLC is compounded by the very emotive and challenging scenarios for all involved [3].

This paper outlines the pre-design stage of research, in which the author, a design researcher, was involved, scoping the issues, evaluating new developments, identifying opportunities for the subsequent design phases for new or improved care package materials (CPMs) to support EoLC. This work formed one work stream of a larger programme of research led by a professor of primary care and ageing and involving a multi-disciplinary team of 15 investigators who were funded to support sharing excellence in EoLC for PwD (SEED) [4]. The project commenced as guidance for EoLC changed.

2 Background

2.1 A Change in Priorities

The Liverpool Care Pathway for the Dying Patient (LCP) had been developed to support palliative care in the 1990s. Although an independent review of the LCP [5] found evidence of both good and poor care, the LCP was found to have become a generic protocol used largely as a 'tick box' exercise tending to standardise care irrespective of individual circumstances and preferences. The review's findings resulted in the LCP being phased out in July 2014, replaced by the new approach detailed in the report of the Leadership Alliance for the Care of Dying People (LADCP) [6]. This states, briefly, that care should be individualised and should reflect the needs and preferences of the dying person and those who are important to them. It proposes five priorities (recognise; communicate; involve; support; and plan and do), recognising variation in need together with a number of commitments to ensure all care given in the last days and hours meets these priorities.

2.2 Opportunities for New Care Package Materials

The discontinuation and replacement of the LCP by the LACDP model allows for the reconsideration of existing and the opportunity to create new CPMs to support EoLC for PwD. CPMs are defined by this author, in this EoLC context, as the broad spectrum of materials and tools which support EoLC which can include, e.g., record of treatment (including, e.g., drugs prescribed) and variance in treatment, team notes, instructions (e.g., not to resuscitate), guidance (e.g., for physicians, paid carers, families, PwD and others), as well as innovative materials and tools to facilitate the sharing of information, initiate and support discussion, and assist decision-making.

2.3 *Questions Driving the Pre-Design Research*

The main questions driving this pre-design research stage are: What are the strengths and weaknesses of existing CPMs? What CPMs are appropriate for use in EoLC for PwD given the new LADCP priorities and the SEED team's own findings? What opportunities are there for improving and innovating CPMs and for (all of) whom should these be designed? What new or emerging developments might be useful in this context?

3 Method

As a precursor to the co-development and trialling of new CPMs which will follow in later stages of this 5 year programme of research, the questions in 2.3 above helped drive the initial requirements capture to inform the design statement and design specification for CPMs with a view to supporting all involved at EoL, i.e. PwD themselves, physicians, paid carers, family (or close friends or other persons important to the PwD), and others (such as, e.g., paramedics, out-of-hours physicians, or clergy) in the many, often uncertain and rapidly changing scenarios during EoLC, and to determine the nature, content and formats of these. Initial scoping and review was facilitated using the methods now described.

Evaluation of CPMs. Prior to the LACDP report, CPMs had been modelled on and adapted from the LCP and the Gold Standards Framework (GSF) [7] by different healthcare boards and regions to suit individual practices and preferences. It was essential to review and evaluate current (i.e. pre-LACDP) CPMs and observations arising from these. An analysis was made, by this author, of a sample of three CPMs, recommended by the primary and palliative care members of the SEED team, from: a national 'last days of life' pathway; a city-wide palliative care network; and a nursing home basing its CPMs on the GSF [7]. A matrix was populated and circulated by the author to the SEED team members to allow easy sight and comparison of the content of each of these CMPs.

Exploring Insights from the Research Team. The research team had, between them, considerable experience in the study area including primary care, ageing, dementia, geriatric care, EoLC; nursing; and long-term illness management. However, the study was structured into a number of separate work-packages, limiting the potential for cohesive synergy amongst the individual team members on sharing the implications and application of research findings with respect to developing new or improved CPMs. Consequently, team workshops were introduced with a view to discussing on-going findings and implications of the research for new or improved CPMs. The workshops were designed and facilitated by the author, their activities and content being developed and agreed with the team prior to the workshops. The team's views of and insights into a number of issues were explored using visual-based group workshop methods and activities, such as EoLC scenarios which are particularly problematic. Findings from the team's own reviews of literature and evidence from their research were discussed along with, e.g., the definition of CPMs, the various needs of the different stakeholders in EoLC scenarios, and the content and formats of CPMs. To date, two workshops involving 10 team members have been held. These are now seen as an ongoing feature of the team-building process, and will also include workshops with the patient and public involvement (PPI) group prior to the co-development stages.

Survey of Recent Innovations. A survey was made, by the author, to identify and evaluate recent innovations for opportunities to address some problems associated with existing CPMs and which might assist with the new LACDP and SEED team priorities. The survey scoped dementia care-related innovations, electronic patient record systems concerned with coordinating care, and communication tools associated with EoLC and dementia.

4 Findings

4.1 Issues Associated with Existing CPMs Derived from the LCP Model

Content. The three CPMs reviewed contained (with some variation between the different CPMs): details about the client, their next of kin and contact details; the client's advanced wishes; advanced care plans; DNACPR (do not attempt cardiopulmonary resuscitation) record; the multidisciplinary team's contact details; medical and nursing on-going assessments; care after death; pathway outcome (bereavement and care after death); multidisciplinary team notes; variance from treatment guidance; medication; symptom management; out-of-hours notes; community nursing service notes; doctors' and nurses' notes on drugs prescribed; pain assessment; physical symptom assessment; syringe-driver check chart; and information sheets for clients and families.

Format. Existing CPMs are largely text- and/or tabular-based, paper documents requiring manual (handwritten) input largely by medical and nursing staff. In use their quality can be degraded, e.g., by repeated photocopying. The three CPMs surveyed, typical of CPMs generally, were all paper-based A4 documents, largely concerned with governance and physicians' needs, recording treatment and consent, and had the appearance of an assemblage of a disparate, rather than a coherently designed, set of forms—largely, if not exclusively, oriented to clinical and nursing staff, and to provide an audit trail. Additional guidance materials fell largely into two broad categories: (i) guidance for boards or regions to develop, monitor and improve the 'integrated care pathway' for EoLC (the term 'pathway' is now discredited and has since been dropped in usage due to its multiple interpretations including a perception that once on the LCP, this was a one-way 'descent towards death'); and (ii) information for clients (patients), their families and carers.

The SEED team also felt it useful that other formats for CPMs should be explored, e.g., visual materials to illustrate 'patient journeys' and electronic or on-line formats to assist sharing essential information or promoting discussion.

Access. Different records, information, guidance and instructions are required at different times by different individuals (physician/paid carer/family/PwD/other) for different purposes, in often rapidly changing, unpredictable and highly individualised scenarios sometimes involving many different individuals (frequently with little continuity) delivering medical and palliative care, and often in emotive circumstances. Locating and accessing the relevant CPMs by all relevant individuals in all situations, if and as required, can be problematic.

Conclusion. From the above it was felt important to understand and distinguish, through audit and from the evidence-base, which (all) kinds of materials work well, for whom, in which formats, in which scenarios, from those that don't work well, need significant adjustment, or are completely absent. Additionally, it was felt that new developments and media could be explored for their relevance to new or improved CPMs.

4.2 Recent Findings from the Team's EoLC Research

It is intended that findings from research conducted by other work streams in the research team would feed into the design of these CPMs. For example, Barclay et al. [1] provide case studies presented in visual diagrammatic form of the different trajectories of dying individuals' last months and days through care, illustrating, e.g., their symptoms and treatment, physicians' visits, their admittance to and discharge from care home to hospital into care home or hospice, logging with each incident or change in condition the important decisions required for, e.g., treatment, site of treatment or care, pain reduction, and quality of life.

4.3 Survey of Recent Innovations

There is insufficient space to be exhaustive here but, for illustrative purposes, a few examples are outlined and thematically grouped below for both their strengths and their limitations.

Facilitating Discussions with PwD. As the new LACDP model prioritises the needs and preferences of the dying person and those who are important to them, this presents a significant challenge if that dying person has moderate to severe dementia. However, 'talking mats' [8], now available as an app, has been reported beneficial for helping to elicit and convey the views of people with moderate to late stage dementia. Although the findings in the report by Murphy, Gray and Cox [9] are positive in this regard, the question remaining for those researchers was of how helpful the tool is in helping PwD make *key* decisions (e.g., such as might be required at EoL).

Knowing the Individual. Given the number, and sometimes high, turn-over of, different individuals who may be involved, across a number of services, in delivering EoLC for a PwD, knowledge of the person is important for individualised care. The Alzheimer's Society has developed 'This is Me' [10] a low-tech paper-based tool that PwD can use 'to tell staff about their needs, preferences, likes, dislikes and interests'. In the same vein, software has been developed to act as a communication bridge between carers and PwD. 'Portraits' [11] contains important but limited personal and social information about PwD for their care staff to access where PwD's biographies are presented on a combination touch screen computer system. It has been designed specifically targeting the 'real life' work schedules and usability needs of care staff and provides what is required in a few minutes.

Guidance. Physicians will require LACDP guidance to hand and app-based tools may be a way of making available LACDP priorities in easy-to-access formats. To this end HELIX [12] has provided 'a strong, clean and simple visual identity, using appropriate formats to present the LACDP guidance to clinicians on the front line, to include posters, leaflets and apps. However, findings from other analysis by this author underline the need for tools to be developed not only for clinicians but also those which can be accessed—and are usable—by all involved, including PwD.

EoL Care Journeys. There is often the desire to map or provide an overview of the patient trajectory or 'pathway' of care. As previously mentioned, Barclay et al. [1] found four types of trajectory. The designers of Hospitaltohome [13], a digitally interactive visualised pathway, have been working with health and social care practitioners, older people, their families and informal carers 'to identify and improve care pathways from hospital to home with the aim of enabling a more positive experience for all'. However, Samsi and Manthorpe [14] discuss the seductiveness of the concept of a neat 'care pathway', advising caution in taking shared understandings of this for granted in scenarios characterised by their complexity and uncertainty, an issue underlined in Barclay et al. [1].

Coordinating Care. One of the challenges in the EoL scenario, as highlighted in Barclay et al. [1], is the dynamic and uncertain trajectory of the health, care and treatment of PwD at EoL. The issue of information sharing, management and coordination of care between all individuals and services involved can be problematic. A pilot clinical service, 'Coordinate My Care' [15, 16], sharing information between healthcare providers coordinating care, and recording wishes of how patients would like to be treated and cared for, has been developed and trialled. This ensures their wishes and personalised care plan is available to view by all those who care for them, i.e. those who have a legitimate relationship with the patient, e.g., the out-of-hours GP, NHS 111, the ambulance service, or community, primary or acute care.

5 Discussion

The above outlines some aspects of the pre-design scoping phase of this work. The early identification and discussion of issues and potential directions for appropriate innovations will inform future team workshop activities and the means and modes of stakeholder engagement, e.g., 'talking mat' style apps [8] could potentially assist in the engagement of PwD in participant workshops, and visualised EoLC trajectories based on Barclay et al's work [1] and the use of scenario methods could assist discussion of which tools could improve communication, understanding and joint decision-making processes, and between whom.

5.1 PPI and Co-Design

Patient and Public Involvement (PPI) is a term commonly used within healthcare for what the design community broadly refers to as participatory design, co-creation and co-development. Savory [17] provides a useful model for design-healthcare collaborations as it distinguishes levels of PPI 'engagement'. Within the context of the research described in this paper, dementia adds another level of challenge in a number of senses. One is with regard to the sensitivity of conducting research at the EoL. A second is around the challenges of involving PwD and their families, as two of the many stakeholder groups, in the 'co-design' of CPMs. However, thinking and practice has moved on substantially in both the design and healthcare fields since the LCP was designed in the 1990s. In design, the greater democratization of designing through the participatory, co-design and service design movements has brought stakeholders into the centre of the process. In this regard, findings from approaches embracing co-design principles, such as Experience Based Co-Design (EBCD) [18, 19], have proved positive and significant, albeit limited in the types of intervention they can generate, and would suggest that modified aspects of these approaches could used in the co-development stage. The SEED team membership includes a patient and public involvement group who are being integrated into the project team workshop schedule in the initial stages, in advance of the later co-development phase for ne CPMs which will itself involve all the main stakeholder groups, namely: people with mild/moderate dementia, family carers: primary care professionals; community nurses; secondary care professionals involved in old age psychiatry, geriatrics, palliative and social care; care home staff; and commissioners. A further stage beyond this co-development process will see these new CPMs being trialed in two different settings.

5.2 *Care 2.0?*

One of the findings in Barclay et al. (2014) [1] was that EoLC tools 'were used infrequently'. An understanding of why will be essential, particularly anticipating the move of CPMs into the technological realm. One of the points made about the apparent success of the 'Coordinate My Care' [CMC] system is that the CMC "*... was never conceived as an IT project; the IT was always led by the clinical need... We tried to develop our solution with Connecting for Health using the summary care record, but that was a technology-led project which restricted it severely. With CMC it is the other way round and as a result the solution is very intuitive and easy to use and fits in nicely with the way clinicians work everyday*" [20]. The examples provided in 4.3 above are predominantly electronic/digital tools. Whilst introducing IT systems in healthcare has been fraught with set-backs [21] and there is the problematic issue of 'platform fatigue' [22], i.e. the learning of new interfaces and new procedures for accessing and logging into multiple systems, one has to ask whether, given the complexities and uncertainties of EoLC scenarios, the need for continuity between the many individuals and services involved, and the need for ready access to essential information including the PwD's wishes, if we can afford not to move these CPMs (or at least some aspects of them) into the digital-electronic realm? However, we need be cautious about how these are developed and by whom, so that these can be used intuitively, and so that they will be used by all who need—and should be able—to access them, as a matter of course within everyday EoLC practice, and particularly, with the concerns of this current SEED project, involving people with dementia.

6 Conclusion

With the new LACDP model's repositioning of the priorities of the patient and all 'individuals important to them' to the centre of EoLC, how should these and the findings from the SEED team's own research be manifest in the design of new CPMs? What are the challenges, opportunities and priorities for design here? This author's survey of existing CPMs found, as stated previously, that the design of CPMs primarily addressed physicians' and nurses' recording and auditing needs. However, in this highly complex and unpredictable stage of life, CPMs need to support all those concerned: PwD, their families, paid carers, clinicians, and others (e.g., ambulance, clerical, and out-of-hours GPs). It is therefore felt vital that the nature and type of CPMs be expanded, and their formats better considered to, e.g., better assist coordination of care, help acknowledge the uncertainties, help anticipate and deal quickly with changing and unpredictable scenarios, be available to provide information, initiate or assist important discussions, and communicate and develop better understanding of consequences of decisions made for all parties involved. To achieve this will require the iterative design, co-development, prototyping and evaluation of improved or new CPMs based on emerging evidence from the types of scoping activities described in 3 above whilst recognising new, perhaps under-exploited opportunities (e.g., digital documents, apps, etc.) and from the findings from others in this SEED team.

Acknowledgements For the background material for this paper, the authors acknowledge the guidance of the SEED (Supporting Excellence in End of life care in Dementia) team members in work streams 1 and 2. This paper presents independent research funded by the National Institute for Health Research (NIHR) under its Programme Grants for Applied Research programme (Grant Reference Number RP-PG-0611-20005). The views expressed are those of the author(s) and not necessarily those of the NHS, the NIHR or the Department of Health.

References

1. Barclay, S., Froggatt, K., Crang, C., Mathie, E., Handley, M., Ilife, S., Manthorpe, J., Gage, H., Goodman, C.: Living in uncertain times: trajectories to death in residential care homes. Br. J. Gen. Pract. (2014). doi:10.3399/bjgp14X681397
2. S.E.E.D.: Supporting Excellence in End-of-life Care in Dementia (SEED programme). In: Application for NIHR Programme Grant for Applied Research, RP-PG-06211-20005 (2012)
3. Chast, R.: Can't We Talk About Something More Pleasant: a Memoir. Bloomsbury, New York (2014)
4. SEED. WWW. (2014) http://research.ncl.ac.uk/seed/. Accessed 11 Oct 2014
5. Neuberger, J., Guthrie, C., Aaronovitch, D., Hameed, K., Bonser, T.: Lord Harries of Pentregarth, et al.. More care, less pathway: a review of the Liverpool Care Pathway. [WWW]. (2011) https://www.gov.uk/government/uploads/system/uploads/attachment_data/file/212450/Liverpool_Care_Pathway.pdf. Accessed 14 Oct 2014
6. Leadership Alliance for the Care of Dying People (LACDP). One chance to get it right. [WWW]. https://www.gov.uk/government/…/One_chance_to_get_it_right.pdf. Accessed 11 Oct 2014
7. The National Gold Standards Framework Centre in End of Life Care. WWW. www.goldstandardsframework.org.uk. Accessed 5 Jan 2015
8. Talking Mats. [WWW]. http://www.talkingmats.com/. Accessed 15 Dec 2014
9. Murphy, J., Gray, C.M., Cox, S.: Communication and Dementia: How Talking Mats Can Help People with Dementia to Express Themselves. University of Stirling, Stirling (2007)
10. Alzheimer's Society. (2014). This is me. [WWW]. http://alzheimers.org.uk/thisisme. Accessed 15 Dec 2014
11. Portait: [WWW]. http://www.portraitsystem.co.uk/ Accessed 25 Jan 2015
12. HELIX Centre [WWW]. http://www.helixcentre.com/ Accessed 28 Dec 2014
13. IRISS: [WWW]. http://content.iriss.org.uk/hospitaltohome/ Accessed 15 Dec 2014
14. Samsi, K., Manthorpe, J.: Care pathways for dementia: current perspectives. Clin. Interv. Aging **2014**(9), 2055–2063 (2014)
15. Bakhai, K., O'Sullivan, C., Riley, J.: End-of-life care: identification, communication, training, and commissioning. Editorial, Brit. J. Gen. Pract. (2013). doi:10.3399/bjgp13X660616
16. Read, C.: A Kinder System. Health Serv. J. suppl. **6**, 6–10 (2012)
17. Savory, C.: Patient and public involvement in translative healthcare research. Clin. Govern. Int. J. **15**, 191–199 (2010)
18. Bate, S.P., Robert, G.: Bringing User Experience to Health Care Improvement: The Concepts, Methods and Practices of Experience-Based Design. Radcliffe Publishing, Oxford (2007)
19. Donetto, S., Tsianakas, V., Robert, G.: Using Experience-Based Co-Design to Improve the Quality of Healthcare: Mapping where we are now and Establishing Future Directions. King's College London, London (2014)

20. Smith, C. Hough, L., Cheung, C.C. et al.: Coordinate my care: a clinical service that coordinates care, giving patients choice and improving quality of life. BMJ Support. Palliat. Care **2**, 301–307 (2012). doi:10.1136/bmjspcare-2012-000265
21. Naughton, J.: The NHS's chaotic IT system shows no sign of recovery. Observer 21 December (2014). http://www.theguardian.com/technology/2014/dec/21/nhs-it-system-failings-addenbrookes-john-naughton. Accessed 22 May 2015
22. Jones, P.H.: Design for Care. Rosenfeld, New York (2013)

A Wireless and Autonomous Sensing System for Monitoring of Chronic Wounds in Healthcare

Alex Hariz and Nasir Mehmood

Abstract Chronic wounds, such as venous leg ulcers, can be monitored non-invasively by using modern sensing devices and wireless technologies. The development of such a wireless diagnostic tool may improve chronic wound management by providing evidence on efficacy of treatments being provided. This paper presents a low-power portable telemetric system for wound condition sensing and monitoring. The system aims at measuring and transmitting real-time information of wound-site temperature, sub-bandage pressure and moisture level from within the wound dressing. Commercially available non-invasive temperature, moisture, and pressure sensors are interfaced with a telemetry device on a flexible 0.15 mm thick printed circuit material to construct a light-weight biocompatible sensing device. The real-time data obtained is transmitted wirelessly to a portable receiver which displays the measured values. The performance of the whole telemetric sensing system is validated on a mannequin leg using commercial compression bandages and dressings. A number of trials on a healthy human volunteer are performed where treatment conditions were emulated using various compression bandage configurations. A reliable and repeatable performance of the system is achieved under compression bandage and with minimal discomfort to the volunteer. The system is capable of reporting instantaneous changes in bandage pressure, moisture level and local temperature at wound site with average measurement resolutions of 0.5 mmHg, 3.0 %RH, and 0.2 °C respectively. Effective range of data transmission is 4–5 m in an open environment.

Keywords Chronic wound monitoring · Telemetric sensing · Wound management · Wound diagnostic system

A. Hariz (✉) · N. Mehmood
School of Engineering, University of South Australia, Adelaide, SA 5095, Australia
e-mail: alex.hariz@unisa.edu.au

Y.-W. Chen et al. (eds.), *Innovation in Medicine and Healthcare 2015*,
Smart Innovation, Systems and Technologies 45,
DOI 10.1007/978-3-319-23024-5_48

1 Introduction

Chronic wounds such as venous leg ulcers and diabetic foot ulcers are becoming increasingly costly for healthcare systems around the world [1, 2]. A current estimate shows the economic cost of wound care activities in the world is distributed as 15–20 % materials, 30–35 % nursing time and more than 50 % as hospitalization time [3]. In 2012, approximately 7 million people suffered from chronic wounds in the USA, and the cost for their treatment was estimated at almost $25 billion annually [4].

The most effective and economical treatment of wounds is covering them with a suitable dressing or bandage in order to protect damaged skin from external infections such as those caused by microorganism attacks [5]. For certain chronic wounds such as venous leg ulcers, appropriate compression bandages are applied to increase the healing rate [6, 7]. These bandages may be retention (low pressure), light support (medium pressure), or compression (high pressure) bandages. The method of applying compression bandages on the affected limb is very important as the efficacy and maintenance of sub-bandage pressure depends on it [8]. Compression bandages can produce a pressure up to 60 mmHg at the ankle (extra high pressure), while the recommended high pressure value is 40 mmHg at the ankle [6, 8]. Depending on the applied pressure range and the type of bandage used, the sub-bandage pressure may vary significantly during the physical movement of the patient, thus affecting the healing rate [9]. In addition to compression bandages, healing rates may also be increased by managing moisture produced by the wound (exudate) through moisture-retentive dressings such as Anasept® (hydrogel) and Hydrocolloids [10, 11] for wounds with low exudate and dressings such as Allevyn® (foam) or Melgisorb® (calcium alginate) for wounds with moderate to high exudate. In addition to moisture levels, the temperature and pH under the dressing may change as a result of an infection [12, 13]. Unfortunately, these parameters associated with the dressings are not currently monitored in clinical practice. There is an opportunity for advanced sensor technologies to contribute to improved wound monitoring and diagnostics.

In this paper, we demonstrate a flexible wireless telemetric system for continuous sensing and monitoring of the wound environment, proposed in our earlier review article [14]. Preliminary results indicate that the system is capable of measuring and transmitting real-time information on temperature, moisture, and sub-bandage pressure from under the bandage or within the wound dressing at programmable transmission intervals [15]. The selection of sensors and their calibration processes have been discussed in our recent article [16]. The sensing system is fabricated on a flexible printed circuit material, while the sensors are micro-sized and flexible, thus making the system minimally invasive to wounds and the human body. The receiver is portable with the capability to receive data accurately within a distance of 4–5 m. The system has been tested on a human volunteer using various compression bandages and moisture-retentive dressings. The results from these trials confirm the clinical utility of this system in a wound environment.

2 Methods and Materials

For chronic wound monitoring application, the diagnostic device is required to perform reliably in a delicate environment involving human skin and wound fluid. In addition to satisfy the essential criteria of flexibility, protection from wound chemicals, and bio-compatibility, the device needs to fulfil certain performance requirements as well, which sets the foundation for minimum measurement resolutions. For meaningful temperature measurements, the device must be able to detect changes in temperature of less ±0.5 °C. The cases with pressure and moisture are different. Although, the aim of compression bandages and stockings is to maintain a constant sub-bandage pressure at certain positions on limb, however, it may be anticipated that a ±5 mmHg variation in bandage pressure would not have a significant impact on wound healing. Similarly, a ±5 % RH resolution could be expected for moisture measurements. The wireless device for this application does not need to transmit continuously, as the wound conditions do not change rapidly. A complete packet of information transmitted twice an hour would be sufficient. The proposed sensing system satisfies all of the above mentioned medical and performance requirements as explained in the following sections.

2.1 Selection and Calibration of Sensors

For wound monitoring application, the sensors and their assemblies need to be biocompatible and minimally invasive to the human body, as the sensors would be placed within a wound dressing or compression bandage over a human limb [16]. Having metallic inflexible structures, the sensors and circuit components would create discomfort to the patients. It has been revealed through online surveys that the majority of available sensors do not qualify for this particular application because of their large size, invasive structure, complex principle of measurement, and the need for additional on-board circuit components for operation [17].

The sensors needed to be carefully selected, calibrated and characterized for the intended environment in order to capture reliable information. Any error in the sensor's measurement would spread through the whole system and in some scenarios might get amplified. This would create ambiguities and false diagnosis by clinicians and health practitioners. For wound-site temperature monitoring, we chose the LM94021B (Texas Instruments, USA) temperature sensor for its small size and reliable performance. This ultra-low power sensor typically consumes just 9 μA current at a rated 5 V supply voltage. With a size of 2.15 × 2.40 × 1.1 mm (L × W × H) and a nominal accuracy of ±1.5 °C in the temperature range 20–40 °C [18], the sensor is quite suitable for our wound monitoring system.

For moisture sensing, Honeywell HIH4030 piezo-electric and Multicomp's HCZ-D5 piezo-resistive moisture sensors were calibrated, characterized, and used with a prototype wireless sensing system. The piezo-resistive sensor (HCZ-D5) was found the most suitable sensor for this application because of its small size (10 × 5 × 0.5 mm). The sensor was calibrated and characterized using a dedicated experimental setup. An interface circuit was also designed to properly operate the moisture sensor.

For sub-bandage pressure measurement, we used the Interlink Electronics' FSR406 piezo-resistive pressure sensor with a square sensing area of 38 × 38 mm. This sensor is non-invasive, flexible and is only 0.5 mm in thickness. The pressure sensor was calibrated using a clinical-grade pressure meter HPM-KH-01 for validation of pressure measurements up to 40 mmHg which is regarded as the desired value for high sub-bandage pressure [8]. An interface circuit was also designed to properly operate the pressure sensor. A commercial compression bandage system (Coban™ 2) was used to create pressure over the sensor placed on a mannequin leg.

2.2 *Flexible Wireless Sensing System*

A number of System-on-Chip (SoC) devices are commercially available with telemetry functions. Most of these devices use standard wireless transmission protocols, such as WiFi®, Bluetooth®, Bluetooth Low Energy®, and ZigBee®. Some examples of such SoCs are CC2530/31 (ZigBee), CC2540/41 (Bluetooth Low Energy), CC2560/64 (Bluetooth), CC3000/3100/3200 (WiFi), EM358x (ZigBee), 88MZ100 (ZigBee), ATMega128RFA1 (ZigBee) etc. In our proposed system, we have chosen ZigBee® for its simplicity, reasonable range, and low power operations. For this purpose, we have used Atmel's ATMega128RFA1 RF transceiver in our sensing system [19]. The transceiver is of small size (9 × 9 × 1 mm) and operates at 2.45 GHz ISM (industrial, scientific, medical) frequency band using IEEE 802.15.4 ZigBee® protocol. It has a −100 dBm sensitivity and a 3.5 dBm programmable output power. It also contains a programmable serial interface and a 10-bit analog-to-digital (ADC) converter, thus the hardware overhead would be minimized.

The information captured by the sensors was first converted into digital format and then stored into the TX frame buffer register. The first byte of TX frame buffer register was written with frame length information followed by the sensors' data [19]. Before transmitting, the transmitter was passed through a set of pre-defined states i.e. RESET → TRX_OFF → PLL_ON → TX_ON. After transmitting one packet of information, the transmitter was turned off (TRX_OFF) to save battery energy.

The net weight of the sensing system is 1.938 g without sensors, 6.709 g with all sensors attached and, 9.740 g with sensors and an alkaline battery having dimensions 14 × 10 mm (length × diameter). The nominal and maximum current consumptions of the sensing system were measured as 13.58 and 17.4 mA, respectively. Hence, the peak power consumption of the sensing system is 57.4 mW at 3.3 V supply voltage. As most of the power is consumed in the RF circuits, reducing the RF switching frequency could save a considerable battery power. In a chronic wound monitoring application, even a very low data transmission rate (e.g. one packet of information per quarter an hour) would be sufficient because changes in wound parameters are very slow. A high data transmission rate would only mean a high switching rate of RF components resulting in unnecessary loss of battery power.

2.3 *Interfacing the Sensors with the Radio Transmitter*

The result of ADC conversion was stored in two 8-bit registers; ADCH for high byte and ADCL for low byte. The maximum reference voltage for the ADC was 1.8 V, which was internally generated and stabilized. All the sensors in our system work at a 5.0 V supply for all input values exceeding its reference voltage and would not be able to detect any input signal above 1.8 V. This problem was resolved by reducing the ADC input voltage range such that the maximum input voltage of any sensor was less than the ADC reference voltage. For this purpose, a simple voltage divider circuit was designed using two surface mount resistors R_1 and R_2 for each sensor (Fig. 1b).

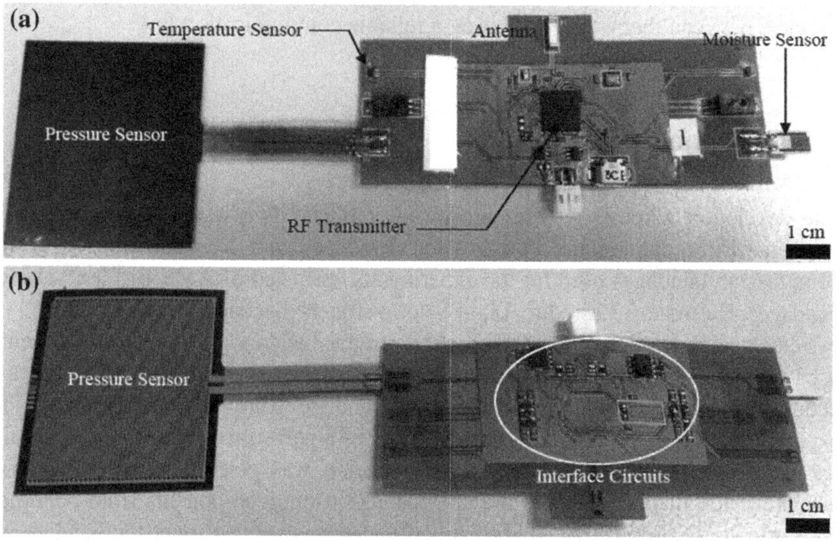

Fig. 1 **a** Photo of the wireless sensing system fabricated on a 0.15 mm thickness 2-layer flexible printed circuit board. The diagram shows various parts of the sensing system (**b**) Rear side of the sensing system showing the voltage divider network used as interface circuits between the sensors and the ADC

2.4 Information Display Module

The transmitted data in ZigBee® 802.15.4 protocol was received by the handheld receiver, processed by the T6963C LCD controller, and displayed on a 10 cm × 8 cm LCD screen [20]. The LCD controller was programmed through the receiver module (ATMega128RFA1) by sending the appropriate commands with required timings as recommended in the datasheet of T6963C [21]. The first transmitted byte consists of frame length information followed by the temperature, moisture and sub-bandage pressure data, respectively. Upon reception, the sensor's data was stored in a 128-byte frame buffer register. This data was then sent to the LCD controller (T6963C) through a parallel interface for processing and display. The LCD controller was also programmed to display the device ID (TX device), frequency channel (2405–2480 MHz in 5 MHz steps), and received signal strength (i.e. RSSI) in dBm.

The TX device ID may be used as a unique identifier for the patient under observation. In a hospital environment where a number of patients would be using these devices, unique frequency channels may be allocated to all devices to avoid any interference between devices or corruption of data. The RSSI level could be indicative of how trustworthy the information of measured parameters is. Information associated with much lower RSSI levels (e.g. −90 dBm) may be discarded on the grounds that the TX device might be too far away from the RX or there might be some obstacle between them, thus inhibiting a reliable communication link.

3 Experiments and Results

The developed wireless wound sensing system was first tested in a room environment using commercial compression bandages and a mannequin leg. The compression bandages used for the experiments consisted of AMS Bi-Flex® elastic bandage, Hartmann Lastodur Light® long-stretch bandage, 3 M Coban™ 2 two-layer, and Hartmann Lastolan® short-stretch bandages. Adjunct components used in the application of compression bandage systems such as Soffban® undercast padding and Idealcrepe® crepe retention bandage were also used. Using the experimental setup, a number of experiments were performed using the mannequin leg in a room environment. The sensing system was placed flat on the central portion of the mannequin to avoid any damage to the components from bending. After the application of dressing, distilled water was sprayed over the bandage in the proximity of the moisture sensor. The measurements were taken with an interval of 5 min by the handheld receiver placed 3 m apart in line of sight to the wireless transmitter. The experiment was performed at 25 °C. The average values of received energy level, temperature, and sub-bandage pressure were calculated as −79.92 dBm, 23.21 °C and 15.14 mmHg, respectively. The average errors in temperature, moisture, and sub-bandage pressure measurements were calculated as

0.93 °C, 3.0 % RH, and 1.50 mmHg, respectively. However, the error in sub-bandage pressure measurements is expected to increase on human leg because of flexible morphology and muscle movements. The errors in moisture and temperature measurements are immune to these factors.

The manufactured wound sensing and monitoring system was extensively tested for its performance on a healthy volunteer. The objectives of these trials were to validate the performance of the sensing system under various clinical scenarios and to determine the optimum placement of the system and sensors on the human body. These scenarios were realized using different compression-bandage systems and various possible postures, both believed to influence the real-time measurements. These trials and their results are discussed in detail in the following sections.

3.1 Establishing Reliability of Measurements

In the first experiment the reliability of measurement results was tested, particularly the sub-bandage pressure measurements as they are prone to variations due to body movements. The sensing system was covered with a transparent adhesive silicone gel on both sides. The trial was performed using a 4-layer compression system Profore® (Smith and Nephew©) as well as a 2-layer inelastic bandage system Coban™ 2 (3 M©) for sub-bandage pressure measurements. The bandages in all experiments were applied by a Wound Management Nurse Practitioner adept in managing chronic wounds and bandaging techniques. The sub-bandage pressure and moisture measurements were performed in two separate experiments. During the sub-bandage pressure measurements, the moisture sensor was placed directly on exposed skin with the sensor facing the skin while the pressure sensor was placed over the flat area of the exposed skin, directly above the medial malleolus (ankle), with the sensor facing the skin. Initial measurements were taken in each experiment prior to applying bandages in order to find and nullify any offset readings. The bandages were applied in accordance with the manufacturer's instructions, achieving 40 mmHg starting pressure. The measurement results are plotted in Fig. 2 for a 4-layer type, at one minute interval using various common postures. Variations in sub-bandage pressure readings are measured by calculating the standard deviation (SD), shown as a red horizontal line in graphs with sub-bandage pressure measurements.

As the moisture and the temperature measurements are independent of posture changes, different setups were used from those used for sub-bandage pressure measurement. For moisture measurements, a moisture-retentive foam dressing Allevyn™ Adhesive (Smith and Nephew) was used. A small slit was made to insert micro-volume extension set tubing in one corner, and another slit was made to insert the moisture sensor in the opposite corner of the dressing. Fluid was then injected through the tubing after every five minutes until the sensor was soaked and started providing moisture values. After that, the dressing was placed upside down so that the fluid moved away from the sensor until it was completely depleted of moisture. Moisture results are plotted in Fig. 3a.

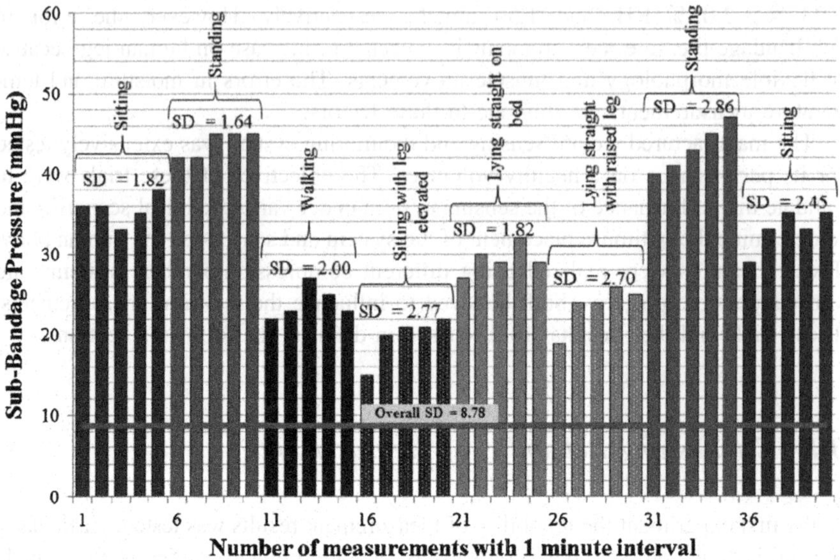

Fig. 2 Graphical plots of pressure measurements during the first trial using 4-layer compression bandage system. The measurements are recorded in various routine movements and postures

For temperature measurements, the sensing system was placed over the lower leg area with the temperature sensor facing skin, and then various temperature readings were recorded continuously for more than 15 min. The experiment was performed at 23 °C room temperature, and with 40 % humidity. The temperature measurements are plotted in Fig. 3b. The average value of the measured skin temperature was 35 ± 1 °C while the standard deviation (SD) was 0.93 °C for skin temperature measurements.

The sub-bandage pressure measurement results (Fig. 2) for both bandages have shown a reliable and repeatable performance of the sensing system under required sub-bandage pressure. In each posture, five consecutive pressure readings were taken over a period of 5 min. For the 4-layer bandage system, the maximum deviation (SD value) observed was 2.86 mmHg during standing, while the same for the 2-layer bandage system was 3.35 mmHg during walking. The moisture level measurement results (Fig. 3a) have also shown a reliable system performance. A steep rise in moisture level was observed as the injected fluid reached in proximity of the sensor. After that, a gradual and consistent drop in the measured moisture level was observed as the sensor was placed in an upward position to allow backward flow of the fluid. In about six hours, the moisture level dropped to zero when the sensor was completely depleted of the fluid. Thus, the first trial concludes that the measurement of temperature, moisture, and sub-bandage pressure with the developed sensing system is reliable, repeatable and consistent with the changes in experimental conditions.

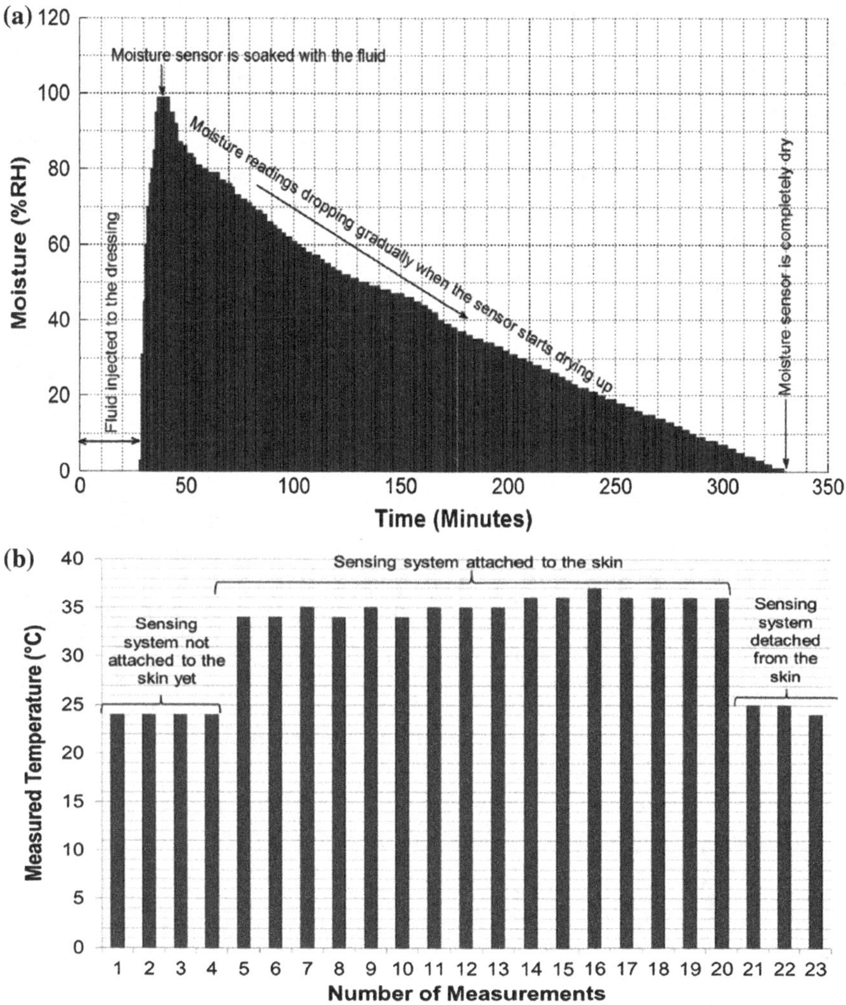

Fig. 3 **a** Graphical plot of moisture values measured using moisture-retentive dressing. Fluid was injected into the dressing through micro-volume extension tubing. The graph indicates a natural rise and fall of moisture level over time (**b**) Graph showing temperature measurements using the flexible sensing system. The graph shows almost constant readings of the room and the skin temperatures

3.2 Measurements at Ankle Level with a 4-Layer Bandage

In this trial, a 4-layer bandage system known to apply 40 mmHg at ankle was used. Bandages were applied as per manufacturer's instructions. A small slit was made in the outermost cohesive bandage (layer 4) to allow battery connection. Allevyn™ Adhesive (Smith and Nephew) 12.5 cm × 12.5 cm dressing was applied to the lower calf and a small cut was made in the back of the dressing. A micro-volume extension set tubing was attached to the dressing and the slit sealed with film tape to allow injection of fluid (As genuine wound fluid was not available soy sauce diluted with water was used). The fluid was injected under the dressing to mimic wound exudate and soy sauce was chosen so that the spread of fluid was visible during experiments. The sensing system was then attached to the lower leg. The pressure sensor was placed proximal to the medial malleolus between exposed skin and bandages. The moisture sensor was placed at the bottom corner of the Allevyn™

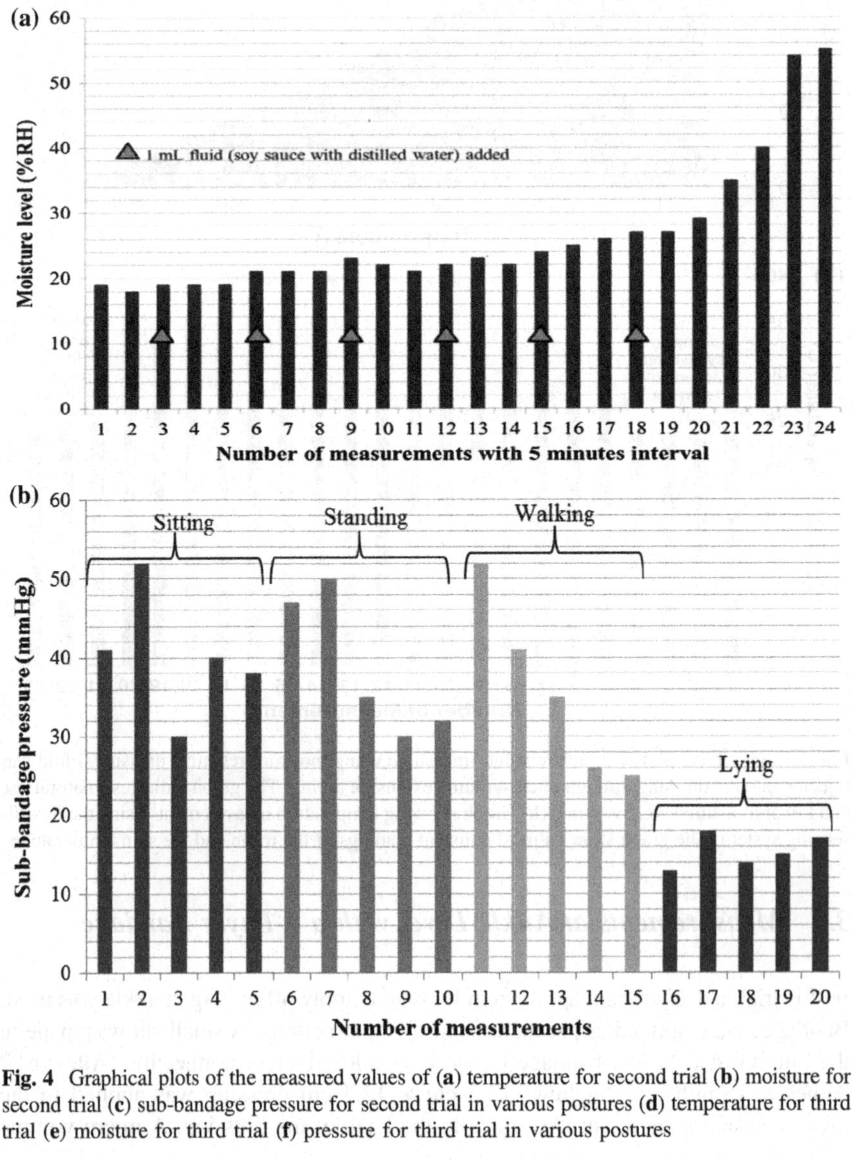

Fig. 4 Graphical plots of the measured values of (**a**) temperature for second trial (**b**) moisture for second trial (**c**) sub-bandage pressure for second trial in various postures (**d**) temperature for third trial (**e**) moisture for third trial (**f**) pressure for third trial in various postures

dressing between the exposed skin and the dressing. The results of second trial are plotted in Fig. 4. The average value of temperature during this trial was 33 ± 1 °C. The moisture values were increasing gradually as more fluid was injected to the dressing until the sensor was soaked with the fluid, the point from where the readings started rising up (readings 21–24 in Fig. 4a). The sub-bandage pressure values (Fig. 4b) were dependent on posture, being higher during walking and standing and lower during sitting or lying. It can also be observed from the graph that the pressure readings were consistently dropping over time. This phenomenon can be attributed to loosening of bandage layers with movement.

4 Discussion

In the first trial, the measurements for pressure, moisture, and temperature were taken separately using distinct experimental setups. The measurements were reliable and consistent with the applied conditions as can be observed in all the figures. The sub-bandage pressure values are expected to fluctuate with the movement, and the graphs in Figs. 2 and 4 have verified this phenomenon. The overall fluctuation of sub-bandage pressure values measured as standard deviation was 8.69 mmHg for the 4-layer and 7.27 mmHg for the 2-layer bandage system. The postures were changed in a cyclic fashion (i.e. starting from 'sitting' and ending in 'sitting') to isolate the source of fluctuations in measurements.

The average sub-bandage pressure values recorded during the first and last 'sitting' postures for the 4-layer were 35.6 and 33.0 mmHg respectively for the 4-layer bandage, and were 42.0 and 43.2 mmHg respectively for the 2-layer bandage. Similarly, the average sub-bandage pressure values during both 'standing' postures were recorded as 43.8 and 43.2 mmHg respectively for the 4-layer bandage, and were 45.8 and 44.0 mmHg respectively for the 2-layer bandage. The twin average values during respective postures for each bandage system were pretty close to each other. These measurements proved that the major source of fluctuations was not the sensing system but the movement of the subject. The variations in measured moisture level over time verified that the measured values were consistent with the dry, wet and intermediate condition of the moisture sensor. Similarly, the body temperature measurement results were also reliable and stable measuring an average value of 35 ± 1 °C. Hence, the reliability and consistency of readings performed on a healthy human volunteer were established during the first trial.

In all trials, variations in sub-bandage pressure can be attributed to muscle movement, blood flow direction, and the type and properties of the bandage used. The temperature and moisture measurements did not manifest any dependency on these factors. However, the moisture readings may be strongly affected by the combined effect of the gravity pull and the location of moisture sensor with respect to fluid entry point. In a clinical scenario, a consistent rise in measured temperature could mean infection at wound site. A gradual decrease in moisture level might indicate the start of healing and the opposite might mean the worsening of healing state. A consistently increasing sub-bandage pressure could be a sign of infection or excessive swelling in the limb, and a gradual decrease in sub-bandage pressure might mean loosening of the bandage layers.

Using this device, a clinician would be able to visualize the state of healing of a chronic wound remotely without disturbing the wound, a phenomenon which was never possible in chronic wound management before. However, the device needs further miniaturization and performance improvements, such as enhancing measurement resolutions, in order to have a significant impact on chronic wound monitoring. Although, the moisture and temperature sensors could be used for any wound, however, the pressure sensing capability is useful only for venous leg ulcers. The device works with an external battery which needs to be attached at all times. The sensing system and sensors are re-usable on a single patient after proper sterilization. The cost incurred by the system will be compensated by reduced frequency of dressing changes, reduced nursing time, and reduced use of hospital resources.

5 Conclusions

Traditional tools and methods have proven insufficient to effectively monitor the chronic wound healing progress. Inaccuracies in chronic wound measurements are responsible for a significant loss in healthcare budgets e.g. a 30 % loss in the US healthcare budget [2]. Engaging an integrated measurement approach (i.e. measuring other critical parameters [12] in addition to wound dimensions) is believed to be more effective to provide stronger evidence of healing than using one kind of measurement only. Though, the wound area and volume calculations over time, and 3D surveillance techniques are useful for this purpose, the proposed sensing system would be a valuable addition to these approaches to mitigate the losses incurred by human errors in chronic wound measurements.

In this paper, we have presented a novel wireless chronic monitoring system which is flexible, biocompatible, and reliable in performance. The sensing system has been fabricated on a flexible circuit material, enabling it to adapt to human limb contours. Low-power profile of the sensing device enables it for being operated continuously under a compression bandage over a longer time period (e.g. 3–4 days) without any disturbance to the bandaged wound. Battery life-time can be further enhanced (e.g. 2–3 weeks) by reducing the frequency of wound data transmission. An effective data transmission range of 4–5 m would enable clinicians and nurses to visualize the current wound state from a distance in a hospital environment.

Experimental results on a healthy human volunteer ascertained that the sensing system was capable of accurately measuring the instantaneous changes in sub-bandage pressure, moisture, and temperature under compression bandages and dressings. Gradual changes in measured wound parameters could reveal the status of healing progress e.g. a consistent rise in sub-bandage pressure might be an indication of infection or swelling. However, the device needs to be tested on patients with chronic wounds to analyze its performance in real environment. The device needs to be tested further even after successful clinical trials to determine its clinical and financial impacts on chronic wound management. The suitability and efficacy of the sensors could be determined during these clinical trials. Nonetheless, the light weight, reliable performance on human limb, flexible and non-invasive structure, low-power consumption and wireless connectivity of the sensing system make it a strong candidate for use in continuous wound sensing and monitoring applications. Future works will incorporate miniaturization of the telemetric sensing system, and its communication with smart phones and display of information on screens using a smart phone application. The system would also incorporate WiFi or 3G communication technologies to share the measured wound parameters to the clinician remotely. This would enable clinicians to gather information on the state of a chronic wound while the patient stays at home.

Acknowledgments We are thankful to the Wound Management Innovation Cooperative Research Centre (CRC) Australia for funding this work. The contents in this paper are part of a pending International Patent (PCT) lodged in the Australian Patent Office on 20th Oct, 2014.

References

1. Cadogan, J., et al.: Identification, diagnosis and treatment of wound infection. Nurs. Stand. **26**, 44–48 (2011)
2. Mark, N.M.D., Christine, M.: Evidence-Based Wound Surveillance-A 3-Dimensional Approach To Measuring. Imaging and Documenting Wounds, Aranz Medical (2014)
3. The Economic Cost of Wounds. http://www.smith-nephew.com/about-us/what-we-do/advanced-wound-management/economic-cost-of-wounds/ (2014)
4. Higher Wound Care Costs are Driving Treatment Research (McKnight's Long-Term Care News, published in June Issue). http://www.mcknights.com/higher-wound-care-costs-are-driving-treatment-research/article/244578/ (2012)
5. Abdelrahman, T., Newton, H.: Wound dressings: principles and practice. Surgery (Oxford) **29**, 491–495 (2011)
6. Partsch, H.: Classification of compression bandages: practical aspects. Dermatol. Surg. Official Publ. Am. Soc. Dermatol. Surg. **34**, 600–609 (2008)
7. Fletcher, A., et al.: A systematic review of compression treatment for venous leg ulcers. Br. Med. J. **315**, 576 (1997)
8. Hopkins, A.: How to apply effective multilayer compression bandaging, Wound Essentials (Wounds UK) **1,** 13 (2006)
9. Kumar, B., et al.: Analysis of sub-bandage pressure of compression bandages during exercise. J. Tissue Viability **21**, 115–124 (2012)
10. Ovington, L.G.: Advances in wound dressings. Clin. Dermatol. **25**, 33–38 (2007)
11. Lagana, G., Anderson, E.H.: Moisture Dressings: The New Standard in Wound Care. J. Nurse Pract. **6**, 366–370 (2010)
12. Harding, K.: Diagnostics and Wounds, A Consensus Document. World Union of Wound Healing Societies (WUWHS) (2007)
13. Dargaville, T.R., et al.: Sensors and imaging for wound healing: a review. Biosens. Bioelectron. **41**, 30–42 (2013)

14. Mehmood, N. et al.: Applications of modern sensors and wireless technology in effective wound management. J. Biomed. Mater. Res. Part B: Appl. Biomater. (2013)
15. Mehmood, N. et al.: An innovative sensing technology for chronic wound monitoring. In: Australian Biomedical Engineering Conference, Canberra, Australia, 20–22 Aug (2014)
16. Mehmood, N., et al.: Calibration of sensors for reliable radio telemetry in a flexible wound monitoring device. Sens. Bio-Sens. Res. **2**, 23–30 (2014)
17. Ochoa, M., et al.: Flexible Sensors for Chronic Wound Management. Biomedical Engineering, IEEE Reviews in **7**, 73–86 (2014)
18. Online datasheet Texas Instruments temperature sensor LM94021. http://www.ti.com/lit/ds/symlink/lm94021.pdf (2013)
19. Online datasheet of RF transceiver ATMega128RFA1. http://www.atmel.com/devices/ATMEGA128RFA1.aspx (2013)
20. Online datasheet of DS-G160128STBWW LCD module. https://www.sparkfun.com/datasheets/LCD/DS-G160128STBWW.pdf (2013)
21. Online datasheet of Toshiba T6963C dot matrix LCD controller. http://www.mikroe.com/downloads/get/1910/t6963c_spec.pdf (2013)

Maturity Models for Hospital Information Systems Management: Are They Mature?

João Vidal de Carvalho, Álvaro Rocha and José Braga de Vasconcelos

Abstract This paper introduces the concepts related with maturity models and analyses the evolution of maturity models for Information Systems Management and mainly the evolution of maturity models focused on the management of Hospital Information Systems. We concluded that current maturity models in the field of Hospital Information Systems management are still in an early development stage, and especially because they are poorly detailed, do not provide tools to determine the maturity stage nor structure the characteristics of maturity stages according to different influencing factors. Consequently, we consider opportune the development of a comprehensive maturity model to improve the Hospital Information Systems management.

Keywords Stages of growth · Maturity models · Hospital information systems · Strategy · Management

1 Introduction

Health care institutions and governmental organizations are starting to understand that the reasons underlying a certain inadequacy in the management of health processes directly relates to infrastructural limitations and their inefficient management

---

J.V. de Carvalho (✉)
ISCAP, Instituto Politécnico Do Porto, Porto, Portugal
e-mail: j.vidal.carvalho@gmail.com

Á. Rocha
Departamento de Engenharia Informática & LIACC, Universidade de Coimbra, Coimbra, Portugal
e-mail: amrocha@dei.uc.pt

J.B. de Vasconcelos
Universidade Atlântica, Oeiras, Portugal
e-mail: jose.braga.vasconcelos@gmail.com

Y.-W. Chen et al. (eds.), *Innovation in Medicine and Healthcare 2015*,
Smart Innovation, Systems and Technologies 45,
DOI 10.1007/978-3-319-23024-5_49

[16, 54]. Hospital Information Systems (HIS) managers usually contemplate the errors that occurred in these organizations and wonder what could have been done to avoid them. They conclude that these errors are usually a natural growth and maturation symptom of organizations, and are often the result of the development that brought the organization to its current maturity stage [51]. This phenomenon of change fits the principles behind the growth stages theory and in the current context surrounding Information Systems (IS) of health organizations.

Based on this presupposition which highlights the relevance of Maturity Models in the HIS fields, this research work is intended at the development of a comprehensive maturity model that is especially adapted to the needs of Hospital Information Systems Management. To develop this new model, we carried out firstly a preliminary literature review on IS Maturity Models and respective specificities.

Besides this section, this article is organized in three more. Accordingly, the second section proposes a preliminary systematization of the state of the art concerning maturity models in IS Management and HIS Management. The third section defines the problem underlying this research work. And, finally, the fourth section offers some final remarks concerning this study.

2 Review of Literature

Information Systems Management (ISM) is the activity responsible for the tasks of an organization pertaining to Information Management, Information Systems and the adoption of Communication and Information Technologies (CIT) [1]. The maturity of this activity is a key factor for the success of organizations, to the extent that an IS is fundamental for their survival, competitive edge and success. In this context, there are several instruments that help the ISM achieve an enhanced maturity, namely the so called Maturity Models. Indeed, maturity models provide organization managers an important model for the identification of the maturity stage of an IS in order to plan and implement actions that will allow them to move towards an enhanced maturity stage, and thus achieve the proposed goals [50]. Maturity Models can be perceived as conceptual models, comprised by discreet stages that are used to identify "anticipated, typical, logical or desired evolution paths towards maturity" [4]. We observe that these models have been used in multiple areas to describe a wide variety of phenomena [9, 12, 28, 29, 35].

Maturity Models are sustained by the principle that people, organizations, functional areas, processes, etc., evolve, towards an enhanced maturity and following a development or growth process, which covers a number of different stages [50]. That is, Maturity Models are based on the theory of cyclic stages of growth, where the changes observed in an IS over the course of time occur in a sequential and predictable mode, covering a certain number of cumulative and hierarchically sequential stages, which can be described and linked to a specific level of maturity [6, 43, 50, 51]. In the same sense, Caralli and Knight [10] argue that maturity models provide organizations with a tool to address their problems and challenges in a structured way, offering both a reference point to evaluate their capabilities and a guide to improve them.

Over the last four decades several maturity models have been proposed, with differences as to the number of stages, influencing factors and intervention areas. Each one of these factors identifies the characteristics that typify the focus of each maturity stage, that is, these factors work as reference descriptors or variables to characterize each stage and provide the necessary criteria to achieve a specific maturity stage [4].

2.1 Evolution of Maturity Models in IS Management

Richard Nolan is considered the mentor of the IS maturity approach. Indeed, after studying/researching the use of IS in the biggest US organizations, Nolan proposed a maturity model that initially included 4 stages [43]. Later, with a view to improve his first proposal, Nolan included two additional stages to the initial model [44]. In this second version, Nolan suggests that organizations start slowly in the Initiation stage, followed by a rapid spread in the use of ITs during the Contagion stage. Subsequently, the need for Control emerges, and this stage is followed by the Integration of different technological solutions. Data Management allows for development without increasing IS related costs and, finally, constant growth promotes the achievement of Maturity.

Although this approach to the maturity models developed by Nolan, has been recognized as significantly ground breaking, it also raised a lot of debate and controversy within the scientific community. Several researchers have published studies that, on the one hand, validated and, on the other hand, expanded the model proposed by Nolan. Indeed, resulting from the researches in this field several researchers have proposed new models [e.g.: 14, 17, 24, 27, 34].

Amongst these new models proposed after the initial approach developed by Nolan, the most widely accepted, detailed and comprehensive is the Revised Model of Galliers and Sutherland [9, 50]. This model provides an improved perspective of how an organization plans, develops, uses and organizes an IS and offers suggestions towards an enhanced maturity stage. This model involves six stages of maturity (Table 1) and assumes that an organization can occupy different maturity stages in any given moment and be conditioned by influencing factors. Moreover, it presents the characteristics of the stages aligned with modern network organizations and offers a data collection tool to evaluate maturity [50].

More recently, after the model proposed by Galliers and Sutherland [17], other models have been resealed [e.g.: 3, 26, 28, 39], including a new Nolan model with nine stages of maturity [45], developed as an answer to the technological evolution in the IS field and its management. As to the field of IS Management, another solid example of a Maturity Model is the model developed by de Khandelwal and Ferguson [26], proposing nine stages of maturity and combining stages theory with Critical Success Factors. Notwithstanding, the model proposed by Galliers and

Table 1 Revised model of maturity stages of Galliers and Sutherland [17]

Factors	Stage I	Stage II	Stage III	Stage IV	Stage V	Stage VI
	"Ad hocracy"	Foundations	Centralized	Cooperation	Entrepreneurial	Harmonious
Strategy	Acquisition of hardware, software, etc	IT audit; find out and meet user needs (reactive)	Top-down IS planning	Integration, coordination and control	Environmental scanning and opportunity seeking	Maintain comparative strategic advantage; monitor futures; interactive planning
Structure	None	IS often subordinate to accounting or finance	Data processing department; centralized DP shop; End-users running free at Stage 1	Information centers, library records, etc. in same unit; information services	SBU coalition(s) (many but separate)	Centrally coordinated coalitions (corporate and SBU views concurrently)
Systems	Ad hoc unconnected; operational; manual and computerized IS; uncoordinated; concentration in financial systems; little maintenance	Many applications; many gaps; overlapping systems; centralized; operational; mainly financial systems; many areas unsatisfied; large backlog; heavy maintenance load	Still mostly centralized; uncontrolled end-user computing; most major business activities covered; database systems	Decentralized approach with some controls, but mostly lack of coordination; some DSS-ad hoc; integrated office technology systems	Decentralized systems but central control and coordination; added value systems (more marketing oriented); more DSS-internal, less ad hoc; some strategic systems; (using external data); lack of external and internal data integration of communications technologies with computing	Inter-organizational systems (supplier, customer, government links); new IS-based products; external-internal data integration

(continued)

Table 1 (continued)

Factors	Stage I	Stage II	Stage III	Stage IV	Stage V	Stage VI
	"Ad hocracy"	Foundations	Centralized	Cooperation	Entrepreneurial	Harmonious
Staff	Programmers/contractors	Systems analysts; DP manager.	IS planners; IS manager; data base; administrator; data administrator; data analysts	Business analysts; information resources manager (Chief information officer)	Corporate/business/IS planners (one role)	IS director/member of board of directors
Style	Unaware	Don't bother me (I'm too busy)	Abrogation/delegation	Democratic dialectic.	Individualistic (product champion)	Business team
Skills	Technical (very low level), individual expertise	Systems development methodology	IS believes it knows what the business needs; project management	Organizational integration; IS knows how the business works; Users know how IS works (for their area); Business management (for IS staff)	IS manager—member of senior executive team; knowledgeable users in some IS areas; entrepreneurial marketing skills	All senior management understand IS and its potentialities
Super-ordinate goals	Obfuscation	Confusion	Senior management concerned DP defensive	Cooperation	Opportunistic; entrepreneurial; entrepreneurial	Interactive planning

Sutherland [17] is still perceived as the most complete and updated in IS management [51].

Additionally, these maturity models are still being used and implemented in multiple types of organizations and to different areas inside them. Mutafelija and Stromberg [38] refer that the concept of maturity has been applied to more than 150 areas inside IS. In fact, there are several examples of maturity models focused on different organization and IS areas, namely the maturity model for Intranet implementation, by Damsgaard and Scheepers [11]; the maturity model for ERP systems by Holland and Light [22]; and the CMMI maturity model for the software development process [53]. We can also mention maturity models for fields such as Software Management [2], Business Management [30], Project Management [8, 25], Project Portfolio and Program Management [37], Information Management [55], IS/ICT Management [48], e-Business [14, 15, 18, 31], e-Learning [32], Knowledge Management [5, 33], BPM—Business Process Management [52], Enterprise Architecture [13, 40], etc.

2.2 Maturity Models for HIS Management

Health related organizations, and more specifically Hospital IS Management organizations, are also increasingly adopting maturity models. This use is connected to a growing provision of health care services based on electronic systems, supported by enhanced computer capacity and an increased ability to seize and share knowledge in a digital format. It is widely agreed that ISs offer significant opportunities for health care providers and health provision in general, as well as access to information required by users [51].

In this context, some maturity models emerged, namely the Quintegra Maturity Model for electronic Healthcare [54], proposed as a model that goes beyond the limits of an organization, incorporating every service linked to the medical process applied to each health care provider in each maturity stage. Another example of a maturity model in the health field is the HIMSS Maturity Model for Electronic Medical Record, which identifies different maturity stages in the Electronic Medical Record (EMR) of hospitals [19]. IDC (Health Industry Insights) has also developed a maturity model which describes the five stages of development in Hospital ISs (Table 2). This maturity model has been used all over the world by IDC, both to evaluate the maturity of IS in hospitals and to compare maturity average differences between regions and countries in different continents [23]. To these models we can add the Maturity Model for Electronic Patient Record, directed to the system that manages every patient related information, that is, a system that manages the EPR (Electronic Patient Record) [47] and the maturity model for PACS by Wetering and Batenburg [56].

National health services from several countries have also started to develop and adopt Maturity Models. That is the case of the model created by the National E-health Transition Authority of Australia (NEHTA) [41] and baptized

Table 2 IDC maturity model for HIS [23]

Stage I	Stage II	Stage III	Stage IV	Stage V
Basic HIS	*Advanced HIS*	*Advanced HIS core clinicals*	*Digital hospital*	*Digital virtual enterprise*
Patient registration/inpatient admission discharge and transfer	Electronic claims submission	Laboratory information	Patient appointment scheduling	Secure email (provider-provider/provider-patient)
Patient billing and accounts receivable HRIS/payroll	Electronic payment processing	RIS/radiology results reporting	Computerized physician order entry	Participation in regionalized patient CDR
General ledger /financial reporting	Inventory, supply requisitioning, and distribution	PACS	Nursing documentation	Home health case management
Purchasing/accounts payable	Basic order communications	Pharmacy	Emergency department management	Remote patient monitoring / telemedicine
	E-mail	Operating room scheduling and management	Cardiology department management	
	Internet access		Physician portal	
	Intranet		Patient portal	
			Wireless infrastructure	
			Inpatient electronic medical record (EMR)	
			Ambulatory EMR	
			Enterprise master patient index	

Interoperability Maturity Model (IMM). This model focuses on interoperability associated with technical, informational and organizational capabilities of the different players involved in health care services. Another example concerns the Maturity Model of the NHS Infrastructure Maturity Model (NIMM) [42]. This is a maturity evaluation model that helps NHS organizations carry out an objective self-assessment in terms of technological infrastructures.

3 The Problem

Health care institutions and governmental organizations are starting to understand that the reasons underlying a certain inadequacy in the management of health processes directly relates to infrastructural limitations and their inefficient management [49, 54]. An analysis to the current health context clearly reveals the weight of the technological transition problem [54]. Moreover, operational information technologies have increased in complexity to answer the demands of the sector. This increase in complexity, in its turn, led to the integration of several new enterprise integration systems, processes and approaches, and the emergence of new companies providing services in this field. Consequently, many underdeveloped products and services are being consumed by HISs undergoing a process of change and demanding, more than ever, a degree of performance and effectiveness that will answer their needs. In this scenario, several questions that require a convincing answer emerge:

- How can we know if we are doing a good job when managing these changes and monitoring their progress on an ongoing basis?
- How can we manage the interactions of systems and processes in constant evolution?
- How can we manage the impact of low interoperability, security, reliability, efficiency and effectiveness processes?
- How can we evaluate the impact of current clinical and hospital software applications in the maturity development of their respective IS?

We observe that the benefits brought by modern technology to the health field, and supported by better methods and tools, cannot be obtained via undisciplined and chaotic processes [20, 21]. That is why we believe that IS Management in health organizations must be carried out based on maturity models.

Several maturity models have been proposed in the course of time, for personal evolution purposes, for the general evolution of organizations and for the evolution of the IS Management task in particular. The differences in these models lie specifically in the number of stages, evolution variables and focus areas [35, 51]. Each of these models identifies certain characteristics that typify the target of different growth or maturity stages and are implemented in different organizations. Where health related organizations are concerned, several maturity models are also proposed. Notwithstanding the specificities of these models that distinguish them from the models of other areas, these are still in an early development stage [35, 51]. In the research that was carried out, we observed that the models pertaining to the health field are poorly detailed, do not provide maturity measuring tools and do not structure the characteristics of maturity stages according to influencing factors. This reality offers an opportunity for the development of new maturity models focused on IS management in the health field that are capable of filling the previously identified gaps. Within the universe of the maturity models that we know, we believe that the model of maturity stages reviewed by Galliers and Sutherland [17] can serve as an inspiration and reference, both to define influencing factors and to develop a measuring instrument for Hospital IS maturity.

Additionally, the very concept of Maturity Model is not devoid of criticism. For instance, Pfeffer and Sutton [46] argue that the purpose of maturity models is to identify a gap that can be filled with subsequent improvement measures. However, most of these models fail to describe how to effectively carry out these actions, as the closing of such gaps can be extremely difficult to illustrate. The strongest point of criticism, where maturity models are involved, is their weak theoretical basis [7]. Most of these models are based on "best practices" or "success factors" connected with processes from organizations that have shown favorable results. Therefore, although these practices are compatible with the maturity model, they provide no guarantee as to the success of the organization. There is no agreement surrounding the "real path" that will ensure a positive result [36]. According to deBruin and Rosemann [12] the reasons for the, sometimes, ambiguous results obtained with the maturity models stem from the insufficient testing of the models in terms of validity, reliability and generalization, as well as from the lack of documents addressing the design and development process behind this type of model. For this reason, it is fundamental to describe the work underlying the development of a maturity model based on an approach sustained by DSR (Design Science Research) principles.

4 Final Remarks

This paper introduced the concepts associated with maturity models and analyzed the evolution of maturity models for Information Systems Management and mainly the evolution of maturity models focused on the management of Hospital Information Systems.

From these analysis it is possible to conclude that current maturity models in the field of Hospital Information Systems management are still in an early development stage, and especially because they are poorly detailed, do not provide tools to determine the maturity stage nor structure the characteristics of maturity stages according to different influencing factors. Thus, it is opportune to develop a comprehensive maturity model which addresses the gaps of the actual maturity models.

Our future work will involve systematic reviews of the available literature concerning maturity models for information systems management in general and hospital information systems management in particular, which will allow us to identify, among others, a set of potential influencing factors that should be considered during the initial development stage of the new comprehensive maturity model.

References

1. Amaral, L., Varajão, J.: Planeamento de Sistemas de Informação, 4th edn. FCA, Lisboa (2007)
2. April, A., Abran, A., Dumke, R.: Assessment of software maintenance capability: a model and its architecture. In: Proceedings of the 8th European Conference on Software Maintenance and Reengineering (CSMR2004), (pp. 243–248). IEEE Computer Society Press, Los Alamitos, CA (2004)
3. Auer, T.: Beyond IS implemention: a skill-based approach to IS use. Paper presented at the 3rd European conference on information systems. Athens, Greece (1995)
4. Becker, J., Knackstedt, R., Pöppelbuß, J.: Developing maturity models for IT management. Bus. Inf. Syst. Eng. **1**(3), 213–222 (2009)
5. Berztiss, A.T.: Capability maturity for knowledge management. In: DEXA Workshop, IEEE Computer Society, pp. 162–166 (2002)
6. Bhidé, Amar V.: The Origin and Evolution of New Businesses. Oxford University Press, New York (2000)
7. Biberoglu, E., & Haddad, H.: A survey of industrial experiences with CMM and the teaching of CMM practices. Journal of Computing Sciences in Colleges, 18(2), (2002)
8. Brookes, N., Clark, R.: Using maturity models to improve project management practice. In: POMS 20th Annual Conference. Orlando, Florida, USA, 1–4 May 2009
9. Burn, J.M.A.: Revolutionary staged growth model of information systems planning. In: Proceedings of the International Conference on Information Systems, Vancouver, British Columbia, Canada, pp. 395–406 (1994)
10. Caralli, R., Knight, M.: Maturity Models 101: A Primer for Applying Maturity Models to Smart Grid Security, Resilience, and Interoperability. Software Engineering Institute, Carnegie Mellon University, Pittsburgh (2012)
11. Damsgaard, J., Scheepers, R.: Managing the crises in intranet implementation: a stage model. Inf. Syst. J. **10**(2), 131–149 (2000). doi:10.1046/j.1365-75.2000.00076.x
12. de Bruin, T., Rosemann, M.: Understanding the main phases of developing a maturity assessment model. In: Proceedings of the 16th Australasian Conference on Information Systems, Sydney, Australia (2005)
13. Doc, I.T.: Architecture Capability Maturity Model. Department of Commerce, USA Government Introduction (2003)
14. Earl, M.J.: Management Strategies for Information Technologies, Upper Saddle River. Prentice Hall, New Jersey (1989)
15. Earl, M.J.: Evolving the e-business. Bus. Strategy Rev. **11**(2), 33–38 (2000)
16. Freixo, J., Rocha, Á.: Arquitetura de Informação de Suporte à Gestão da Qualidade em Unidades Hospitalares. RISTI—Revista Ibérica de Sistemas e Tecnologias de Informação **14**, 1–18 (2014). doi:10.17013/risti.14.1-18
17. Galliers, R.D., Sutherland, A.R.: Information systems management and strategy formulation: the 'stages of growth' model revisited. J. Inf. Syst. **1**(2), 89–114 (1991). doi:10.1111/j.1365-2575.1991.tb00030.x
18. Gardler, R., Mehandjiev, N.: Supporting component-based software evolution. In: Aksit, M., Mezini, M., Unland, R. (eds.) Objects, Components, Architectures, Services, and Applications for a Networked World, Series: Lecture Notes in Computer Science, vol. 2591, pp. 103–120. Springer (2003)

19. Garets, D., Davis, M.: Electronic Medical Records versus Electronic Health Records: Yes, there is a difference, Chicago. HIMSS Analytics, IL (2006)
20. Gonçalves, J., Rocha, Á.: A decision support system for quality of life in head and neck oncology patients. Head & Neck Oncology **4**(3), 1–9 (2012). doi:10.1186/1758-3284-4-3
21. Gonçalves, J., Silveira, A., Rocha, Á.: A platform to study the quality of life in oncology patients. Int. J. Inf. Syst. Change Manage. **5**(3), 209–220 (2011). doi:10.1504/IJISCM.2011.044501
22. Holland, C., Light, B.: A stage maturity model for enterprise resource planning systems. Data Base Adv. Inf. Syst. **32**(2), 34–45 (2001)
23. Holland, M., Piai, S., Dunbrack, L.A.: Healthcare IT Maturity Model: Western European Hospitals—The Leading Countries (Tech. Rep. No. HI210231). IDC Health Insights, Framingham, MA (2008)
24. Huff, Sidney L., Munro, Malcolm C., Martin, Barbara H.: Growth stages of end-user computing. Commun. ACM **31**(5), 542–550 (1988)
25. Kerzner, H.: Using the Project Management Maturity Model: Strategic Planning for Project Management, 2nd edn. Wiley, New York (2005)
26. Khandelwal, V., Ferguson, J.: Critical Success Factors (CSFs) and the growth of IT in selected geographic regions. In: Proceedings of 32nd Hawaii International Conference on Systems Sciences (HICSS-32), USA (1999)
27. King, J., Kraemer, K.: Evolution and organizational information systems: an assessment of Nolan´s stage model. Commun. de ACM **27**(5), 466–475 (1984)
28. King, W.R., Teo, T.S.H.: Integration between business planning and information systems planning: validating a stage hypothesis. In: Decis. Sci. **28**(2), 123–139 (1997)
29. Kohlegger, M., Maier, R., Thalmann, S.: Understanding maturity models results of a structured content analysis. In: Proceedings of I-KNOW and I-SEMANTIC 09. University of Innsbruck, School of Management, Information Systems, Graz, Austria (2009)
30. Levin G., Nutt, H.: Achieving Excellence in Business Development: The Business Development Capability Maturity Model (2005)
31. Ludescher, G., Usrey, M.: Towards an ECMM (E-commerce maturity model). In: Proceedings of the First International Research Conference on Organizational Excellence in the Third Millennium. Colorado State University, Estes Park (2000)
32. Marshall, S.: E-l0earning maturity model (2007). http://www.utdc.vuw.ac.nz/research/emm/. Accessed Set/2014
33. Maybury, M.T.: Knowledge management at the MITRE corp (2002). http://www.mitre.org
34. McKenney, James L., McFarlan, Franklin W.: The Information Archipelago – Maps and Bridges. Harvard Bus. Rev. **60**(5), 109–119 (1982)
35. Mettler, T.: A Design Science Research Perspective on Maturity Models in Information Systems. University of St. Gallen, St. Gallen (2009)
36. Montoya-Weiss, M.M., Calantone, R.J.: Determinants of new product performance: a review and meta-analysis. J. Prod. Innov. Manage. **11**(5), 397–417 (1994)
37. Murray, A.: Capability maturity models—using P3M3 to improve performance, vol. 2, issue 0616-01-12 (2006). www.outperform.co.uk. Accessed Set/2014
38. Mutafelija, B., Stromberg, H.: Systematic process improvement using ISO 9001:2000 and CMMI. Artech House, Boston (2003)
39. Mutsaers, E., Zee, H., Giertz, H.: The evolution of information technology. Inf. Manage. Comput. Secur. **6**(3), 115–126 (1998)
40. Nascio: NASCIO enterprise Architecture Maturity Model, Version 1.3. National Association of State Chief Information Officers. December (2003)
41. NEHTA: NEHTA Interoperability Maturity Model. 2007 edn. Level 25, 56 Pitt Street, Sydney, NSW, 2000, National EHealth Transition Authority Ltd, Australia (2007)
42. NHS: National Infrastructure Maturity Model (Online) (2011), Available: http://www.connectingforhealth.nhs.uk/systemsandservices/nimm (Retrieved in Set/2014)
43. Nolan, R.: Managing de computer resource: a stage hypotesis. Commun. de ACM **16**(7), 399–405 (1973)

44. Nolan, R.: Managing the crisis in data processing. Harvard Bus. Rev. **57**(2), 115–126 (1979)
45. Nolan, R., Koot, W.: Nolan stages theory today: a framework for senior and it management to manage information technology. Holland Manage. Rev. **31**, 1–24 (1992)
46. Pfeffer, J., Sutton, R.: Knowing "what" to do is not enough: turning knowledge into action. Calif. Manag. Rev. **42**(1), 83–108 (1999)
47. Priestman, W.: ICT strategy 2007–2011 for the Royal Liverpool and Broadgreen University Hospitals NHS trust. Trust Board Meeting 6th November (2007)
48. Renken, J.: Developing an IS/ICT management capability maturity framework. In: Research conference of the South African Institute for Computer Scientists and Information Technologists (SAICSIT), Stellenbosch, pp. 53–62 (2004)
49. Rocha, Á., Rocha, B.: Adopting nursing health record standards. Inform. Heal. Soc. Care **39** (1), 1–14 (2014). doi:10.3109/17538157.2013.827200
50. Rocha, Á., Vasconcelos, J.: Os Modelos de Maturidade na Gestão de Sistemas de Informação. Revista da Faculdade de Ciência e Tecnologia da Universidade Fernando Pessoa **1**, 93–107 (2004)
51. Rocha, Á.: Evolution of information systems and technologies maturity in healthcare. Int. J. Healthc. Inf. Syst. Inform. (IJHISI) **6**(2), 28–36 (2011). doi:10.4018/jhisi.2011040103
52. Rosemann, M., deBruin, T.: Business process management maturity—a model for progression. In Proceedings of the 13th ECIS, May, Regensburg (2005)
53. SEI Software Engineering Institute. CMMI® for Development, Version 1.3, Improving processes for developing better products and services, (Tech. Rep. No. CMU/SEI-2010-TR-033), Carnegie Mellon University (2010)
54. Sharma, B.: Electronic Healthcare Maturity Model (eHMM). Quintegra, India (2008)
55. Venkatesh, V., et al.: User acceptance of information technology: Toward a unified view. MIS Q. **27**(3), 425–478 (2003)
56. Wetering, R., Batenburg, R.: A PACS maturity model: a systematic meta-analytic review on maturation and evolvability of PACS in the hospital enterprise. Int. J. Med. Inform. **78**, 127–140 (2009). doi:10.1016/j.ijmedinf.2008.06.010

Why Cannot Control Your Smartphones by Thinking? Hands-Free Information Control System Based on EEG

Yuanyuan Wang, Tomoki Hidaka, Yukiko Kawai and Jiro Okuda

Abstract Smartphones are the most frequently used devices for acquiring information, but people should operate the smartphones still using hands, even though wearable devices, e.g., Google Glass, are rapidly spreading. Meanwhile, electroencephalogram (EEG) is commonly used for recording brain activity, to translate the brain signals into computer commands; it is widely used for aiding disabled people. EEG has a potential to enable people to control information directly by brain activity. So, why cannot you control smartphones by thinking? EEG can enable people to control information directly. For example, your favorite song can be played without browsing by brain activity, even your smartphone in the pocket; and it can also prevent risks while driving or walking. We have developed a hands-free brain computer interface of practical use for controlling applications based on user intentions and feelings by adopting a wearable EEG device and smartphones.

Keywords Intentions · Feelings · EEG-based information control system

1 Introduction

Brain-computer interface (BCI) technology has a potential to enable disabled people to control external devices such as computers, wheelchairs or virtual environments

Y. Wang (✉)
Nagoya University, Nagoya 464-8601, Japan
e-mail: circl.wang@gmail.com

T. Hidaka
Yamasa Corporation, Okayama, Fukutomihigashi 702-8033, Japan
e-mail: i1358086@gmail.com

Y. Kawai · J. Okuda
Kyoto Sangyo University, Kyoto 603-8555, Japan
e-mail: kawai@cc.kyoto-su.ac.jp

J. Okuda
e-mail: jokuda@cc.kyoto-su.ac.jp

Y.-W. Chen et al. (eds.), *Innovation in Medicine and Healthcare 2015*,
Smart Innovation, Systems and Technologies 45,
DOI 10.1007/978-3-319-23024-5_50

directly by brain activity rather than by physical means. However, disabled people need to wear high restriction headgear for acquiring high-quality EEG based on many standard positions on the surface of the brain. Currently, smartphones and car navigation systems are the most frequently used convenient devices for acquiring information in daily lives of people, especially for disabled people. By accessing various applications or services on smartphones, people can quickly and easily obtain information in a wide variety of situations, but they still use hands, even though wearable devices, e.g., Google Glass [6], Apple Watch [1], are rapidly spreading. For instance, there is considerable concern that using a smartphone while driving makes an accident risk, to the driver and other people on the road, because it distracts the driver, impairs his control of the vehicle, and reduces his awareness of what is happening on the road around him.

So, why cannot you control smartphones by thinking? We considered that EEG has a potential to enable people to control information on smartphones directly by brain activity. In this way, your favorite song can be played without browsing any information on your smartphone, even it is in a pocket. In this research, we aim to develop a hands-free information controllable system based on a smartphone of practical use for controlling applications (apps) or contents (e.g., Websites) on smartphones without browsing anything, but based on human EEG at anytime and anywhere. The system enables users to automatically control information on smartphones by deliberate control and habitual control. The deliberate control indicates that the users control information for their explicit purposes. We define user intentions as user's purposes, that is what the user actually wants to do with an interaction with an app on a smartphone. Therefore, the deliberate control is determined by extracting the users' most frequently used apps in personal from their usage history of smartphones and the user intentions through their EEG states. Then, the system automatically recommends the most frequently used apps by different time periods, they can be automatically controlled on smartphones by the extracted user intentions. The habitual control indicates that the users perform the control same as their usual behavior. In general, feelings are users' emotions; we define user feelings as users' brain states, referring to where and when of their surrounding situation. Then, the system automatically controls the users' habitually-used apps by extracting their feelings and acquiring similar feelings in the past through the EEG states and their situations (i.e., location and time), for example, starting users' habitually-used apps, or playing music according to users' situations.

Although several techniques for voice-based and vision-based methods for hands-free control of devices or software have been studied [3], these studies have focused on the hands-free feature; they do not solve the aforementioned issues on information control on smartphones. To achieve our goal, we utilize EEG instead of hands. B-Bridge developed a wearable EEG measurement device, called B3 Band [2], it is a low restrain headband equipment at a low price that are good for health care for disabled people. As depicted in Fig. 1, our novel EEG-based information controllable system makes two primary research contributions:

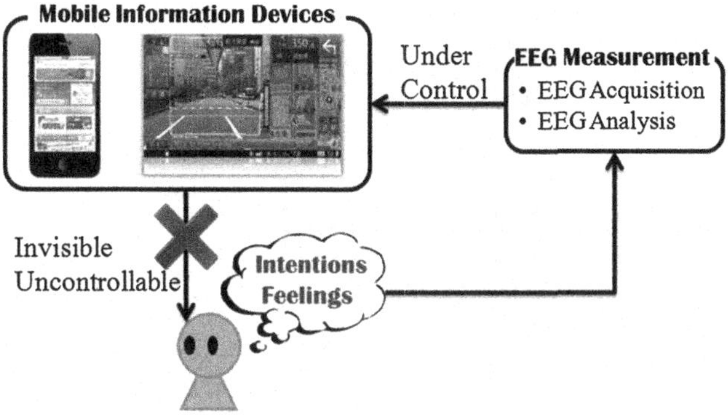

Fig. 1 Proposed EEG-based information control system

1. Users can automatically control apps on smartphones by extracting user intentions through voice guidance. It is possible to measure EEG states with a simple EEG measurement device (only 3 electrodes) and smartphones.
2. Users can automatically control their habitually-used apps by extracting their current feelings that are similar to the past feelings. In order to extract users' feelings by acquiring spatio-temporal information, the system measures EEG states that are affected by the surrounding situations of them.

For example, a user is frustrated in a traffic jam, when he drives a car on the road. Our system extracts his feeling and assumes he is in the traffic jam by measuring his EEG, and compares the past similar feelings by acquiring situations of him. Therefore, it enables playing a music to soften his feeling, since he habitually plays the music in the same situation. Specially, our system can learn EEG features of disabled people, to help them automatically control their purposes about what they want to do according to their surrounding situations.

2 System Overview and Related Work

2.1 System Overview

As depicted in Fig. 2, we propose two methods to control apps or contents of smartphones based on human EEG. In the system, we connect the smartphone to a simple EEG device via a Bluetooth. EEG data are acquired by the smartphone. As an initial learning of users' brain states in advance, the system measures their EEG under a concentration or relaxation state. Then, we developed a classifier by the initial learning that is stored in a server.

In order to control all apps (e.g., mails, SNS) or contents on smartphones by extracting user intentions, they are firstly announced by voice guidance to users.

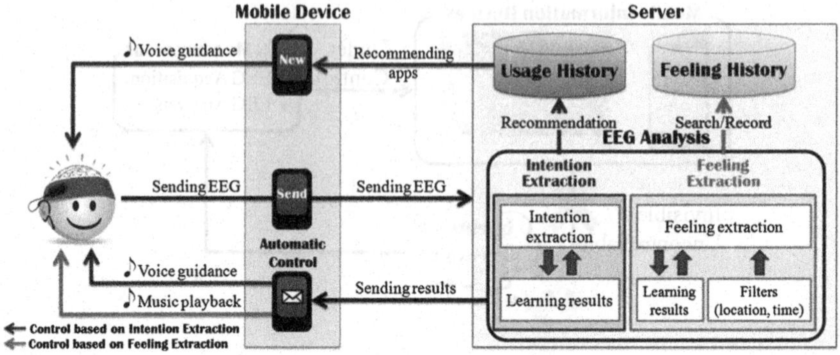

Fig. 2 System configuration diagram

Next, users express their intentions (thought) to the announced information from EEG with two states, i.e., concentration and relaxation; then, our system measures and learns their EEG under these states. The measured EEG data is sent to the server through the smartphone. In the server side, the system inputs the received EEG into a classifier to determine the EEG states. Then, the system automatically controls apps or contents on smartphones, according to the determined results, and announces the results to the users by voice guidance.

In order to control apps or the contents on smartphones in the same situations as before by extracting user feeling, our system acquires users' locations and time information in advance, to measure the EEG that is affected by situations of the users and to search for the similar EEG in the past. Furthermore, the acquired location, time information and the controlled histories are stored in a database, called a feeling history. Next, the measured EEG data is sent to a server through the smartphone. In the server side, the system accesses the feeling history database, and searches for the similar EEG data in the past, then, the system controls apps through his EEG when he is in the same situations.

2.2 Related Work

Several techniques of hands-free control system have been studied. VoiceBot [7] is a voice controlled robotic arm, using the Vocal Joystick inference engine. This study based on voice controls needs high-quality speech recognition techniques, which is not suitable for outdoor use, since a lot of outside noise may affect the quality of the voice. In this work, we aim to develop a hands-free information control system to recommend users' required information according to their surrounding situations by measuring EEG states.

Lampe et al. [9] presented an Internet-based brain-computer interface (BCI) for controlling an intelligent robotic device with autonomous reinforcement-learning.

EEG-based brain-controlled wheelchair has been developed for use by completely paralyzed patients [12]. The proposed design includes a novel approach for selecting optimal electrode positions, a series of signal processing algorithms and an interface to a powered wheelchair. These studies have focused on hands-free device control for patients, and they measured brain activity by using high price and high restrain equipments e.g., headgear and MRI (magnetic resonance imaging), at homes or hospitals. In this work, we use a simple headband type EEG measurement device for not only patients, but also general users to automatically control apps or the contents on smartphones.

3 EEG Measurement

We aim to develop a hands-free information controllable system for operating apps or the contents on smartphones without using hands. For this, the system was designed to extract user intentions and feelings by measuring EEG data.

3.1 Classifier Configuration

We developed an application of EEG measurement on smartphones to acquire a sample learning data for each individual user in advance. We adopted a simple EEG measurement device, B3 Band (see Fig. 4a). The application first makes a connection between the smartphones and the B3 Band via a Bluetooth. Then, all the EEG data can be measured and sent to the server. The processing flow is shown in Fig. 3, (a) Explaining how to measure EEG in 7 s. (b) Selecting CONNECT button to connect the B3 Band with a Bluetooth. (c) Starting a task by START button. (d) Indicating a user's state, i.e., concentration or relaxation.

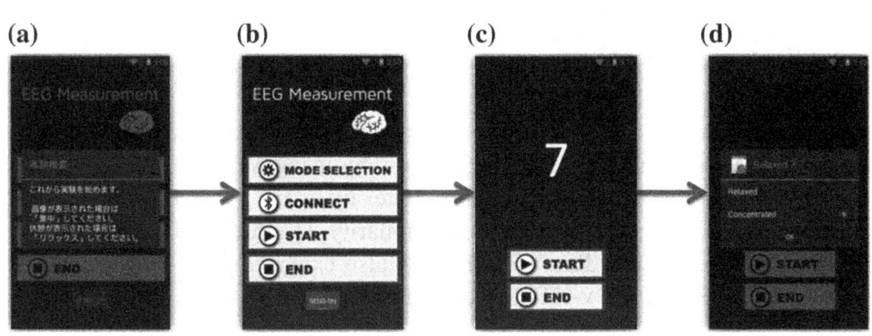

Fig. 3 Screenshot of processing flow of our application

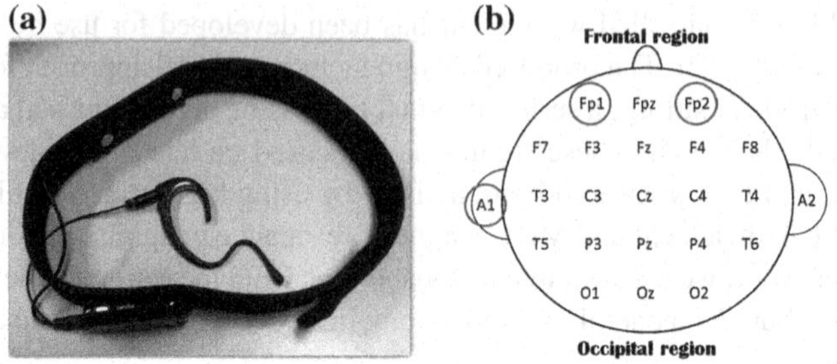

Fig. 4 B-Bridge B3 Band and electrode placements

3.2 Simple EEG Measurement Device

Electric potentials were recorded from the scalp surface by an EEG measurement device; it mainly reflects postsynaptic potentials that occurred in dendritic spines of pyramidal neurons of the cerebral cortex. Figure 4b shows electrode placements for the International 10–20 Standard [8]. Since eye-blink affects EEG during measurement [11], we adopted an algorithm by B3 Band, which enabled to identify and remove artifacts, i.e., signals caused by eye blinks and ocular movements. The size of the B3 Band is 54 mm(L) × 25 mm(W) × 17 mm(H), the weight of it about 100 g. It is a compact, low restraint device. The metal part of the left ear in the B3 Band corresponds to A1 location, and electrodes are mounted on the band part which corresponded to Fp1 and Fp2 locations. Eight indicators of EEG are considered to be correlated with the user's states, e.g., levels of alertness and relaxation. EEG powers of eight frequency bands are believed to be correlated with the mental state, e.g., levels of alertness and relaxation. Degrees of Attention (concentration) and Mediation (relaxation) are calculated, which can be acquired once per second by taking a value of $0 \sim 100$.

4 Analysis of EEG Data

In order to extract user thoughts or behaviors, we used two analysis methods. One is analyzing user thought or behavior patterns by using Support Vector Machine (SVM), the other one is determining brain states by taking a threshold value of the similarity of EEG are calculated by cosine similarity. The threshold value is decided by using Half Total Error Rate (HTER). We also extended these two methods to v-SVM (voting-SVM) and v-HTER (voting-HTER).

4.1 SVM-Based Analysis

Since the generalization capability of SVM is high in class determination [5], we then use it to determine concentration and relaxation states of users with two manners. One is SVM that used EEG indices (Attention and Meditation) per second as inputs into a classifier, which are acquired by a simple EEG device. The other one is o-SVM (order-SVM) that used EEG indices per user's thought time as inputs into a classifier. Outputs of them are concentration and relaxation states. If acquired EEG data are unknown data, its states are determined by using a classifier. Else if acquired EEG data are known learning data, its states are determined by using cross-validation. The determination of the acquired EEG data by using the classifier per second is described as follows:

$$\begin{cases} \textit{concentration if } y_1 > y_2 \\ \quad \textit{relaxation} \qquad \textit{else} \end{cases}$$

Here, the output value of concentration is y_1, the output value of relaxation is y_2, both of them take the real value of $0 \sim 1$.

4.2 HTER-Based Analysis

Chuang et al. [4] proposed an authentication method based on EEG, and confirmed that it has high accuracy. We then used this method to determine concentration and relaxation states of users. Therefore, we first calculate the cosine similarity of each EEG data and its center of gravity, and determine a temporary threshold value by multiple cosine similarities. Each temporary threshold value is calculated by error rate, and the temporary threshold value with the minimum error rate of a classifier is chosen. EEG states are determined by using a group of EEG when users are concentrated or relaxed as follows:

1. Calculating a center of gravity coordinate g_C (g_R) of a group of concentrated (relaxed) EEG by Eq. (1).

$$g_{C(R)} = \left(\frac{\sum_{i=1}^{k} a_i}{k}, \frac{\sum_{i=1}^{k} m_i}{k} \right) \tag{1}$$

   Here, k denotes each data in a group of concentrated (relaxed) EEG. a_i is a value of Attention, and m_i is a value of Meditation.

2. Calculating a cosine similarity of each data $d(k, C)$ ($d(k, R)$) in a concentration (relaxation) group and its g_C (g_R) by Eq. (2).

$$\cos(g_{C(R)}, d(k, C(R))) = \frac{g_{C(R)} \cdot d(k, C(R))}{|g_{C(R)}||d(k, C(R))|} \tag{2}$$

3. Assuming a threshold value Th_{Ck} (Th_{Rk}) of each k of cosine similarity from 2., and the cosine similarity of each data and each center of gravity coordinate is determined by a temporary threshold. The determined results are measured in terms of their *False Acceptance Rate* (FAR_{Ck} or FAR_{Rk}) and *False Rejection Rate* (FRR_{Ck} or FRR_{Rk}).

$$FAR_{Ck(Rk)} = \frac{\#\text{incorrect data are determined as correct}}{\text{Total number of incorrect data}}$$

$$FRR_{Ck(Rk)} = \frac{\#\text{correct data are determined as incorrect}}{\text{Total number of correct data}}$$

4. Calculating the average $HTER_{Ck}$ ($HTER_{Rk}$) of FAR_{Ck} and FRR_{Ck} (FAR_{Rk} and FRR_{Rk}) from 3. by Eq. (3), and the minimum of error rate $HTER_{Ck}$ ($HTER_{Rk}$) as a threshold value $Th2_C$ ($Th2_R$) is decided in a concentration (relaxation) group.

$$HTER_{Ck(Rk)} = \frac{FAR_{Ck(Rk)} + FRR_{Ck(Rk)}}{2} \tag{3}$$

5. Calculating the cosine similarity of measurement data, g_C (g_R) of the concentration (relaxation) group, and a concentration (relaxation) state to be determined if the cosine similarity is more than the decided $Th2_C$ ($Th2_R$) from 4. Here, a threshold value with a low error ratio.

4.3 SVM and HTER Based on Voting Principle

We newly propose a determination method that is based on voting of multiple EEG states by taking a majority decision in whole thought time after determining the EEG state per second. v-SVM utilized voting of the determined results of SVM in one second, and v-HTER utilized voting of the determined results of HTER in one second. The procedure of them is described as follows:

1. We determined EEG states by SVM or HTER in one second.
2. We re-determined the results by using the results from the whole thought time, when the determined number of concentration or relaxation states is max and the voting rate is more than a threshold value Th_v from 1.

5 Evaluation

The purpose of this evaluation was to verify whether our proposed user intention extraction method was useful for helping users to control apps or the contents on smartphones based on their EEG. 7 college students (4 males, 3 females) completed all experiments in a general environment without substantial noisy.

5.1 User Intention Extraction Based on Voice Guidance

We first conducted an experiment to evaluate the performance of our proposed intention extraction method in a condition of voice guidance. In this experiment, our developed EEG measurement application notified information to users by means of voice guidance, and the users did not browse any information on smartphones. There are 6 steps of this experiment as follows:

1. Presenting background images, and running voice guidance
2. Measuring the subjects' EEG for 7 s after voice guidance
3. Extracting EEG for 5 s ($2 \sim 6$) out of the 7 s measurement
4. Labeling the EEG state into concentration or relaxation
5. Determining EEG state per second by using SVM and HTER
6. Re-determining the results of 6. By voting

A black picture was used in order to make no differences for ease of concentration and relaxation. Our developed application provided three kinds of voice guidance, *Do you want to see emails?*, *Do you want to play music?*, and *Do you want to search Web pages?*. All subjects participated in this experiment. In one set of measurement, voice guidance was played 3 times. Then, we acquired 15 EEG data (= 5 s × 3) in one set. We measured a total of 300 EEG data (concentration: 150, relaxation: 150) in twenty sets. Table 1 shows the classification results.

We also used scenery pictures were shown in Fig. 5, since our assumed environment was not only indoor but various outdoor situations. Although a sound is necessary in a real environment, it may introduce unwanted noise into the EEG. Therefore, we only presented scenery pictures to subjects in this experiment as a first step for the study. 4 subjects (*A*, *B*, *C*, *D*; males) participated in this experiment. In one set of measurement, voice guidance was played 3 times, and background images were presented 4 times. Therefore, we acquired 60 EEG data (=5 s × 3 × 4) in one set. We measured a total of 360 EEG data (concentration: 180, relaxation: 180) in six sets. Table 2 shows the classification results by each determination method, and the results can be summarized as follows:

- The accuracy rates of v-SVM in all subjects with a black picture and scenery pictures were higher than those of SVM. The results suggest that v-SVM is useful for improving the accuracy rates.

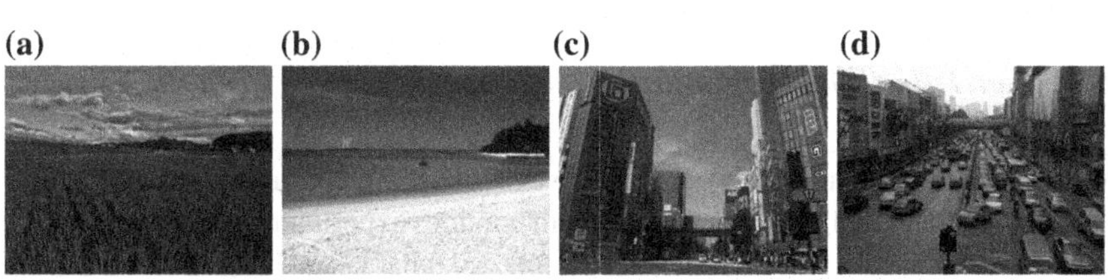

Fig. 5 Examples of scenery pictures

Table 1 Results of intention extraction by presenting a black picture

Subject	SVM (%)	o-SVM (%)	v-SVM (%)	HTER (%)	v-HTER (%)
A	61.0	60.0	**68.3**	60.0	66.7
B	63.3	61.7	**73.3**	59.7	58.3
C	64.0	68.3	**71.7**	63.0	65.0
D	70.0	73.3	**85.0**	63.0	66.7
E	54.0	53.3	**63.3**	60.3	60.0
F	64.7	68.3	**76.7**	61.7	66.7
G	61.0	63.3	**75.0**	66.3	65.0
Average	64.8	64.1	**74.6**	61.4	64.8

Table 2 Results of intention extraction by presenting scenery pictures

Subject (%)	SVM (%)	o-SVM (%)	v-SVM (%)	HTER (%)	v-HTER (%)
A	61.1	56.9	**66.7**	50.0	50.0
B	69.7	70.8	**88.9**	60.0	58.3
C	65.8	63.9	**79.2**	57.2	58.3
D	62.5	61.1	**72.2**	57.2	54.2
Average	64.8	63.2	**76.7**	56.1	55.2

- The accuracy rates of *A* and *D* were higher for the black picture, and those of *B* and *C* were higher for the scenery pictures. This may indicate that the black picture could easily make *A* and *D* concentrated and relaxed, and the scenery pictures could easily make *B* and *C* concentrated and relaxed.
- Compared average accuracy rates of HTER and SVM with a black picture and scenery pictures, the average accuracy rate of HTER was lower than that of SVM. Because we determined the threshold that is corresponded to all data including noise data.

This experiment indicated that our method can identify which picture easily makes the subjects concentrated and relaxed. Our method still has a problem about the determination of the threshold for HTER. Therefore, we conducted the following experiments without the methods using HTER.

5.2 User Intention Extraction Based on Mental Arithmetic

We confirmed that our method was able to extract user intentions by measuring concentration and relaxation states from EEG in previous experiments. In order to realize concentration and relaxation states of subjects, Mizuhara et al. [10] combined simultaneous fMRI (functional magnetic resonance imaging) and EEG measurements

Table 3 Results of intention extraction while walking and standing

Subject	While walking		While standing	
	SVM (%)	v-SVM (%)	SVM (%)	v-SVM (%)
A	80.0	**100.0**	71.7	**91.7**
C	61.7	**75.0**	71.7	**91.7**
G	70.0	**100.0**	83.0	**100.0**
Average	70.6	**91.7**	75.7	**94.5**

during a mental arithmetic task. Since beta synchronization was related to the concentration state, in this experiment, we evaluated user intention extraction during the mental arithmetic task that may easily make users concentrated. For this experiment, there are 4 steps under the eyes closed.

1. Ringing a mental arithmetic start sound
2. Measuring the subjects' EEG (concentration state) for 7 s in a mental arithmetic task (serial subtraction of a random constant from 1000)
3. Ringing a mental arithmetic end sound
4. Measuring the subjects' EEG (relaxation state) for 7 s in a break

In order to verify whether our system can control information at anytime and anywhere. We evaluated our proposed user intention extraction method during a mental arithmetic task while subjects are walking and standing, and compared the accuracy rates across these conditions. Subjects (*A*, *C*; males, *G*; female) participated in this experiment. We extracted only 5 s of EEG from 7 s, and we acquired 10 EEG data (=5 s × 2) in one set. We measured a total of 60 EEG data (concentration: 30, relaxation: 30) in six sets. Measurement environment for *A* and *C* was quiet and less crowded indoor and *G* was quiet and less crowded outdoor.

The experimental results are shown in Table 3. Compared the average accuracy rates of SVM and v-SVM in all subjects between the conditions of walking and standing, the accuracy rate for standing was higher in all subjects, and the results suggest that it is difficult for subjects to control their EEG in the mental arithmetic task while they were moving (e.g., walking).

6 Conclusion and Future Work

In this paper, we developed a novel EEG-based automatic control system for controlling all apps and the contents on smartphones without hands. The experimental results shown that the system has a potential to automatically control information on smartphones by the user intentions from the EEG states.

For future work, we plan to enhance the system based on the experimental results, and the experiments should be carried out in many situations (e.g., driving) with many more subjects of different age groups.

Acknowledgments This work was partially supported by JSPS KAKENHI Grant Numbers 26280042, (C) 15K00162.

References

1. Apple Watch. https://www.apple.com/watch/
2. B-Bridge International B3 Band. http://www.neuro-bridge.com/#!untitled/c4ty
3. Biswas, P., Langdon, P.: A new input system for disabled users involving eye gaze tracker and scanning interface. J. Assit. Technol. **5**(2), 58–67 (2011)
4. Chuang, John, Nguyen, H., Wang, C., Johnson, B.: I think, therefore i am: usability and security of authentication using brainwaves. In: Proceedings of the Financial Cryptography Workshops 2013, pp. 1–16 (2013)
5. Cortes, C., Vapnik, V.: Support vector networks. Mach. Learn. **20**, 273–297 (1995)
6. Google Glass. https://www.google.com/glass/start/
7. House, B., Malkin, J.: The voicebot: a voice controlled robot arm. In: Proceedings of the CHI 2009, pp. 183–192 (2009)
8. Kandel, E.R., Schwartz, H.J., Jessell Thomas, M., Siegelbaum, S.A., Hudspeth, A.J.: Principles of neural science. McGraw-Hill Professional, New York (2012)
9. Lampe, T., L.D.J., Fiederer, M., Voelker, A., Knorr, M., Riedmiller, T., Ball.: A brain-computer interface for high-level remote control of an autonomous, reinforcement-learning-based robotic system for reaching and grasping. In: Proceedings of the IUI 2014, pp. 83–88 (2014)
10. Mizuhara, H., Wang, L., Kobayashi, K., Yamaguchi, Y.: Long-range EEG phase synchronization during an arithmetic task indexes a coherent cortical network simultaneously measured by fMRI. NeuroImage **27**(3), 553–563 (2005)
11. Nakanishi, Isao, Baba, S., Miyamoto, C., Li, S.: Person authentication using a new feature vector of the brain wave. J. Commun. Comput. **9**(1), 101–105 (2012)
12. Yazdani, N., Khazab, F., Fitzgibbon, S., Luerssen, M., Powers, D., Clark, C.R.: Towards a brain-controlled wheelchair prototype. In: Proceedings of the BCS 2010, pp. 453–457 (2010)

Comparative Analysis of Retinal Fundus Images with the Distant Past Images Using a Vessel Extraction Technique

Toshio Modegi, Yoichi Takahashi, Tae Yokoi, Muka Moriyama, Noriaki Shimada, Ikuo Morita and Kyoko Ohno-Matsui

Abstract There are ophthalmological diseases accompanied with remarkable deformation or expansion of posterior shape of eyeballs such as high myopia. We proposed a three-dimensional quantitative analysis tool for posterior shape of eyeballs without invasion using 3D-MRI. In order to progress a further research of this disease, a long-term follow-up study is important. We have tried to analyze a collection of retinal images including several photographs shot about 20–30 years ago. However, it is difficult to correct the past images more than 20 year ago for comparing them with recent images of the same case, only by photographical parameters. Therefore, we have developed a registration tool for retinal images by aligning vessel patterns extracted from retinal images for comparative analysis. Using this tool, we have tried 150 pairs of retinal images in high myopia cases, and vessel patterns of 136 pairs could be properly extracted and used for registration.

Keywords Retinal fundus image · Temporal subtraction · Comparative analysis · Vessel extraction · Long-term follow-up · High myopia

1 Introduction

There are ophthalmological diseases accompanied with remarkable deformation or expansion of posterior shape of eyeball such as the high myopia. We proposed a three-dimensional quantitative analysis tool for posterior shape of eyeballs without

T. Modegi (✉) · Y. Takahashi
Advanced Business Center, Dai Nippon Printing Co.Ltd, 1-1-1, Ichigaya-Kagacho Shinjuku-Ku, Tokyo 162-8001, Japan
e-mail: Modegi-T@mail.dnp.co.jp

T. Yokoi · M. Moriyama · N. Shimada · I. Morita · K. Ohno-Matsui
Department of Ophthalmology and Visual Science, Tokyo Medical and Dental University Graduate School of Medicine and Dental Sciences, 1-5-45, Yushima, Bunkyo-Ku Tokyo 113-8510, Japan

Y.-W. Chen et al. (eds.), *Innovation in Medicine and Healthcare 2015*,
Smart Innovation, Systems and Technologies 45,
DOI 10.1007/978-3-319-23024-5_51

invasion using 3D-MRI [1]. Using this tool, we can classify eyeballs of high myopia by 4 kinds of three-dimensional measured parameters as axial length, posterior roundness, horizontal or vertical symmetry [1]. In order to progress a further research of this disease, a long-term follow-up study is also important. As it is difficult to carry out a retrospective study using 3D-MR images, we have tried to use a collection of retinal images including several photographs shot about 20–30 years ago. Although there have been several retrospective trials of temporal subtraction of retinal images, their follow-up period has been limited to less than 10 years [2]. By the Littman's method [3], we can correct each retinal image to the standard scale for measurement of some area or comparison with the others. But in order to apply this correcting method, we need optical parameters of the eyeballs shot in the analyzing images such as an axial length, a kerato-level and a corneal curvature. Moreover, there is a limitation that refraction index of the eyeball must be less than—12D (diopter) for the scaling correction to work properly. This condition makes difficult to apply it to retinal images of high myopia cases. Therefore it is difficult to correct the past images more than 20 year ago for comparing them with recent images of the same case, only by photographical parameters.

We have prototyped a registration tool for retinal images by overlaying two kinds of gray-scale images converted from full-color retinal images for comparative analysis [4]. We assume that outline of major vessel patterns in a retina will not be changed for lifelong unless an eyeball is externally injured. Using this tool we can align two retinal images by adjusting interactively duplicated vessel patterns viewed in gray-sale images [4]. However, it is difficult to determine properly aligned conditions, which are scale, angle and position parameters of either of two comparing images, and we cannot obtain numerical matched levels of two kinds of vessel patterns duplicated. In this paper, we propose an improved registration tool for retinal images by overlaying two kinds of vessel patterns extracted from full-color retinal images for comparative analysis. From the following sections, we describe an overview of our developed tool, an algorithm of our proposing vessel extraction and experimental results by using this tool.

2 Overview of Proposed Method

Figure 1 shows a basic structure of our developed registration tool for retinal images, and an example of registration of two retinal images of the same patient's eyeball. This example indicates trying to align the past image shown in right, which was the image scanned from the 35-mm film recorded in 1989, with the recent image shown in the left, which has been shot in digital in 2014. In order to compare these images we have proposed using a vessel extraction for registration as shown in the flow-chart at the left of Fig. 1. There have been several works using a vessel extraction for registration between fundus images and OCT images such as [5, 6],

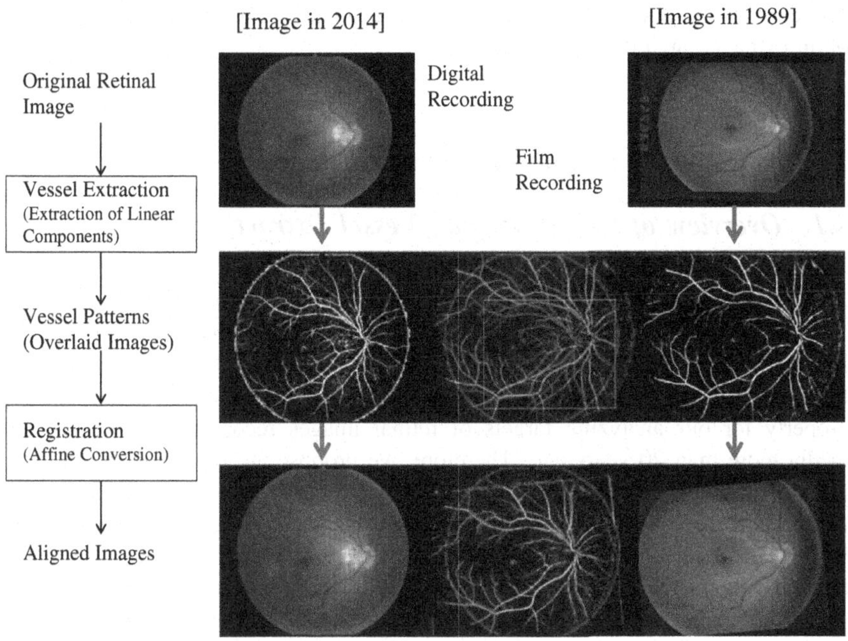

Fig. 1 Proposing registration tool for retinal images by aligning vessel patterns

but the temporal interval of shooting between images was not so long as what we are trying to.

The specific algorithm of the vessel extraction shown at the first part of the flow-chart in Fig. 1, will be described in next section. The registration process shown at the second part of the flow-chart in Fig. 1 is basically using the affine conversion proposed in [4], which is correcting the past image by scaling in the X-axis or Y-axis direction, rotating and moving in the X-Y plane in order to align it with the recent image. In order to carry out these aligning operations interactively, we have proposed creating overlaid image from two kinds of vessel extracted images as shown in the two pseudo-color images located at the middle in the two sets of three-series images in Fig. 1. These pseudo-color images are mixed by the left extracted image colored in red with the right extracted image colored in green. Therefore, duplicated areas of two extracted images can be recognized as yellow parts.

During or after interactive aligning operations, we can evaluate numerically matched level of duplicated areas in these pseudo-color images. We provide two kinds of numerical parameters of matched level as a matched ratio and a correlation coefficient. The matched ratio is defined as a ratio of a duplicated extracted area by a total extracted area of either image with less extracted area. The correlation coefficient is known as a normalized correlation coefficient in duplicated areas between two images. The latter calculated value is generally less influenced by size of an extracted area than the former one.

3 Proposing Algorithm of a Vessel Extraction

3.1 Overview of Our Proposing Vessel Extraction

As for the vessel extraction, there have been several proposals such as [7–9], and two major development projects of vessel extraction named as the STARE [10] in the U.S. and DRIVE [11] in the K.N. have been promoted. However, we have found these previously proposed algorithms of extraction were not working properly for our analyzing targets of retinal images recorded in miscellaneous media more than 20 years ago. Therefore, we propose an improved algorithm of the vessel extraction as shown in Fig. 2. In the first process of (A) Gray-scale Conversion from a full-color retinal image consisting of RGB components, we have tried to include blue-components, which most of the previously proposed method ignored [7–11]. More specifically, as a gray-scale value, we use a geometric mean-value of a green-component and a negative blue-component instead of using only a green-component. The second process of the (B) Top-hat

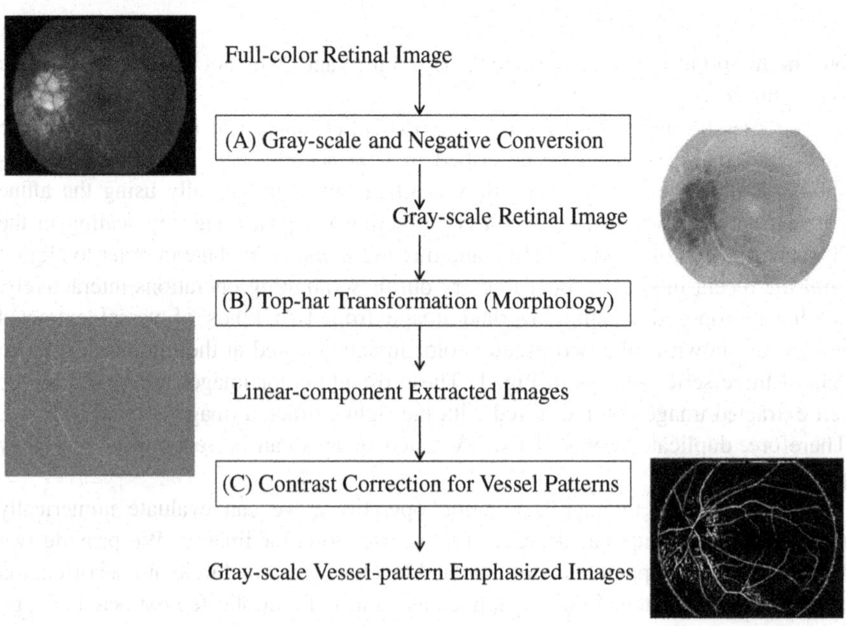

Fig. 2 Proposing algorithm of vessel extraction for retinal images

Transformation consists of emphasizing of linear components and deemphasizing of granular components, whose basic idea is based on the morphology filter-bank proposed in [7]. We have originally designed the structuring elements for these morphology operations in more effective way. The specific algorithm will be described in the next sub-section. In the third process of (C) Contrast Correction for vessel patterns, we propose extracted patterns by expressing 256-level gray-scale image, in order for level of each pixel to indicate probability of included level in vessel areas, based on histogram calculations of pixel values.

3.2 Proposing Top-Hat Transformation

Figure 3 shows detailed algorithm of the (B) Top-hat Transformation shown in Fig. 2. At first, the Linear-component Emphasized Image L is created from the Gray-scale Converted Retinal Image by a morphology process of the (B1) Opening Operation by Linear Structure. This morphology process is based on the proposed in [7, 8], but we use our designed set of linear structuring elements described later. As the created image L includes a lot of granular components, we extract non-linear

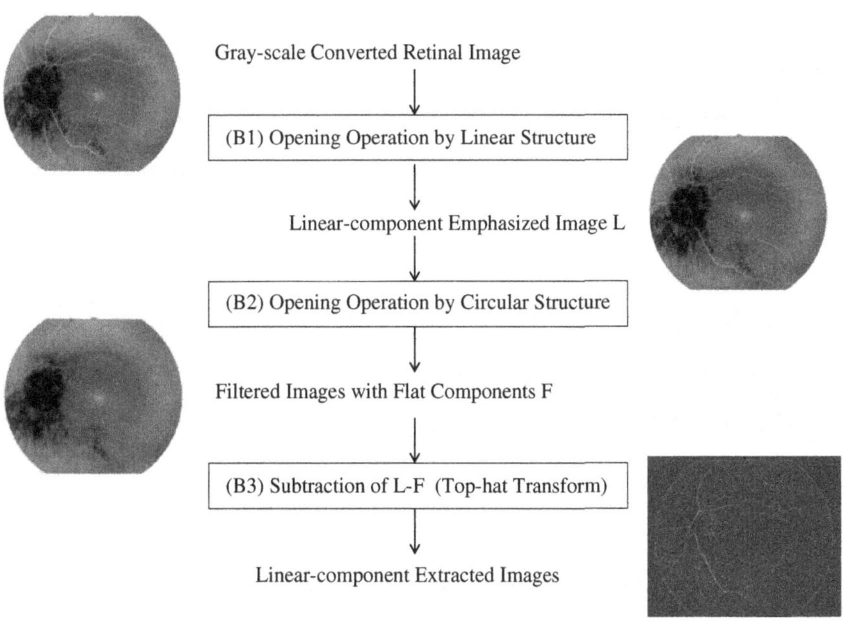

Fig. 3 Proposing algorithm of top-hat transformation for vessel extraction

component from it in the morphology process of the (B2) Opening Operation by Circular Structure. In this process we use a set of circular structuring elements described later, and create the Filtered Images with Flat Components F. Finally, by subtraction of the secondly created image F from the firstly created image L, granular components included in the Linear-component Emphasized Image L can be reduced. Thus we can obtain the Linear-component Extracted Images.

3.3 Proposing Opening Operations

The two opening operations shown in Fig. 3 are specifically illustrated as Fig. 4, which is a detailed flow-chart description of Fig. 3. An opening operation is generally known as a set of erosion-operations and dilation-operations. An erosion-operation is replacing value of a target pixel with the minimum value of the near pixels inside the defined region such as $\pm 7 \times \pm 7$ pixels. A dilation-operation is replacing value of a target pixel with the maximum value of the near pixels inside the defined region such as $\pm 7 \times \pm 7$ pixels. By these consecutive two operations, tiny granular noises less than 7×7 pixels can be removed. The near pixels referred to these operations are controlled by a set of structuring elements.

In case of the (B1) Opening Operation by Linear Structure, we use 8 sets of linear-directed structuring elements shown in Fig. 5. From a single image of the

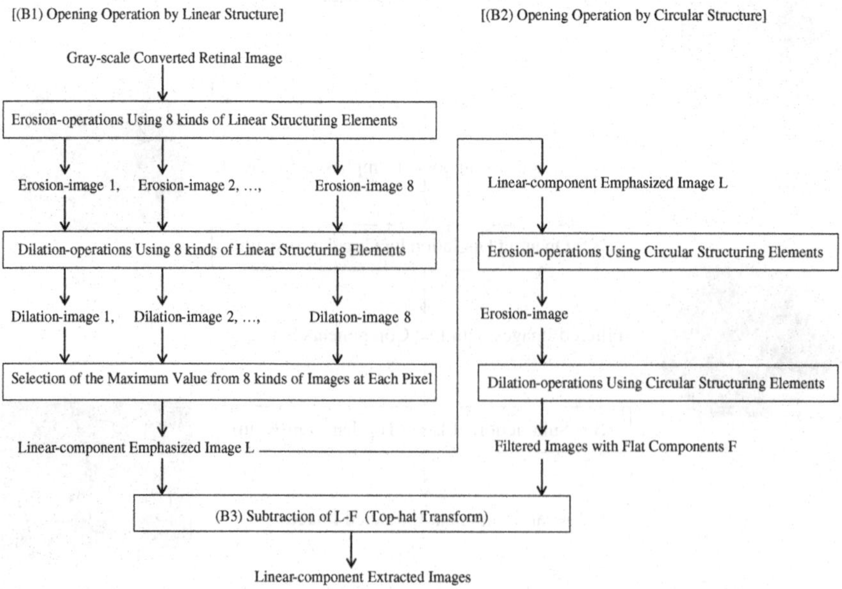

Fig. 4 Detailed algorithm of top-hat transformation for vessel extraction

Fig. 5 Proposing set of hybrid structure elements for vessel extraction

0	0	0	0	0	0	0	110	0	0	0	0	0	0	0
0	0	0	0	120	100	100	110	100	100	108	0	0	0	0
0	0	0	100	120	100	100	110	100	100	108	100	0	0	0
0	0	100	140	100	120	100	110	100	108	100	104	100	0	0
0	180	180	100	140	120	100	110	100	108	104	100	102	102	0
0	100	100	180	180	140	120	110	108	104	102	102	100	100	0
0	100	100	100	100	180	1E0	110	10E	102	100	100	100	100	0
101	101	101	101	101	101	101	1FF	101	101	101	101	101	101	101
0	100	100	100	100	102	10E	110	1E0	180	100	100	100	100	0
0	100	100	102	102	104	108	110	120	140	180	180	100	100	0
0	102	102	100	104	108	100	110	100	120	140	100	180	180	0
0	0	100	104	100	108	100	110	100	120	100	140	100	0	0
0	0	0	100	108	100	100	110	100	100	120	100	0	0	0
0	0	0	0	108	100	100	110	100	100	120	0	0	0	0
0	0	0	0	0	0	0	110	0	0	0	0	0	0	0

Gray-scale Converted Retinal Image, 8 kinds of erosion-images and dilation-images referring to 8 kinds of structuring elements are created respectively. By selection of the maximum value from 8 kinds of dilation-images at each pixel, a single image of the Linear-component Emphasized Image L is generated. In case of the (B2) Opening Operation by Circular Structure, we use a set of circular structuring elements shown in Fig. 5. From a single image of the Linear-component Emphasized Image L, a set of an erosion-image and a dilation-image referring to a set of structuring elements are created respectively. Thus we can obtain the Filtered Images with Flat Components F.

Figure 5 shows our designed structuring elements for $\pm 7 \times \pm 7$ nearest pixel-operations, which function as both 8 sets of linear-directed structuring elements and a set of circular structuring elements. By logical AND operations of given control value with each hexadecimal value of the 15×15 matrix, we can determine whether the corresponding pixel should be referred or not during morphology operations such as erosion or dilation. More specifically, if value of logical AND of each element with given control value is not zero, the corresponding pixel of the element is referred to a morphology operation, otherwise it is not referred to. In case of the (B1) Opening Operation by Linear Structure, we give 8 kinds of hexadecimal control values as 1, 2, 4, 8, 10, 20, 40, and 80, and 8 kinds of matrices are generated for linear-directed structuring elements. Whereas, in case of the (B2) Opening Operation by Circular Structure, we give a single hexadecimal control value of 100, and a single matrix is generated for circular structuring elements.

3.4 Evaluation of Proposing Method by Comparison with the Previously Proposed Methods

Figure 6 shows 4 kinds of vessel extracted images from the full-color retinal image shown at the top-left in Fig. 2, processed by the 3 kinds of previously proposed methods and by our proposed method in this paper. Figure 6a is an extracted image using the software tool developed by the STARE project [10]. In this method, all of vessel patterns are converted to thin lines whose width is a single pixel including excessively extracted granular patterns. For this type of a binary image, it is difficult to evaluate numerically extracted vessel patterns. Figure 6b is an extracted image by our developed tool based on the conventional gray-scale conversion methods [7–11], which are using only green components in a full-color retinal image. As shown in Fig. 6b, these methods are likely to be influenced by lighting bias, and it is difficult to extract vessels located in the outskirts of the image. Figure 6c is an extracted image by our developed tool based on the simple top-hat transformation proposed by [8]. There are more granular components left than the image of Fig. 6d, which is extracted by our proposed method in this paper.

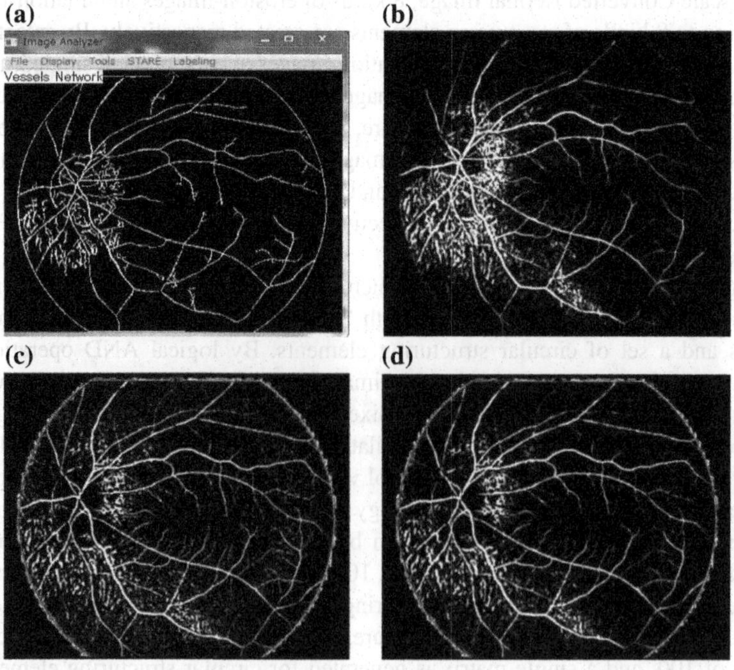

Fig. 6 Evaluation of proposing method by comparison with 3 kinds of vessel extracted, **a** Extracted using by the softwaretool of the STARE Project [10], **b** Extracted based on the gray-conversionusing only green components [7–11], **c** Extracted by the simple Tophattransformation [8], **d** Extracted by the proposedmethod in this paper

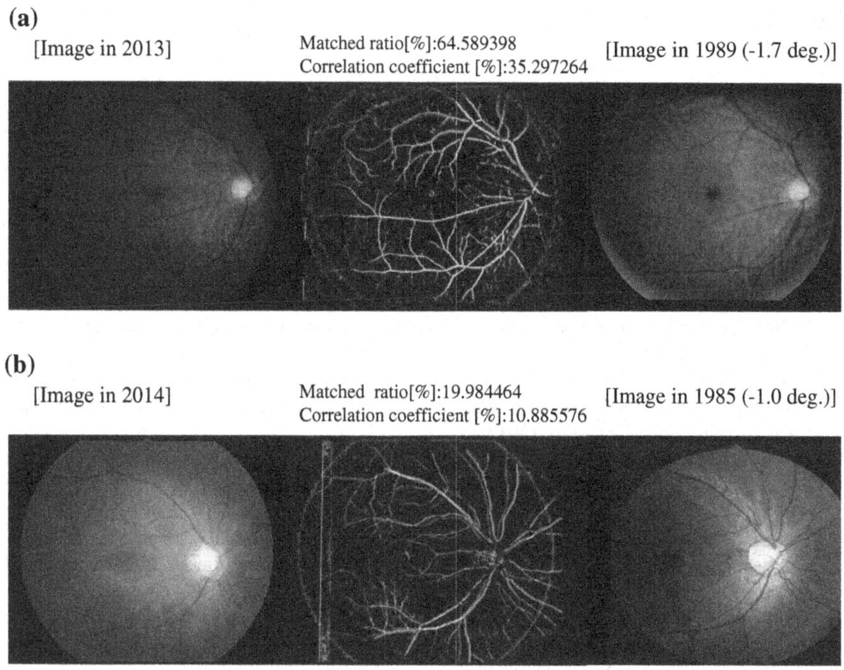

Fig. 7 Two analyzed examples of a well matched case and an Ill matched case, **a** Well matched case, **b** Ill matched case

4 Conclusions

Using this tool, we have tried 150 pairs of retinal images in high-myopia cases and 22 pairs of retinal images in non high-myopia cases, whose pairs consist of a recently shot image and a past image shot 20–30 years ago. Figure 7 shows two analyzed examples of a well matched case and an ill matched case chosen from the 150 analyzed pairs. As shown in the upper-right of the two pairs of images, each of the past images has been rotated −1.7°and −1.0° for alignment, respectively. The two pairs of numerical data shown in the middle of Fig. 7 are calculated values of the matched ratio and the correlation coefficient, whose definitions have been described in the former Sect. 2.

Vessel patterns of 136 pairs in the total 150 high-myopia cases and all 22 pairs of retinal images in non high-myopia cases could be properly extracted and used for registration. Although it seems to be difficult to extract vessel patterns from all of given retinal images completely, we are going to improve our developed analysis tool in order for some of 14 pairs failed in this experiment to be properly analyzed in the future.

References

1. Modegi, T., Kondo J., Takahashi, Y., Moriyama, M., Ohno-Matsui, K., Morita, I.: Trial of high myopia disease classification using MRI and prototyping of image analysis software. In: Proceeding of SICE Annual Conference, pp. 1841–1848, (2012)
2. Nakazawa, M., Kurotaki, J., Ruike, H.: Longterm findings in peripapillary crescent formation in eyes with mild or moderate myopia. Acta Opthalmologica **86**, 626–629 (2008)
3. Bengtsson, B., Krakau, C.: Correction of optic disc measurements on fundus photographs. Graefe's Arch. Clinical Exp. Ophthalmol. **230**, 24–28 (1992)
4. Modegi, T., Kondo J., Takahashi, Y., Yokoi, T., Moriyama, M., Ohno, K., Morita, I.: Image correction techniques for time series analysis of fundus photographs. In: Proceeding Of the 127th Conference of Japanese Society of Printing Science and Technology, A-17, pp. 78–83, (2012) (in Japanese)
5. Golabbakhsh, M., Rabbani, H: Vessel-based registration of fundus and optical coherence tomography projection images of retina using a quadratic registration model. IET J. Mag. Image Process. **7**(8), 768–776, (2013)
6. Fang, B., Hsu, W., Lee, M.L.: Techniques for temporal registration of retinal images. In: Porceeding of IEEE International Conference on Image Processing, vol. 2, pp. 1089–1092, (2004)
7. Uruma, S., Uchiyama, Y., Prochazka, Z.,Hatanaka, Y., Muramatsu, C., Hara. T., Fujita, H., Shiraishi, J.: Computerized extraction of vessel regions in retinal fundus images. In: IEICE Technical Report, MI2011-134, vol. 111, No. 389, pp. 315–318, (2012) (in Japanese)
8. Tohma, E., Misawa, H., Suetake, N., Uchino, E.: Extraction of blood vessels in retinal images by black-top-hat transformation using structuring elements with various radii. In: Proceeding of 28th Fuzzy System Symposium, FL2-2, pp. 137–140, (2012) (in Japanese)
9. Salazar-Gonzalez, A., Kaba, D., Yongmin, L., Xiaohui, L.: Segmentation of the blood vessels and optic disk in retinal images. IEEE J. Biomed. Health Inform. **18**(6), 1874–1886 (2014)
10. STARE (STructured Analysis of the Retina): Project, by U.S. National Institutes of Health. http://www.ces.clemson.edu/~ahoover/stare/. Accessed March 2015
11. DRIVE (Digital Retinal Images for Vessel Extraction) Project. http://www.isi.uu.nl/Research/Databases/DRIVE/. Accessed March 2015

Interactive Segmentation of Pancreases from Abdominal CT Images by Use of the Graph Cut Technique with Probabilistic Atlases

Takenobu Suzuki, Hotaka Takizawa, Hiroyuki Kudo and Toshiyuki Okada

Abstract This paper proposes a method of interactive segmentation of pancreases from abdominal CT images based on the anatomical knowledge of medical doctors as well as the statistical information of pancreases. This method is composed of two phases: training and testing. In the training phase, pancreas regions are manually extracted from sample CT images, and then a probabilistic atlas of pancreases is constructed from the extracted regions. In the testing phase, a medical doctor selects seed voxels for a pancreas and background in a test image. The probabilistic atlas is translated so that the atlas and the seeds are fitted as much as possible. The graph cut technique whose data term is weighted by the probabilistic atlas is applied to the test image. The seed selection, the atlas translation and the graph cut are executed iteratively. This doctor-in-the-loop segmentation method is applied to actual abdominal CT images, and experimental results are shown.

Keywords Abdominal CT image · Pancreas · Interactive organ segmentation · Probabilistic atlas · Graph cut

1 Introduction

Pancreatic diseases, such as pancreas cancers, have high mortality rate worldwide [1]. In order to decrease the mortality rate, such diseases should be detected by medical doctors in their early stages, and then treated adequately. Abdominal CT images are widely used for their early detection, but it is difficult for medical doctors to

T. Suzuki (✉)
Department of Computer Science, Graduate School of Systems and Information Engineering, University of Tsukuba, Ibaraki, Japan
e-mail: suzuki@mibel.cs.tsukuba.ac.jp

H. Takizawa · H. Kudo
Faculty of Engineering, Information and Systems, University of Tsukuba, Ibaraki, Japan

T. Okada
Faculty of Medicine, University of Tsukuba, Ibaraki, Japan

Y.-W. Chen et al. (eds.), *Innovation in Medicine and Healthcare 2015*,
Smart Innovation, Systems and Technologies 45,
DOI 10.1007/978-3-319-23024-5_52

diagnose a large amount of abdominal CT images in a limited time. Therefore, it is necessary to build a computer-aided diagnosis (CAD) system that has functions to assist medical doctors in diagnosing abdominal CT images. One of the most important functions is to segment pancreas regions from abdominal CT images.

There are two types of segmentation method: automatic segmentation [2] and interactive segmentation. Park et al. proposed an automatic segmentation method that extracted a target organ from a test CT image by using a probabilistic atlas constructed from training CT images [3]. Heimann et al. proposed a method that constructed a statistical shape model from training CT images, and then used the model as a priori information to segment a target organ [4]. These automatic segmentation methods can work well if the target organ in a test CT image have the similar properties (e.g., sizes, shapes and intensities) to organs in training CT images. However, if they have different properties, they would fail to extract the target organ from the test image.

In an interactive method, on the other hand, a medical doctor can flexibly deal with such irregular organs by giving several clues, such as seed voxels, to a CAD system on the basis of his/her anatomical knowledge. The CAD system can use such information for more accurate segmentation. In a live wire technique [5], a user puts seed points along the boundary of a target object. Then, the Dijkstra's algorithm is executed to obtain the shortest path between each defined points. This technique can be applied only to two-dimensional images, and requires many seed points when an object boundary is subtle or noisy. Another live wire technique [6] can be applied to three-dimensional images by use of automatic interpolation, but this method requires a lot of interactive specifications. The active contour model is introduced by Kass et al. [7]. In this method, an energy function is defined to evaluate the fidelity between a target object and a contour model in an image. This method often provides the sub-optimal contour which corresponds to a local minimum of the energy function. The level set [8] also provides the sub-optimal contour, and it is difficult to modify the sub-optimal contour intuitively. Grady [9] proposed an interactive segmentation method based on a random walk technique. In this method, first, a user defines voxels for K-labels. The probabilities that unlabeled voxels reach each of the defined labels are calculated, and a label with the greatest probability for each unlabeled voxels is determined as the segmentation result. This method can obtain arbitrary contours through user-system interaction, and perform well even with ambiguous or discontinuous boundaries. However, the segmentation result is still sub-optimal.

The graph cut methods [10–12], which are focused in this paper, can obtain the globally optimal contour from seed voxels which are interactively selected by a user. The problem of the conventional graph cut method is that it doesn't make use of a priori knowledge of the properties of target objects. For example, pancreases have particular sizes and shapes though their variety is very wide. By using such a priori knowledge adequately, the segmentation accuracy can be increased.

This paper proposes a method of interactive segmentation of pancreases from abdominal CT images based on the anatomical knowledge of medical doctors as well as the statistical information of pancreases. This method is composed of two phases: training and testing. In the training phase, pancreas regions are manually extracted from sample CT images, and then a probabilistic atlas of pancreases is constructed from the extracted regions. In the testing phase, a medical doctor selects seed voxels for a pancreas and background in a test image. The probabilistic atlas is translated so that the atlas and the seeds are fitted as much as possible. The graph cut technique whose data term is weighted by the probabilistic atlas is applied to the test image. The seed selection, the atlas translation and the graph cut are executed iteratively. This doctor-in-the-loop segmentation method is applied to actual abdominal CT images.

2 Method

Figure 1 shows the algorithm of the proposed method. First, a probabilistic atlas of a pancreas is constructed from training CT images. A medical doctor selects seed voxels for a pancreas and background from a test image. The probabilistic atlas is fitted to the seed voxels by translating the atlas. The graph cut technique whose data term is weighted by the probabilistic atlas is applied to the test image. These processes are iterated until the target region is segmented sufficiently.

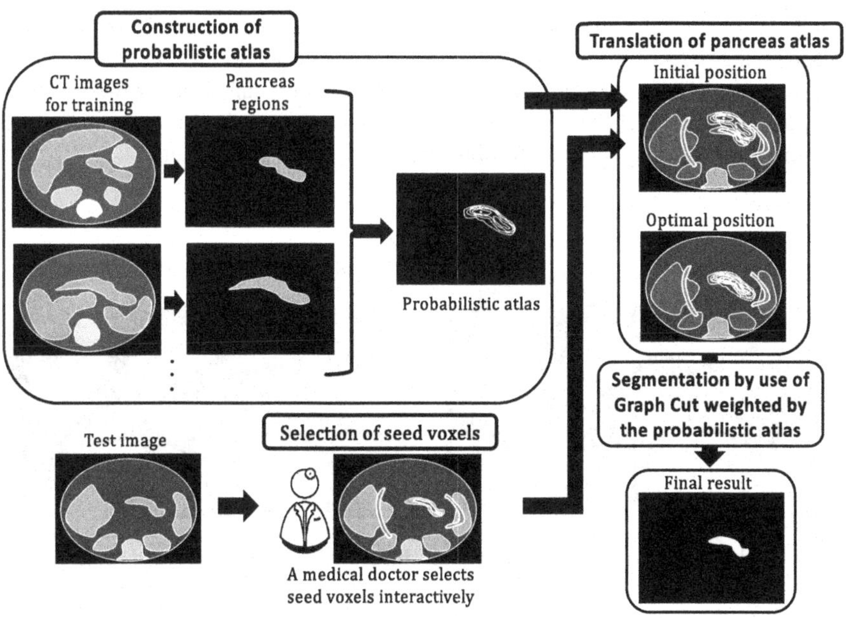

Fig. 1 The algorithm of the proposed method

2.1 Construction of Probabilistic Atlas

A probabilistic atlas is an image each of whose voxels contains the probability of a hypothesis that the voxel is inside a target organ. First, pancreas regions are manually extracted from training CT images. Rectangular-solid volumes of interest (VOIs) which circumscribe the pancreas regions are set to the CT images. The images are resampled so that the VOI sizes are $S_x \times S_y \times S_z$ voxels. By applying the signed distance transform filter to the normalized images, positive and negative values are assigned to voxels of pancreas and background, respectively. The probability of each voxel being inside a pancreas is calculated by the following Sigmoid function:

$$\varsigma_a(d) = \frac{1}{1 + e^{-ad}}, \qquad (1)$$

where d is a signed distance value, and a is a gain parameter. Finally, a probabilistic atlas is obtained by averaging the probability values of the corresponding voxels over the training CT images.

2.2 Selection of Seed Voxels

A medical doctor selects the seed voxels of a pancreas and background from a test CT image on the basis of his/her anatomical knowledge of organs. We build a graphical user interface (GUI) software by which a medical doctor can easily browse an arbitrary slice in a test CT image and select seed voxels. Figure 2a shows an abdominal CT image for testing, and Fig. 2b shows the examples of seed voxels.

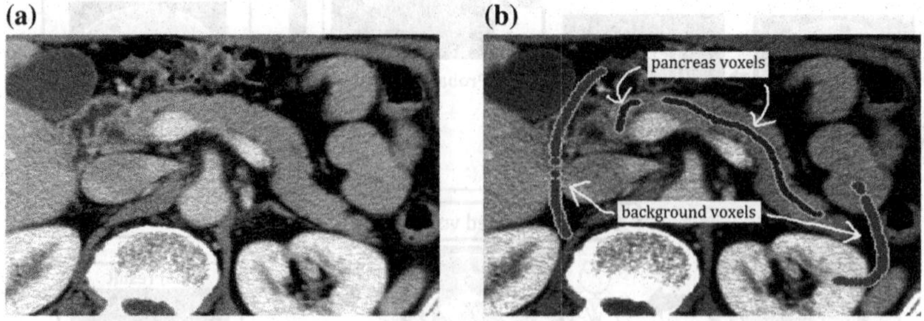

Fig. 2 Seed voxels on a test image. **a** Test image. **b** Seed voxels of a pancreas and background

2.3 Translation of Pancreas Atlas

The probabilistic atlas is fitted to the seed voxels by translating the atlas along the x, y, and z directions. Let $A(x, y, z)$ denote the value of a voxel at (x, y, z) in the probabilistic atlas. $S(x, y, z)$ is defined as

$$S(x,y,z) = \begin{cases} -1 & if\ (x,y,x)\ \in pancreas\,seeds, \\ \alpha & if\ (x,y,x)\ \in background\,seeds, \\ 0 & otherwise, \end{cases} \tag{2}$$

where α is a coefficient for background. First, the probabilistic atlas is translated so that the gravity point of the atlas is set to the center point of the pancreas seeds. From this initial position, the atlas is further translated by minimizing the following energy function:

$$E(t_x, t_y, t_z) = \sum_{x,y,z} A(x + t_x, y + t_y, z + t_z) \cdot S(x, y, z), \tag{3}$$

where t_x, t_y, t_z are the translation along the x, y, and z directions, respectively. The energy function evaluates the fidelity between the atlas and the seeds. As the overlapped areas between the atlas and the seeds are larger, the energy becomes smaller. The optimal translation is obtained by updating the following function:

$$\begin{bmatrix} t_x^{(n+1)} \\ t_y^{(n+1)} \\ t_z^{(n+1)} \end{bmatrix} = \begin{bmatrix} t_x^{(n)} \\ t_y^{(n)} \\ t_z^{(n)} \end{bmatrix} - \gamma \cdot grad\ E^{(n)}(t_x, t_y, t_z), \tag{4}$$

where γ is a coefficient. $grad\ E^{(n)}(t_x, t_y, t_z)$ is obtained by

$$grad\ E^{(n)}(t_x, t_y, t_z) = \left(\frac{\partial E}{\partial t_x}, \frac{\partial E}{\partial t_y}, \frac{\partial E}{\partial t_z} \right)^T$$

$$= \begin{bmatrix} \sum_{x,y,z} S(x,y,z) \cdot \frac{\partial A(x+t_x, y+t_y, z+t_z)}{\partial t_x} \\ \sum_{x,y,z} S(x,y,z) \cdot \frac{\partial A(x+t_x, y+t_y, z+t_z)}{\partial t_y} \\ \sum_{x,y,z} S(x,y,z) \cdot \frac{\partial A(x+t_x, y+t_y, z+t_z)}{\partial t_z} \end{bmatrix}. \tag{5}$$

$\frac{\partial A(x+t_x, y+t_y, z+t_z)}{\partial t_x}$ represents an image obtained by applying the differential filter with respect to the x direction. The optimally translated atlas is denoted by $A^*(x, y, z)$.

Figure 3 shows an example of atlas translation. The probabilistic values are represented by contours in the figures. Figure 3a, b shows the atlas at the initial and the

(a) (b)

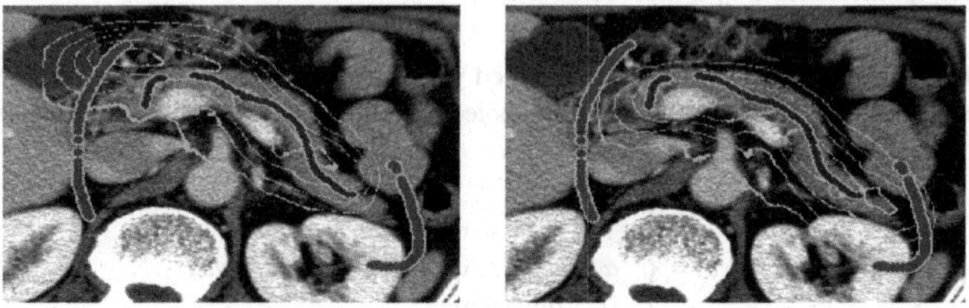

Fig. 3 Translation of a probabilistic atlas. **a** Probabilistic atlas at the initial position. **b** Probabilistic atlas at the optimal position

optimal positions, respectively. The figure demonstrates that the probabilistic atlas can be well fitted to the pancreas seeds by the translation.

2.4 Segmentation by Use of Graph Cut Technique

Let $p \in P$ denote a voxel in a test CT image, and $\omega_p = \{pnc, bkg\} \in \Omega$ denote a label assigned to a voxel p. *pnc* and *bkg* represent a pancreas and background, respectively. The energy function of graph cut [11, 12] is defined as

$$E(\Omega) = B(\Omega) + \lambda \cdot R(\Omega). \tag{6}$$

$B(\Omega)$ is a smoothing term defined as follows:

$$B(\Omega) = \sum_{\{p,q\} \in N} B_{\{p,q\}} \cdot \delta(\omega_p, \omega_q), \tag{7}$$

where,

$$B_{\{p,q\} \in N} = \exp\left(-\frac{(v_p - v_q)^2}{dist(p,q)} \right), \tag{8}$$

$$\delta(\omega_p, \omega_q) = \begin{cases} 1 & if\ \omega_p \neq \omega_q, \\ 0 & otherwise. \end{cases} \tag{9}$$

N represents the neighborhood relationship between voxels, and v_p is the value of a voxel p. $R(\Omega)$ is a data term defined as follows:

$$R(\Omega) = \sum_{p \in P} R_p(\omega_p), \tag{10}$$

and $R_p(\omega_p)$ is defined by

$$R_p(pnc) = -ln\ Pr(v_p|\ pnc\ ), \tag{11}$$

$$R_p(bkg) = -ln\ Pr(v_p|\ bkg\ ). \tag{12}$$

$Pr(v_p|\ pnc\ )$ and $Pr(v_p|\ bkg\ )$ are the conditional probabilities of the voxel values given a pancreas and background, respectively. These conditional probabilities are calculated from the histograms of pancreas and background seeds, respectively.

2.5 Data Term Weighting with Probabilistic Atlas

The graph cut whose data term is weighted by the optimal probabilistic atlas $A^*(x, y, z)$ is applied to the test CT image. The atlas is used as a priori probability to obtain posteriori probabilities of pancreases and background given v_p in the following formulas:

$$Pr(pnc\ |v_p) \propto Pr(v_p|\ pnc) \cdot A^*(x, y, z), \tag{13}$$

$$Pr(bkg\ |v_p) \propto Pr(v_p|\ bkg) \cdot \{1 - A^*(x, y, z)\}. \tag{14}$$

By replacing the conditional probabilities in Eqs. (11) and (12) with posterior probabilities in formulas (13) and (14), respectively, the probabilistic atlas is used as a weighting factor in the data term in the graph cut based segmentation.

3 Experiment and Results

We use fifteen abdominal CT scans, which are provided by the Japanese Society of Medical Imaging Technology [13]. Pancreas regions are manually extracted by the authors, and are used as ground truth in this study. We use the leave-one-out method to compare the segmentation accuracy between the conventional graph cut technique and the proposed method. The segmentation accuracy is evaluated by use of the following Jaccard index:

$$JI(A, B) = \frac{|A \cap B|}{|A \cup B|}, \tag{15}$$

where A is the ground truth and B is an extracted region. The JI value is 1 if A and B are the same, and 0 if A and B are completely different from each other. In this paper, the segmentation of the two methods are conducted by using the same seed voxels. Figure 4a shows the ground truth, Fig. 4b is the result of the conventional graph cut, and Fig. 4c is the result of the proposed method. Figure 4 indicates that

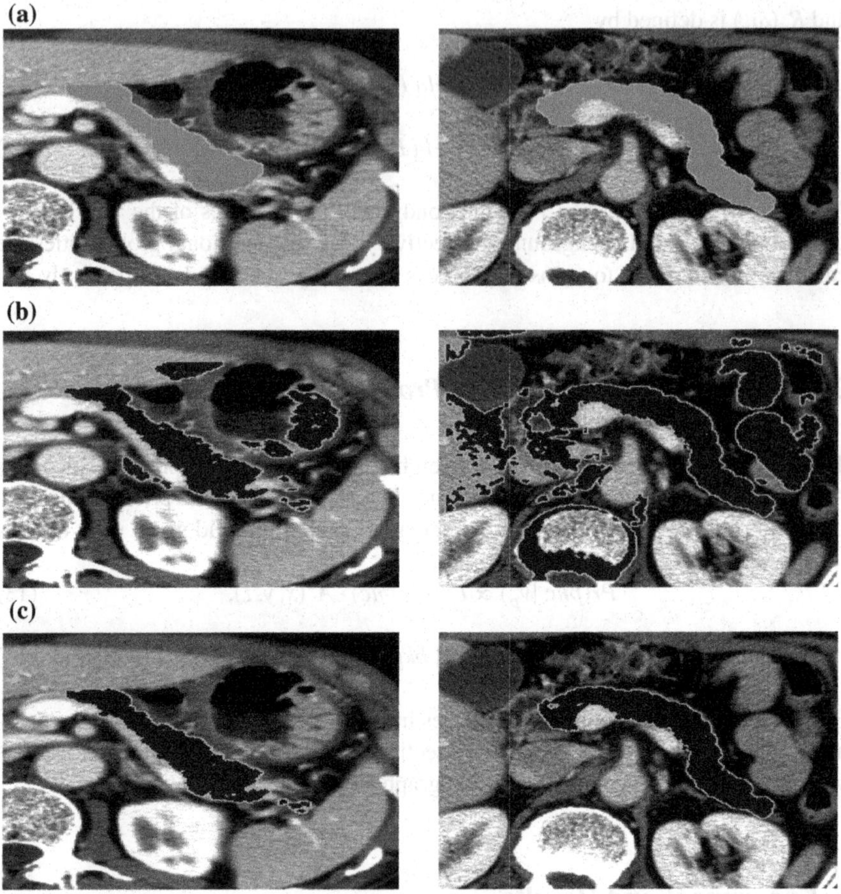

Fig. 4 Comparison of the results between the conventional graph cut and the proposed method. **a** Ground truth. **b** Results of the conventional graph cut (*left* JI = 0.4, *right* JI = 0.16). **c** Results of the proposed method (*left* JI = 0.78, *right* JI = 0.78)

the result of the proposed method is more accurate than that of the conventional graph cut. Figure 5 shows the Jaccard indexes of the conventional graph cut and the proposed method for fifteen subjects. The proposed method is more accurate than the conventional graph cut in every CT scans. The mean Jaccard index of the conventional graph cut is $0.433(\sigma = 0.158)$, whereas that of the proposed method is $0.705(\sigma = 0.054)$. The Jaccard index of the proposed method is significantly higher than that of the conventional graph cut ($p < 0.001$).

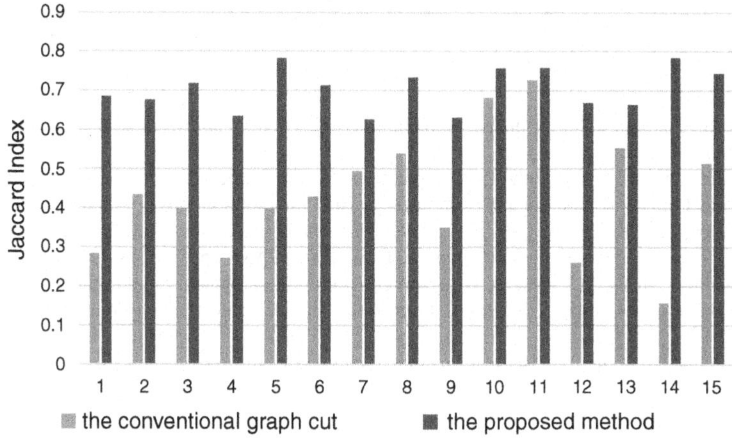

Fig. 5 Comparison of JI between the conventional graph cut and the proposed method

4 Conclusion

This paper proposed a method of interactive segmentation of pancreases from abdominal CT images based on the anatomical knowledge as well as the statistical information of pancreases. The proposed method used the graph cut algorithm whose data term was weighted by the probabilistic atlas constructed beforehand. The proposed method was applied to actual CT images, and compared with the segmentation method based on the conventional graph cut. The experimental results demonstrated that the proposed method was more accurate than the conventional graph cut.

One of our future works is to evaluate the tradeoff between the segmentation accuracy and the costs for seed selection.

References

1. Ghaneh, P., Costello, E., Neoptolemos, J.P.: Biology and management of pancreatic cancer. Postgrad. Med. J. **84**(995), 478–497 (2008)
2. Computational Anatomy for Computer-aided Diagnosis and Therapy, http://www.comp-anatomy.org
3. Park, H., Bland, P., Meyer, C.: Construction of an abdominal probabilistic atlas and its application in segmentation. IEEE TMI **22**(4), 483–492 (2003)
4. Heimann T., Meinzer H.-P.: Statistical shape models for 3D medical image segmentation: a review. Med. Image Anal. **13**(4), 543563 (2009)
5. Barrett, W., Mortensen, E.: Interactive live-wire boundary extraction. Med. Image Anal. **4**, 331–341 (1997)
6. Schenk A., Prause G.P.M., Peitgen H.O.: Efficient semiautomatic segmentation of 3D obects in medical images. In: Proceedings of the Third International Conference on Medical Image Computing and Computer-Assisted Intervention (MICCAI 2000), pp. 186–195, Springer (2000)

7. Kass, M., Witkin, A., Terzopoulos, D.: Snakes: active contour models. Int. J. Comput. Vis. **1**(4), 321–331 (1988)
8. Sethian, J.A.: Level Set Methods and Fast Marching Methods. Cambridge University Press, Cambridge (1999)
9. Leo G.: Random walks for image segmentation. IEEE Trans. Pattern Anal. Mach. Intell. 28(11) (2006)
10. Boykov, Y., Jolly, M.P.: Interactive organ segmentation using graph cuts. In: Proceedings of Medical Image Computing and Computer-Assisted Intervention, pp. 276–286 (2000)
11. Boykov, Yuri, Kolmogrov, Vladimir: An experimental comparison of min-cut/max-flow algorithms for energy minimization in vision. IEEE Trans. PAMI **26**(9), 1124–1137 (2004)
12. Boykov, Y., Jolly, M.P.: Interactive graph cuts for optimal boundary and region segmentation of objects in N-D images. In: Proceedings of Internation Conference on Computer Vision, pp. 105–112 (2001)
13. The Japanese Society of Medical Imaging Technology, http://www.jamit.jp

Validation of Knot-Tying Motion by Temporal-Spatial Matching with RGB-D Sensor for Surgical Training

Yoko Ogawa, Nobutaka Shimada, Yoshiaki Shirai, Yoshimasa Kurumi and Masaru Komori

Abstract We propose a method for validating surgical knot-tying motions for self-training of surgical trainee. Our method observes their hands by a RGB-D sensor and describes the point cloud as a SHOT feature. We use the features for matching an input point cloud sequence to that of an expert by dynamic programming. On the basis of the matched frames, the method validates relative positions of both hands and each hand shape in each input frame. Then the system detects and shows inappropriate parts in each frame. This paper shows the results of our method on a knot-tying motion dataset of a novice and an expert surgeon.

1 Introduction

Medical trainees usually learn surgical procedures under face-to-face teaching by skillful surgeons. The skillful surgeons are much busy for their own medical duties and have very limited time for teaching. For keeping the trainee's learning chances, an automatic system validating trainee's surgical procedure can be one of the solutions. We first target knot-tying procedures and propose a method that automatically visualizes and indicates inappropriate parts of trainee's motions.

In general, recognition of hand gesture from a movie consists of feature extraction and matching the input to motion models. Hand feature extraction can be roughly divided into 3D-parametric-model-based approach [1] and appearance-based approach [2]. Although the latter needs more parameters than the former, it is more robust to complicated hand shape with strong self-occlusion than the former for the recognition. Li et al. [3] proposed a method for recognizing hand actions

Y. Ogawa (✉) · N. Shimada · Y. Shirai
Ritsumeikan University, 1-1-1 Noji-Higashi, Kusatsu, Shiga, Japan
e-mail: ogawa@i.ci.ritsumei.ac.jp

Y. Kurumi · M. Komori
Shiga University of Medical Science, Seta Tsukinowa-Cho, Otsu, Shiga, Japan

Y.-W. Chen et al. (eds.), *Innovation in Medicine and Healthcare 2015*,
Smart Innovation, Systems and Technologies 45,
DOI 10.1007/978-3-319-23024-5_53

such as suturing and tying in suture operations. Their method concentrates to recognition of action types but treats neither indication of inappropriate parts nor temporal-spatial matching. In this study, we employ a customized SHOT (Signature of Histograms of Orientations) [4] feature for a frame-wise feature representing the 3D point distribution of both hands. We take modified CDP for frame-wise matting of input sequences and models. On the basis of the matching, our method evaluates appropriateness of hand postures in each input frame.

Finally, it visualizes the inappropriate parts of the trainee's procedure. This paper shows the results of our method by testing on a knot-tying motion dataset of a novice and an expert surgeon.

2 Structure of Knot Tying Motion

Surgical operators should tie as fast and correct as possible in surgical operations. The correctness of a knot-tying motion is evaluated based on both making knot and tightening knot techniques. We divide a knot-tying motion into three steps: closing, tying and tightening. Figure 1 shows a knot-tying motion and the corresponding steps. The hand postures in the tying step are the most important for evaluation of making knot technique. In this paper, we use the tying step for validation of the motions.

3 Detection of Hand Point Clouds

The system observes point clouds by a RGB-D sensor. The observed points have RGB color information and XYZ position information. In order to describe the hand motion, hand regions should be extracted from the input point clouds. First, our method extracts skin points by thresholding the input position and color which converted from RGB to HSV. Next, it chooses left and right hand-arm areas based on the area sizes. Finally, it finds wrist points and divides the extracted skin points into arm and hand points.

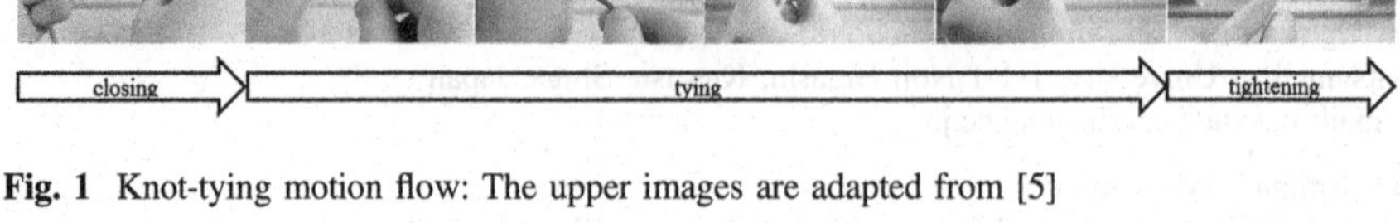

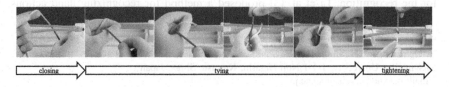

Fig. 1 Knot-tying motion flow: The upper images are adapted from [5]

4 Feature Description and Model Construction

We employ a SHOT feature to describe shapes of both hands in each frame. The feature is relative histograms of normals of a point cloud. The feature consists of Local Reference Frame (LRF) and SHOT descriptor. LRF is a local coordinate system for the feature description. SHOT descriptor shows local shapes based on normals of the points in sphere of radius R around the origin of LRF **P**. In this study, we assign a gravity center of the hand points in every frame to **P**, and we fix the coordinate system of LRF to the camera's one. Furthermore, we set R to 150 mm in order to enclose both hands. We prepare 6 model sequences of typical tying-motion types and extract their features.

5 Frame-to-Frame Matching

The system observes known type tying-motions and describes them as SHOT feature sequences. We divide the input sequences into each tying-motion section by our method in [6]. We define the frame difference d between an input and a model as $d = \sum_{k} |f_k^I - f_k^M|$. f_k^I is the k-th dimensional value of the feature vector of the input frame. f_k^M is the one of the model frame. The system matches each tying section with the model using CDP matching. We minimize the average cost along the path regardless of time passage in order to evaluate equally all frames in the tying motion. The given path represents the corresponding frame pairs.

6 Validation of Knot-Tying Motion

Our method detects the inappropriate relative hand positions based on thresholding the feature differences between matched frames. The method also detects inappropriate hand shapes by alignment of each hand points with ICP algorithm. If the distance between the corresponding points more than a threshold, the method extracts the points for inappropriate spatial parts. If many inappropriate parts are detected in left or right hand, the system issues a notice for users. In Figs. 2 and 3, left columns are input frames and right columns are corresponding model frames. Red rectangles show inappropriate frames, and red pixels indicate inappropriate spatial parts. Figure 2 shows matched frames with detected inappropriate relative hand positions and spatial parts of one sequence. Figure 3 shows detected frames in several input sequences. Our method detected both the differences of hand shapes and those of relative hand positions.

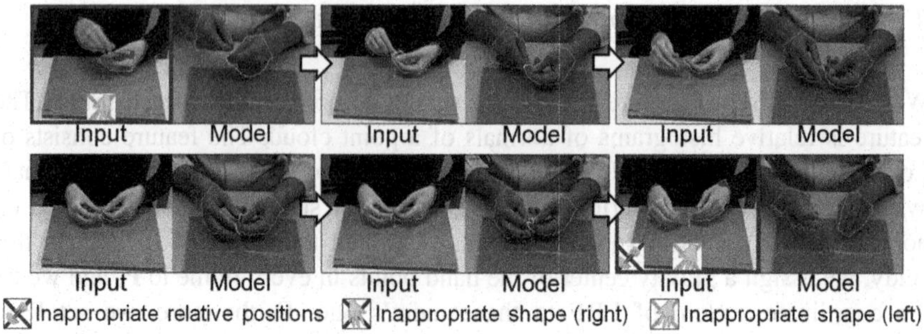

Fig. 2 Examples of matching and detection of one sequence

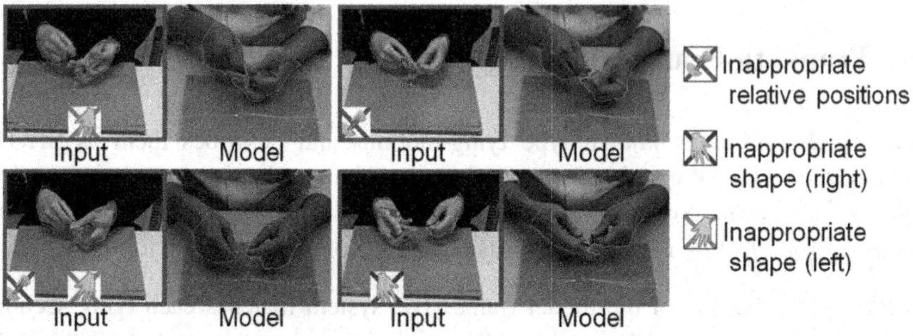

Fig. 3 Examples of detected frames of several input sequences

7 Conclusion

In this paper, we propose a system which validate knot-tying procedure by temporal-spatial matching for self-training of surgical procedures. Our method matches an input sequence and the models frame-to-frame by modified CDP, and then matches them point-to-point by ICP. Our future work includes detection of unknown motions.

Acknowledgement This work was supported by JSPS KAKENHI Grant Number 15H02764.

References

1. Oikonomidis, I., Kyriazis, N., Argyros, A.A.: Tracking the articulated motion of two strongly interacting hands. In: 2012 IEEE Conference on Computer Vision and Pattern Recognition (CVPR), IEEE, pp. 1862–1869 (2012)
2. Biswas, K.K., Basu, S.K.: Gesture recognition using microsoft kinect®. In: 2011 5th International Conference on Automation, Robotics and Applications (ICARA). IEEE, pp. 100–103 (2011)

3. Li, Y., Ohya, J., Chiba, T., Xu, R., Yamashita, H.: Study of recognizing hand actions from video sequences during suture surgeries based on temporally-sectioned sift and sliding window based neural networks. IEICE Tech. Rep. **113**(493), 151–156 (2014)
4. Tombari, F., Salti, S., Stefano, L.D.: Unique signatures of histograms for local surface description. In: Computer Vision-ECCV 2010. Springer, Berlin, Heidelberg, pp. 356–369 (2010)
5. Ethicon Inc., 'Knot Tying Manual'. Accessed April 2015 from: http://academicdepartments.musc.edu/surgery/education/resident_info/supplement/suture_manuals/knot_tying_manual.pdf, 2005
6. Ogawa, Y., Shimada, N., Shirai, Y., Kurumi, Y., Komori, M.: Temporal-spatial validation of knot-tying procedures using Rgb-D sensor for training of surgical operation. In: IAPR International Conference on Machine Vision Applications (MVA2015), 18–22 May 2015 (accepted for publication)

Erratum to: Prediction of Clinical Practices by Clinical Data of the Previous Day Using Linear Support Vector Machine

Takashi Nakai, Tadamasa Takemura, Risa Sakurai, Kenichiro Fujita, Kazuya Okamoto and Tomohiro Kuroda

Erratum to:
Chapter 1 in: Y.-W. Chen et al. (eds.), *Innovation in Medicine and Healthcare 2015*, Smart Innovation, Systems and Technologies 45, DOI 10.1007/978-3-319-23024-5_1

The original version of the below mentioned sections in Chapter-1 titled as "Prediction of Clinical Practices by Clinical Data of the Previous Day Using Linear Support Vector Machine" were inadvertently published with an incorrect content.

The online version of the original chapter can be found under DOI 10.1007/978-3-319-23024-5_1

T. Nakai (✉) · T. Takemura · R. Sakurai · K. Fujita
Graduate School of Applied Informatics University of Hyogo, Kobe, Japan
e-mail: ab14h405@ai.u-hyogo.ac.jp

T. Takemura
e-mail: takemura@ai.u-hyogo.ac.jp

R. Sakurai
e-mail: ab14v403@ai.u-hyogo.ac.jp

K. Fujita
e-mail: kfujita@kuhp.kyoto-u.ac.jp

K. Fujita · K. Okamoto · T. Kuroda
Division of Medical Information Technology and Administration Planning,
Kyoto University Hospital, Kyoto, Japan
e-mail: kazuya@kuhp.kyoto-u.ac.jp

T. Kuroda
e-mail: tomo@kuhp.kyoto-u.ac.jp

Y.-W. Chen et al. (eds.), *Innovation in Medicine and Healthcare 2015*,
Smart Innovation, Systems and Technologies 45,
DOI 10.1007/978-3-319-23024-5_54

Abstract
3.2. Experiment
3.3. Result
3.4. Discussion

The correct content appears as follows.

Abstract

For preventing mistakes and guaranteeing quality, Clinical Decision Support System (CDSS) is expected to support decision-making of healthcare professionals. Until now, there had been many studies of CDSS based on rule-based production system. However practical use of CDSS had been limited because of the complexity of medical care. On the other hand, the machine learning that required huge amounts of data is used to make data-driven predictions or decisions in computer science recently. We considered that this method was effective in practical care. Firstly, we constructed a model based on the hypothesis that clinical practices of a day might determine them of next day for the same patients. Next, we created predictors using linear support vector machines and clinical actions on Diagnosis Procedure Combination/Per-Per Diem Payment System introduced for medical billing in Japan. Finally we evaluated predictive performance by cross validation. As a result, the clinical actions whose frequency of appearance were higher trend to have higher predictive performance. Thus, it was suggested that predictive performance was improved by preparing sufficient amount of data and ensuring the frequency of appearance.

Experiment

The purpose of the proposed model is the clinical practices a day could determine the clinical practice next day. Linear SVM handles data as vector as described in Sect. 2.3, therefore we handle data as 5279-dimensional vectors in this experiment. Each element of the vector is mapped to 5279 clinical practices as shown in Table 3.

We make the experimental data set for each clinical practice. We evaluate the predictive performance.

1. Make lists of clinical practices for each patient by the day from DPC data

Make vectors from lists of step 1 as shown in Fig. 2. The value of vector elements is 1 if the clinical action is done. The value of vector elements is 0 if the clinical action is not done.

Table 3 Elements of vector for linear svm

Element number of feature vector	Data category code	Receipt computerized system code	Medical specification name
1	11	111000110	first consultation fee (hospital)
2	11	111000370	first consultation fee (infants)
3	11	111000570	first consultation fee (overtime)
4	11	111000670	first consultation fee (holiday)
:			
4543	60	160101210	Arterial blood sampling
:			
5278	97	197000470	special diet fee (per one meal)
5279	97	197000570	diet fee in dining room

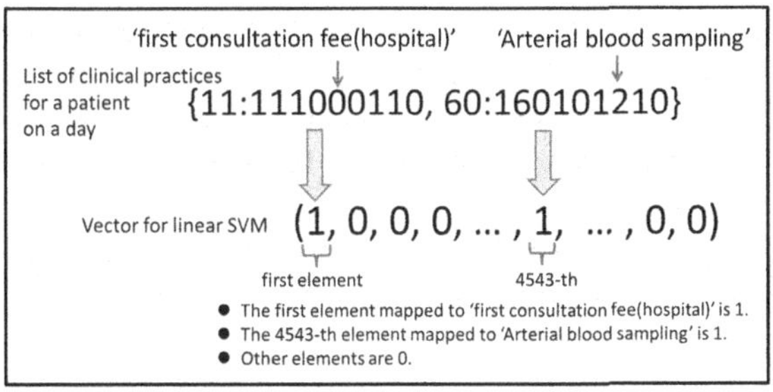

Fig. 2 Conversion of list of clinical practices to vectors

2. Classify vectors of step 0 into class 1 if the target clinical practice is done on the day after. Classify vectors into class 0 if not. For example, Table 4 shows the example of experimental data whose target clinical practice is 'Arterial blood sampling'. The 4543-th element is mapped to 'Arterial blood sampling' as shown in Table 3. Therefore we classify the vector into class 1 if the 4543-th element of vector of the day after is 1. We classify the vector into class 0 if not. We remove the vectors for discharge date from the experimental data because none of clinical practices on the next day. As a result we got 111,705 vectors as experimental data of each clinical practice of prediction target.
3. Divide experimental data into 10 parts. Use one of parts as test data in rotation and use other parts as teacher data. Create the classifier by using teacher data, and evaluated prediction performance for teacher data by 10-fold cross validation [5]. We used Liblinear [6] to create classifiers and to predict for test data.

Table 4 Image of experimental data for 'Arterial blood sampling'

Patient ID	Date	List of clinical actions provided (feature vector)	Whether 'Arterial blood sampling' has been practiced on the next day	Class
α	dα (admission date)	(1,0,0,0,...,0,...,0,0,0)	Not practiced	0
α	dα+1	(0,0,0,0,...,0,...,0,0,0)	Practiced	1
α	dα+2	(0,0,0,0,...,1,...,0,0,0)	Not practiced	0
		:		
α	dα+x-1	0,0,0)	Not practiced	0
α	dα+x (discharge date)	remove the vectors for discharge date from th		
β	dβ (admission date)	(1,0,0,1,...,0,...,0,0,1)	Practiced	1
β	dβ+1	(1,0,0,1,...,1,...,0,0,1)	Not practiced	0
		:		
β	dβ+x-1	(1,0,0,1,...,0,...,0,0,1)	Not practiced	0
β	dβ+x (discharge date)	remove the vectors for discharge date from the experimental data		
		:		

4543-th element

If 'Arterial blood sampling' practiced on the next day, the vector is classified into class 1. If not, the vector is classified into class 0.

Result

Table 5 shows the result of experiment about 'Arterial blood sampling' by the method described in Sect. 3.2. 'True Positive' is the number of test data of class 1 predicted correctly. 'False Positive' is the number of test data of class 0 predicted to be class 1 by mistake. 'False Negative' is the number of test data of class 1 predicted to be class 0 by mistake. 'True Negative' is the number of test data of class 0 predicted correctly. We calculated precision and recall rate for each 10 test data. Based on cross validation, the average values of these rates are final precision

Table 5 Results of prediction for "Arterial blood sampling"

Target test data	True positive (TP)	False positive (FP)	False negative (FN)	True negative (TN)	Precision = TP/(TP + FP)	Recall = TP/(TP + FN)
1	66	26	186	10893	0.717	0.262
2	99	43	140	10889	0.697	0.414
3	55	25	149	10942	0.688	0.270
4	92	57	161	10861	0.618	0.364
5	68	29	147	10927	0.701	0.316
6	73	37	167	10893	0.664	0.304
7	124	81	207	10758	0.605	0.375
8	97	37	168	10868	0.729	0.366
9	47	19	163	10941	0.712	0.224
10	49	30	134	10957	0.620	0.268
The average precision and recall (result of 10-folds cross validation)					0.675	0.316

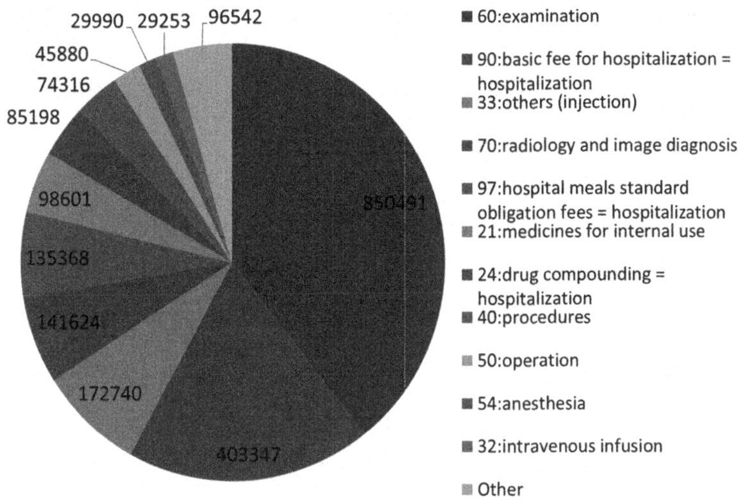

Fig. 3 Number of clinical actions by clinical data category

and recall rate of 'Arterial blood sampling' in this paper. As a result, precision rate was 0.675 and recall rate was 0.316.

We predicted 5279 kinds of clinical practices by the same steps. Figure 3 shows number of clinical actions by clinical data category in experimental data. The number of appearances of clinical actions can be restated as the number of vectors classified into class 1 by the step 4 of 0, and was divided by data category code and by unified electronic receipt code.

The 235 clinical practices only appeared on the first day of admission in total 5279 practices, so this system did not predict these admission date practices. In addition, few clinical practices appeared in this data could not be fitted SVMs because this machine learning method needs a certain amount data to learn and judge the correct answers. Therefore, on 10-fold cross validation, we omitted clinical practices that did not appear on all validation from the total practices. As a result, there were 657 clinical practices could be calculated on 10-fold validation this time. Figure 4 shows a scatter diagram of precision rate versus recall rate. The sizes of circle are proportional to the frequency of appearance.

We shows examples of clinical practices and their precision rate and recall rate of '33 others (injection)' as Table 6 and '21 medicines for internal use' as Table 7. In addition, Fig. 5 shows a scatter diagram of precision rate versus recall rate of '33 others (injection)' as well as Fig. 4. Figure 6 is the same diagram of '21 medicines for internal use'.

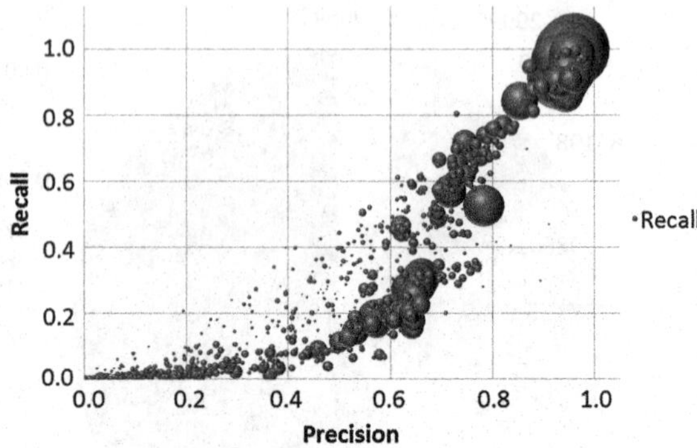

Fig. 4 Scatter diagram of precision rate versus recall rate

Table 6 Examples of precision and recall of others (injection)

Receipt computerized system code	Medical specification name	Number of appearance	Precision	Recall
130004410	Central venous injection	6249	0.896	0.885
640451009	Omepral 20 mg	2862	0.836	0.758
643910067	Stronger Neo-Minophagen C 20 mL	1595	0.806	0.680
620002258	Twinpal 500 mL	1204	0.805	0.721
130000210	Precise continuous intravenous infusion	5797	0.801	0.758
620002191	Glyceol 200 mL	744	0.796	0.624
620001934	Neoparen No. 2 1000 mL	1207	0.790	0.722
620001933	Neoparen No. 1 1000 mL	870	0.789	0.706

Table 7 Examples of precision and recall of medicines for internal use

Receipt computerized system code	Medical specification name	Number of appearance	Precision	Recall
616130532	Cefzon 100 mg	891	0.519	0.167
612320346	Selbex 50 mg	2162	0.435	0.077
611140694	Loxonin 60 mg	1215	0.383	0.043
610411058	Flomox 100 mg	1209	0.377	0.053
612520024	Methergin 0.125 mg	109	0.318	0.108
620003469	Plavix 75 mg	242	0.305	0.093
613330003	Warfarin 1 mg	1494	0.290	0.047
610451009	Prograf 0.2 mg	425	0.227	0.082

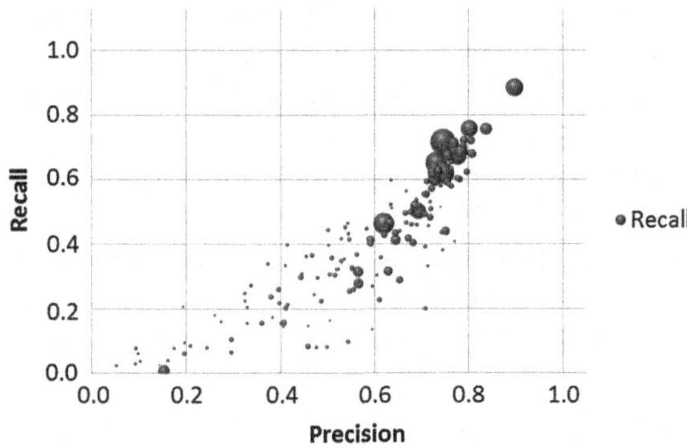

Fig. 5 Scatter diagram of precision rate versus recall rate of others (injection)

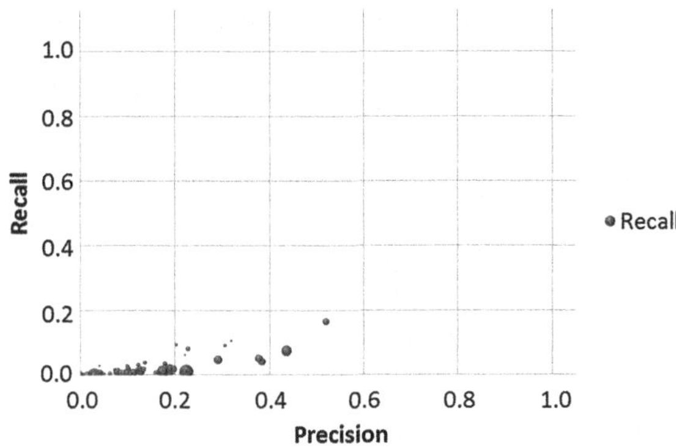

Fig. 6 Scatter diagram of precision rate versus recall rate of medicines for internal use

Discussion

In this study, we used machine learning and all clinical practice data of the day before as teacher data, and evaluated predictability of clinical practices for a patient of a day. Although there are some differences in each data category, some clinical practices have high precision rate and recall rate and others have low precision rate and recall rate. Generally, recall rate seems to be positively correlated with precision rate especially when precision rate is more than 0.4 as shown in Fig. 4. On the other hand, when precision rate is less than 0.4, recall rate trends to be low. Furthermore, from the aspect of the number of data included in each data category (i.e. the number of times that is appeared as a clinical action), the precision rate of the practice with higher frequency tends to be higher. It is assumed that larger amount of data improves the prediction performance. Additionally, the basic codes for medical calculation appear almost every day. It is assumed that it is easy to predict these codes. Concretely, data categories such as ‘injection’ and ‘procedures’ have relatively high precision rate and recall rate as shown in Table 6 and Fig. 5. It is seems that this is the result of prediction by learning quantitatively patterns of practices as training data. On the other hand, data categories such as ‘medicines for internal use', 'potion', 'medicine for external use' and 'examination' have relatively low precision rate and recall rate as shown in Table 7 and Fig. 6. Especially, a lot of medicines are included in categories such as 'medicines for 'internal use', 'potion' and 'medicine for external use'. Therefore, the frequency of appearances of individual code is not relatively high. As a result, it seems that linear svm was not been able to learn in the 10-fold cross-validation sufficiently. In fact, codes for medicine was 1163 types, whereas, codes that were able to be calculated precision rate were only 65 types. The linear svm could predict more types of medicine if we could get more data. On the other hand, the precision rate and recall rate of the codes of 'examination' with high frequency are high relatively but the precision rate and recall rate of the practice which appears rarely is low relatively.

As a result, we consider that the precision rate is high when the frequency of appearance is increased. We intend to improve the prediction performance for more clinical practices by using larger data.

Author Index

Y.-W. Chen et al. (eds.), *Innovation in Medicine and Healthcare 2015*,
Smart Innovation, Systems and Technologies 45,
DOI 10.1007/978-3-319-23024-5